Bailey & Love's
ESSENTIAL CLINICAL ANATOMY

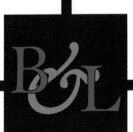

Bailey & Love's

ESSENTIAL CLINICAL ANATOMY

Edited by

JOHN SP LUMLEY DSc (Hon) MS FRCS FMAA (Hon) FGA
Foundation Dean, University of Bolton School of Medicine, Bolton, UK
Emeritus Professor of Vascular Surgery, University of London, London, UK
Past Council Member and Chairman of the Primary Fellowship Examiners,
Royal College of Surgeons of England, London, UK

JOHN L CRAVEN MD FRCS
Formerly Consultant Surgeon, York District Hospital, York, UK
Past Chairman of the Primary Examiners, Royal College of Surgeons of England, London, UK

PETER H ABRAHAMS MB BS FRCS(Ed) FRCR DO(Hon)
Professor of Clinical Anatomy, Warwick Medical School, University of Warwick, UK
Director or Anatomy, West Midlands Surgical Training Centre, UHCW NHS Trust, Coventry, UK
Extraordinary Professor, Department of Anatomy, University of Pretoria, South Africa
Fellow, Girton College, Cambridge, UK
Professor of Clinical Anatomy, St George's University, Grenada, West Indies
Examiner to the Royal College of Surgeons, London, UK
Family Practitioner, Brent, London, UK

RICHARD G TUNSTALL BMedSci PhD PGCLTHE FHEA
Professor and Head of Clinical Anatomy and Imaging, Warwick Medical School, University of Warwick, UK
MBChB Admissions Lead, Warwick Medical School, University of Warwick, UK
Director of Clinical Anatomy, West Midlands Surgical Training Centre, UHCW NHS Trust, Coventry, UK
Examiner to the Royal College of Surgeons, London, UK

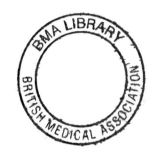
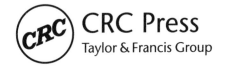

CRC Press
Taylor & Francis Group

CRC Press
Taylor & Francis Group
6000 Broken Sound Parkway NW, Suite 300
Boca Raton, FL 33487-2742

Printed and bound in India by Replika Press Pvt. Ltd.

Printed on acid-free paper

International Standard Book Number-13: 978-1-138-29523-0 (Hardback)
International Standard Book Number-13: 978-1-138-29518-6 (Paperback)

Visit the Taylor & Francis Web site at
http://www.taylorandfrancis.com

and the CRC Press Web site at
http://www.crcpress.com

Contents

Foreword

It goes without saying that anatomical knowledge is the bedrock of clinical surgery and indeed all of medicine. Not only do surgeons in particular need to be fully cognisant of their own specialty requirements but they need to have more far reaching knowledge so as to make thorough clinical examinations, to interpret all modalities of imaging and to deal with trauma and malignancy, which by their very nature know no anatomical barriers. It is therefore a delight to welcome *Essential Clinical Anatomy* as the first publication into the fold of what we envisage will constitute a Bailey and Love compendium of associated titles. As editors of *Bailey and Love's Short Practice of Surgery* we see this anatomy book as very much a companion to the main tome. Although there are snippets of relevant anatomical knowledge in the parent volume, we readily accept that it lacks the detail that is invariably required for a complete understanding of various disease processes and the concomitant therapeutic procedures required to treat them. *Essential Clinical Anatomy* fulfils this need and all undergraduate and postgraduates who are unsure of the relevant anatomy when reading *Short Practice of Surgery* will not put a foot wrong if they keep the former close when perusing the pages of the latter.

Essential Clinical Anatomy covers the modern curricula required by most regulatory medical bodies worldwide and hence provides all that is required for relevant examinations. A constant feature of *Bailey and Love's Short Practice of Surgery* throughout all its editions has been an emphasis on high-quality illustrations and clinical photographs and we are delighted to see this tradition is very much at the fore in this companion volume. The authors are to be congratulated on assembling the information in a most readable and visual format, which will be considerably enhanced by a variety of anatomical teaching videos that can be viewed via the Bailey and Love website.

While we are confident that *Essential Clinical Anatomy* will provide the foundation for all those pursuing a surgical career, we also believe it will be of tremendous benefit for all undergraduate and postgraduate students no matter which branch of medicine they wish to pursue, and we warmly commend this book to you.

Norman S. Williams
Ronan O'Connell
Andrew McCaskie

Preface

The expansion and integration of disciplines within the medical curriculum has reduced time for anatomy teaching, particularly for human dissection, but has not reduced its vital importance. While surgeons need to know the detailed anatomy in their operating field, knowledge of the anatomy that underlies every clinical examination and every radiological/medical image is an essential component of everyday clinical practice.

This text provides a comprehensive cover of most normal and abnormal living anatomy, essential for students across the world. It addresses the knowledge and skills laid down by the General Medical Council (GMC) and the American Association of Clinical Anatomists (AACA; 'A clinical anatomy curriculum for the medical student of the 21st century: gross anatomy', *Clinical Anatomy* 1996;9:71–99; see also Smith *et al.*, 'The Anatomical Society core regional anatomy syllabus for undergraduate medicine', *Journal of Anatomy* 2016;228:15–23).

The regional approach followed corresponds to a typical clinical examination. The nervous system is included, rather than being covered in an additional text; also included is embryology in sufficient detail to explain many common congenital abnormalities. Wherever possible, information, such as muscle attachments, is tabulated and clinical information is highlighted.

The extensive number of illustrations include surface anatomy, coloured labelled diagrams, dissections, a wide range of radiological, laparoscopic and endoscopic images, and clinical pictures of common diseases. A comprehensive index facilitates rapid location of the desired passages. Self-assessment material is included at the end of each chapter; these multiple choice questions (MCQs), single best answer (SBA) questions (used in the USA and also now more widely), extended matching questions (EMQs) and applied questions reflect styles of examination around the world. The answers and explanations can be found in the text, but additional material is included where appropriate.

The authors bring a combined experience of over 150 years of anatomy teaching at all levels, and present this large volume of information in a palatable, interesting and understandable form, emphasizing its relevance to disease and clinical practice.

John Lumley
John Craven
Peter Abrahams
Richard Tunstall

Acknowledgements

We would like to thank Matthew Boissaud-Cooke BMed-Sc(Hons), MBChB, MRCS, Speciality Trainee in Neurosurgery, University Hospital Plymouth NHS Trust, Plymouth, for contributing the text for Chapter 24.

The authors and publisher also thank the following individuals and institutions for kindly supplying figures for this book. Dr Tania Abrahams for tropical pathology. Dr Rosalind Ambrose for tropical radiology. Dr Ray Armstrong and ARC for musculoskeletal cases. Professor JM Boon for dissections from 'The Virtual Procedures Clinic' CD-ROM (www.primalpictures.com 2003). Section of Clinical Anatomy University of Pretoria, Dr L Van Heerden and the following students: Van Jaarsveld M; Joubert AT; Van Schoor AN; Phetla MV; Mbandlwa L; Mahlomoje ID; Deetlefs MEC; Schoonraad B; Van Blerk EM; Gichangi C; Smith AB; Van der Colff FJ; Connell A; Sitholimela SC for their beautiful dissections 2002/3. Mr S Dexter for laparoscopic shots. Professor R Ger for photos from *Essentials of Clinical Anatomy*, Parthenon, 1986. R Hutchings, freelance photographer. Professor Kubrick for lymphatic dissections. Dr Lahiri and the Wellington Hospital Cardiac Imaging and Research Centre for EBCT scans of one of the authors. Miss Gilli Vafidis for ophthalmoscopy views. Dr Alan Hunter for a bronchoscopic view. Professor J Weir and team for images from *Imaging Atlas of Human Anatomy*, 4th edition, Elsevier, 2010. Mr T Welch for tropical pathology. University of Warwick and the West Midlands Surgical Training Centre (UK) for images of their plastinated prosection collection, funded by the West Midlands Strategic Health Authority and produced in Guben (Germany) by von Hagens Plastinations. Professor T Wright for auriscopic views.

The following figures are reproduced with kind permission of Bart's Medical Illustration Collection, previously published in *Hamilton Bailey's: Demonstrations of Physical Signs in Clinical Surgery*, 19th edition. (eds. JSP Lumley, AK D'Cruz, JJ Hob-allah, CEH Scott-Conner) CRC Press, 2016:

1.3, 1.6a, 1.12, 1.18, 1.20a, 2.20, 4.3a, 4.3b, 4.18, 5.8, 5.12, 5.14, 5.15, 6.8, 6.14, 7.8, 10.6, 12.5a, 12.5c, 12.5d, 12.6, 12.19a, 12.21, 14.4b, 14.8. 14.11, 15.6c, 15.7, 15.12c, 15.12d, 15.12e, 15.13, 15.18, 15.26a, 15.26b, 15.32b, 16.3a, 16.3b, 16.3c, 16.3d, 16.11a, 16.11b, 16.11c, 16.12, 17.6a, 17.6b, 17.6c, 17.6d, 17.10, 17.16, 19.6, 19.7b, 19.11, 19.26, 20.8, 20.17, 21.3, 22.12.

Bailey & Love · Essential Clinical Anatomy

Essential Clinical Anatomy · *Bailey & Love*

Bailey & Love · Essential Clinical Anatomy

Introduction

The structure of the body - the systems and organs   2

The structure of the body – the systems and organs

The systems and organs of the body are composed of epithelial, connective, muscular and nervous tissues.

EPITHELIAL TISSUE

Epithelium forms a protective covering over the internal and external surfaces of the body. It is derived from all three primitive embryonic layers. The ectoderm forms the skin; the mesoderm forms the pleura, pericardium and peritoneum; and the endoderm forms the endothelial lining of the blood vessels and gut.

Most glands are epithelial in origin, as they are formed by invagination of an epithelial surface. Epithelium is resistant to physical and chemical damage and the effects of dehydration. It can serve as a selective barrier and can be resistant to harmful metabolites, chemicals and bacteria. It is characterized by a minimal amount of intercellular substance and a tendency to form sheets of cells of one or more layers, having a capability of continuous replacement. It may be simple, transitional or stratified.

Simple epithelium

This consists of a single layer of cells on a basement membrane (Figs. 0.1a–e). It is described as squamous (pavement), cuboidal or columnar, depending on the shape of its cells. Squamous cells are found lining the alveoli of the lungs, the blood vessels (endothelium) and the serous cavities (mesothelium). Cuboidal cells line the ducts of many glands. Columnar cells are often ciliated and may be modified as mucus-forming goblet cells; they line much of the alimentary, respiratory and reproductive tracts. Mucus, a glycoprotein, accumulates in the cell and is discharged from its free (luminal) surface.

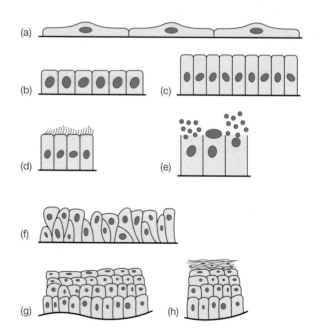

Figure 0.1 Epithelial tissue: (a) squamous; (b) cuboidal; (c) columnar; (d) columnar ciliated; (e) columnar with goblet cells; (f) transitional; (g) stratified epithelium; (h) stratified squamous epithelium

Transitional epithelium

This contains two or three layers of cells, most of which are attached to the basement membrane and are nucleated (Fig. 0.1f). It lines most of the urinary tract, is stretchable and does not desquamate. It contains few glands.

Stratified squamous epithelium

This also has two or more layers of cells (Figs. 0.1g,h). Cells in contact with the basement membrane are columnar cells.

The more superficial cells are flattened, and the surface cells have no nuclei (enucleate) and are continually being rubbed away (desquamated). This form of epithelium covers the exterior of the body, lines both ends of the alimentary tract and is particularly suited to areas exposed to wear and tear. In the upper respiratory tract the differing lengths of the columnar cells gives the appearance of a double layer, and this is known as pseudostratified columnar epithelium; it contains numerous mucous cells.

Skin

This consists of two layers, an outer **epidermis** and an inner **dermis** (corium) (Fig. 0.2). The epidermis is composed of keratinized stratified squamous epithelium. **Hair follicles, sweat and sebaceous glands** and **nails** are modifications of the epidermis. The colour of the skin is determined by blood flow and melanocytes, the pigment-producing cells that lie in the basal layer of the epidermis. The scales on the surface of the skin consist mainly of **keratin**, a sulphur-containing fibrous protein largely responsible for the skin's protective and barrier properties.

The dermis is a layer of vascular connective tissue moulded tightly to the epidermis and merging in its deeper part with the subcutaneous tissues. Lying in the dermis are the coiled tubular sweat glands opening on to the skin surface and hair follicles, to each of which is attached an arrector pili muscle. The roots of the hairs and the sweat glands extend into the subcutaneous tissue.

Mucous and serous membranes

These line the wet internal surfaces of the body and consist of two layers, an epithelium and a corium. The epithelium of mucous membranes is usually of a simple variety with many mucous or serous cells, but the urinary tract is lined by transitional epithelium, and the respiratory tract by pseudostratified columnar ciliated epithelium with mucous cells. The serous membranes line most of the closed body cavities. The corium underlies the epithelium and is composed of connective tissue. In the alimentary tract it contains a thin sheet of smooth muscle – the **muscularis mucosa**.

Glands

These are epithelial ingrowths modified to produce secretions. These secretions may pass on to the epithelial surface (**exocrine** glands) or into the bloodstream (**endocrine** glands). Exocrine glands may be unicellular (goblet) or multicellular. The latter may be simple (containing one duct) or compound (branched) where numerous, small ducts open into a single main duct. The secretory part of the gland may be long and thin (tubular), globular (acinar), oval (alveolar) or intermediate, e.g. tubuloalveolar. The secretions of the exocrine glands may be formed by disintegration of the whole cell (holocrine, e.g. sebaceous glands), disintegration of the free end of the cell (**apocrine**, e.g. mammary glands), or without cellular damage (merocrine or **epicrine**, e.g. most other glands). Most endocrine glands are of the last type.

If the duct of an exocrine gland becomes blocked and the gland continues to secrete, the fluid accumulates and a cyst is formed. A generalized enlargement of glands is termed adenopathy.

CONNECTIVE TISSUE

This is characterized by having a large amount of intercellular substance. It forms areolar tissue, the packing material of the body, the supporting tissues (cartilage, bone) and blood (Fig. 0.3). Embryonic connective tissue is called mesenchyme.

Areolar tissue

The intercellular substance is semisolid and composed of proteins and mucopolysaccharides. Three types of fibres are found: coarse **collagen** fibres, which are white (in bulk), flexible, inelastic and arranged in bundles; **elastic** fibres, which are yellowish (in bulk), less frequent and branching; and **reticular** fibres, which form a very fine silver-staining network throughout the tissues.

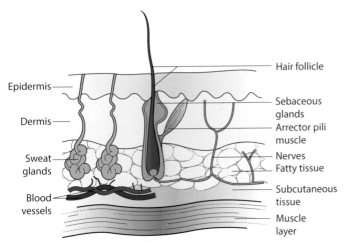

Figure 0.2 Diagram of a cross-section through the skin

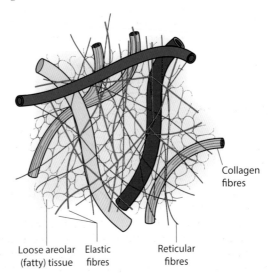

Figure 0.3 Connective tissue

The cells are of five main varieties: large, slender poorly staining fibroblasts, closely concerned with the production of the three types of tissue fibre; tissue macrophages, which are phagocytic and can engulf particulate matter; oval plasma cells with their cartwheel-like staining nucleus, concerned with antibody production; granular basophilic mast cells, concerned with histamine and heparin production; and the cyst-like fat-containing cells.

The relative amounts of cellular and intercellular substance vary throughout the body. Subcutaneous tissue contains a variable amount of fat and loose fibrous tissue. Superficially, fat is usually predominant, but more deeply the fibrous tissue forms a well-defined superficial fascial sheet connecting it to the deep fascia that invests the limbs and trunk. In other places condensations of non-elastic fibrous tissue form **ligaments**, **tendons** and **aponeuroses**, and **retinacula**. Ligaments are usually attached to the bones on each side of a joint, maintaining its stability; tendons join the muscles to the bones by blending with the periosteum; aponeuroses are thin flattened tendinous sheets through which muscles gain wider attachments. Retinacula are usually thickenings of the deep fascia related to joints.

SUPPORTING TISSUE

Cartilage

This is an avascular, firm tissue composed of cells (chondrocytes) in an abundant intercellular substance (matrix) (Fig. 0.4). It is formed from an overlying fibrous layer, the perichondrium, and classified, according to its predominant fibres, into hyaline cartilage, fibrocartilage and yellow elastic cartilage.

- **Hyaline cartilage** contains many cells and a few fine collagen-like fibres, and is found in the rib cartilages and over most articular surfaces. It also forms the precursor in cartilaginous ossification.

- **Fibrocartilage** contains many dense fibrous bundles and fewer cells, and is present in the intervertebral discs, over the articular surface of bones that ossify in membranes, e.g. the mandible, and in intra-articular cartilages, e.g. the menisci of the knee.
- **Yellow elastic cartilage** contains elastic fibres and is found in the auricular, epiglottic and the apices of the arytenoid cartilages of the head.

Bone

This is a hard supporting tissue composed mainly of inorganic calcium salts impregnating a network of collagen fibres (Fig. 0.5). The basic unit, composed of concentric layers around a central vessel, is known as a **Haversian system**. The bone cells (osteocytes) lie within spaces (lacunae) between the layers and their processes pass into canaliculi in the bone. **Compact bone** is dense and strong and forms the outer part of most bones. The **cancellous** (spongy) bone within consists of a network of thin partitions (trabeculae) around intercommunicating spaces; the osteocytes lie within lacunae in the trabeculae. The outer surface of a bone is covered by a thick fibrous layer, the **periosteum**, many of the cells of which are the granular, bone-forming **osteoblasts**. These cells, when enclosed in the hard intercellular substance, become osteocytes. The blood supply of bone is from the periosteum and muscular vessels and, in the case of long bones, from one or two nutrient arteries that enter the shaft.

The shape of the bones of the body, the proportion of compact to cancellous tissue and the architecture of the trabeculae are arranged to give maximum strength along with economy of material. Both genetic and local factors influence the shape and size of a bone. Adjacent muscles or organs (e.g. the brain) mould the bone to some extent. Many of these factors can be investigated in the living person by means of X-rays.

Bones are classified as long, short, flat, sesamoid or irregular (Fig. 0.6).

Long bones are present in the limbs. The body (shaft) is a cylinder of compact bone surrounding a medullary cavity

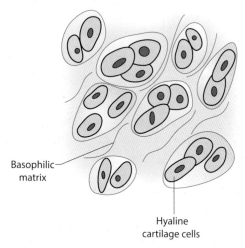

Basophilic matrix

Hyaline cartilage cells

Figure 0.4 Hyaline cartilage

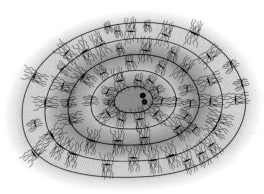

Figure 0.5 Haversian bony systems with osteoblasts in circular layers with central canals carrying nutrient vessels

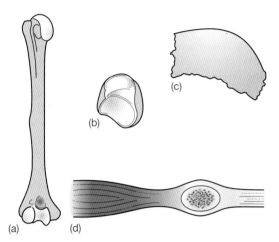

Figure 0.6 Bone types: (a) long bone (humerus); (b) irregular bone (lunate); (c) flat bone (from vault of skull); (d) sesamoid bone, a small pebble-like bone within a tendon, e.g. in the tendon of flexor hallucis longus beneath the head of the first metatarsal

that is filled with some cancellous bone and a large amount of yellow fatty marrow. The two ends are formed of spongy bone with a thin outer shell of compact bone. The trabeculae in the cancellous bone are laid down along the lines of force. In the developing long bone of a child but not normally in the adult, blood-forming tissue is found in the marrow.

The **short bones** are found in the carpus and tarsus. They consist of spongy bone covered with a thin layer of compact bone.

The **flat bones**, e.g. the scapula, give attachment to muscles and form a protective covering (the bones of the skull vault). They consist of two layers of compact bone with a thin intervening spongy layer (the diplöe in the skull).

Sesamoid bones are formed within tendons and serve to relieve friction and to alter the line of pull of a muscle. The largest sesamoid bone is the patella.

The remaining **irregular bones** may contain red, blood-forming marrow (the vertebrae), or air spaces (sinuses) (Fig. 0.7).

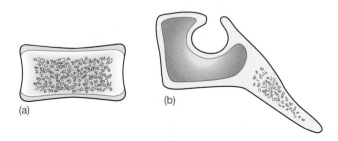

Figure 0.7 (a) Cancellous bone, e.g. within the centre of a vertebral body, surrounded by a layer of compact bone. (b) Pneumatized bone, e.g. the skull sinuses around the nasal cavity

Excessive force applied to a bone may cause it to break (fracture), and in such injuries the adjacent soft tissues may be damaged both by the force and by the broken ends of the bone. Knowledge of the anatomical relations of the bone enables the clinician to predict the likely association of nerve, artery and muscle injury with a fracture. A break in the overlying skin is a serious complication of fractures, as it permits the entry of infecting organisms. In these circumstances the fracture is said to be compound (Fig. 0.8).

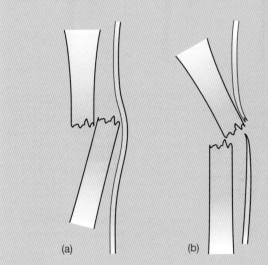

Figure 0.8 Fracture: (a) simple; (b) compound. In the latter the overlying skin has been lacerated. This is much more serious because bacterial infection can enter the bone, with possible long-term sequelae

Ossification

Bone may develop either (i) in a condensed fibrous tissue model, when the process is called **membranous** (mesenchymal) ossification, or (ii) in a cartilage model that has replaced the mesenchyme, when the process is called **cartilaginous** (endochondral) ossification.

Mesenchymal ossification usually starts in the 5th to 6th weeks of intrauterine life and is found in the bones of the skull vault, the bones of the face and part of the clavicle.

Cartilaginous ossification occurs in all long bones except the clavicle. A primary centre appears for the body of a long bone in about the 8th week of intrauterine life, and secondary centres for each end appear between birth and puberty. Fusion of the body and these centres occurs in about the 18th year in males. Secondary centres appear and fuse up to a year earlier in females. Further ossification centres may develop at puberty in areas of major muscle attachment, e.g. the processes of the vertebrae and the crests of the scapula and the hip. They fuse with the rest of the bone by about the 25th year.

Development of a long bone

A long bone develops from a cartilaginous model possessing an outer perichondrium and an irregular cartilaginous matrix; the deep layers of the perichondrium have bone-forming properties (Fig. 0.9).

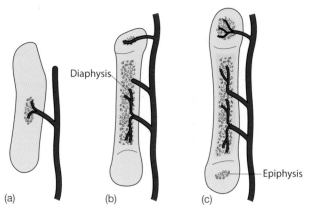

Diaphysis

Epiphysis

(a)   (b)   (c)

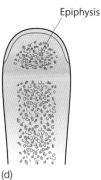

Epiphysis

(d)

Figure 0.9 (a)–(d) Ossification of a long bone. The ossification starts in the shaft of the bone, usually during uterine life. Secondary centres start in the epiphysis, one end often preceding the other, and appear after puberty. (e) Staining techniques show ossification in the fetal long bones and skull. The shafts are already ossified but the secondary epiphyseal centres are not visible as they only appear after birth. Note that the wrist, elbow, shoulder, knee and hip joints are still cartilaginous

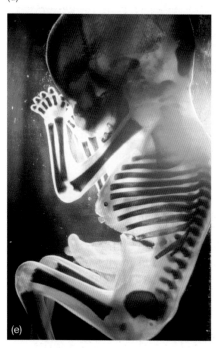

(e)

The first changes occur in the cartilage cells of the middle of the body (the **diaphysis**). They become greatly enlarged and the matrix is correspondingly reduced and calcified. The cells die and undergo shrinkage, leaving spaces known as primary alveoli. The deeper layer of **perichondrium** around the middle of the body starts to produce bone, and is then known as the **periosteum**. Blood vessels and bone cells (the bone-forming osteoblasts and the bone-removing osteoclasts) pass inwards from the periosteum to the calcified zone. The cartilage is not converted into bone but is replaced by it after its removal by the osteoclasts. The multinucleated osteoclasts initiate absorption of the calcified material, producing larger spaces, the secondary alveoli. Osteoblasts come to line the secondary alveoli and layers of bone are deposited. Some osteoblasts are incorporated into the bone, becoming the bone cells (**osteocytes**). Ossification extends up and down the body from this primary centre. The cells of the adjacent cartilage come to lie in parallel longitudinal rows and are subsequently replaced in the manner already described. This form of ossification is known as endochondral (cartilaginous).

Secondary centres of ossification (the **epiphyses**) appear later in life. Osteogenic cells invade the calcified cartilage after the cells have undergone hypertrophy, death and shrinkage. The layer of cartilage left between the epiphysis and the diaphysis is known as the **epiphyseal plate**. The part of the diaphysis bordering the plate is known as the **metaphysis**; the cartilage adjacent to the metaphysis is continually being ossified. New cartilage cells are formed in the epiphyseal plate. Growth in length of the bone continues until the cartilage cells stop multiplying, and fusion of the diaphysis and epiphysis then occurs. The internal architecture of the bone is remodelled by osteoclastic and osteoblastic activity. Simultaneous laying down of layers of bone around the body by the periosteum increases the girth of the bone and is known as **subperiosteal ossification**; it is a form of mesenchymal ossification. Growth and remodelling of the bone continues until adulthood through continuous destruction by osteoclasts and replacement by osteoblasts.

Epiphyses may be classified into three types: **pressure** epiphyses, seen at the ends of weight-bearing bones; **traction** epiphyses occurring at the site of muscle attachments; and 'atavistic' epiphyses, which are functionless skeletal remnants that may show on an X-ray and be mistaken for disease or injury.

Injury in a young person can dislodge the epiphysis from the metaphysis; e.g. a fall on the outstretched arm may produce a slipped epiphysis of the lower end of the radius. This injury may interfere with further growth at that end of the bone.

In summary, most primary ossification centres of long bones appear by the end of the second month of intrauterine life, and most epiphyseal centres before puberty. The epiphyses at the knee joint appear just before birth and are an indication of the age of the fetus. Most long bones cease to grow in length between the 18th and 20th years in men, and a year or so earlier in women.

The skeleton

The skeleton is divisible into an **axial** part (the bones of the head and trunk) and an **appendicular** part (the bones of the limbs). The upper limb is joined to the trunk by the mobile muscular pectoral girdle, and the lower limb by the stable bony pelvic girdle.

JOINTS

These are unions between two or more bones and may be of four types: bony, fibrous, cartilaginous or synovial.

Bony

The three elements of the hip bone are joined by bony union, as are the occipital and the sphenoid in the skull after completion of the second dentition (Fig. 0.10).

Fibrous

The bony surfaces are united by fibrous tissue. These joints comprise the skull sutures, the articulations of the roots of the teeth and the inferior tibiofibular joint (Fig. 0.11).

Cartilaginous

These may be primary or secondary. In the primary cartilaginous joints the bony surfaces are united by hyaline cartilage, as seen in the union of the body and the ends in a developing long bone (Fig. 0.12).

In the secondary cartilaginous joints, the symphyses (Fig. 0.13), the bony surfaces are covered with hyaline cartilage and united by a fibrocartilaginous disc. These joints all lie in the midline and comprise the intervertebral discs, the symphysis pubis and the manubriosternal and xiphisternal junctions.

Synovial

The bony articular surfaces (facets) are covered with **hyaline cartilage** (with the exception of the temporomandibular and sternoclavicular joints, where they are covered with fibrocartilage) (Fig. 0.14). A fibrous **capsule** is attached near to the articular margins of the bones. The surfaces of the interior of the joint, except those covered by cartilage, are lined by a delicate vascular **synovial membrane**, which secretes a lubricating **synovial fluid** into the joint cavity.

The capsule may possess **ligamentous thickenings**, and accessory extracapsular and intracapsular **ligaments** may pass across the joint. Fibrous intra-articular **discs** are present in some joints, occasionally completely dividing their cavity (e.g. temporomandibular joint). **Tendons** occasionally enter the joint cavity by piercing the capsule (biceps brachii), and

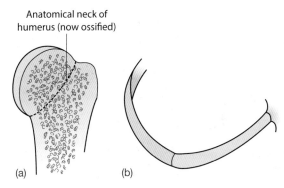

Figure 0.12 Primary cartilaginous joints: (a) union of epiphysis and metaphysis (dotted line); originally hyaline cartilage, now ossified; (b) union between rib and costal cartilage

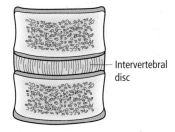

Figure 0.13 Secondary cartilaginous joint where the bone is covered by hyaline cartilage and the two surfaces are joined by a fibrocartilaginous disc. These occur in the midline and include the intervertebral, symphysis pubis and manubriosternal joints

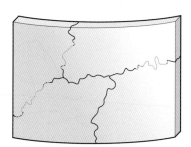

Figure 0.10 Bony joints between the skull bones. These ossify and disappear later in life

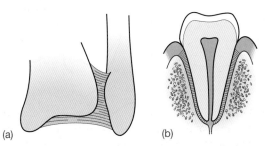

Figure 0.11 Fibrous joints where two bones are attached by fibrous tissue: (a) inferior tibiofibular joint; (b) tooth socket, where the enamel is attached to the surrounding bone by fibres of the periodontal ligament

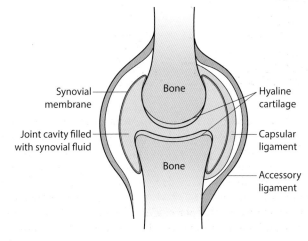

Figure 0.14 Synovial joint

fat pads may be present between the capsule and the synovial lining (knee joint).

Muscles or tendons crossing superficial to the joint may be protected by a synovial sheath or sac whose fluid prevents excessive friction. The sacs are known as **bursae**, and the cavity may communicate with that of the joint.

Functional aspects of joints

Movement

Bony, fibrous and primary cartilaginous joints are immobile, secondary cartilaginous joints are slightly mobile and synovial joints are freely mobile.

Synovial joints are subdivided into a number of varieties according to the movements possible at the joint. These varieties are listed below and the movements are best understood by examining the examples given.

- **Hinge** – elbow, ankle and interphalangeal joints; the knee and temporomandibular joints are modified hinge joints (Fig. 0.15)
- **Pivot** – the proximal radioulnar joint and the dens articulation of the atlantoaxial joint (Fig. 0.16)
- **Condyloid** – metacarpophalangeal joint (Fig. 0.17a)
- **Ellipsoid** – radiocarpal (wrist) joint (Fig. 0.17b)
- **Saddle** – carpometacarpal joint of the thumb (Fig. 0.18)
- **Ball and socket** – hip and shoulder joints (Fig. 0.19)
- **Plane** – intercarpal joints and joints between the articular processes of adjacent vertebrae (Fig. 0.20).

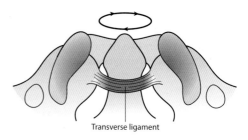

Transverse ligament

Figure 0.16 Pivot joint: horizontal view of the atlantoaxial joint. The odontoid process of the axis rotates with the anterior articular facet of the atlas anteriorly and transverse ligament posteriorly

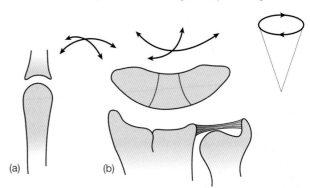

(a)   (b)

Figure 0.17 (a) Condyloid joint, e.g. metacarpophalangeal joint. (b) Ellipsoid joint of the wrist (radiocarpal) joint. These joints move in two planes: flexion–extension and abduction–adduction. Circumduction is a combination of all of these movements where the distal part of the limb can rotate around the pivot point or the centre of the joint

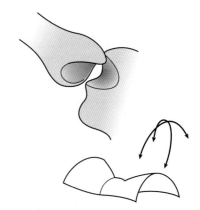

Figure 0.18 Saddle joint. The carpometacarpal joint of the thumb is shaped like the saddle of a horse where the rider can slide off from side to side as well as move backwards and forwards

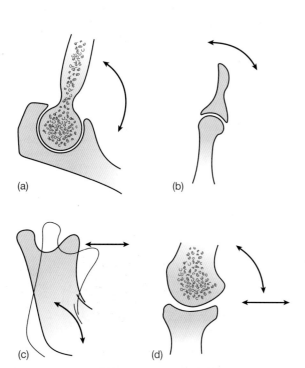

(a)   (b)

(c)   (d)

Figure 0.15 Hinge joints: (a) elbow and (b) interphalangeal joints, allowing flexion–extension in a single plane. The temporomandibular joint (c) and knee joint (d) are modified hinge joints with flexion and extension in a single plane but with a little rotation or gliding in the lax position of the capsules

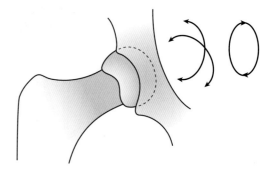

Figure 0.19 Ball and socket joint, e.g. the hip. The hip joint has all the movements of the condyloid joint and in addition the head can rotate within the socket, i.e. there is additional medial and lateral rotation

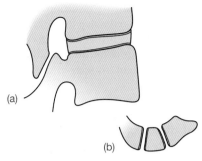

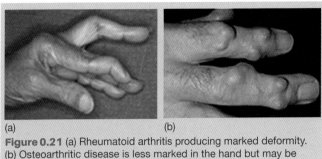

Figure 0.21 (a) Rheumatoid arthritis producing marked deformity. (b) Osteoarthritic disease is less marked in the hand but may be accompanied by skin nodules called Osler's disease

Figure 0.20 Joint movements. (a) In a secondary cartilaginous joint, e.g. in the symphysis pubis or an intervertebral joint, there is the possibility of slight stretching and movement. The symphysis softens in pregnancy and allows slight adaptation of the pelvic form during parturition. (b) Plane joints allow a little gliding of the adjacent joints, e.g. in the carpus

Stability

Stability depends on bony, ligamentous or muscular factors. It is usually inversely related to the mobility of the joint.

Many of these functional aspects of joints may be assessed by radiology. Displacement of the articulating surfaces of a joint is known as dislocation. Partial displacement of the articulating surfaces is known as subluxation. Dislocation of a joint may follow severe injury and is always associated with damage to the capsular and accessory ligaments. There may also be fractures of the bony structures of the joint, and occasionally damage to closely related nerves and vessels. Chronic inflammatory processes are prone to affect the bone ends (osteoarthritis) and synovial membrane (rheumatoid arthritis), and joints thus affected may be deformed and painful (**Figs. 0.21a,b**), with marked limitation of movement.

Nerve supply

The capsule and ligaments of a joint contain pain, proprioceptive and stretch fibres: these provide information on the position of the joint and any abnormal forces. The nerve supply of a joint is from the nerves supplying the muscles acting on the joint.

MUSCULAR TISSUE

This is a contractile tissue. There are skeletal, smooth and cardiac varieties.

Skeletal (striated, voluntary) muscle

This acts mainly on the bony skeleton or as a diaphragm, but it is also found around the pharynx and larynx, and forms some sphincters (**Fig. 0.22**). It is composed of unbranched fibres of sarcoplasm limited by a membrane, the sarcolemma, and contains many nuclei. Each fibre has a motor endplate and contains many contractile units, the myofibrils, which have

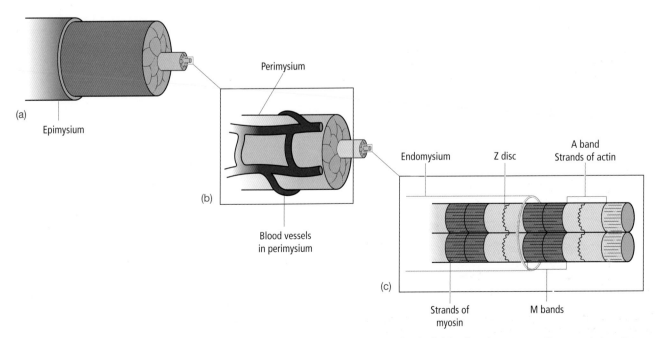

Figure 0.22 Muscle fibres of striated muscle [(a), (b) and (c) showing increasing magnification]: (a) epimysium surrounding muscle bundles; (b) muscle bundles surrounded by perimysium containing nutrient blood vessels and nerves; (c) muscle fibres contained within endomysium. The strands of myosin and actin interlock during muscle contraction in a similar fashion to Velcro

alternating dark (A) and light (I) bands. A dark line (the Z disc) crosses the middle of the I band. The bands of adjacent myofibrils coincide, giving the muscle fibre its striated appearance. Each fibre is enveloped and attached to its neighbour by a fibrous endomysium, and bundles of fibres are enclosed by a fibrous perimysium. A muscle composed of many bundles is surrounded by an epimysium.

The motor nerve supply of the muscle comes from the anterior horn cells of the spinal cord and the motor nuclei of the brainstem. The sensory supply arises in the more specialized spindles and tendon organs as well as the simpler touch and pain endings. Impulses from the sensory endings pass into the posterior horn of the spinal cord.

Skeletal muscles are formed by voluntary fibres. The muscles are usually attached at each end to bone, by the periosteum, either directly or through **tendons** and **aponeuroses**, and cross one or more joints. Occasionally two muscles meet at a common stretchable union known as a **raphé**, e.g. the mylohyoid muscles (**Fig. 0.23g**). Muscles have a very rich blood supply.

Muscle fibres are arranged either **parallel** (**Fig 0.23a**) to the direction of the action (sartorius), or **obliquely** to it (known as **pennate** muscles). **Unipennate** muscles (extensor digitorum longus) have oblique fibres inserted into one side of a side tendon (**Fig. 0.23c**). In **bipennate** muscles (rectus femoris) oblique fibres are inserted into each side of the tendon (**Fig. 0.23d**). A **multipennate** muscle has a number of parallel bipennate tendons (deltoid) or is a circular muscle with a central tendon (tibialis anterior). In muscles of equal volume, a parallel arrangement of fibres gives greater movement but less power than an oblique arrangement. The least mobile attachment of a muscle is often called its **origin**, and the more mobile attachment its **insertion**. However, this is an arbitrary distinction, so reference in the text here is made to muscle **attachments**, rather than to origin or insertion. An **aponeurosis** (**Fig. 0.23f**) is a flat, thin tendinous expansion providing a wide attachment, as seen in the abdominal wall muscles.

When a movement occurs at a joint, the muscles concerned in producing it are known as the prime movers or agonists and those opposing it as antagonists. Muscles contracting to steady the joint across which movement is occurring are known as synergists. A further type of action is known as the action of paradox, in which a muscle gradually relaxes against the pull of gravity, e.g. bending forwards produced by relaxing the back muscles.

Smooth (unstriated, involuntary) muscle

This is present in the walls of most vessels and hollow organs of the body. It is composed of unbranched spindle-shaped cells with a single central nucleus and containing many unstriated myofibrils (**Fig. 0.24**). The fibres are arranged in interlacing bundles and are supplied by the autonomic nervous system.

Cardiac muscle

This is found in the heart. It consists of short, branched cylindrical fibres joined end to end (**Fig. 0.25**). The adherent ends of adjacent fibres form dark intercalated discs. Each fibre contains a single central nucleus and striated myofibrils resembling those of voluntary muscle. It is supplied by the

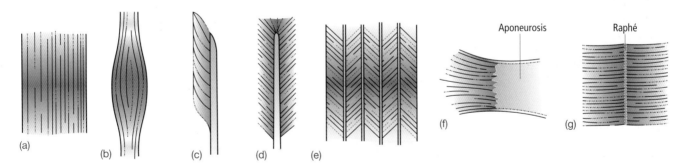

Figure 0.23 Types of striated muscle: (a) parallel (quadrate); (b) fusiform; (c) unipennate; (d) bipennate; (e) multipennate; (f) flat muscle inserted into a tendinous sheet (aponeurosis); (g) two muscles attached to each other along a raphé

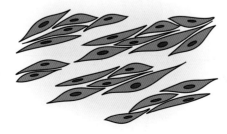

Figure 0.24 Smooth muscle fibres contained within a loose muscle bundle

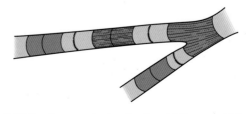

Figure 0.25 Cardiac muscle showing the striations of striated muscle and branching, producing a continuous network of muscle

autonomic nervous system, but heart muscle also has the properties of spontaneous and rhythmic activity. The conducting system of the heart is made up of modified cardiac muscle cells.

NERVOUS TISSUE

This is capable of excitability and conductivity. It consists of excitable cells (**neurons**) (Fig. 0.26) and supporting cells, which in the central nervous system are the **neuroglial cells** and in the peripheral nervous system are the **Schwann cells**.

The neuron is the functional unit of the nervous system and consists of a cell body and processes, usually an **axon** and one or more **dendrites**. The cell bodies are situated in the central nervous system or in peripheral ganglia. They possess a large nucleus and well-marked cellular inclusions. The axon (fibre) begins at a small axon hillock on the cell body and carries impulses away from the cell body. This often long, slender process ends by dividing into many branches that have small terminal knobs, **boutons**, related to the cell bodies or branches of other neurons. The relationship is known as a **synapse** and may be either facilitatory or inhibitory, depending on the neuron of origin, and possibly on the receptor area of the second neuron. A rather specialized synapse is formed when a nerve ends on a muscle fibre at a **motor endplate**.

Axons may give off one or more short collateral branches. They are myelinated or unmyelinated. The myelin is interrupted about every millimetre or so by a constriction called the **node of Ranvier**. In the peripheral nervous system each internodal segment of sheath is produced by a **Schwann cell**, the nucleus of which is seen on its surface. These cells play an important role in peripheral nerve regeneration. Fibres of the peripheral nervous system are also covered by a thin fibrous membrane, the **neurilemma**. In the central nervous system oligodendroglia take the place of the Schwann cells. Dendrites are usually short unmyelinated processes carrying membrane depolarizations to the cell body. The volume over which the dendrites of a single cell extend is known as the dendritic field.

Afferent neurons carry information towards the central nervous system, and efferent neurons carry instructions away from it. Within the central nervous system afferent and efferent neurons are often connected by many intercalated (internuncial or intermediate) neurons.

The neurons are organized to form the central and peripheral nervous systems. The former comprises the brain and spinal cord (Fig. 0.27) and the latter the cranial nerves, spinal nerves and autonomic nervous system (see below). A group of neurons in the central nervous system is called a **nucleus**, and outside the central nervous system (CNS) such a group is known as a **ganglion**. Within the CNS are neuroglial cells, variously known as **astrocytes**, **oligodendroglia** and **microglia**, and these make up almost half of the brain substance.

Astrocytes are stellate cells with large nuclei and numerous processes, which may be of the thick protoplasmic variety, as found mainly in the grey matter, or the thin fibrous variety found mainly in the white matter. Some of the processes end on blood vessels, and the astrocytes are thought to be concerned with fluid balance in the central nervous system and with the nutrition of the neurons. Oligodendroglia are oval dark-staining cells possessing few processes. They produce the myelin of the central nervous system. Microglia are small mobile phagocytic cells and form part of the macrophage system.

Ependymal cells are columnar in shape and line the cavities of the brain and spinal cord. In certain regions the ependyma is modified to form the choroid plexuses of the brain, which produce the cerebrospinal fluid.

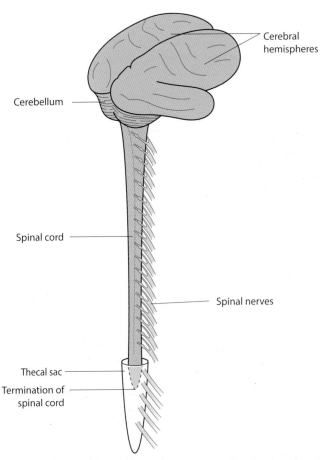

Figure 0.27 Brain and spinal cord

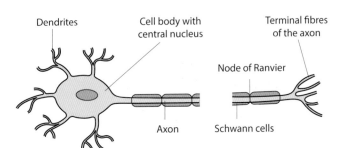

Figure 0.26 Neuron

Cranial nerves

Twelve pairs of nerves are attached to the brain (p. 360). Some are mainly sensory, some mainly motor, and others are mixed sensory and motor.

Spinal nerves

The 31 paired spinal nerves (8 cervical, 12 thoracic, 5 lumbar, 5 sacral and 1 coccygeal) (**Fig. 0.27**) are formed within the vertebral canal, each by the union of a ventral and a dorsal root. The roots are formed from a number of rootlets that emerge from the anterolateral and posterolateral sulci of the spinal cord. The **ventral root** carries efferent (motor) fibres *from* the cord and the **dorsal root** carries afferent (sensory) fibres *to* the cord. The cell bodies of the sensory fibres are situated in a **ganglion** on the dorsal root (**Fig. 0.28**). The spinal nerves are therefore a mixture of motor and sensory fibres. Each nerve leaves the vertebral canal through an intervertebral foramen and soon divides into a large **ventral** and a smaller **dorsal ramus** (branch).

The adjacent ventral rami of most regions communicate to form **plexuses** (cervical, brachial and lumbosacral), whereas those of the thoracic region become the intercostal and subcostal nerves. The dorsal rami pass backwards into the postvertebral muscles and divide into medial and lateral branches. These rami supply the muscles and skin over the posterior aspect of the body, but give no branches to the limbs.

Tumours within the vertebral canal or a protrusion from a degenerate intervertebral disc may compress a spinal nerve and, occasionally, the spinal cord to produce segmental sensory and motor dysfunction. Knowledge of the anatomical distribution of the individual nerves enables the site of the disease to be identified.

Local anaesthetic agents produce reversible regional loss of sensation, reduce pain and thus facilitate surgical procedures. Infiltrative local anaesthetics permit biopsy of skin lesions and excision of skin and subcutaneous lesions. The anaesthetic agent is injected into the skin, which has been sterilized with alcohol or a povidone–iodine solution, over and around the lesion to be biopsied or excised and into the subcutaneous tissue surrounding it. This will allow, after 2 minutes, the procedure to be carried out painlessly. Sensation will return within 2 hours.

Autonomic nervous system

The motor part of this system innervates glands and smooth and cardiac muscle. Its fibres form a fine network on the blood vessels and in the nerves. All its fibres arise from neurons of the visceral columns of the brain and spinal cord and synapse with **peripheral ganglion** cells before reaching the organs they supply. This fine network is divisible into two complementary parts, **sympathetic** and **parasympathetic**, which leave the central nervous system at different sites. They usually have opposing effects on the structure they supply through endings, which are mainly adrenergic or cholinergic.

Sympathetic system

Each ventral ramus from the 1st thoracic to the 2nd lumbar nerve gives a bundle of myelinated (preganglionic) fibres to the **sympathetic chain or trunk** (**Fig. 0.28**). The bundles arise near the formation of a ramus and are called **white rami communicantes**; they form the sympathetic outflow of the central nervous system. Each ventral ramus later receives a bundle of unmyelinated (postganglionic) fibres from the sympathetic trunk – a **grey ramus** communicans. (The myelinated and unmyelinated fibres are also termed the white and grey rami communicantes, respectively.)

The peripheral ganglia of the system lie within the two parallel sympathetic trunks alongside the vertebral column. The trunks extend from the base of the skull to the coccyx and have 3 cervical, 12 thoracic, 4 lumbar and 5 sacral ganglia. The preganglionic fibres from the thoracolumbar outflow

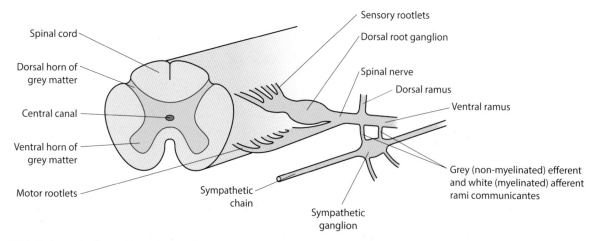

Figure 0.28 Typical spinal nerve formation and connections to the sympathetic ganglia and chain. The ventral motor rootlets unite to form a ventral motor root, joining with the dorsal sensory root, which comes from the sensory rootlets and dorsal root ganglion of each spinal segment. The 'mixed' spinal nerve then divides into a dorsal and a ventral primary ramus. The dorsal rami supply the back whereas the larger ventral rami supply all the limbs and trunk. The sympathetic ganglia are connected to the ventral rami via white (presynaptic) rami communicantes and grey (postsynaptic) rami

may synapse (i) in the adjacent ganglion, (ii) in other ganglia higher or lower in the chain, or (iii) in the collateral ganglia situated in the plexuses around the aorta (e.g. coeliac plexus). Each preganglionic fibre may synapse with 15 or more ganglionic cells, thus giving rise to widespread activity. A number of preganglionic fibres end in the medulla of the suprarenal gland.

Postganglionic (unmyelinated) fibres may (i) return to a spinal nerve in a grey ramus communicans to be distributed to peripheral smooth muscle, e.g. arterial walls, (ii) pass along the major arteries and their branches to be distributed to the organs these supply, or (iii) form named nerves, e.g. cardiac, running to the viscus concerned.

The cell bodies of the sympathetic fibres supplying the upper and lower limbs are situated in ganglia in the cervicothoracic and lumbosacral regions, respectively.

Chemical destruction or surgical removal of these ganglia may be undertaken to improve the cutaneous blood supply of the limb or to reduce excessive sweating.

The visceral branches supply the smooth circular muscle, including the sphincters of the viscera.

Parasympathetic system

This system receives preganglionic fibres from four cranial nerves (oculomotor, facial, glossopharyngeal and vagus) and the 2nd, 3rd and 4th sacral spinal nerves (**craniosacral outflow**). The peripheral ganglia of this system are near the organs they supply, usually in its walls. There are, however, four well-defined, isolated, parasympathetic ganglia associated with the cranial nerves. The postganglionic fibres are usually short and unmyelinated. The visceral branches usually supply the smooth muscle responsible for emptying the organ, and also produce dilatation of the blood vessels. There is little evidence of parasympathetic supply to the limbs.

Afferent (e.g. pain) fibres from the viscera are present in both sympathetic and parasympathetic systems and pass to the central nervous system without synapsing. Their subsequent paths are similar to those of somatic pain. Afferent (reflex) fibres, e.g. from the lungs, heart and bladder, and visceral sensations of nausea, hunger and rectal distension, also reach the central nervous system, probably along parasympathetic pathways.

Most transmitter chemicals can be classified as adrenergic (for the sympathetic system) or cholinergic (for the parasympathetic system).

THE CARDIOVASCULAR SYSTEM

The cardiovascular system comprises the heart and blood vessels, **arteries**, **veins**, **capillaries** and **sinusoids**. The arteries and veins passing to organs and muscles are usually accompanied by the nerves, and together form a compact **neurovascular bundle**.

The walls of the arteries possess three coats (**Fig. 0.29a**): the intima, composed of an **endothelial** lining and a small amount of connective tissue; the **media**, which is composed mainly of elastic tissue in the larger arteries and almost entirely of smooth muscle in the small **arterioles** and medium-sized

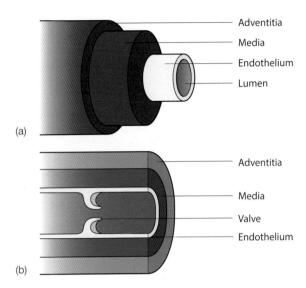

Figure 0.29 Structure of (a) an artery, and (b) a vein

arteries; and the outer fibrous **adventitia**. The coats of the veins correspond to those of the arteries (Fig. 0.29b), but the media contains less smooth muscle and fewer elastic fibres. In the larger veins the adventitia is thicker than the media. In most veins, **valves** are present. These are formed of paired folds of endothelium and help to determine the direction of flow. Medium and smaller arteries are often accompanied by two veins, the **venae comitantes**, rather than one. The smallest, postcapillary veins are termed **venules**. The **capillaries**, which unite the arteries and veins, have walls formed of a single endothelial layer of large angular flattened cells.

The direct union between two vessels is called an anastomosis. **Arteriovenous anastomoses** occur around the nail beds and are an important mechanism in controlling digital blood flow.

They may also exist as congenital abnormalities of the vascular system and can be created surgically when a large vein with an arterialized circulation is required for regular access to the circulation.

Sinusoids are thin-walled, dilated channels uniting arteries and veins and are found in the bone marrow, liver, spleen and suprarenal glands.

In some situations blood passes through two capillary beds before returning to the heart: this constitutes a **portal circulation**. The passage of blood from the stomach, intestine, pancreas and spleen through the liver exemplifies such a system. Short vessels passing through foramina in the skull and joining venous channels (**sinuses**) inside and veins outside are called **emissary** veins.

Reduction of the blood supply to a region is known as ischaemia, and this is of clinical importance in the heart and brain. One important degenerative arterial disease that can affect the vessels is arteriosclerosis, and this is very prevalent in developed countries. The arterial narrowing produced by the disease may cause local intravascular clotting (thrombosis) to occur. A **thrombus** may become detached and flushed into the bloodstream, forming an **embolus** and blocking distal smaller vessels. Local death of an area of tissue or organ owing to reduction of its blood supply is known as an infarction. In situations where bacteria infect the infarcted area it undergoes putrefaction, a condition known as **gangrene**. In some instances it is possible surgically to bypass arterial blockages, thus re-establishing the distal blood supply and preventing infarction and gangrene.

The body responds to an injury, e.g. invading bacteria, by the process known as **inflammation**. The capillaries dilate and white blood cells pass out of the circulation to phagocytose the offending organisms. The area becomes red and hot because of the increased blood supply, and swollen with increased tissue fluid; it is also painful. A collection of dead tissue and dead white blood cells is called an **abscess**.

THE LYMPHATIC SYSTEM

Lymph consists of cells, mainly lymphocytes, and plasma.

The lymphatic system collects tissue fluid and conveys it to the bloodstream. It comprises the **lymph capillaries and vessels**, the lymph nodes, and aggregations of lymph tissue in the spleen and thymus and around the alimentary tract. The system forms an extensive network over the body, although its fine vessels are not easily identified (**Figs. 0.30a,b**).

The lymph capillaries are larger than those of the blood; they are composed of a single layer of **endothelial** cells. The lymph vessels resemble veins and possess many paired valves. The larger collecting vessels open into the venous system near the formation of the brachiocephalic veins.

A **lymph node** (**Fig. 0.30c**) is an aggregation of lymph tissue along the course of a lymph vessel. It is bean-shaped, with a number of afferent vessels (conveying lymph to the node) entering its convex surface and an efferent vessel (carrying lymph away from the node) leaving its hilus (opening). It is surrounded by a fibrous capsule from which fibrous trabeculae pass inwards. It is filled with a reticular network of fine collagen fibres, and the cells are either primitive (lymphocyte precursors) or fixed macrophages. Numerous lymphocytes and a few monocytes lie freely within the meshwork, but they are absent peripherally, leaving a subcapsular lymph space. The cells of the outer part of the node (cortex) are densely packed and known as germinal centres. The centre of the follicle and the hilar (medullary) regions of the node contain loosely packed lymphocytes.

Lymph aggregations elsewhere in the body consist of a mixture of follicles and loosely packed lymphocytes.

Bacterial infections produce inflammatory responses in the regional lymph nodes. In many malignant diseases neoplastic cells spread via the lymph vessels to the regional lymph nodes, and there develop to such an extent as to completely replace the normal tissue of the lymph node and occlude lymph flow. The stagnation of lymph within the tissues due to obstruction of flow produces a swelling of the tissues known as lymphoedema (**Fig. 1.20b, p. 29**). Lymphoedema may also occur in subjects who are born with a defective lymphatic system, this being termed primary lymphoedema; acquired obstruction is called secondary lymphoedema. The term lymphadenopathy is used to describe a generalized enlargement of the lymph nodes, although they are not glands in the strict definition of the term.

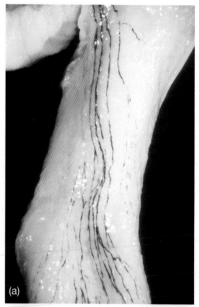

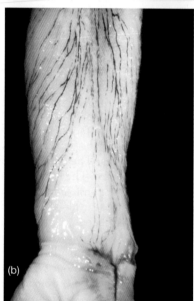

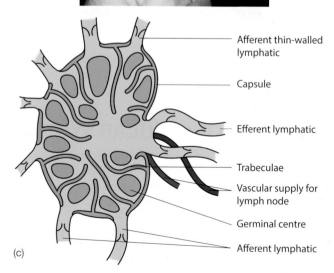

Afferent thin-walled lymphatic

Capsule

Efferent lymphatic

Trabeculae

Vascular supply for lymph node

Germinal centre

Afferent lymphatic

Figure 0.30 (a) and (b) Injection with Indian ink into the palmar skin to show lymphatics of the arm. (c) Lymph node structure

ORIENTATION

The **anatomical position** is that to which all anatomical descriptions refer. It is one in which the person stands upright with feet together, eyes looking forward and arms straight down the side of the body, with the palms facing forward (Fig. 0.31).

Structures in front are termed **anterior** (ventral) and those behind are termed **posterior** (dorsal). In the hands and feet the surfaces are referred to as **palmar** and dorsal and **plantar** and dorsal, respectively. Structures above are **superior** (cranial, rostral) and those below are **inferior** (caudal). Structures may be nearer to (**medial**) or further from (**lateral**) the midline, and those in the midline are called **median**. **Paramedian** means alongside and parallel to the midline. **Superficial** and **deep** denote the position of structures in relation to the surface of the body. A **sagittal** plane passes vertically anteroposteriorly through the body and a **coronal** plane passes vertically at right angles to a sagittal plane. **Transverse** (horizontal) planes pass horizontally through the body and are known radiologically as axial planes.

Proximal and **distal** are terms used to indicate the relation of a structure to the centre of the body. The ankle is distal to the knee joint; the shoulder is proximal to the elbow joint. Blood flows distally (peripherally) in the arteries and proximally (centrally) in the veins.

Movements

Forward movement in a sagittal plane is usually known as **flexion** (Fig. 0.32) and backward movement as **extension** (Fig. 0.33). Owing to rotation of the lower limb during development, backward movement of the leg extends the hip and flexes the knee; downward movement of the toes is flexion. Upward movement at the ankle joint is dorsiflexion (extension) and downward movement is plantar flexion (flexion) (Fig. 0.34). Movement away from the midline in the coronal plane is **abduction** and movement towards the midline is **adduction** (Fig. 0.35). Abduction and adduction of the fingers and toes is taken in relation to the middle finger and second toe. During development of the thumb its axis is rotated in relation to the fingers, therefore movement is described in relation to the plane of the thumbnail. Side-to-side movement of the neck and trunk is termed **lateral flexion**. Circumduction (Fig. 0.35) is the movement when the distal end of a bone describes the base of a cone whose apex is at the proximal end. **Rotation** occurs in the long axis of a bone; in the limbs it may be **medial**, towards the midline, or **lateral**, away from it (Fig. 0.36). Medial and lateral rotation of the forearm occurs through the axis drawn through the heads of the radius and ulna, and is termed **pronation** and **supination**, respectively (Fig. 0.37). Rotation of the thumb and little finger so that their pulps meet is termed **opposition** of the two digits, the movement being particularly marked in the thumb. **Rotation** of the forefoot is termed **inversion** when the sole faces the midline and **eversion** when it is turned away from the midline (Fig. 0.38).

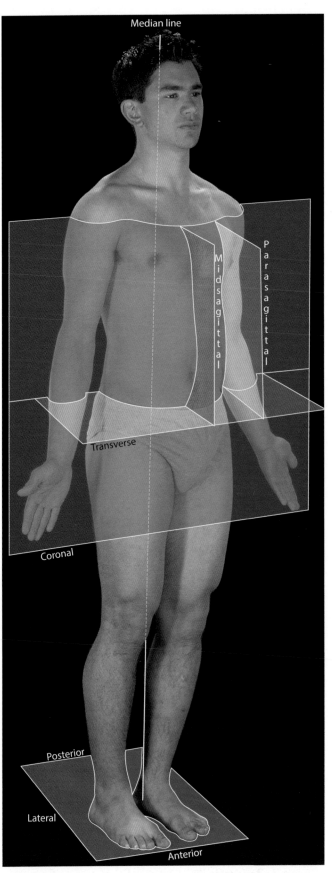

Figure 0.31 Anatomical position. The median line passes from the top of the head to between the ankles

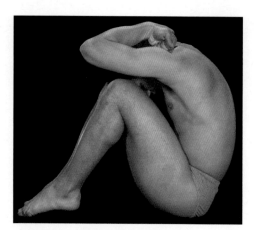

Figure 0.32 Flexion

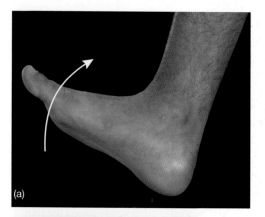

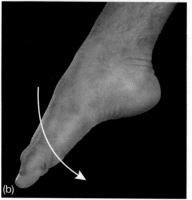

Figure 0.34 (a) Dorsiflexion (true extension). (b) Plantar flexion (true flexion)

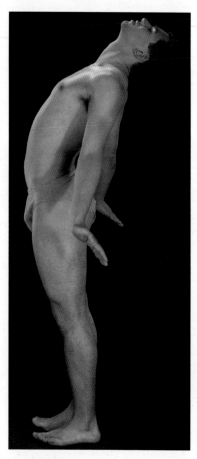

Figure 0.33 Extension

IMAGING – THE ESSENTIALS

Since the discovery of X-rays over 120 years ago, the study of the normal and diseased human body has become one of the most rapidly expanding fields in medicine. In the 21st century, we now have ultrasound (US), computed tomography (CT), contrast studies and radionuclide scans, and, the last 30 years have provided huge advances in magnetic resonance imaging and angiography (MRI and MRA, respectively) and, more recently, electron beam CT (EBCT).

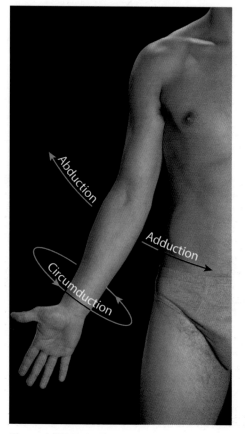

Figure 0.35 Abduction, adduction and circumduction

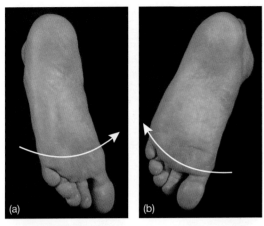

Figure 0.36 Rotation: (a) medial; (b) lateral

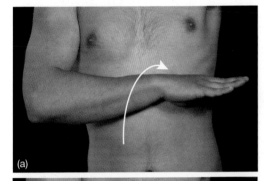

Figure 0.37 (a) Pronation. (b) Supination

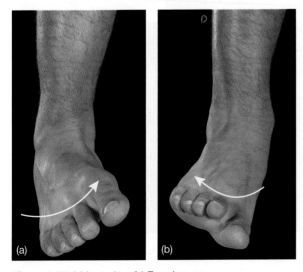

Figure 0.38 (a) Inversion. (b) Eversion

X-rays (Fig. 0.39)

X-rays pass easily through air or fatty tissues (i.e. they are radiotransparent) but substances such as bone, calcium stones and heavy metals absorb most of the X-rays (i.e. they are radiopaque). X-rays that do not pass through to the X-ray plate release their energy inside the body, damaging the molecules they collide with. This is the mechanism by which X-rays are harmful – the effect is seen particularly on rapidly dividing cells, especially fetal and gonadal cells. Caution is therefore taken to shield the fetus when radiographing pregnant women and the gonads of those of reproductive age.

The direction that the beam passes through the subject determines the name of the view, e.g. a posteroanterior chest X-ray is taken with the subject's back towards the beam and the chest on the 'cold' X-ray plate. This view is ideal for judging heart size and lungs, whereas the anteroposterior chest X-ray is much better for viewing the vertebral bodies.

Contrast media

Body cavities, the lumen of vessels (e.g. arteries and veins), ureters or hollow viscera (e.g. bowel) can be outlined by using suspensions of heavy metals or halogens. These contrast media can be introduced in a variety of ways: by direct introduction (barium enema); by injection (arteriograms and venograms); or by injection into the bloodstream and then concentration by specific organs (e.g. in an intravenous urogram for outlining the kidneys and urinary tract; Fig. 0.40). Nowadays, the use of digital, computerized images allows the 'removal' of the images of soft tissues in the background and easier visualization of the system under investigation (digital subtraction angiography – DSA). More recently, the advent of non-invasive angiography, such as magnetic resonance angiography, will help to reduce the use of many invasive procedures.

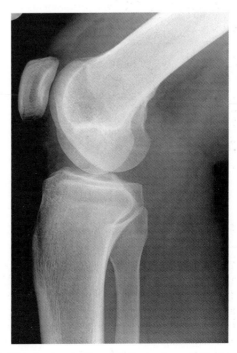

Figure 0.39 Lateral projection plain X-ray of an adult knee

Nuclear medicine (Fig. 0.41)

Nuclear medicine uses radioactive isotopes, mainly for diagnosis but occasionally for therapeutic uses such as in hyperthyroid disease. In the diagnostic field, myocardial perfusion imaging, lung scans to detect pulmonary embolism and bone scans to find widespread metastases are now routine procedures.

Ultrasound (Fig. 0.42)

Much more easily performed, however, are ultrasound techniques that use high-frequency sound waves and their interaction with biological tissues to produce 'echograms'. Modern ultrasound hardware now allows real-time tomographic images, and the addition of the Doppler principle has led to duplex scanning, which measures movement and blood flow in real-time and has the added attraction of providing easily interpreted colour images. Another really important advantage of ultrasound is that the technique is multi-planar and can be used at the bedside. These advantages now mean that many interventional procedures (e.g. biopsy and drainage of cysts or abscesses) can be done under ultrasound guidance. Usage of a variety of different transducers has improved the range of ultrasound imaging, but this technique is still totally operator-dependent and, as it is a real-time interactive process, it is not best seen with hard-copy images. This explains why so few ultrasound images are included in this book.

Computed tomography (Fig. 0.43)

CT obtains a series of different angular X-ray projections that are processed by a computer to give X-ray views of a section or slice of specified thickness. The CT machine consists of a rigid metal frame with an X-ray tube sited opposite a set of detectors. All of the views per slice are collected simultaneously so that the tube and detectors rotate around the patient. One slice takes 15–30 seconds.

No specific preparation is required for examinations of the brain, spine, musculoskeletal system and chest. Studies of the abdomen and pelvis often require opacification of the gastrointestinal tract using a solution of dilute contrast medium (either a water-soluble or a barium compound). CT

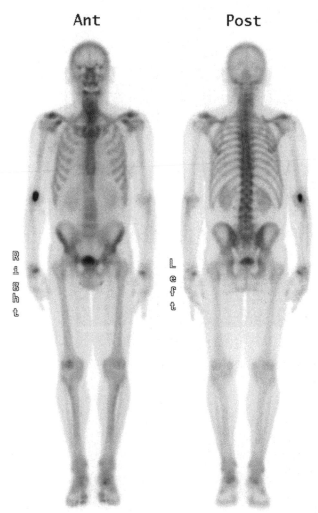

Figure 0.41 Whole-body bone scan

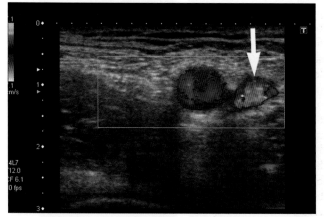

Figure 0.42 Colour Doppler ultrasound of the femoral vessels – the arrow points to the femoral artery, which is red due to the direction of flow

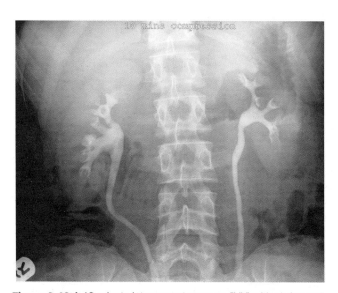

Figure 0.40 A 10-minute intravenous urogram (IVU) with abdominal compression

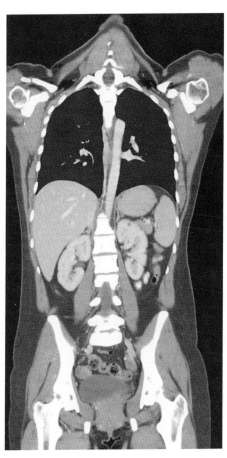

Figure 0.43 Coronal CT scan of the female thorax, abdomen and pelvis

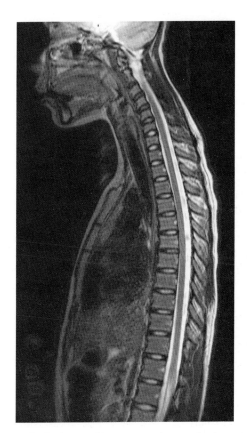

Figure 0.44 Sagittal magnetic resonance image of spine

is especially useful in the analysis of bony structures, and the most modern 64-slice units provide fantastically detailed 3D reconstructions that are prized by surgeons for their accurate preoperative assessment.

Magnetic resonance imaging (Fig. 0.44)

MRI combines a strong magnetic field and radio-frequency energy to study the distribution and behaviour of hydrogen protons in fat and water. MRI systems are graded according to the strength of the magnetic field they produce. High-field systems are those capable of producing a magnetic field strength of 1–2 Tesla. MRI does not cause any recognized biological hazard, but patients who have any form of pacemaker or implanted electroinductive device must not be examined using MRI because of risks to its function. Other prohibited items include ferromagnetic intracranial aneurysm clips, certain types of cardiac valve replacement and intraocular metallic foreign bodies. It is generally safe to examine patients who have extracranial vascular clips and orthopaedic prostheses, but these may cause local artefacts. Loose metal items must be excluded from the examination room, and beware of your credit cards being wiped clean!

The real advantage of MRI is that it provides a vastly superior visualization of the soft tissues than CT. It also provides especially detailed imaging of soft tissues such as muscles, brain, fascial planes and intervertebral discs. An intravenous injection of contrast medium (a gadolinium complex) may be given to enhance tumours and inflammatory and vascular abnormalities. In recent years there has been an increase in the use of MRA in which the flow of blood in vessels is picked up without the use of contrast medium or any interventional procedure.

New techniques and future developments

Invasive techniques such as injections of contrast are unpopular with patients so it is only natural that non-invasive procedures quickly gain approval. However, it is not only this aspect that has pushed back the boundaries – it is also the ability to see images in three dimensions and perform reconstructions of the body in real-time that have brought us new imaging modalities. Modern machines are increasingly fast with their investigations: an electron beam CT with high-speed sequencing of the cardiac cycle enables 3D chest reconstructions to be performed in a few minutes. A 64-slice CT machine has the ability to perform a whole-torso scan in less than 15 seconds. This is particularly useful in trauma cases where there may be damage to more than one system. Resolution has now also improved as the computer-generated slices get thinner – down to 0.35 mm resolution; and with greater computer power, the ability to reconstruct images in three dimensions is ever advancing.

EMQs

Each question has an anatomical theme linked to the chapter, and a list of 10 related items (A–J) placed in alphabetical order: these are followed by five statements (1–5). Match **one or more** of the items A–J to each of the five statements.

Structure of the body
A. Ciliated columnar epithelium
B. Collagen fibre
C. Columnar epithelium
D. Elastic fibre
E. Endothelium
F. Osteoblast
G. Schwann cell
H. Squamous epithelium
I. Stratified squamous epithelium
J. Transitional epithelium

Answers
1 A, 2 E, 3 G, 4 J, 5 B

Match the following statements with the appropriate item(s) from the above list.
1. Lines the trachea
2. Lines the aortic arch
3. Surrounds peripheral nerves
4. Stretches without desquamation
5. A component of hyaline cartilage

Joints
A. Ball and socket
B. Bony
C. Condyloid
D. Ellipsoid
E. Fibrous
F. Hinge
G. Primary cartilaginous
H. Saddle
I. Secondary cartilaginous
J. Synovial

Answers
1 E, 2 HJ, 3 E, 4 I, 5 I

Match the following joints to the appropriate item(s) in the above list.
1. Inferior tibiofibular
2. Carpometacarpal of thumb
3. Sutures of the skull
4. Intervertebral disc
5. Manubriosternal

Bailey & Love · Essential Clinical Anatomy

Essential Clinical Anatomy · Bailey & Love

Bailey & Love · Essential Clinical Anatomy

PART 1

The thorax

Chapter 1

The thoracic wall and diaphragm

INTRODUCTION

The bony–cartilaginous skeleton of the thorax protects the heart, lungs and great vessels. It is conical, with a narrow inlet superiorly and a wide outlet inferiorly, and is formed of 12 thoracic vertebrae posteriorly, the sternum anteriorly, and 12 pairs of ribs with costal cartilages medially. The **thoracic inlet**, 10 cm wide and 5 cm anteroposteriorly, slopes downwards and forwards and is bounded by the 1st thoracic vertebra posteriorly, the upper border of the manubrium anteriorly, and the first rib and costal cartilage anteriorly. It transmits the oesophagus, the trachea and the great vessels of the head and neck, and on each side lies the dome of the pleura. The **thoracic outlet** too is widest from side to side, and is bounded by the 12th thoracic vertebra posteriorly, the 11th and 12th ribs posteriorly, and the costal cartilages of the 7th, 8th, 9th and 10th ribs, which ascend to meet the sternum anteriorly (Fig. 1.1). The diaphragm separates the thorax from the abdomen.

The **sternum** is a flat bone, palpable throughout its length, with three parts, the manubrium, the body and the xiphoid process (**Fig. 1.1**). The **manubrium** is the thickest part, bearing on its upper border the **jugular notch** between the two lateral facets for articulation with the clavicles. Its inferior border articulates with the body at the palpable **sternal angle** (the **angle of Louis**; **Fig. 1.2**).

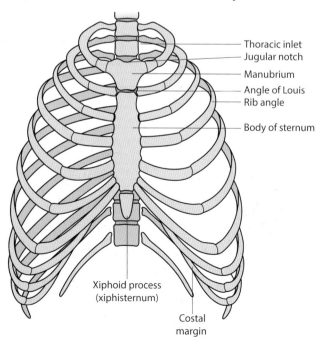

Thoracic inlet
Jugular notch
Manubrium
Angle of Louis
Rib angle
Body of sternum
Xiphoid process (xiphisternum)
Costal margin

Figure 1.1 Thoracic cage

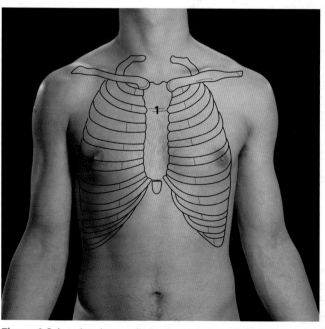

Figure 1.2 Anterior chest wall showing the sternal angle (1)

This readily palpable protuberance is an important landmark: here the 2nd costal cartilage articulates on the same plane as the 4th thoracic vertebra, the bifurcation of the trachea, and the beginning and end of the aortic arch.

The **body** of the sternum is some 10 cm long and articulates on its lateral borders with the 2nd to 7th costal cartilages. Behind the body lie the heart valves, in the order from above downwards: pulmonary, aortic, mitral and triscupid (PAMT, **Fig. 2.1b**, p. 35). The narrow lower end articulates with the **xiphoid cartilage**, which is cartilaginous in early life and gives attachment to the diaphragm and rectus abdominis.

In later life the xiphoid calcifies and can be mistaken for a gastric tumour by the inexperienced clinician. Sternal fractures have become more common because of the frequency of car accidents in which the driver's chest forcibly hits the steering column – less common with seat belts. Pericardial, cardiac or aortic damage may then follow. A flail chest may also result from multiple rib fractures, when a whole section of the chest wall moves paradoxically during respiration (**Fig. 1.3**). Air bags and safety belts reduce the incidence of this injury. Although the procedure is less popular nowadays, the sternum is still a useful site for bone marrow aspiration in adults if using the iliac crest is unsuccessful.

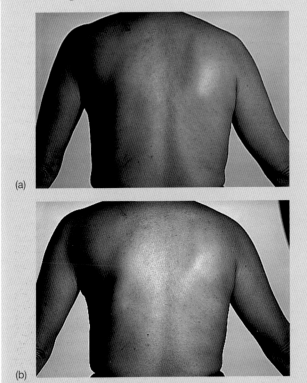

(a)

(b)

Figure 1.3 (a) and (b) Multiple rib fractures, flail chest: note drawing in of the left side of the chest during inspration

The **ribs**, usually 12 on each side, all articulate posteriorly with the thoracic vertebrae; the upper 7, known as true ribs, articulate through their costal cartilages with the sternum; the 8th to 10th ribs, 'false ribs', articulate through their cartilages with the cartilage above; and the 11th and 12th, the 'floating ribs', have free anterior ends (**Fig. 1.1**).

The costochondral and costosternal joints are tiny synovial joints reinforced with fibrous bands. Painful inflammation of these joints, sometimes known as Tietze's syndrome, can easily be misdiagnosed as cardiac disease. A special form of costochondritis known as the 'clicking-rib' syndrome is due to subluxation of a rib casing irritating the underlying intercostal nerve, and the pain it produces is easily confused with abdominal pathology.

A **typical rib** has a head, neck, tubercle and body (**Fig. 1.4**). The **head** articulates with adjacent vertebrae and is attached to the intervertebral disc. The **neck** gives attachment to the costotransverse ligaments and the **tubercle** articulates with the transverse process. The flattened curved **body** has a rounded upper border and a sharper lower border, on the inside of which is the costal groove within which lie the intercostal nerve and vessels.

The 1st, 10th, 11th and 12th ribs are not typical. All articulate with only one vertebra. The **1st rib** is short, wide, and has superior and inferior surfaces (**Fig. 1.5**). The lower smooth surface lies on the pleura; the upper surface has two grooves separated by the **scalene tubercle**, to which scalenus anterior is attached; the anterior groove is for the subclavian vein and the posterior groove for the subclavian artery and the lower trunk of the brachial plexus. The **11th and 12th ribs** are short and have neither necks nor tubercles. Their costal cartilages lie free within the abdominal wall musculature.

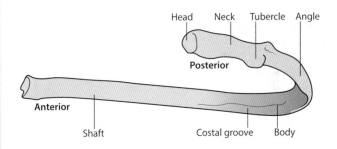

Figure 1.4 Typical right rib viewed from behind

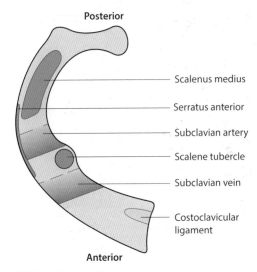

Figure 1.5 First rib – superior view

The weakest part of the rib is the body anterior to the angle, and it is here that most fractures occur after blunt trauma. Direct trauma may produce fracture in any part of the rib. In both cases, the fracture fragments may damage adjacent structures, such as intercostal vessels, pleura, lung or spleen. A pneumothorax, air in the pleural cavity, is a common complication of serious rib fractures rupturing the underlying lung (Fig. 1.6). In certain circumstances, the valvular nature of the tear in the lung tissue causes air to accumulate in the pleural cavity with each inspiration, and this accumulation will cause the mediastinum to shift across to the opposite side (tension pneumothorax; Fig. 1.6b).

THE THORACIC CAGE

Note that:

- The cavity is kidney-shaped in cross-section because the vertebral column intrudes into the thoracic cage posteriorly.
- The ribs increase in length from the 1st to the 7th, and thereafter become shorter.
    - The ribs lie at an angle of about 45° to the vertebral column, the maximum obliquity being reached by the 9th rib.
    - The costal cartilages increase in length from above downwards – from ribs 1 to 10.

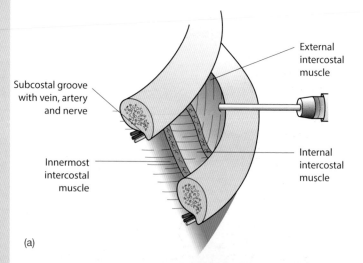

(a)

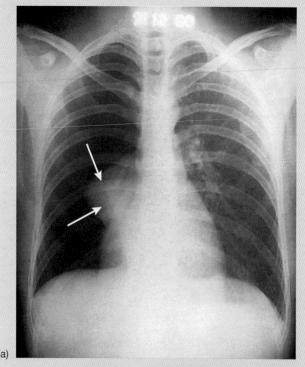

(a)

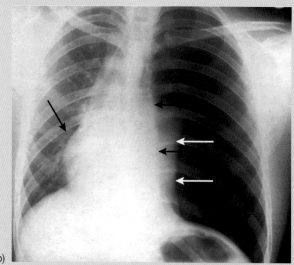

(b)

Figure 1.6 (a) Right pneumothorax: note the dark shadow cast by air and the absence of lung markings in the right chest. The right lung is collapsed (arrows). (b) Left tension pneumothorax with mediastinal shift. The heart is displaced to the right (arrowed). White arrows show collapsed lung, black arrows the left border of the heart

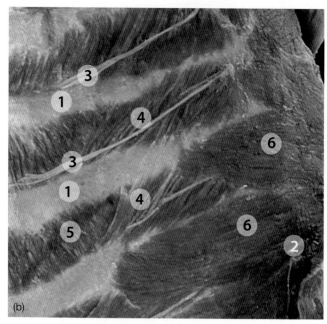

(b)

Figure 1.7 (a) Intercostal space showing the aspirating needle passed just above the rib, thus avoiding the vessels in the subcostal groove above. (b) Left thoracic wall showing details of intercostal muscles: 1, rib; 2, intercostal nerves; 3, lateral cutaneous branch of intercostal nerve; 4, external intercostal muscle; 5, internal intercostal muscle; 6, serratus anterior muscle

- The cage gives attachment to the muscles of the upper limb, the abdominal wall muscles, the extensor muscles of the back, the diaphragm and the intercostal muscles.

The **intercostal spaces**, bounded by ribs and costal cartilages, contain the intercostal vessels and nerves. The pleura lies deep to them. The spaces contain three layers of muscles from without inwards: the external, the internal and the innermost intercostal muscles. They are supplied by their adjacent intercostal nerve and move the ribs (Fig. 1.7). When the 1st rib is anchored by contraction of the scalene muscles, approximation of the ribs by the intercostal muscles **raises** the sternum and air is drawn into the lungs. When the lower ribs are anchored by the abdominal muscles, approximation of the ribs **lowers** the sternum and air is forced out of the lungs.

Intercostal vessels and nerves

The **intercostal vessels and nerves** form a neurovascular bundle that passes forwards in the subcostal groove deep to the internal intercostal muscle, separated from the pleura only by the innermost intercostal muscle.

Each intercostal space is supplied by posterior and anterior **intercostal arteries**, which anastomose in the space. The first and second posterior arteries arise from branches of the subclavian artery, and the remainder all arise directly from the descending aorta; the anterior arteries are branches of the internal thoracic artery, a branch of the subclavian artery. The **intercostal veins**, lying above their arteries in the costal groove, drain to the internal thoracic and azygos veins.

The **intercostal nerves** are formed from the ventral rami of the upper 11 thoracic spinal nerves. Each is attached to the spinal cord by ventral and dorsal roots. The dorsal root bears

a sensory ganglion in the intervertebral foramen. Once the roots have united, the nerve divides into dorsal and ventral rami (Fig. 1.8). Each dorsal ramus supplies the extensor muscles of the back and, by cutaneous branches, the skin of the back. The ventral ramus forms the intercostal nerve, and this runs forwards in the costal groove below the artery to supply the intercostal muscles and the skin of the lateral and anterior chest wall.

Insertion of a needle to obtain fluid or blood from the pleural cavity will be undertaken safely if the needle is introduced into the lower part of the intercostal space away from the intercostal neurovascular bundle lying in the subcostal groove (Figs. 1.7a and 1.9).

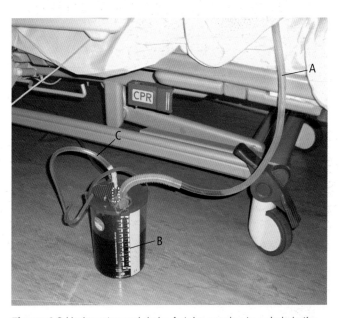

Figure 1.9 Underwater seal drain: A, tube passing to a drain in the patient's anterior mediastinum; B, tube passing below the waterline of the container (white dashed line); C, exit tube above the water line at atmospheric pressure (white dotted line). NB: the container must never be raised above the level of the patient, as fluid may otherwise siphon in the opposite direction

DERMATOMES

Through the cutaneous branches of the ventral and dorsal rami each spinal nerve supplies a **dermatome** – a strip of skin between the posterior and anterior midlines. These are arranged in segmental fashion because of their origin from segments of the spinal cord. There is overlapping of adjacent dermatomes.

Clinicians need a working knowledge of the dermatomal innervation of the skin in order to establish the normality or otherwise of the function of a particular segment of the spinal cord (Figs. 1.10 and 1.11; see also Figs. 12.17b, 17.12 and 17.13, pp. 198 and 295). Herpes zoster (shingles) is a viral infection of the dorsal root ganglia. Infection produces a sharp burning pain in the dermatome supplied by the infected segment. Several days later, the affected dermatome becomes reddened and vesicular eruptions appear (Fig. 1.12).

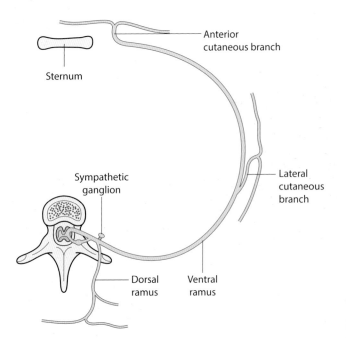

Figure 1.8 Typical spinal nerve

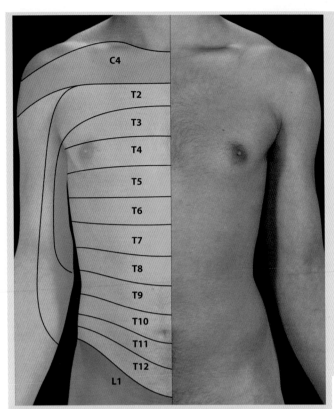

Figure 1.10 Cutaneous innervation of the anterior trunk showing dermatomes: note the umbilicus is innervated by T10 and the groin by L1

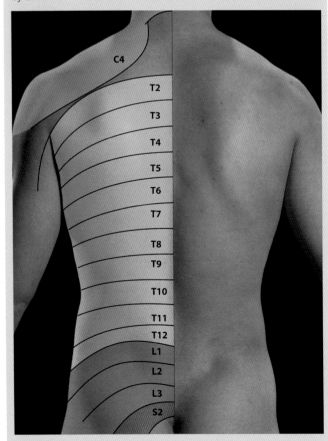

Figure 1.11 Cutaneous innervation of the posterior trunk showing dermatomes

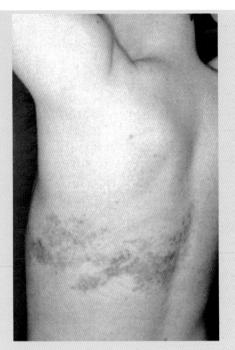

Figure 1.12 Lower thoracic herpes zoster (shingles)

THE MEDIASTINUM

For the purposes of description, the mediastinum is divided into:

- The superior mediastinum extending from the thoracic inlet (Fig. 1.13) to the transverse plane, T4
- The posterior mediastinum below the plane and behind the heart
- The anterior mediastinum below the plane and anterior to the heart
- The middle mediastinum containing the pericardium, heart and main bronchi.

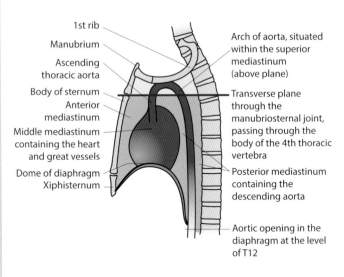

Figure 1.13 Thorax: sagittal section showing divisions of the mediastinum

THE DIAPHRAGM

This musculotendinous septum separates the thoracic and abdominal cavities; it has a central tendinous part and a peripheral muscular part. It has peripheral attachments around the outlet of the thoracic cavity:

- **Sternal** – from the back of the xiphoid process
- **Costal** – from the inner surfaces of the lower six costal cartilages
- **Vertebral** – from the sides of the upper lumbar vertebrae by two crura, and from medial and lateral arcuate ligaments.

The **right crus** arises from the bodies of the upper three vertebrae and the **left crus** from the first two. The **medial arcuate ligament**, the thickened upper edge of the psoas fascia, passes between the body of the 1st lumbar vertebra and its transverse process; the **lateral arcuate ligament** lies anterior to quadratus lumborum and extends between the 12th rib's transverse process and the tip of the 12th rib. Its central attachment is to the periphery of a trefoil central tendon. The diaphragm is the principal muscle of respiration. Contraction flattens the dome of the diaphragm and makes it descend, thereby increasing the vertical diameter of the chest; air is then drawn into the lungs. In expiration, the diaphragm relaxes. The diaphragm curves upwards on each side, reaching the 5th intercostal space on the left side and slightly higher on the right (Figs. 4.1 and 4.2, pp. 63 and 64).

Nerve supply

The two halves of the diaphragm are each supplied by a phrenic nerve, and its periphery receives sensory branches from the lower intercostal nerves.

Openings

There are three large openings in the diaphragm (Fig. 1.14):

- The **caval opening** – at the level of the 8th thoracic vertebra. This transmits the inferior vena cava and the right phrenic nerve.

- The **oesophageal opening** – in the right crus, to the left of the **midline** at the level of the 10th thoracic vertebra. It transmits the oesophagus, the gastric branches of the vagus nerves and the gastric vessels.
- The **aortic opening** – between the diaphragmatic crura in front of the 12th thoracic vertebra. It conveys the aorta, the thoracic duct and the azygos vein.

The left phrenic nerve pierces the dome of the left diaphragm. The heart and lungs, within the pericardial and pleural sacs, lie on its upper surface. The fibrous pericardium is firmly attached to its upper surface. Inferiorly on the right lie the liver, the right kidney and the suprarenal gland; on the left are the left lobe of the liver, gastric fundus, spleen, left kidney and suprarenal gland.

Respiration

Inspiration and expiration are produced by increasing and decreasing the volume of the thoracic cavity. In quiet respiration, only the diaphragm is involved, and inspiration is aided by the weight of the liver attached to the underside of the diaphragm.

- **Inspiration** – the diaphragm contracts and descends and the height of the thoracic cavity thus increases. The upper ribs are fixed by the scalene muscles, and contraction of the intercostals thus raises the ribs, thereby increasing the anteroposterior and transverse diameters of the chest.
- **Expiration** – largely produced by relaxation of the diaphragm and elastic recoil of the lungs and the costal cartilages. Simultaneous contraction of the abdominal muscles forces the diaphragm upwards in forced expiration, such as in coughing and sneezing.

The diaphragm also helps in defecation. Straining involves deep inspiration and fixation of the contracted diaphragm and prevention of expiration by closure of the glottis. This action also assists in lifting heavy objects from the ground.

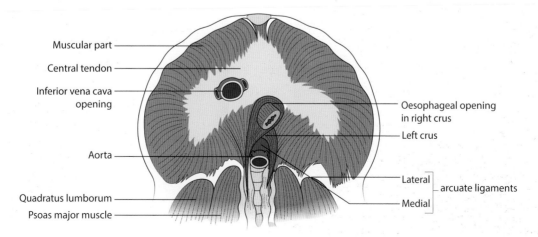

Figure 1.14 Inferior surface of the diaphragm. The anterior chest wall has been removed and the diaphragm lifted upwards to show its under surface while retaining its posterior attachments

THE BREAST

The adult female breast is a soft, hemispherical structure. It is composed of glandular tissue and a variable amount of fat and fibrous tissue and lies in the superficial fascia of the upper anterior thoracic wall. The fascia invests it and forms radial septae, the suspensory ligaments (Cooper), which traverse the gland from the underlying fascia to be attached to the overlying skin. They divide the gland into 15–20 lobules. From the alveoli of each lobule, the ducts unite to form a lactiferous duct. The breast lies on the fascia over pectoralis major but is separated from it by loose connective tissue. The male breast is a rudimentary organ comprising small ducts but no alveoli. It is, however, susceptible to all the diseases that afflict the female breast.

The female breast extends over the 2nd to the 6th ribs just lateral to the sternum as far as the midaxillary line, and lies mainly on the pectoralis major muscle (Fig. 1.15). For descriptive purposes, it is divided into four quadrants; the upper outer quadrant extends laterally into the axilla as the **axillary tail**. Each of the 15 or so breast lobules drains by a lactiferous duct into the **nipple**, which is surrounded by thin pigmented skin, the **areola**, containing modified sebaceous glands and smooth muscle (**Figs. 1.15–1.17**).

Blood supply is via branches of the internal thoracic, intercostal and lateral thoracic arteries.

Lymph drains from the gland along vascular tributaries via two lymphatic plexuses: the subcutaneous subareolar plexus and the submammary plexus on pectoralis major. Although there is communication between lymphatics from these plexuses, they mainly drain laterally to the axillary nodes, superiorly to infraclavicular and lower deep cervical nodes, inferiorly to lymphatics in the anterior abdominal wall and medially to nodes around the internal thoracic artery. A small

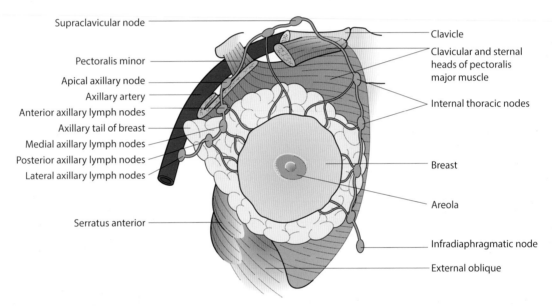

Figure 1.15 Relations and lymphatic drainage of female breast

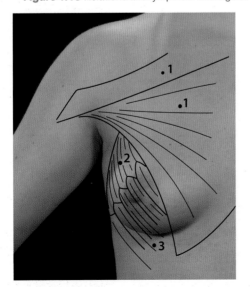

Figure 1.16 Surface anatomy of the breast: 1, clavicular and sternocostal parts of pectoralis major; 2, serratus anterior; 3, external oblique

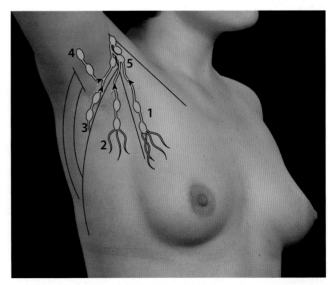

Figure 1.17 Lymphatic drainage of the breast. Axillary lymph nodes: 1, anterior; 2, medial; 3, posterior; 4, lateral; 5, apical

amount of lymph drains from the medial side of the breast into the opposite breast.

Supernumerary breasts or nipples may be formed anywhere along the 'milk line', which extends from axilla to groin (Fig. 1.18).

Pregnancy and lactation promote marked glandular proliferation, an increased pigmentation of the areola and nipple, and an increase in blood supply.

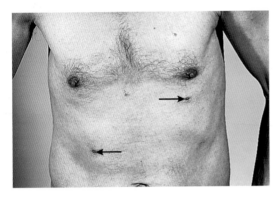

Figure 1.18 Accessory nipples (arrows)

A lactating breast is susceptible to infection. Abscess drainage should be by a radial incision to avoid damage to the duct system. A breast cancer that has spread by infiltration may invade and become attached to the fascia and the pectoralis major muscle beneath it. If the suspensory ligaments are invaded, these contract and may produce retraction of the nipple (Fig. 1.19). If the spread has invaded and blocked the lymphatics of the breast, skin oedema will occur – **peau d'orange** (Fig. 1.20a). Cancerous infiltration of the axillary lymph nodes may produce arm swelling (lymphoedema) (Fig. 1.20b).

It is now realized that the former treatment of breast cancer – the attempted surgical removal of the whole breast with its contained cancer along with pectoralis major and all possibly involved lymph nodes – was based on the wrong assumption that it was possible to excise most breast cancers and the local lymphatic spread by surgical means. Nowadays it is accepted that, in most cases, the spread of the disease is wider than any possible surgical field could contain, so the surgical approach is limited to removal of the breast (or, in small cancers, the tumour and surrounding tissue) and the axillary nodes. Treatment of the wider spread of the cancer is undertaken with chemotherapy and/or radiotherapy.

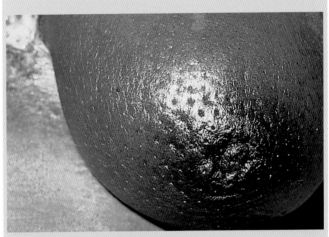

(a)

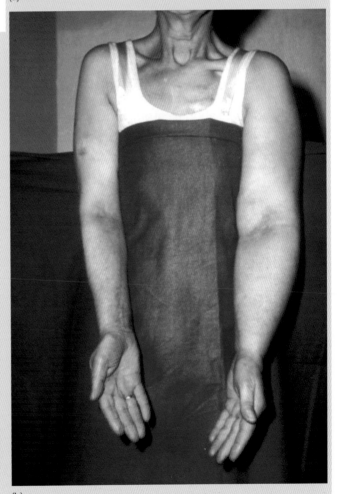

(b)

Figure 1.20 (a) Peau d'orange due to lymphatic obstruction. (b) Lymphoedema of the left arm due to breast malignancy

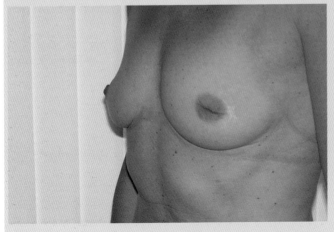

Figure 1.19 Retracted nipple

DEVELOPMENT OF THE DIAPHRAGM

The diaphragm is formed by the fusion of five separate embryonic membranes, and myoblasts from the C3–C5 somites, which explains its cervical spinal nerve innervation. A single midline ventral mass of splanchnic mesenchyme, the septum transversum, forms the anterior part of the diaphragm, including the central tendon (Fig. 1.21a,b). The septum transversum does not fully separate the thoracic and abdominal cavities, especially in the region of the pericardioperitoneal canals. The diaphragm is completed via the growth of paired transverse dorsolateral folds of tissue, the left and right pleuroperitoneal membranes or folds, from the body wall; these fuse with the posterior border of the septum transversum and the mesentery of the distal oesophagus. The diaphragm is completed peripherally by tissue contributions from the developing body wall (Fig. 1.21b).

Congenital diaphragmatic hernia

Due to the complexity of diaphragmatic formation, structural defects can occur (1:2000 incidence), which generally result in a congenital diaphragmatic hernia. The Bochdalek hernia, the most common type of congenital diaphragmatic hernia, represents an absence of a pleuroperitoneal membrane, usually on the left side of the diaphragm (Figs. 1.21b and 1.22). Consequently, adjacent abdominal organs can enter the thorax, where they may compress the lungs and move the heart anteriorly.

A congenital diaphragmatic hernia may also occur in the para/retrosternal region, leading to a Morgagni parasternal hernia. This hernia is rare (around 2% of congenital diaphragmatic hernias), may be asymptomatic, most often occurs on the right side of the diaphragm and is due to muscular deficits in the sternocostal triangles (foramina of Morgagni), which are located between the sternal and costal attachments of the diaphragm (Figs. 1.21b and 1.22). A hiatus hernia can occur via an abnormally large oesophageal hiatus, although many are acquired.

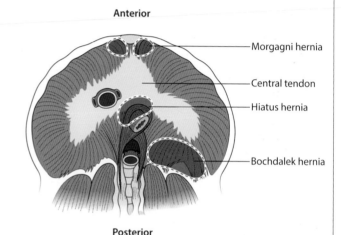

Figure 1.22 The formed diaphragm (inferior view) showing the central tendon, muscular region and normal orifices, and the most likely locations of the defects resulting in Bochdalek, Morgagni and hiatus hernias

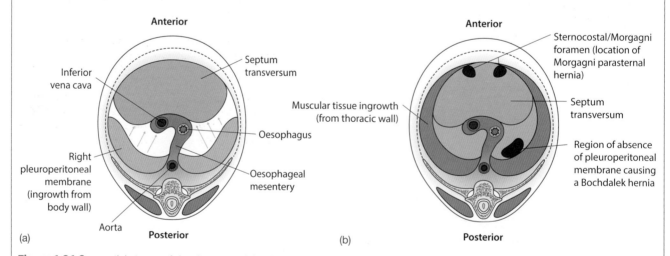

Figure 1.21 Sequential stages of development of the diaphragm from multiple different regional tissues (inferior view). (a) Early stage (~week 5). (b) Late stage (~week 20) showing the potential locations of defects and diaphragmatic hernias

MCQs

1. A typical rib:
		T/F
a	articulates with two vertebral bodies	(___)
b	is attached to an intervertebral disc	(___)
c	bears three facets for articulation with the vertebral column	(___)
d	has a costal cartilage that articulates with the sternum by a synovial joint	(___)
e	is grooved superiorly by the costal groove	(___)

Answers

1.

a **T** – *Each typical rib bears two facets on its head for articulation with its own vertebra...*

b **T** – *... and the one above. The intervening crest is attached by an intra-articular ligament to the intervertebral disc.*

c **T** – *Two facets for articulation with two vertebral bodies and one for the transverse process.*

d **T** – *The joint between the 1st rib (which is not typical) and the sternum is a cartilaginous joint, but the joints between the 2nd to 7th costal cartilages and the sternum are synovial.*

e **F** – *The costal groove, conveying the intercostal vessels and nerve, lies inferiorly on the rib's inner surface.*

2. A typical intercostal nerve:
		T/F
a	is the ventral ramus of a thoracic spinal nerve	(___)
b	lies, for most of its course, deep to the internal intercostal muscle	(___)
c	lies, for the most part, in the subcostal groove	(___)
d	supplies, among other structures, the skin of the back	(___)
e	may supply the skin of the abdominal wall	(___)

Answers

2.

a **T** – *It has cutaneous and muscular branches.*
b **T** – *Much of it is lying against the pleura.*
c **T** – *The artery and vein separate it from the rib.*
d **F** – *The skin of the back is supplied by branches of the dorsal rami.*
e **T** – *Anterior abdominal wall skin is supplied segmentally by the 7th to 12th intercostal nerves.*

3. The diaphragm:
		T/F
a	is attached in part to the sternum	(___)
b	is supplied by the phrenic and intercostal nerves	(___)
c	increases the horizontal diameter of the chest when contracting	(___)
d	has an opening in its central tendon for the inferior vena cava	(___)
e	contracts during micturition	(___)

Answers

3.

a **T** – *It gains attachment to the back of the xiphoid, the lowest six cartilages, the lateral and medial arcuate ligaments and, by the right and left crura, to the upper two or three lumbar vertebrae.*

b **T** – *Only the phrenic nerve is motor; the intercostal nerves supply sensory branches to the periphery of the diaphragm.*

c **F** – *Contraction flattens the diaphragm, thereby increasing the vertical diameter of the chest.*

d **T** – *The opening is slightly to the right of the midline and also conveys the right phrenic nerve.*

e **T** – *Expulsive acts, such as micturition and defecation, require a rise in intra-abdominal pressure that is usually produced by simultaneous contraction of the diaphragm and anterior abdominal wall.*

SBA

1. An adult was admitted to the emergency department. He was the driver of a car that had sustained a head-on collision. He had not been wearing a seat belt and had suffered severe trauma to his sternum. Which part of the heart is most likely to have been injured?

   a apex of left ventricle
   b right ventricle
   c left ventricle
   d anterior part of left atrium
   e left atrium
   f aortic root

   b The right ventricle is the part lying adjacent to the deep surface of the sternum and is often injured in sternal fractures. The aorta can be avulsed in certain stretch injuries.

2. A woman is admitted with the diagnosis of a pleural effusion. Draining this effusion requires a chest tube to be inserted through an intercostal space. Which part of the intercostal space lying over the effusion must the doctor try to insert the tube into?

   a into the midpoint of the space
   b between the external and internal intercostal muscles
   c immediately below the lower border of the rib
   d between the internal intercostal muscle and the posterior intercostal membrane
   e immediately above the upper border of the rib

   e The chest tube must be inserted away from the neurovascular bundle of vein, artery and nerve, which lie in a groove on the internal aspect of the lower border of the rib. The pleural cavity will not be gained by placing the tube to lie either between the internal and external intercostal muscles or between the internal intercostal muscle and the posterior intercostal membrane.

EMQs

Each question has an anatomical theme linked to the chapter, and a list of 10 related items (A–J) placed in alphabetical order: these are followed by five statements (1–5). Match **one or more** of the items A–J to each of the five statements.

Thoracic cage

A. 1st rib
B. 2nd rib
C. 5th rib
D. 7th rib
E. 9th rib
F. 10th rib
G. 12th rib
H. Body of sternum
I. Manubrium
J. Xiphisternum

Match the following statements with the appropriate item(s) from the above list.

1. Articulates at the sternal angle
2. Typical rib
3. Related to the subclavian artery
4. Atypical rib
5. Related to the right ventricle

Answers
1 BHI; 2 CDEF; 3 A; 4 ABG; 5 H

Diaphragm

A. Central tendon
B. Lateral arcuate ligament
C. Left crus
D. Left gastric nerve
E. Median arcuate ligament
F. Opening at the level of the 8th thoracic vertebra
G. Opening at the level of the 10th thoracic vertebra
H. Opening at the level of the 12th thoracic vertebra
I. Right crus
J. Right phrenic nerve

Match the following statements with the appropriate item(s) from the above list.

1. Gives passage to the inferior vena cava
2. Attached to the 12th rib
3. Overlies the aorta
4. Gives passage to the oesophagus
5. Attached to the 3rd lumbar vertebra

Answers
1 AF; 2 B; 3 CEHI; 4 GI; 5 I

APPLIED QUESTIONS

1. Where do ribs fracture? What may be the consequences?

1. The region of the angle of a rib is its weakest part, and crushing injuries tend to fracture ribs just anterior to their angles. A direct blow may fracture the rib anywhere. Broken ends of fractured ribs may, when driven inwards, puncture the pleural sac and damage underlying viscera such as the lung, heart, spleen or kidney. The ribs of children, being mainly cartilaginous, are rarely fractured. A severe blow to the anterior chest may fracture the sternum and/or multiple ribs to produce a 'flail' anterior segment of the chest wall and respiratory embarrassment.

2. At which vertebral levels do the jugular notch, manubriosternal joint and inferior angle of the scapula usually lie?

2. These three palpable skeletal landmarks are reasonably constant and lie at T2, T4/5 and T7, respectively. The manubriosternal joint, also known as the sternal angle (of Louis), is also palpable and a useful point from which to count ribs – the 2nd rib articulates with the sternum at this point – and in this way provides a reliable method of identifying intercostal spaces.

3. Intradermal swelling and pitting of the skin may be seen in breast cancers. What is the anatomical explanation for this?

3. This is due to skin oedema and is known as peau d'orange. It is a classic sign of advanced breast cancer and is caused by blockage of the lymphatic drainage of the skin by cancer cells.

4. What special features may you see on examining the breasts of a pregnant woman?

4. The whole breast is enlarged and the axillary tail possibly noticed for the first time. Many dilated veins can be seen under the breast skin. The nipple and areola are more deeply pigmented and the areolar glands (Montgomery) larger and more numerous. Their function is to lubricate the nipple during lactation.

Bailey & Love · Essential Clinical Anatomy · Bailey & Love · Essential Clinical Anatomy
Essential Clinical Anatomy · Bailey & Love · Essential Clinical Anatomy · Bailey & Love
Bailey & Love · Essential Clinical Anatomy · Bailey & Love · Essential Clinical Anatomy

Chapter 2

The thoracic cavity

The thoracic cavity is divided into right and left pleural cavities by the central mediastinum. The mediastinum is bounded behind by the vertebral column and in front by the sternum; it extends from the diaphragm below to become continuous above with the structures in the root of the neck. It contains the heart, great vessels, oesophagus, trachea and lymphatics.

THE HEART

The heart is the muscular pump of the systemic and pulmonary circulations. It has four chambers: two atria and two ventricles (Figs. 2.1a and 2.17a) The direction of blood flow is controlled by unidirectional valves between the atria and ventricles and between the ventricles and the emerging aorta and pulmonary trunk. The heart, the size of a clenched fist, weighs about 300 g and is the shape of a flattened cone with a base and an apex. It lies obliquely across the lower mediastinum behind the sternum within the pericardial sac, suspended by it from the great vessels.

Its square base faces posteriorly and is formed from the left atrium and the four pulmonary veins (Fig. 2.2). The tip of the left ventricle forms the apex and is at the lower left extremity of the heart. The anterior surface is formed by the right atrium and the ventricles, separated by the anterior interventricular grooves. The inferior surface rests on the central tendon of the diaphragm and is formed of both ventricles (mainly the left), separated by the posterior interventricular groove. The left surface, in contact with the left lung, is formed by the left ventricle and a small part of the left atrium. The right surface, in contact with the right lung, is formed by the right atrium, into which enter the superior and the inferior vena cavae.

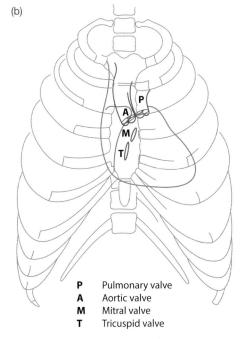

(b)

P	Pulmonary valve
A	Aortic valve
M	Mitral valve
T	Tricuspid valve

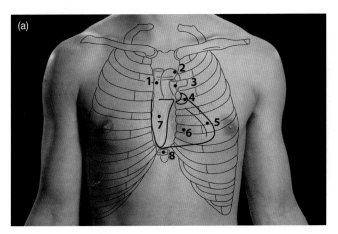

(a)

Figure 2.1 (a) Surface anatomy of chambers of the heart: 1, superior vena cava; 2, arch of aorta; 3, pulmonary trunk; 4, left auricle; 5, left ventricle; 6, right ventricle; 7, right atrium; 8, inferior vena cava. (b) Great vessels and position of valves

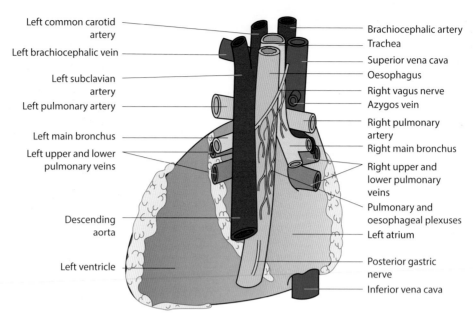

Figure 2.2 Posterior view of the heart and great vessels and their relationship to the oesophagus and trachea. Note that the posterior aspect of the heart contains the left atrium and pulmonary veins, with the oesophagus in direct contact with the left atrium

Surface markings (Fig. 2.1b)

The right border of the heart extends between the 3rd and 6th right costal cartilages, projecting just beyond the right sternal border. Its inferior border runs from the right 6th cartilage to the apex, situated in the 5th intercostal space in the midclavicular line. The left border extends from the apex to the left 2nd costal cartilage about 2 cm from the sternal edge.

THE CHAMBERS OF THE HEART

The right chamber pumps blood through the lungs and the left pumps blood through the systemic circulation (Fig. 2.3).

The **right atrium**, a thin-walled chamber, receives blood from the superior and inferior venae cavae and the coronary sinus. Superomedially, its small projection, the right auricle, overlaps the root of the aorta. On the right side, a vertical ridge, the crista terminalis, passes between the cavae. The atrial wall behind the caval openings, the atrial septum, separates it from the left atrium, is smooth and bears a shallow central depression, the **fossa ovalis**. The wall is thicker anteriorly and formed of parallel muscular ridges that pass transversely to the vertical ridge that is the crista terminalis. The superior caval orifice has no valves; that of the inferior vena cava has a rudimentary valve anteriorly, and between them, posteriorly, is the smaller opening of the coronary sinus.

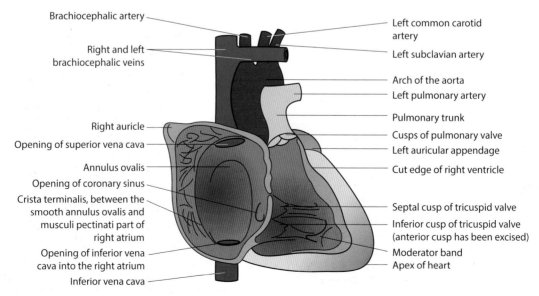

Figure 2.3 Anterior view of the heart and great vessels to show the main chambers of the right side of the heart. The right atrial wall has been opened to reveal the internal structures and vessels draining into this chamber. The opened ventricle reveals the tricuspid valve and musculature

The **right ventricle**, a thick-walled chamber, projects forwards and to the left of the right atrium. An interventricular septum separates it from the left ventricle and bulges into the right cavity (Fig. 2.4). The ventricular walls are marked by interlacing muscular bands, except superiorly, where the smooth-walled infundibulum leads to the pulmonary orifice. The atrioventricular orifice lies posteroinferiorly and is guarded by the **tricuspid valve**, which has three cusps. Their ventricular surfaces are rough and anchored to the ventricular walls by fine tendinous cords arising from the ventricular septum or from two conical **papillary muscles**, which arise from the anterior and inferior ventricular walls. These cords and papillary muscles prevent eversion of the valve cusps into the atrial cavity during ventricular contraction, and thus prevent regurgitation of blood into the atrium. The **pulmonary valve**, which lies at the upper end of the infundibulum, has three semilunar cusps; these are concave when viewed from above.

The **left atrium** is a rectangular chamber and lies behind the right atrium. Its appendix, the left auricular projection, overlies the left side of the pulmonary trunk. Four pulmonary veins enter its posterior surface, two on each side; their orifices possess no valves. The left atrioventricular orifice is on the anterior atrial wall. The posterior wall lies anterior to the oesophagus, left bronchus and descending thoracic aorta (Figs. 2.2 and 2.5).

The **left ventricle** (Fig. 2.6), extending forwards and to the left of the left atrium, lies mainly behind the right ventricle. Its very thick walls (Fig. 2.4) are covered on the inside by muscular ridges, except for the smooth area below the aortic orifice, the vestibule. It has two orifices, the left atrioventricular posteriorly and the aortic superiorly. The left atrioventricular orifice is guarded by the **mitral valve**, which has two cusps, each anchored to papillary muscles by tendinous cords. The **aortic valve** has three cusps, above which are small dilatations, the aortic sinuses. The surface anatomy of the valves is shown in Fig. 2.7, and their relationships in Fig. 2.8.

The interventricular septum is thick, except for a thin membranous portion between the infundibulum and the vestibule. Both ventricular and atrial muscle fibres are anchored to a fibrous framework around the four valvular orifices, the fibrous skeleton of the heart (Fig. 2.8).

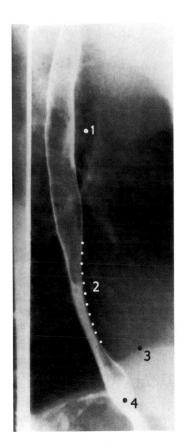

Figure 2.5 Barium swallow, right lateral view: 1, trachea (revealed by its translucency); 2, cardiac impression (left atrium); 3, diaphragm; 4, gastro-oesophageal junction

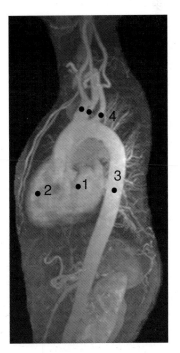

Figure 2.6 Arteriogram of the left side of the heart. A catheter (not outlined) has been passed retrogradely though the brachial artery into the left atrium and contrast medium injected. This shows the left atrium (1), the ventricle (2), the aorta (3), and branches arising from the aortic arch (4)

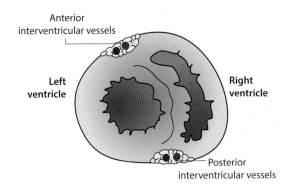

Figure 2.4 Transverse section through the ventricles, showing the relative thickness of the walls

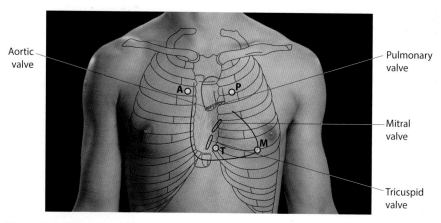

Figure 2.7 Surface markings of the four heart valves. The sites where the sounds coming from these valves are best heard with a stethoscope are indicated by a small circle with a corresponding letter

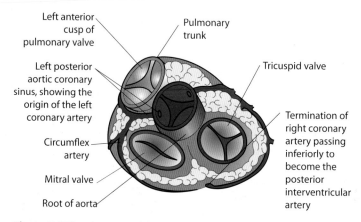

Figure 2.8 Upper aspect of the heart with the atria removed, showing the aortic root, pulmonary trunk, mitral and tricuspid valves, fibrous skeleton and right and left coronary arteries

BLOOD SUPPLY

This is derived from the right and left coronary arteries. The **right coronary artery** (Figs 2.9. and 2.10) arises from the anterior aortic sinus and descends to the heart's anterior surface in the atrioventricular groove, supplying atrial and ventricular branches. It gains the posterior surface, where it gives off a marginal and a posterior interventricular artery, which may anastomose with the anterior interventricular branch of the left coronary artery. The **left coronary artery** (Figs. 2.8, 2.9 and 2.11) is larger and arises from the left posterior aortic sinus. It passes forwards to supply atrial and ventricular branches. Its most important branch is the **anterior interventricular artery** (known clinically as the left anterior descending artery – LAD), which descends in the anterior interventricular groove to the apex and the lower border to anastomose with the posterior interventricular branch of the right coronary artery. The circumflex branch passes posteriorly to supply much of the left ventricle. The right ventricle is usually supplied by the right coronary artery, the left by the left, the interventricular septum by both, and the atria in a variable manner. The sinoatrial node and atrioventricular node are usually supplied by the right coronary artery (Figs. 2.10 and 2.12).

The **mitral valve** is the most frequently diseased heart valve; fibrosis causes the cusps to shorten and causes incompetence and/or stenosis of the valve. Congenital stenosis of the pulmonary and the aortic valves may occur and result in hypertrophy of the right and left ventricles, respectively, and eventual cardiac decompensation. Although anastomoses exist between the two **coronary arteries**, sudden occlusion of a major branch may result in ischaemia and death of some heart muscle (**myocardial infarction**), and if the area affected includes the conducting system or is large, the patient may die. Lesser degrees of ischaemic damage diminish the heart's work capacity, and pain (angina) may be felt on exertion. Narrowing of the coronary arteries may, by diminishing blood supply to the cardiac muscle, also cause angina, a pain usually felt in the substernal region. Ischaemia of the myocardium stimulates nerve endings within it. Sensory impulses are carried, largely on the left side, in the sympathetic branches to the thoracic segments T1–T4. Pain arising in the heart is felt substernally but is often referred to the left arm and neck. This coronary narrowing is sometimes amenable to treatment

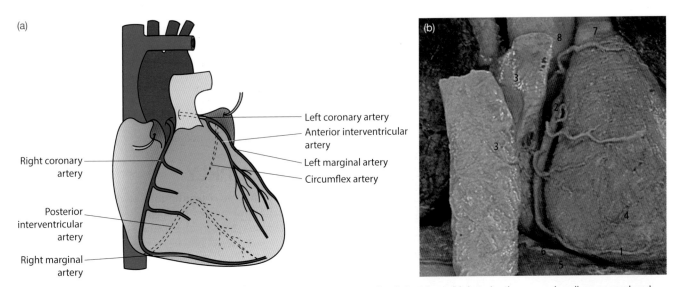

Figure 2.9 (a) Coronary arteries of the heart; those lying posteriorly are shown by dotted lines. (b) Anterior thorax, pericardium opened and retracted to the right: 1, right coronary artery, marginal branch; 2, right coronary artery; 3, retracted double layer of pericardium, shining parietal serous layer; 4, right ventricle, covered with visceral serous pericardium; 5, diaphragm; 6, fibrous pericardium attachment to central tendon of diaphragm; 7, pulmonary trunk; 8, aorta

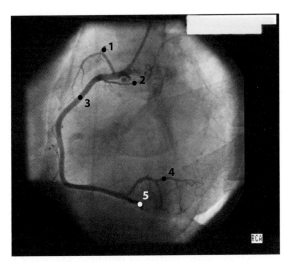

Figure 2.10 Right coronary arteriogram: 1, conus branch; 2, sinoatrial nodal artery; 3, right main coronary artery; 4, posterior interventricular artery; 5, origin of atrioventricular nodal branch

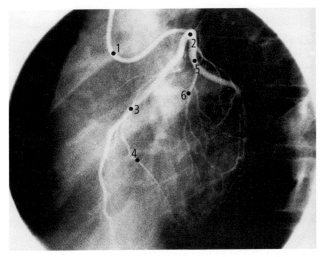

Figure 2.11 Left coronary arteriogram: 1, catheter; 2, common origin of left and right coronary arteries; 3, left anterior descending artery; 4, diagonal branch; 5, left main coronary artery; 6, anterior interventricular artery

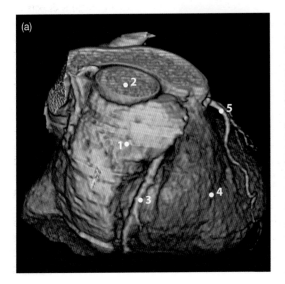

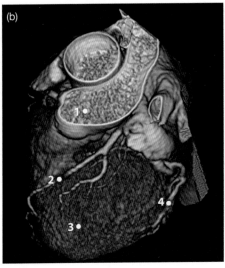

Figure 2.12 Electron beam CT. (a) Anterior view: 1, right atrium; 2, superior vena cava; 3, right coronary artery; 4, right ventricle; 5, anterior descending interventricular branch of left coronary artery (left anterior descending artery). (b) Left lateral superior view: 1, aortic root; 2, anterior descending interventricular branch of the left coronary artery; 3, left ventricle; 4, circumflex branch of left coronary artery

by balloon dilatation, stenting (Fig. 2.13) or surgical bypass of the occlusion (CABG – coronary artery bypass grafting). Rupture of a papillary muscle, for instance after ischaemic damage, may result in incompetence of the mitral or tricuspid valve. Valvular stenosis or incompetence may require surgical replacement of the valve.

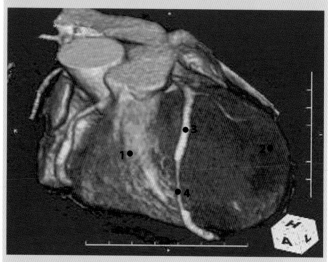

Figure 2.13 Electron beam CT scan of a patient following insertion of a stent (a small tube to open up a blocked artery): 1, right ventricle; 2, left ventricle; 3, stent in descending interventricular branch of the left coronary artery; 4, stenosis (narrowed segment) of coronary artery even after stenting

Venous drainage

This is largely via the **coronary sinus**, which drains into the right atrium near to the opening of the inferior vena cava (Fig. 2.14). It is about 3 cm long and receives the **great cardiac vein**, which ascends the anterior interventricular groove, the **middle cardiac vein** running in the posterior interventricular groove, a **small cardiac vein** that reaches it in the coronary sulcus, and branches from the posterior of the left ventricle

and atrium. **Anterior cardiac veins**, several in number, draining the anterior right ventricle, drain directly into the right atrium. **Venae cordis minimae** drain much of the heart wall. They are small and open directly into the heart's chambers.

LYMPHATIC DRAINAGE

This is to the tracheobronchial nodes.

NERVE SUPPLY

This is from the vagus (cardio-inhibitory) and sympathetic (cardio-excitatory) nerves through the cardiac plexus (see p. 71). The fibres pass with the branches of the coronary arteries. Parasympathetic ganglia lie in the heart wall. The vagus conveys sensory fibres; pain fibres run with the sympathetic nerves and traverse the cervical and upper thoracic sympathetic ganglia before entering the spinal nerves T1–T4.

Cardiac pain is produced by ischaemic heart tissue. Because the afferent sensory fibres pass through the cervical and upper thoracic ganglia before entering the upper thoracic spinal cord segments, the visceral pain produced by ischaemia is commonly referred to those somatic structures with the same nerve supply, i.e. the left upper limb, the precordium and the left neck.

The conducting system of the heart is formed of specialized cardiac muscle cells and initiates, coordinates and regulates the complex pattern of contraction in the cardiac cycle. It consists of the **sinoatrial (SA) node**, the **atrioventricular (AV) node**, the **AV bundle of His**, its right and left branches, and the terminal subendocardial plexus of Purkinje fibres (Fig. 2.15). The **sinoatrial node** (known as the pacemaker) is a small area of conducting tissue in the right atrial wall anterior to the opening of the superior vena cava. Impulses from it are conducted by the muscle of the atrial wall to the **atrioventricular node**, a similar nodule lying on the right of the atrial septum close to the entry of the coronary sinus. From it, the **atrioventricular bundle** descends the inter-

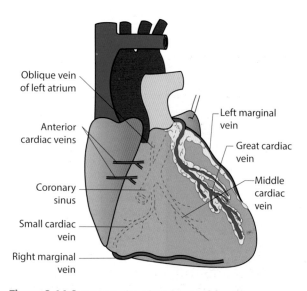

Figure 2.14 Coronary veins of the heart – those lying posteriorly are shown by dotted lines

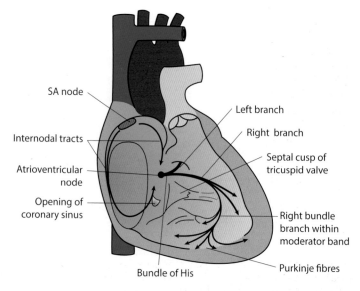

Figure 2.15 Conducting system of the heart – arrows show the anatomical arrangement. SA, sinoatrial

ventricular septum and divides into right and left branches, mainly supplying the corresponding ventricle, which ramify as the subendocardial plexus supplying the ventricular walls and papillary muscles.

THE PERICARDIUM

The pericardium is a fibroserous membrane that surrounds the heart and the adjacent parts of the large vessels entering and

leaving it. It consists of an outer fibrous and an inner serous layer; the latter is divided into two layers, the visceral and parietal, between which is the pericardial sac (Figs. 2.17–2.19).

The **serous pericardium** is a closed serous sac, invaginated by the heart and enclosing within its layers a thin pericardial cavity. Visceral pericardium, which covers the outer surface of the heart, is continuous with the parietal pericardium that lines the inside of the fibrous pericardium.

Electrocardiogram (ECG)

The ECG is a record of the electrical potential detected at the body surface. Ten electrodes are placed as shown in Fig. 2.16a – four limb leads are positioned on the muscular parts of each forearm and lower leg, and six precordial leads, named V_1–V_6, are placed:

V_1 – right side of sternum, 4th intercostal space
V_2 – left side of sternum, 4th intercostal space
V_3 – midway between V_2 and V_4
V_4 – midclavicular line, 5th intercostal space
V_5 – anterior axillary line horizontal to V_4
V_6 – midaxillary line horizontal to V_4

The ECG traces measure the electric potential resulting from the heart muscle contraction: each trace corresponds to a specific region of heart muscle, and abnormalities can thus be identified and localized. Each component of the waveform (labelled P, Q, R, S, T and U) indicates the specific electrical events of one heart beat (Fig. 2.16b)

- P wave – indicates atrial contraction
- QRS complex – usually begins with a short downward deflection, Q, followed by a peak, R, and then a downwards-pointing S wave. It represents ventricular contraction.
- PR interval – shows the transit time for the electrical signal to travel from the sinus node to the ventricular muscle.
- T wave – a slight upwards wave indicating ventricular repolarization.

The ECG is of great importance in detecting cardiac irregularities and the site of cardiac ischaemia. If the atrioventricular bundle is damaged, for instance after a coronary artery thrombosis, total heart block may occur; in this, the ventricles beat slowly at their own rate independent of the atria, which continue to contract at the rate determined by the sinoatrial node. Atheroma may cause ischaemia or myocardial infarction, which may damage the atrioventricular node, resulting in a delay in impulse propagation (heart block). This is treated by insertion of a cardiac pacemaker whose electrode is placed to lie in the right ventricle.

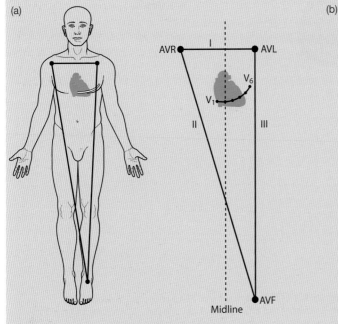
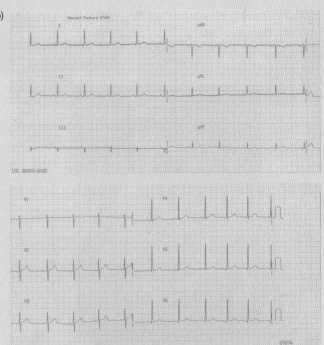

Figure 2.16 (a) The electrocardiogram records the electrical activity of the heart. Leads, attached by adhesive pads, are placed on the shoulders and left leg, and around the chest (V_1–V_6). Leads I, II and III record the voltage between two limb leads; AVR, AVL and AVF between one limb and the other two; and V_1–V_6 between a point on the chest and an average of the three limb leads. AVR and V_1 are oriented towards the cavity of the heart; II,III and AVF face the inferior surface; I, AVL and V_6 face the lateral wall of the left ventricle; V_1 and V_2 are directed at the right ventricle, V_3 and V_4 at the interventricular septum, and V_5 and V_6 at the left ventricle. (b) Normal electrocardiogram

(a)

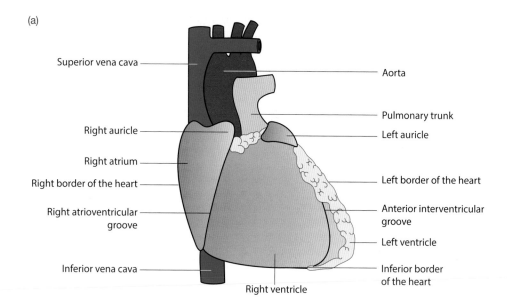

Superior vena cava

Right auricle

Right atrium

Right border of the heart

Right atrioventricular groove

Inferior vena cava

Right ventricle

Aorta

Pulmonary trunk

Left auricle

Left border of the heart

Anterior interventricular groove

Left ventricle

Inferior border of the heart

(b)

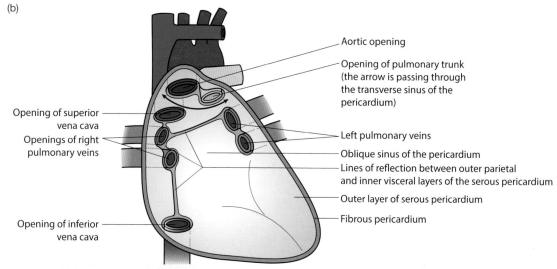

Opening of superior vena cava

Openings of right pulmonary veins

Opening of inferior vena cava

Aortic opening

Opening of pulmonary trunk (the arrow is passing through the transverse sinus of the pericardium)

Left pulmonary veins

Oblique sinus of the pericardium

Lines of reflection between outer parietal and inner visceral layers of the serous pericardium

Outer layer of serous pericardium

Fibrous pericardium

(c)

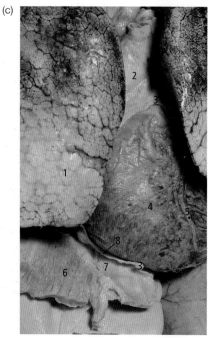

Figure 2.17 (a) Anterior view of heart and great vessels. (b) Pericardial sac after removal of the heart. (c) Anterior thorax revealing opened pericardium *in situ*: 1, lung; 2, pericardium covering the great vessels of the superior mediastinum; 3, cut edge of fibrous and serous parietal layers of pericardium; 4, right ventricle; 5, left coronary artery, anterior interventricular branch; 6, diaphragm; 7, attachment of fibrous pericardium to central tendon of the diaphragm; 8, pericardial cavity

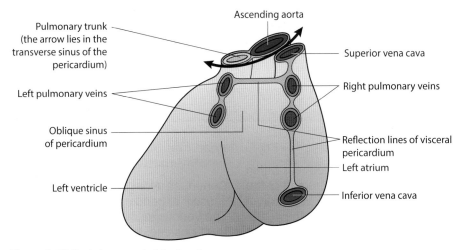

Pulmonary trunk
(the arrow lies in the
transverse sinus of the
pericardium)

Ascending aorta

Superior vena cava

Left pulmonary veins

Right pulmonary veins

Oblique sinus
of pericardium

Reflection lines of visceral
pericardium

Left atrium

Left ventricle

Inferior vena cava

Figure 2.18 Posterior aspect of the heart

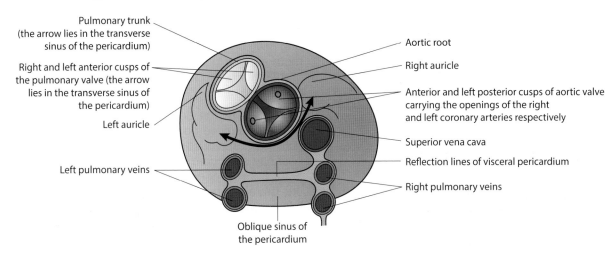

Pulmonary trunk
(the arrow lies in the transverse
sinus of the pericardium)

Right and left anterior cusps of
the pulmonary valve (the arrow
lies in the transverse sinus of
the pericardium)

Left auricle

Left pulmonary veins

Aortic root

Right auricle

Anterior and left posterior cusps of aortic valve
carrying the openings of the right
and left coronary arteries respectively

Superior vena cava

Reflection lines of visceral pericardium

Right pulmonary veins

Oblique sinus of
the pericardium

Figure 2.19 Superior aspect of the heart showing the site of origin of the great vessels and the pericardial reflections

Fluid in the pericardium, as the result of trauma or infection (Fig. 2.20), limits the filling and output of the heart (cardiac tamponade). This causes the veins of the face and neck to become congested, and eventually the cardiac output decreases as the pressure of the fluid in the inextensible pericardial sac rises. In these circumstances, it is necessary to aspirate the fluid. The pericardial sac is most easily entered by a needle inserted between the xiphoid process and the left costal margin, directed headwards, backwards and medially through the central tendon of the diaphragm (Fig. 2.21).

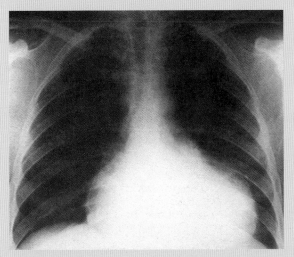

Figure 2.20 Chest X-ray showing pericardial effusion

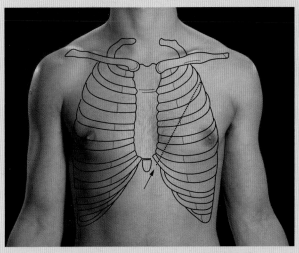

Figure 2.21 Anterior chest wall – the arrow and dotted line show the needle direction for pericardial aspiration

The **fibrous pericardium** is a strong flask-shaped sac surrounding the heart and serous pericardium, which blends below with the central tendon of the diaphragm and the adventitia of the inferior vena cava, above with the adventitia of the aorta, pulmonary trunk and superior vena cava, and behind with that of the pulmonary veins.

DEVELOPMENT OF THE HEART

Heart tube formation (approximately days 18–21)

The heart develops from progenitor cardiac cells within the embryonic mesoderm, cranial to the region of the future mouth and brain and ventral to the pericardium (Fig. 2.22). Initially, a pair of heart tubes form; these subsequently merge and remodel to form a single heart tube that quickly expands (Fig. 2.23). The folding of the embryonic disc moves the heart tube into the thoracic region, dorsal to the pericardium. The heart tube later grows to become surrounded by the pericardial layers (Fig. 2.24). The venous inflows and arterial outflows of the developing heart anchor it to the diaphragm and pharyngeal arches, respectively. The heart tube continues to grow and lengthen after it has formed. A disruption of this process can lead to outflow tract defects, including ventricular septal defects, double-outlet right ventricle or tetralogy of Fallot.

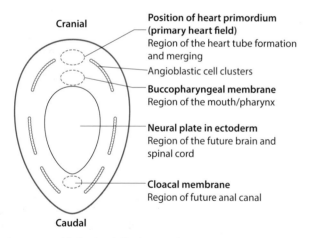

Figure 2.22 View onto the superior/upper surface of the embryonic disc, as if looking down on the disc from within the amniotic cavity. The position of the heart primordium and angioblastic/progenitor cell clusters within the mesodermal layer are shown projected onto the ectodermal layer

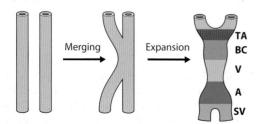

Figure 2.23 Merging, fusion and remodelling of the paired heart tubes to form the singular heart tube. TA, truncus arteriosus; BC, bulbus cordis; V, ventricle; A, atria; SV, sinus venosus

Heart tube differentiation, folding and rotation (approximately days 22–35)

Continued elongation and growth of the heart tube cause it to bend and form the cardiac loop (Fig. 2.25). The venous inflow/atrial region moves dorsocranially to sit posterior to the cranially located arterial outflow. During heart tube looping, a series of five expanded regions develop: the sinus venosus, atria, ventricle, bulbus cordis and truncus arteriosus. Continued growth and movement results in structures that were originally on the right side of the heart moving into a more anterior position and vice versa, explaining the 'right' and 'left' nomenclature used in relation to the developed heart.

The cusps of the developing aortic and pulmonary valves also move position, making their naming difficult. The three cusps of the aortic valve are therefore best named according to which coronary artery originates from the coronary sinus above, or not. The cusps are therefore named right coronary (anterior cusp), left coronary (left posterior cusp) and non-coronary (right posterior cusp); since there is no associated coronary artery (Fig. 2.29b). The cusps of the pulmonary valve are named according to their relationship with the cusps of the aortic valve, with two being adjacent (right and left adjacent) and one non-adjacent.

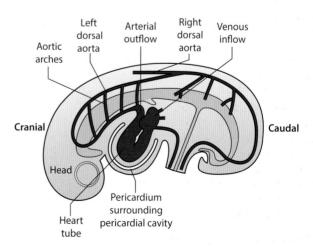

Figure 2.24 Left lateral view of day 34 embryo showing the developing cardiovascular system. The heart tube has begun to fold and become surrounded by the pericardium and pericardial cavity

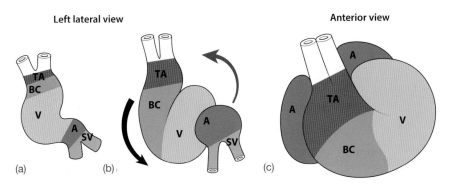

Figure 2.25 The heart tube and formation of the cardiac loop from 24 days (a) to 28 days (c). The atria initially move dorsally, cranially and leftwards (blue arrow), whereas the bulbus cordis and ventricle moves caudally, ventrally and to the right (black arrow). TA, truncus arteriosus; BC, bulbus cordis; V, ventricle; A, atria; SV, sinus venosus

Heart tube septation (from the middle of week 4 to the end of week 8)

The heart tube is divided into left and right sides by the formation of membranous and/or muscular septa (Figs. 2.26–2.28). Initially, two endocardial cushions grow towards each other within the centre of the atrioventricular canal. The cushions meet each other and divide the atrioventricular canal into left and right channels. The mitral valve develops in the left channel and the tricuspid valve in the right. The endocardial cushion also contributes to the formation of the atrial and ventricular septa.

In-utero blood shunting and circulation

Blood is shunted from the right to the left circulation *in utero* in order to bypass the developing lungs. Right-to-left shunting occurs via the atrial septum (through foramina ovale and secundum) and the ductus arteriosus, which connects the pulmonary trunk to the aortic arch.

Atrial septum formation

Atrial septum formation begins at the end of week 4 from two separate sheets of tissue and is complete early in week 6 (Figs. 2.26, 2.27). Initially, the membranous septum primum grows from the roof of the atrium towards the endocardial cushion. Before closure of the foramen primum (the gap between the septum primum and the endocardial cushion), a hole forms in its upper region (foramen secundum), which permits a continuous right-to-left shunting of blood. The muscular septum secundum grows on the right side of the septum primum, passing down from the roof of the atrium towards the endocardial cushion and overlapping the foramen secundum. Part of the lower region of the septum secundum remains incomplete, leaving an oval-shaped hole, the foramen ovale.

The paired atrial septa form a simple valve mechanism through which blood can shunt, with the membranous septum primum acting as a valve leaflet/cusp. As the pressure in the right side of the heart is higher than that

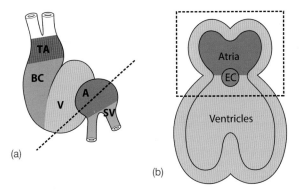

Figure 2.26 Development of the interatrial septum. (a) Left lateral view of the folded heart tube showing the plane of the cross-section (black dashed line) used to visualize (b). (b) Coronal cross-section through the developing atria, ventricle and atrioventricular canal viewed from an anterior perspective. The endocardial cushion (EC) divides the atrioventricular canal into left and right sides. The black rectangle shows the region drawn in Fig. 2.27. A, atria; V, ventricle

in the left *in utero*, due to the high pulmonary vascular resistance, blood shunts from the right atrium into the left atrium via the foramen ovale and foramen secundum, bypassing the lungs. Defects can occur in different parts of the atrial septum, the most common being a patent foramen ovale (due to a large foramen secundum) and foramen/ostium secundum defects (due to septum primum or secundum defects). Small defects may be inconsequential, but large defects may require surgical correction.

Smooth and rough atrial walls

The smooth-walled parts of the left and right atria are formed by venous-type tissues. The left atrium incorporates parts of the pulmonary veins into its wall, whereas the right atrium incorporates the sinus venosus and parts of the venae cavae. The primitive atria contribute to the rough-walled/trabeculated parts of the atria and the auricular appendages.

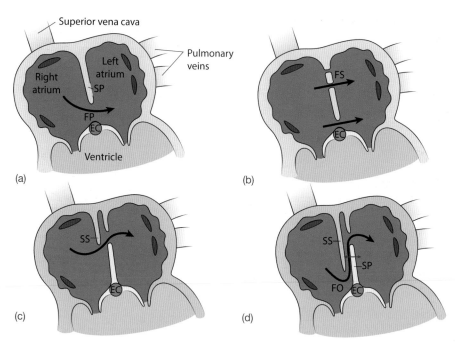

Figure 2.27 Formation of the interatrial septum. (a) Formation of the septum primum (SP) and foramen primum (FP). (b) Partial breakdown of the upper part of the septum primum to form the foramen secundum (FS). (c) Closure of the foramen primum and formation of the more rigid septum secdundum to the right side of the septum primum. (d) Septum secundum grows to meet the endocardial cushion (EC) but leaves an oval shaped hole, the foramen ovale (FO), through which blood can pass. The more mobile septum primum (SP) forms a valve cusp, which moves towards or away from the septum secundum (SS) (red arrow) allowing only a one way (right-to-left) shunting of blood (black arrow)

Intracardiac pressure changes at birth

Lung inflation following birth reduces pulmonary vascular resistance, enabling a greater flow of blood to the lungs and a greater venous return to the left atrium. This consequently causes the blood pressure on the left side to exceed that on the right. The altered pressure differential pushes the septum primum against the septum secundum, sealing off the foramen ovale. Over time, the two septa usually fuse, although some (around 25%) do not, resulting in a probe-patent foramen ovale. This can predispose to a transient ischaemic attack or stroke if the blood pressure in the right side exceeds that in the left (e.g. during a Valsava manoeuvre) and venous clots/emboli pass directly into the left atrium.

Ventricular septum formation (weeks 5–8)

Formation of the ventricular septum requires four pieces of tissue to join together in the region of the arterial outflow tract and endocardial cushion (Fig. 2.28a,b). A muscular septum grows from the floor of the ventricle towards the endocardial cushion but does not fully separate the ventricles, leaving the interventricular foramen. The foramen is later completed by contributions from the membranous tissues of the aorticopulmonary septum and endocardial cushion. Ventricular septal defects most commonly occur in the membranous region owing to the complexity of its formation; they are often associated with a failure of the

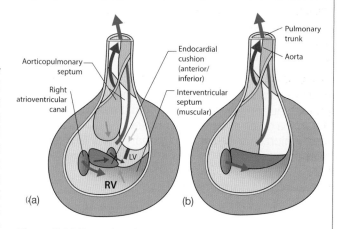

Figure 2.28 Formation of the intraventricular septum via contributions from muscular tissue of the ventricular wall (blue), the aorticopulmonary septum (green and yellow) and the endocardial cushion (purple). (a) The different tissues grow toward each other (week 7), separating the right (RV) and left (LV) ventricles. The interventricular foramen is still present. (b) The fully formed interventricular septum (week 8) requires multiple tissues to grow and join in the region of the interventricular foramen. This point of union (the membranous part of the septum) is therefore the most likely location for ventricular septal defects

contribution from the endocardial cushion. Muscular ventricular septal defects are less common and can be singular or multiple.

Much of the smooth-walled infundibular and vestibular parts of the ventricles is formed from parts of the bulbus cordis. The rough muscularly walled regions are formed by what was originally the primitive ventricle.

Septum formation in the truncus arteriosus and bulbus cordis (weeks 5-7)

The aorticopulmonary septum divides the common arterial outflow (bulbus cordis and truncus arteriosus) of the heart. This formed from pairs of bulbar and truncal ridges that appear opposite, and grow to meet, each other in the bulbus cordis and truncus arteriosus, respectively (Fig. 2.29a,b). The aorticopulmonary septum divides the truncus arteriosus into the aorta and the pulmonary trunk (Fig. 2.28) and while doing so rotates through 180 degrees, explaining the final disposition of the aorta and pulmonary trunk. Malformation of the aorticopulmonary septum is associated with membranous ventricular septal defects. Absence of the septum results in a common truncus arteriosus (arterial outflow) with a ventricular septal defect (Figs. 2.30a-c). Unequal division of the arterial outflow region can lead to tetralogy of Fallot. Failure of spiralling of the septum results in transposition of the great vessels, in which the aorta arises from the right ventricle and the pulmonary trunk from the left ventricle.

Aortic arches

The embryonic aortic arches join, regress and/or remodel to form the recognizable great vessel vascular tree of the thorax (Table 2.1, Figs. 2.31 and 2.33). Defects in aortic arch formation and remodelling can lead to aortic coarctation (Fig. 2.34), double aortic arch or an abnormal origin of the right subclavian artery (Figs. 2.32a,b).

Five pairs of aortic arch arteries arise from the aortic sac and pass via their correspondingly numbered pharyngeal arch into the cranial end of either the right or left dorsal aorta. Caudally, the paired dorsal aortae join to form a single vessel. Five pharyngeal arches and arch arteries (I, II, III, IV and VI) develop. Arch V regresses or fails to develop. The first and second arch arteries have mostly regressed before the fourth and sixth appear.

TABLE 2.1 Derivatives of the aortic arch arteries

Arch	Side	Main Arterial Derivative
1	L & R	Mainly regress. Remnants form the maxillary arteries
2	L & R	Mainly regress. Remnants form the hyoid and stapedial arteries
3	L & R	Form the common carotid artery and proximal part of the internal carotid artery (distal part of the internal carotid artery formed by dorsal aortae)
4	L	Segment of the aortic arch running between the left common carotid and left subclavian arteries
4	R	Proximal part of the right subclavian artery (completed distally by the right dorsal aorta and 7th intersegmental artery)
5	L & R	Regress or do not develop
6	L	Forms the ductus arteriosus and left pulmonary artery
6	R	Forms the right pulmonary artery

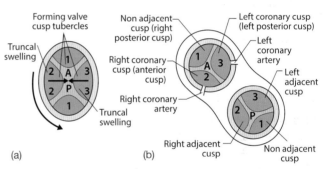

(a)   (b)

Figure 2.29 Formation of the aortic and pulmonary valves in the dividing truncus arteriosus. (a) Three mesenchymal swellings/tubercles (labelled 1-3) normally appear in both the aorta and pulmonary trunk, each of which remodels and thins to form a valve cusp. The truncal swellings meet in the midline. (b) Disposition and naming of the formed aortic and pulmonary valve cusps, and the origins of the right and left coronary arteries. A, aorta; P, pulmonary trunk

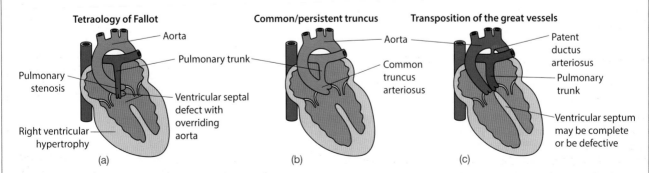

(a)   (b)   (c)

Figure 2.30 Cardiac outflow defects related to malformation of the aorticopulmonary septum. There is inadequate oxygenated blood reaching vital organs, and the neonate will be cyanotic. The defects have to be corrected for long-term survival. (a) Unequal division of the bulbotruncal region resulting in tetralogy of Fallot (pulmonary stenosis, ventricular septal defect, large aorta sat over the ventricular septal defect and hypertrophy of the right ventricular wall). (b) Failure of aorticopulmonary septum formation resulting in a common arterial outflow sat over a large ventricular septal defect. (c) Failure of aorticopulmonary septum spiralling resulting in transposition of the great vessels. The patent ductus arteriosus permits mixing of oxygenated (red) and deoxygenated (blue) blood. Purple, Mixed oxygenated and deoxygenated blood

Following septum formation in the truncus arteriosus, the sixth arch arteries are continuous with the pulmonary trunk.

The recurrent laryngeal nerves are located inferior to left and right sixth aortic arch arteries. The distal part of the right sixth aortic arch regresses, allowing the right recurrent laryngeal nerve to move superiorly and sit inferior to right aortic arch 4 (the right subclavian artery) (Figs.

2.33a,b). The left sixth aortic arch forms the ductus arteriosus *in utero*, leaving the left recurrent laryngeal nerve trapped inferior to both it and the aortic arch.

Shortly after birth the tissue of the left sixth aortic arch (ductus arteriosus) contracts to seal off the ductus arteriosus. Coarctation (a narrowing) of the aorta in children may occur if some of the contractile tissue is incorporated into the aortic arch. Coarctation can be classified relative to its positional relationship to the ductus arteriosus, with preductal, juxtaductal or postductal forms observed (Figs. 2.34a–c).

Following formation of the aorticopulmonary septum, the aortic sac divides into the left and right horns. The right horn forms the brachiocephalic trunk, and the left horn, together with the left fourth arch and left dorsal

Figure 2.31 Development of the aortic arches. Each of the six pharyngeal arches initially has a pair of arteries passing from the ventral to the dorsal aortas. The fifth quickly disappears and the others are modified to match organ development (ghosted vessels have regressed)

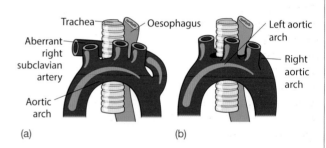

Figure 2.32 Defects of the aortic arch and associated great vessel tree (left lateral view). (a) Aberrant right subclavian artery passing posterior to the oesophagus and trachea (b) Double arch aorta encircling and compressing the trachea and oesophagus

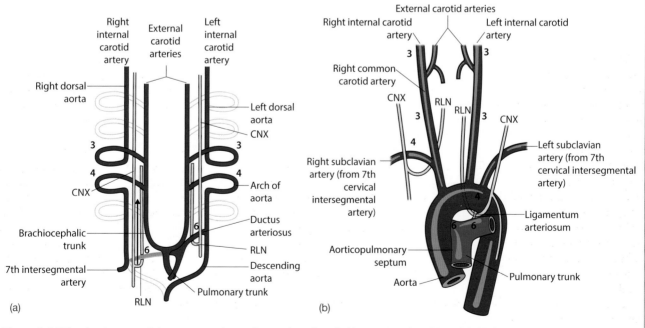

Figure 2.33 The development of the great vessel vascular tree from the primitive aortic arches (Fig. 2.31). (a) Growth and remodelling stage. Regression of the distal part of the right 6th arch artery enables the right recurrent laryngeal nerve to ascend and sit under the 4th arch artery, the future right subclavian artery. The distal part of the left 6th arch artery persists to form the ductus arteriosus, therefore the left recurrent laryngeal nerve loops under the ligamentum arteriosum and aortic arch. (b) Adult arterial system and final disposition of the recurrent laryngeal nerves. CNX, cranial nerve X; RLN, recurrent laryngeal nerve; the numbers indicate the aortic arch artery derivation of a given vessel

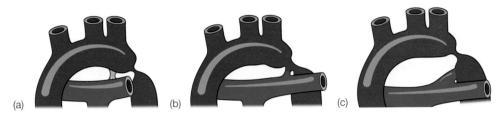

Figure 2.34 Coarctation of the aorta. (a) Postductal coarctation of the aorta with a non-patent ductus arteriosus (more common type). (b) Juxtaductal coarctation with patent ductus arteriosus. (c) Preductal coarctation of the aorta with a patent ductus arteriosus

aorta, forms the ascending, arch and descending parts of the aorta. In some cases, the aortic arch is duplicated or aberrant vessels may form, both of which can compress the trachea and/or oesophagus (Figs. 2.32a,b). Children tend to present with respiratory symptoms and adults with problems swallowing.

Cardiac valves

The semilunar valves initially develop as swellings of subendocardial tissue in the pulmonary and aortic region of the truncus arteriosus (Figs. 2.29a,b). Remodelling and thinning of the swellings forms the valve cusps. Differing numbers of valve cusps, for example a bicuspid aortic valve (normally asymptomatic), can result from a variation in this process. The atrioventricular valves develop in a similar manner within the atrioventricular canals.

Fetal circulation

Oxygenated blood from the placenta passes from the umbilical vein to the inferior vena cava via the ductus venosus, thereby mostly bypassing the liver. The angle of entry of the inferior vena cava into the right atrium directs blood towards the foramen ovale and into the left atrium. Much of the blood passing in the pulmonary trunk is shunted into the aortic arch via the ductus arteriosus, bypassing the lungs and joining the aorta distal to the points of emergence of the cephalic blood flow. Blood passes to the placenta via the umbilical arteries, which are connected to the internal iliac arterial system. The venous return from the body enters the inferior vena cava and mixes with the blood coming from the placenta through the umbilical vein and ductus venosus.

After birth, changes in left-to-right pressure differentials result in closure of the valve of the foramen ovale. The ductus arteriosus closes within 24–72 hours of birth due to increased oxygen tension and reduced levels of prostaglandin E2. A patent ductus arteriosus commonly causes a left-to-right shunt, resulting in hyperperfusion of the lungs and pulmonary hypertension, and hypoperfusion of the distal body.

Congenital cardiac abnormalities are quite common, and some are incompatible with long-term survival. Bicuspid aortic valves are among the most common but are often symptom-free. A patent ductus arteriosus, atrial septal defects (ASD) (caused by a persistent foramen ovale) and ventricular defects usually require surgical correction, especially if a clinically significant left-right shunting of blood occurs. If the ductus fails to close, pulmonary hypertension results from the shunting of higher pressure systemic blood into the pulmonary circulation, and cardiac failure usually follows. Surgical correction is required. Aortic coarctation is congenital narrowing of the aorta in the region of the ductus. Usually, if the coarctation is short, the circulation of the lower body and limbs is maintained by anastomoses between the scapular and intercostal, and the internal thoracic and inferior epigastric, vessels.

In 25% of people, fusion of the septum primum and septum secundum is incomplete but the septa overlap; this condition, known as probe patent foramen ovale, is usually of no functional significance unless a right to left shunting of blood occurs (e.g. during the valsava maneuver) thus increasing the risk of venous emboli entering the left circulation. This condition is a potential cause of transient ischaemic attack (TIA). Ventricular septal defects (VSDs) are usually sited in the membranous part of the interventricular septum (a region of complex developmental origin). They vary in size and clinical significance, but the larger ones cause a shunt of blood from the left to the right ventricle and a consequent increase in pulmonary blood flow, pulmonary hypertension and cardiac failure. Congenital pulmonary stenosis may occur, and if this is associated with a ventricular septal defect, various syndromes may result, such as tetralogy of Fallot (Fig. 2.30a). This consists of a combination of a VSD, an overriding aorta, pulmonary stenosis and right ventricular hypertrophy.

MCQs

1. The right atrium: T/F

a is related to the central tendon of the (___)
   diaphragm at the level of the 8th thoracic
   vertebra
b has a thin anterior endocardial fold 'guard- (___)
   ing' the superior vena cava
c has an auricle situated superolaterally (___)
d has the coronary sinus opening near the (___)
   fossa ovalis
e has a fossa ovalis on the atrioventricular (___)
   wall

Answers

1.
a **T** – The inferior vena cava enters the atrium at this point.
          The wall of the atrium between the inferior and superior
          venae cavae forms the right border of the heart.
b **F** – The superior vena cava has no valve. There is an
          anterior fold 'guarding' the entry of the inferior vena
          cava.
c **F** – The auricle lies superomedially against the root of
          the aorta. On the inner surface, a ridge, the crista
          terminalis, separates the rough-walled auricle from
          the smooth-walled atrium.
d **T** – The sinus opening lies between the fossa ovalis and
          the opening into the right ventricle. The sinus opening
          is 'guarded' by an endocardial fold.
e **F** – The fossa, a remnant of the fetal foramen ovale, lies
          on the interatrial wall.

2. The coronary arteries: T/F

a arise from the inferior aspect of the aortic (___)
   arch
b each give atrial and ventricular branches (___)
c anastomose extensively with each other (___)
d supply the conducting system of the heart (___)
e supply the papillary muscles of the tricuspid (___)
   and mitral valves

Answers

2.
a **F** – The right coronary artery arises from the anterior
          aortic sinus and the left from the left posterior sinus
          immediately above the aortic valve.
b **T** – The right artery supplies most of the right side of the
          heart and the left the left, but ...
c **T** – ... although they anastomose in the septum and at the
          apex, sudden occlusion of a ...
d **T** – ... large branch may result in death of cardiac muscle.
          The conducting system is supplied by coronary
          vessels ...
e **T** – ... and coronary artery occlusion may cause death of
          a papillary muscle and its rupture.

3. The atrioventricular bundle: T/F

a forms part of the conducting system of the (___)
   heart
b is formed of nervous tissue (___)
c lies in the interventricular septum (___)
d divides into two branches that end in the (___)
   subendocardial plexus
e bridges the atrial and ventricular muscles (___)

Answers

3.
a **T** – The system comprises the sinoatrial node,
          atrioventricular node, atrioventricular bundle and
          subendocardial plexus.
b **F** – It is formed of specialized cardiac muscle cells.
c **T** – It lies in the membranous part of the interventricular
          septum.
d **T** – It divides as it descends the interventricular wall and
          ramifies to form the subendocardial plexus.
e **T** – The atrioventricular bundle is the only continuity
          between the atria and ventricles, whose muscles are
          separated by the fibrous tissue on which are mounted
          the atrioventricular valves.

4. The right atrium is innervated by the: T/F

a left recurrent laryngeal nerve (___)
b XIIth cranial nerve (___)
c sinus nerve (___)
d Xth cranial nerve (___)
e right phrenic nerve (___)

Answers

4.
a **F** – The left recurrent laryngeal nerve loops around the aortic
          arch and ascends to supply the laryngeal muscles.
b **F** – The XIIth cranial nerve supplies the intrinsic and
          extrinsic muscles of the tongue.
c **F** – The sinus nerve is a branch of the glossopharyngeal
          nerve supplying the carotid baroreceptors and
          chemoreceptors.
d **T** – The Xth cranial nerve innervates the right atrium
          through the cardiac plexus. The denervated heart also
          has innate myocardial contractility.
e **F** – The right phrenic nerve supplies the right half of the
          diaphragm.

SBA

An atrial septal defect is caused by the incomplete closure of the:
   a   foramen ovale
   b   ductus arteriosus
   c   ligamentum arteriosus
   d   coronary sinus
   e   sinus venarum

Answers

a   *During the formation of the wall separating the right and left atria, the opening of the foramen secundum or foramen ovale usually closes at birth. If the closure fails to occur, an atrial septal defect results.*

EMQs

Each question has an anatomical theme linked to the chapter, and a list of 10 related items (A–J) placed in alphabetical order: these are followed by five statements (1–5). Match **one or more** of the items A–J to each of the five statements.

Surface anatomy of heart and great vessels
A. Left 5th intercostal space in the anterior axillary line
B. Left 5th intercostal space in the midclavicular line
C. Left 7th costosternal junction
D. Medial end of the 3rd left intercostal space
E. Medial end of the 2nd right intercostal space
F. Medial to the 4th left intercostal space
G. Medial to the 4th right costosternal junction
H. Midsternal at the level of the 4th intercostal space
I. Right of the costoxiphoid junction
J. Right sternal border in line with the 4th intercostal space

Answers
1 E; 2 B; 3 I; 4 H; 5 D

Match the following structures to the appropriate surface marking(s) in the above list.
1. Superior vena cava
2. Apex of the heart
3. Inferior vena cava
4. Tricuspid valve
5. Pulmonary valve

Blood supply of the heart
A. Anterior interventricular artery
B. Circumflex artery
C. Coronary sinus
D. Great cardiac vein
E. Left coronary artery
F. Left marginal artery
G. Middle cardiac vein
H. Posterior interventricular artery
I. Right coronary artery
J. Right marginal artery

Answers
1 BCI; 2 C; 3 I; 4 I; 5 I

Match the following statements with the appropriate vessel(s) in the above list.
1. Lies in the atrioventricular groove
2. Opens into the right atrium
3. Lies in the anterior atrioventricular groove
4. Usually supplies the sinoatrial node
5. Opens in the anterior aortic sinus

APPLIED QUESTIONS

1. What are the surface markings of the heart valves, and why does one not listen at these sites to hear them best?

1. The heart valves lie on a diagonal line from approximately the 3rd left costosternal joint to the 6th right costosternal junction. They are arranged in the following order, from above downwards: pulmonary, aortic, mitral and tricuspid – PAMT. To hear the valves closing, one must listen to where the sound is transmitted along the vessel through which the blood flows after valve closure. Thus the aortic valve is heard best over the ascending aorta in the 2nd right intercostal space, and the mitral valve is heard best over the apex of the heart.

2. On a plain posteroanterior chest X-ray, what structures form the borders of the heart shadow?

2. The right heart shadow is formed, from above downwards, by the right brachiocephalic vein, superior vena cava, right atrium and inferior vena cava. The left border is formed from the aortic arch, pulmonary trunk, auricular appendage of the left atrium and left ventricle.

3. Why is the pain of a myocardial infarction not felt over the apex beat?

3. The heart is a visceral organ, so pain arising in its sensory innervation is experienced as referred pain in the dermatomes corresponding to the nerves that supply the heart. It is supplied bilaterally from the upper four or five thoracic nerves, and hence pain originating from it, e.g. from a myocardial infarction, is felt deeply in the anterior upper chest, with spread to the inner arm(s) and the neck and jaw. If a patient complains of pain over the apex, it is originating either in the chest wall or the pleurae, or is hysterical in origin.

The mediastinal structures

THE AORTA

This, the main arterial trunk of the systemic circulation, arises from the left ventricle and ascends briefly before arching backwards over the root of the left lung to descend through the thorax and abdomen. Descriptively, it is divided into the ascending part, the arch, a descending thoracic part and an abdominal part.

The ascending aorta

The ascending aorta is a wide vessel some 5 cm long. It begins at the aortic orifice behind the 3rd right costal cartilage below the level of the sternal angle and ascends to the right, around the pulmonary trunk, to the level of the sternal angle. At its base above each of the semilunar valvules of the aortic valve is a dilatation, an aortic sinus.

Relations

The ascending aorta is enclosed in a sheath of serous pericardium common to it and the pulmonary trunk within the fibrous pericardium. Its lower part lies behind the infundibulum of the right ventricle and the origin of the pulmonary trunk, and above this the sternum is anterior. Posterior, from below upwards, are the left atrium, the right pulmonary artery and the right main bronchus. On its left lie the left auricle and pulmonary trunk, and to the right the right auricle and superior vena cava.

Branches

The right and left coronary arteries arise from the anterior and left posterior aortic sinuses (p. 37).

Aortic arch

The **arch** of the aorta passes upwards from the sternal angle behind the manubrium to arch backwards and to the left over the left lung root, and then descends to the left side of the 4th thoracic vertebra (Fig. 3.1). From the convexity of the arch arise the three arteries supplying the head, neck and upper limbs.

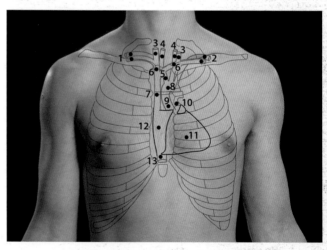

Figure 3.1 Surface markings of the great vessels of the superior mediastinum: 1, right subclavian vessels; 2, left subclavian vessels; 3, internal jugular veins; 4, common carotid arteries; 5, brachiocephalic artery; 6, brachiocephalic veins; 7, superior vena cava; 8, aortic arch; 9, ascending aorta; 10, pulmonary trunk; 11, ventricles; 12, right atrium; 13, inferior vena cava

Relations

To the left of the arch of the aorta lie the mediastinal pleura and lung, the left phrenic nerve and the left vagus nerve. To its right lie the superior vena cava, the trachea and left recurrent laryngeal nerve, the oesophagus and thoracic duct and, finally, the 4th thoracic vertebra. Inferiorly, the aortic arch crosses the bifurcation of the pulmonary trunk, the ligamentum arteriosum and the left main bronchus. Superiorly are its three branches (Fig. 3.2). The arch is connected inferiorly to the left pulmonary artery by the ligamentum arteriosum, a fibrous remnant of the ductus arteriosus. The left recurrent laryngeal nerve passes posteriorly around the ligamentum and the arch. The cardiac plexus is closely related to the ligamentum. Remnants of the thymus gland may be found in front of the arch.

Branches

The first branch, the brachiocephalic artery, arises behind the manubrium and ascends as far as the right sternoclavicular joint, there to divide into two terminal branches, the right subclavian and right common carotid arteries (Fig. 3.3). Anteriorly, the left brachiocephalic vein and thymus separate it from the manubrium; posteriorly lies the trachea. To its right lie the right brachiocephalic vein and superior vena cava, and to its left is the left common carotid artery. The left common carotid artery arises from the arch just behind the brachiocephalic artery and passes upwards alongside the left side of the trachea into the neck. The left subclavian artery arises behind the left common carotid artery and arches to the left over the dome of the left pleura behind the left sternoclavicular joint and over the first rib (Fig. 3.3).

The descending aorta

The descending aorta descends from the left of the 4th thoracic vertebra, inclining medially to the front of the 12th, where it passes through the diaphragm to become the abdominal aorta (Fig. 3.3).

Relations

Anteriorly, from above downwards, are the left lung root, the left atrium, covered by pericardium, the oesophagus and the diaphragm. Posteriorly are the 4th to 12th thoracic vertebrae. The left side of the descending aorta is in contact with the left pleura and lung, and its right side with the oesophagus above and the right lung and pleura below. The thoracic duct and azygos vein are also on its right side.

Branches

These are the 3rd to 11th posterior intercostal arteries, a pair of subcostal arteries, two or three small bronchial arteries, several small oesophageal arteries and arteries to the diaphragm.

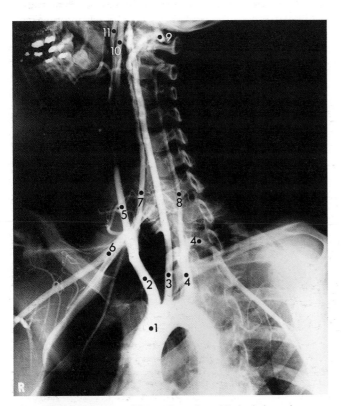

Figure 3.2 Arteriogram of the aortic arch and its main branches: 1, aortic arch; 2, brachiocephalic artery; 3, left common carotid artery; 4, left subclavian artery; 5, right common carotid artery; 6 right subclavian artery; 7, right vertebral artery; 8, left vertebral artery; 9, loop of left vertebral artery as it passes around the lateral mass of the atlas; 10, right internal carotid artery; 11, right external carotid artery

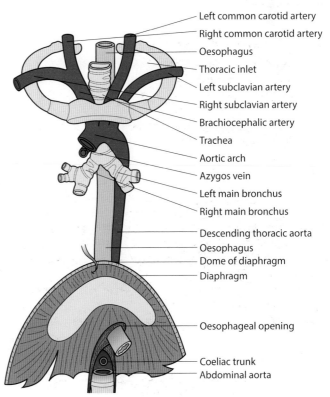

Left common carotid artery
Right common carotid artery
Oesophagus
Thoracic inlet
Left subclavian artery
Right subclavian artery
Brachiocephalic artery
Trachea
Aortic arch
Azygos vein
Left main bronchus
Right main bronchus
Descending thoracic aorta
Oesophagus
Dome of diaphragm
Diaphragm
Oesophageal opening
Coeliac trunk
Abdominal aorta

Figure 3.3 Diagram showing the thoracic inlet and structures in the superior and posterior aspects of the mediastinum

THE PULMONARY TRUNK

This wide vessel, about 5 cm long, originates at the pulmonary orifice and ascends posteriorly to the left of the aorta to end at its bifurcation into right and left pulmonary arteries under the concavity of the aortic arch (Figs. 3.4 and 3.5). It is contained within a common sleeve of serous pericardium with the ascending aorta and lies in front of the transverse sinus of the pericardium. The two auricles and both coronary arteries surround its base. These mediastinal structures can be conveniently studied by radiological techniques (Fig. 3.6).

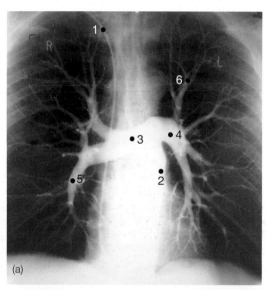

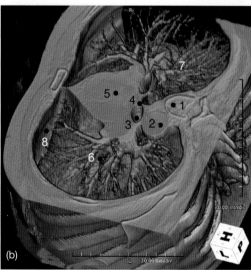

Figure 3.4 (a) Pulmonary arteriogram – performed by passing a catheter, 1, through the venous system, right atrium, right ventricle and onwards into, 2, the pulmonary trunk. The contrast medium is then injected to outline the anatomical features: 3, right pulmonary artery; 4, left pulmonary artery; 5, right basal segmental arteries; 6, left superior lobe segmental arteries. (b) Electron beam CT of the thorax showing the three-dimensional anatomy. This is part of a video sequence that rotates round the whole chest for detailed examination, having only taken a few minutes to acquire the data: 1, vertebral body; 2, desending thoracic aorta; 3, left main bronchus; 4, carina; 5, heart chamber; 6, pulmonary segmental vessels; 7, segmental bronchial 'tree'; 8, diaphragm – left dome

Branches

The right pulmonary artery passes to the right lung hilus behind the ascending aorta and superior vena cava and in front of the oesophagus and right main bronchus. The left pulmonary artery passes in front of the left bronchus and descending aorta to its lung hilus. It is connected by the ligamentum arteriosum to the lower aspect of the aortic arch. Branches of the pulmonary arteries accompany the bronchi and bronchioles.

THE GREAT VEINS

The pulmonary veins are paired, short wide vessels lying in the hilus of each lung, anterior and inferior to the artery (Fig. 3.6).

Brachiocephalic veins

The brachiocephalic veins (Fig. 3.6) form behind the sternoclavicular joint by the union of the internal jugular and subclavian veins of each side and, after a short course, unite to form the superior vena cava behind the right side of the manubrium. The right brachiocephalic vein is some 3 cm long, with the right phrenic nerve lateral to it, descending behind the right margin of the manubrium anterolateral to the brachiocephalic artery. The longer left brachiocephalic vein descends obliquely behind the manubrium, above the arch of the aorta, and anterior to its three large branches and the trachea.

Tributaries

These are the vertebral veins draining the neck muscles, the inferior thyroid veins, which unite in front of the trachea

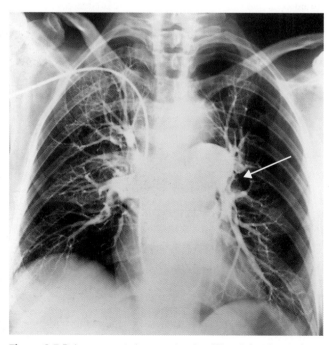

Figure 3.5 Pulmonary arteriogram showing filling defect in arteries (arrow) due to an embolus arising from a thrombus in the deep veins of the leg (p. 245)

and drain into the left brachiocephalic vein, and the internal thoracic vein draining the anterior chest wall. The thoracic duct drains into the left brachiocephalic vein, and the smaller right lymph duct drains into the right brachiocephalic vein) (Fig. 4.16, p. 71).

Superior vena cava

The superior vena cava, 1.5 cm wide and about 7 cm long, is formed by the union of the two brachiocephalic veins behind the right border of the manubrium and descends behind the body of the sternum to enter the right atrium at the level of the 3rd costal cartilage. It has no valves.

Relations

Its lower half, covered by fibrous and serous pericardium, lies behind the right lung, pleura and manubrium, and anterior to the right lung root. The ascending aorta and right brachiocephalic artery are medial to it; the pleura and right lung are lateral. Its only tributary, the azygos vein, enters posteriorly.

Determination of **right atrial pressure** is important in the management of the critically ill patient; this can be measured by a catheter introduced into the internal jugular or subclavian vein via the superior vena cava into the right atrium (central venous pressure line; Fig. 23.5b, p. 392). **Obstruction of the superior vena cava** by a tumour leads to diversion of its venous blood into subcutaneous veins of the chest wall and, via them, into veins of the anterior abdominal wall. From there, the diverted blood drains into the inferior vena cava and azygos system of veins.

Azygos vein

The azygos vein is formed in the abdomen in front of the 2nd lumbar vertebra and passes into the chest via the aortic opening in the diaphragm, lying to the right of the aorta. It ascends the posterior mediastinum on the vertebral bodies. At the level of the 4th thoracic vertebra, it arches over the right lung root anteriorly to enter the superior vena cava (Figs. 3.6d,e).

Tributaries

The azygos vein and the smaller left-sided hemiazygos vein drain the intercostal spaces and the right bronchial veins.

The inferior vena cava has a very short intrathoracic course. It pierces the central tendon of the diaphragm and directly enters the right atrium.

NERVES

The phrenic nerves

The phrenic nerves arise from the ventral rami of C3, C4 and C5 and descend from the neck through the thorax in front of each lung root (Fig. 3.6g). The right phrenic nerve enters the thorax lateral to the right brachiocephalic vein, descends on the pericardium over the superior vena cava, right atrium and inferior vena cava, and passes through the caval opening of the diaphragm. Throughout, it is covered laterally by mediastinal pleura. The left phrenic nerve enters between the left subclavian artery and left brachiocephalic vein, descending across the aortic arch and pericardium over the left ventricle to reach and pierce the left diaphragm. It is covered laterally by mediastinal pleura.

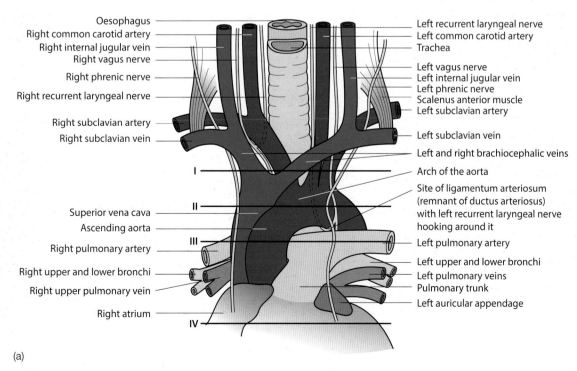

(a)

Figure 3.6 (a) Anterior aspect of the thorax showing mediastinal structures: I, II, III and IV are axial planes as shown in parts (b)–(i) (*overleaf*)

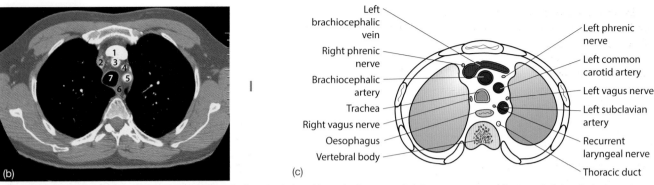

(b) 1, Left brachiocephalic vein; 2, right brachiocephalic vein; 3, brachiocephalic artery; 4, left common carotid artery; 5, left subclavian artery; 6, oesophagus; 7, trachea

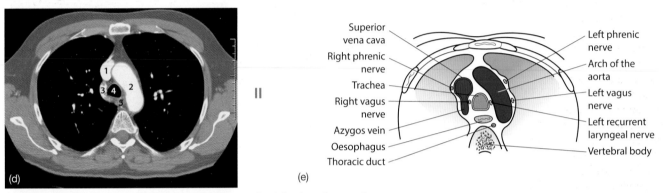

(d) 1, Superior vena cava; 2, arch of aorta; 3, azygos vein; 4, trachea; 5, oesophagus

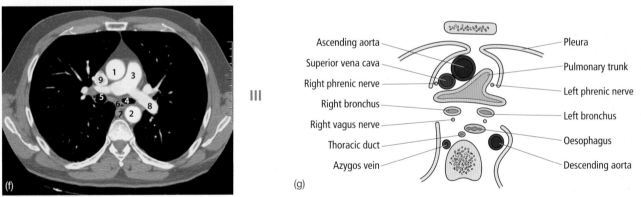

(f) 1, Ascending aorta; 2, descending aorta; 3, pulmonary trunk (artery); 4, left bronchus; 5, right bronchus; 6, oesophagus; 7, azygos vein; 8, left pulmonary artery; 9, superior vena cava

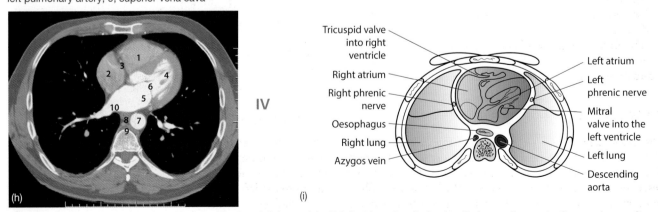

(h) 1, Right ventricle; 2, right atrium; 3, tricuspid valve; 4, left ventricle; 5, left atrium; 6, mitral valve; 7, descending aorta; 8, oesophagus; 9, azygos vein; 10, right pulmonary vein

Figure 3.6 (*continued*) (b)–(i) transverse sections (CT scans and accompanying diagrams) at levels I–IV (shown on (a)) through the mediastinum

Both nerves are motor to the diaphragm and supply sensory branches to the mediastinal and diaphragmatic pleura, the pericardium and the peritoneum.

Pain arising from inflammation of the diaphragmatic pleura is classically referred to skin over the shoulder tip, which is supplied by nerves derived, like the phrenic nerve, from the C4 spinal segment.

The vagus nerves

The right vagus enters the thorax posterolateral to the right brachiocephalic artery and descends lateral to the trachea under the mediastinal pleura to the back of the right main bronchus, where it gives branches, first to the pulmonary plexus and then to the oesophageal plexus. The left vagus enters the thorax between the left common carotid and subclavian arteries and descends across the left of the aortic arch, where it gives off its recurrent laryngeal branch, before passing behind the left lung root to the oesophagus. The two vagi form the oesophageal plexus, from which emerge anterior and posterior gastric nerves (anterior and posterior vagal trunks) containing fibres of both vagi and sympathetic nerves, which descend to pass through the oesophageal opening of the diaphragm. The nerves supply the stomach, duodenum, pancreas and liver, and contribute branches via the coeliac plexus to other viscera (pp. 71–73).

Branches

The left recurrent laryngeal nerve winds around the ligamentum arteriosum and aortic arch and ascends between the trachea and oesophagus into the neck (Fig. 3.6a), providing cardiac branches to the cardiac plexus (p. 71) and branches to the pulmonary and oesophageal plexuses (Fig. 2.2, p. 36 and p. 71).

THE THYMUS

The thymus, a bilobed mass of lymphoid tissue, lies in front of the trachea, extending downwards posterior to the manubrium. It may enlarge into the lower neck and upper thorax. Larger at birth, it atrophies after puberty, but is variable in size and so may extend down below the aortic arch to the anterior mediastinum (Fig. 3.7).

The **thymus** occasionally develops a tumour – a thymoma – which may be associated with myasthenia gravis and require surgical removal.

THE OESOPHAGUS

The oesophagus begins at the level of the cricoid cartilage (Figs. 3.3 and 3.6b–i). Its cervical portion lies in the midline on the prevertebral fascia (see also p. 371), and then it descends through the thorax mainly to the left of the midline. Initially close to the vertebral column, it curves forwards in its lower part and pierces the diaphragm surrounded by fibres of its right crus at the level of the 10th thoracic vertebra. Its intra-abdominal portion is about 2 cm long and the overall length is 25 cm.

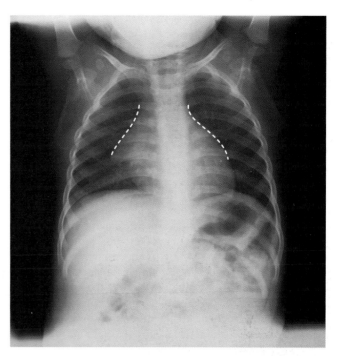

Figure 3.7 Chest X-ray of a child, showing a normal variant of a relatively large thymus (dashed lines)

Relations

In the upper mediastinum, the oesophagus lies between the vertebral column posteriorly and the trachea anteriorly, the left recurrent laryngeal nerve lying in the groove between it and the trachea. Below, it is separated from the vertebral column by the thoracic duct, the azygos and hemiazygos veins, and the aorta. Anteriorly, below the trachea it is crossed by the left bronchus, and below this it is separated from the left atrium by the pericardium. On the right, it is covered by mediastinal pleura and the azygos vein; on the left, from above, the aortic arch, the subclavian artery and the descending aorta separate it from mediastinal pleura. Its lower part is in contact with the pleura.

During development, both the trachea and the oesophagus develop from the tracheo-oesophageal septum, which lies between them. Failure of development of the septum results in a congenital tracheo-oesophageal fistula, and the newborn child quickly regurgitates any milk that is drunk, the child becoming cyanotic as milk enters the respiratory tract. Urgent surgery is required.

Lymphatic drainage

The cervical oesophagus drains to the deep cervical lymph nodes, the thoracic portion drains to the tracheobronchial and posterior mediastinal nodes and its abdominal portion drains to the left gastric nodes.

Radiological examination of the oesophagus is achieved by having the patient swallow barium (Fig. 2.5, p. 37). This usually reveals slight constrictions where the oesophagus is crossed by the aortic arch and the left bronchus, and as it passes through the diaphragm. In patients with heart failure, the oesophagus will be seen to be compressed by the enlarged left atrium. More direct examination of its luminal surface is obtained by endoscopy (Fig. 6.2, p. 95). **Oesophagoscopy**, whether performed with a rigid or a flexible oesophagoscope, is facilitated by knowledge that, in the adult, the origin of the oesophagus is 15 cm from the incisor teeth, and the oesophagogastric junction is usually 40 cm from that point.

THE THORACIC TRACHEA AND BRONCHI

The trachea commences in the neck just below the cricoid cartilage; it lies in the midline and descends into the superior mediastinum, bifurcating into two main bronchi at the upper border of the 5th thoracic vertebra. Its cervical portion is described on page 377. In the chest, the left recurrent laryngeal nerve lies in the groove between the trachea and the oesophagus. Its walls, like those of the main bronchi, are strengthened by U-shaped incomplete rings of cartilage. Anteriorly, the brachiocephalic artery and the left brachiocephalic vein cross it; on its left lie the common carotid and subclavian arteries, and below them the aortic arch; on the right, the right vagus nerve and azygos vein separate it from the pleura.

The tracheal bifurcation (carina) lies at the level of the sternal angle and the lower border of the 4th thoracic vertebra, anterior to the oesophagus and to the right of the pulmonary trunk bifurcation (Figs. 3.6a,g).

The extrapulmonary bronchi

The right and left main bronchi arise at the bifurcation and descend laterally to enter the hilus of the lung, where they divide to form the intrapulmonary bronchial tree. The right bronchus, 3 cm long, is wider and more vertical than the left. The right upper lobe bronchus arises before it enters the hilus.

Relations

Anteriorly, the left pulmonary artery separates the carina from the left atrium; the aortic arch lies above it, and posteriorly lie the oesophagus and descending thoracic aorta.

Because the **trachea** contains air, it is recognized on chest X-rays as a radiolucent (dark) structure descending backwards and slightly to the right in the upper mediastinum. It may be compressed or displaced by enlargement of the thyroid gland. Widening or distortion of the carina may result from enlargement of the tracheobronchial lymph nodes or secondary spread of lung cancer. Inhaled foreign bodies tend to pass more frequently to the wider, more vertical right bronchus (Fig. 3.8). Direct viewing of the trachea and proximal bronchi is possible endoscopically. Instillation of a radiopaque medium, e.g. Lipiodol, into the bronchi, permits a radiograph of the bronchial tree to be obtained (Figs. 4.9 and 4.10, p. 67). Bronchial cancer commonly produces symptoms of ulceration and bleeding, obstruction of the bronchi and production of blood-stained sputum.

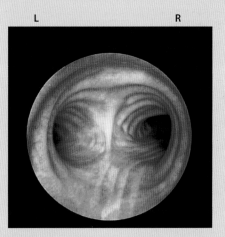

Figure 3.8 The cartilaginous rings indent the mucosa of the trachea and carina, as seen down the endoscope. Note that the wider right bronchus lies more vertically, and thus descends more directly and less obliquely. It is in this bronchus that inhaled foreign bodies get lodged

MCQs

1. The left phrenic nerve: **T/F**

  a arises from the dorsal rami of the C3, C4   (____)
     and C5 cervical nerves

  b descends through the thorax in the left   (____)
     pleural cavity

  c conveys sensory fibres from the mediastinal   (____)
     and diaphragmatic pleura, and from the
     diaphragmatic peritoneum

  d leaves the abdomen through the caval   (____)
     opening of the diaphragm

  e descends the thorax posterior to the root of   (____)
     the lung

Answers

1.

a ***F*** *– It arises from the ventral rami of these nerves.*

b ***F*** *– It descends within the mediastinum covered by the left mediastinal pleura.*

c ***T*** *– It also supplies motor branches to the diaphragm.*

d ***F*** *– The left phrenic nerve pierces the dome of the diaphragm, giving branches to its undersurface. It is the right phrenic nerve that passes through the caval opening of the diaphragm.*

e ***F*** *– Both phrenic nerves pass anterior to the root of the lung.*

2. The pulmonary trunk: **T/F**

  a lies anterior to the aortic root   (____)

  b is contained with the ascending aorta in a   (____)
     common sleeve of serous pericardium

  c bifurcates anterior to the aortic arch   (____)

  d is in contact with the left pleura   (____)

  e is closely related to both right and left coro-   (____)
     nary arteries

Answers

2.

a ***T*** *– It then ascends posteriorly and to the left …*

b ***T*** *– … and both are also within the fibrous pericardium.*

c ***F*** *– It lies within the concavity of the aortic arch and hence posterior and to the left of the ascending aorta.*

d ***T*** *– Both its anterior and left surfaces are covered, with the left pleura covering the lung.*

e ***T*** *– Both vessels surround its base.*

3. The thoracic oesophagus: **T/F**

  a is posterior to the trachea   (____)

  b is directly related to the vertebral column   (____)
     throughout its course

  c is related to the left atrium   (____)

  d pierces the central tendon of the diaphragm   (____)
     at the level of the 8th thoracic vertebra

  e is crossed anteriorly by the left bronchus   (____)

Answers

3.

a ***T*** *– With the left recurrent laryngeal and right vagus nerves lying between it and the trachea.*

b ***F*** *– It is so related in its upper part, but inferiorly it is separated from the vertebral column by the thoracic duct, the azygos and hemiazygos veins, and the thoracic aorta.*

c ***T*** *– It is only separated from it by the pericardium.*

d ***F*** *– The oesophagus pierces the right crus of the diaphragm to the left of the midline at the level of the 10th thoracic vertebra.*

e ***T*** *– The left bronchus crosses the middle of the oesophagus anteriorly.*

SBA

A newborn baby swallows milk, has a bout of coughing and becomes cyanotic for a short time. The next day she is found to have pneumonia. A tracheo-oesophageal fistula is suspected. If this is the case, in which structure has a failure of development occurred?

a the oesophagus

b the trachea

c the tongue

d the pharynx

e the tracheo-oesophageal septum

Answer

e *In the early stages of development, the tracheo-oesophageal septum separates the trachea and oesophagus. However, if it fails to develop further, these two structures will fail to separate and a tracheo-oesophageal fistula will occur. Swallowed milk will enter the trachea, respiratory embarrassment follows and lung infections inevitably ensue.*

EMQs

Each question has an anatomical theme linked to the chapter, and a list of 10 related items (A–J) placed in alphabetical order: these are followed by five statements (1–5). Match **one or more** of the items A–J to each of the five statements.

Mediastinal structures
A. Aortic arch
B. Ascending aorta
C. Brachiocephalic artery
D. Descending thoracic aorta
E. Left brachiocephalic vein
F. Left carotid artery
G. Left vagus nerve
H. Right phrenic nerve
I. Right subclavian artery
J. Superior vena cava

Answers
1 AB; *2* AFG; *3* DG; *4* D; *5* CF

Match the following statements with the appropriate item(s) from the above list
1. Related to the medial side of the superior vena cava
2. Related to the left side of the trachea
3. Lies to the left of the oesophagus
4. Posterior to the oesophagus
5. Posterior to the left brachiocephalic vein

APPLIED QUESTIONS

1. During a barium swallow, what anatomical structures, in their normal or pathological states, may cause indentation of the oesophagus on an oblique view?

   1. Oblique X-rays of a barium swallow may reveal three normal impressions on the oesophageal silhouette, caused by the aortic arch, the left main bronchus and the right crus of the diaphragm. Each impression indicates where swallowed foreign objects may lodge and where a stricture may develop after accidental or suicidal swallowing of a caustic liquid. Pathological compressions may be observed from a dilated left atrium, an aberrant aortic arch or an aberrant right subclavian artery passing retro-oesophageally.

2. Why do the trachea and the main bronchi not collapse during the negative pressure of inspiration?

   2. The consistent diameters of the trachea and main bronchi are due to the strengthening cartilaginous bands and incomplete rings, which maintain their shape even during inspiration. The walls of the trachea are supported by 15–20 U-shaped bands of hyaline cartilage.

Bailey & Love · Essential Clinical Anatomy · Bailey & Love · Essential Clinical Anatomy
Essential Clinical Anatomy · Bailey & Love · Essential Clinical Anatomy · Bailey & Love
Bailey & Love · Essential Clinical Anatomy · Bailey & Love · Essential Clinical Anatomy

Chapter 4

The pleura and lungs

THE PLEURA

The pleura is a fibroelastic serous membrane lined by squamous epithelium forming a sac on each side of the chest. Each pleural sac is a closed cavity invaginated by a lung. Parietal pleura lines the chest wall and visceral (pulmonary) pleura covers the lungs. These two pleural layers are continuous around the root of the lung and are separated by a thin film of serous fluid, permitting them to glide easily on each other. The layers are prevented from separating by the fluid's surface tension and the negative pressure in the thoracic cavity. Thus, when the thoracic cage expands, the lung also must expand and air is inhaled.

Parietal pleura lines the ribs, costal cartilages, intercostal spaces, lateral surface of the mediastinum and upper surface of the diaphragm. Superiorly, it extends above the thoracic inlet into the neck as the cervical dome of pleura; inferiorly, around the margin of the diaphragm, it forms a narrow gutter, the **costodiaphragmatic recess**; anteriorly, the left costal and mediastinal surfaces are in contact, extending in front of the heart to form the **costomediastinal recess**. Mediastinal pleura invests the main bronchi and pulmonary vessels and passes on to the surface of the lung to become visceral pleura, which covers the lung and extends into its interlobar fissures.

The **surface markings** of the pleural sacs should be noted (Figs. 4.1 and 4.2). On both sides, the upper limit lies about 3 cm above the medial third of the clavicle. From here, the lines of pleural reflections descend behind the sternoclavicular joints to almost meet in the midline at the level of the 2nd costal cartilage. At the 4th costal cartilage, whereas the left pleura deviates laterally and descends along the lateral border of the sternum to the 6th costal cartilage, the right pleural reflection continues down, near to the midline, to the 6th costal cartilage. At this point, on both sides, the pleural reflections pass laterally behind the costal margin to reach the 8th rib in the midclavicular line and the 10th rib in the midaxillary line, and along the 12th rib and the paravertebral line (lying over the tips of the transverse processes, about 3 cm from the midline).

Visceral pleura has no pain fibres, but the parietal pleura is richly supplied by branches of the somatic intercostal and phrenic nerves. Lymph from the pulmonary pleura passes to a superficial plexus in the lung and then to the hilar nodes. Parietal pleura drains to the parasternal, diaphragmatic and posterior mediastinal nodes.

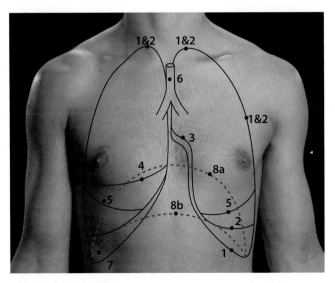

Figure 4.1 Surface markings of the pleura and lungs, anterior aspect: 1, pleural markings; 2, lung markings; 3, cardiac notch; 4, horizontal fissure; 5, oblique fissure; 6, trachea; 7, costodiaphragmatic recess; 8, diaphragm, (a) expiration, (b) inspiration

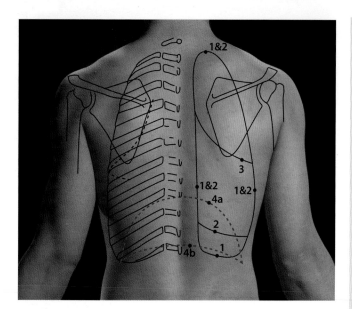

Figure 4.2 Surface markings of the pleura and lungs, posterior aspect: 1, pleural markings; 2, lung markings; 3, oblique fissure; 4, diaphragm, (a) expiration, (b) inspiration. The black dotted line shows the incision for opening the chest through 5th intercostal space

The pleural sac is a potential space that can in pathological conditions fill with fluid or air; with blood after intrathoracic haemorrhage (**haemothorax**); with inflammatory exudate (pleural **effusion**) or pus (**pyothorax**) (Fig. 4.3); or with air (**pneumothorax**) (Fig. 1.6, p. 24) after chest wall trauma that has torn the lung or after the rupture of a lung bulla that has burst the visceral pleura. A distended pleural cavity may interfere with lung expansion. Fluid may be drained from the pleural cavity by insertion of a needle or tube, attached to an underwater seal, into the 7th intercostal space in the midaxillary line (Fig. 1.7, p. 24). Insertion below this level runs the risk of the needle penetrating the diaphragm and the underlying liver or spleen. To avoid danger to the neurovascular bundle, it is best to insert the needle along the top of the rib, which avoids the vessels lying in the subcostal groove. Emergency aspiration of air is most safely achieved by inserting a needle, attached to an underwater seal or flutter valve, into the 2nd or 3rd intercostal space in the midclavicular line.

Punch biopsy needles inserted through the intercostal space allow specimens of pleura to be obtained for histological examination. **Pleurisy** – inflammation of the pleura – causes pain that is magnified by respiratory movements. The pain is referred by sensory fibres within the parietal pleura to the cutaneous distribution of the nerve supplying it. Thus costal inflammation is referred to the chest wall or, in the case of lower nerves, to the upper abdominal wall, and inflammation of the diaphragmatic pleura is referred to the area supplied by the nerve root (C4) from which originates the phrenic nerve, i.e. to the tip of the shoulder.

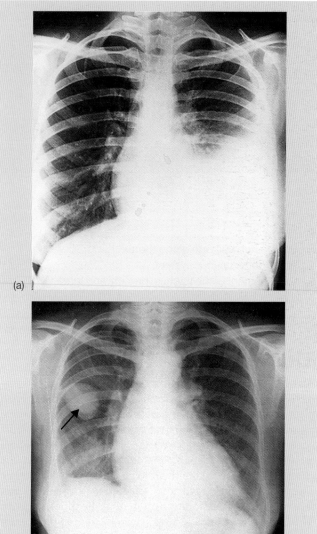

Figure 4.3 (a) Left pleural effusion obliterating much of the lower lung markings; (b) localized interlobar fluid collection (arrow)

THE LUNGS

These paired organs lie in separate pleural sacs attached to the mediastinum at the hila (Fig. 4.1, and Figs. 4.6 and 4.7 below). Spongy and elastic in composition, they conform to the contours of the thoracic cavity. The right lung weighs about 620 g, and the left about 560 g. They have a characteristic mottled appearance on x-rays – lung tissue is clear; denser shadows at the hilus are caused by hilar lymph nodes and radiating shadows by blood vessels. A posteroanterior (PA) chest X-ray will also reveal the normal aortic arch (knuckle), the inferior vena cava and the outline of the heart. A lateral view reveals details of the mediastinal structures (Figs. 4.4 and 4.5).

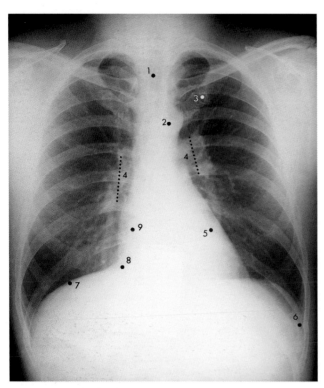

Figure 4.4 X-ray of the chest: 1, trachea; 2, aortic knuckle; 3, 1st costochondral junction; 4, hilar shadows; 5, left ventricle; 6, left costodiaphragmatic recess; 7, right dome of diaphragm; 8, inferior vena cava; 9, right atrium

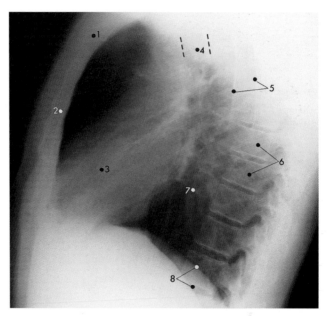

Figure 4.5 Lateral chest X-ray showing mediastinal structures: 1, manubriosternal joint; 2, sternum; 3, cardiac shadow; 4, trachea; 5, border of scapula; 6, vertebral bodies; 7, retrocardiac space; 8, domes of diaphragm

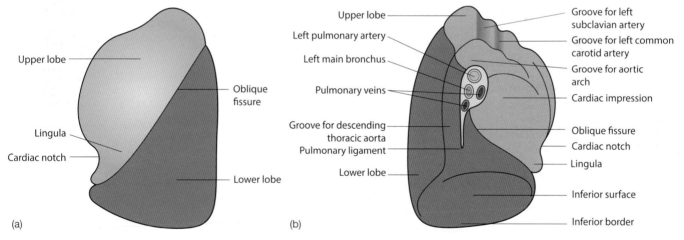

(a)   (b)

Figure 4.6 Left lung: (a) lateral surface; (b) medial surface

Each lung has an apex in the root of the neck and a base resting on the diaphragm. The base is separated by a sharp inferior border from a lateral convex costal surface and a medial concave mediastinal surface, in the centre of which are the structures of the lung root surrounded by a cuff of pleura (Figs. 4.6 and 4.7). The deeper concavity of the left lung accommodates the heart's left ventricle. The left lung's anterior border is deeply indented by the heart to form the cardiac notch; the rounded posterior border of each lung lies in the paravertebral sulcus.

The lungs are each divided by fissures extending deeply into their substance. An **oblique fissure** divides the left lung into an upper and lower lobe (Fig. 4.6); **oblique and horizontal fissures** divide the right lung into upper, middle and lower lobes (Fig. 4.7). The oblique fissure on each side can be marked by a line around the chest wall from the spine of the 3rd thoracic vertebra to the 6th costochondral junction. The horizontal fissure is marked by a horizontal line passing from the 4th right costal cartilage to the oblique line previously drawn (Figs. 4.1 and 4.2). The **lower lobes** of both lungs lie below and behind the oblique fissure and comprise most of the posterior and inferior borders. The **upper lobe** of the left lung is above and anterior to the oblique fissure, and includes the apex and most of the mediastinal and costal surfaces. The

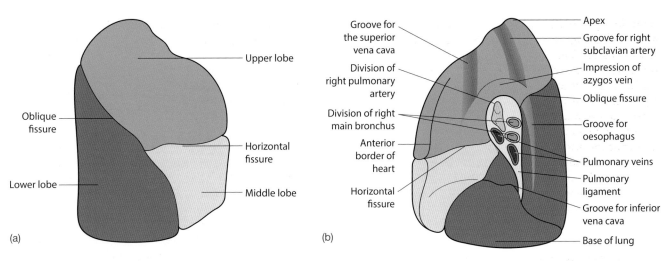

Figure 4.7 Right lung: (a) lateral surface; (b) medial surface

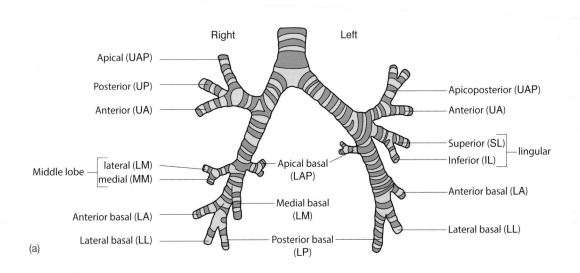

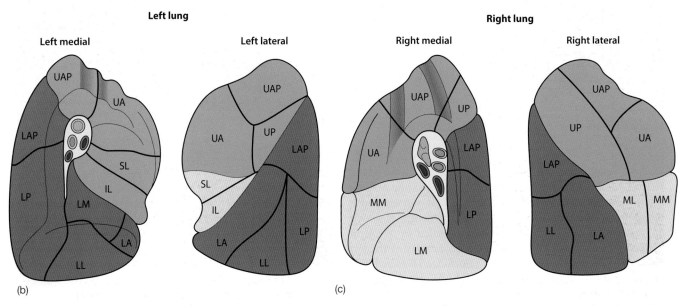

Figure 4.8 (a) Bronchial tree. (b) and (c) Bronchopulmonary segments; (b) right lung – mediastinal and costovertebral surfaces; (c) left lung – medial and lateral surfaces

equivalent part of the right lung is divided by the horizontal fissure into a large upper lobe and a smaller, anterior, wedge-shaped **middle lobe**, which lies deep to the right breast. A thin anteroinferior part of the left upper lobe, adjacent to the cardiac notch, is known as the **lingula** and is the left-sided equivalent of the middle lobe. Fissures may be incomplete or absent, and additional lobes are occasionally present.

The **hilum** or root of each lung contains a main bronchus, a pulmonary artery, two pulmonary veins, the pulmonary nerve plexus and lymph nodes, all enveloped by the pleural cuff; an inferior narrow extension of the cuff is known as the pulmonary ligament (**Figs. 4.6** and **4.7**). The bronchus lies behind the pulmonary artery and the two veins are below and anterior.

The intrapulmonary bronchi and bronchopulmonary segments

Each main bronchus descends to enter the hilum of the lung: that of the right side is shorter, wider and more vertical than that of the left, with the result that aspiration of foreign bodies is more common on the right side. Each main bronchus divides into **lobar bronchi**, which further divide into **segmental bronchi**, each supplying **bronchopulmonary segments**. Each lung contains 10 such segments. The right upper lobe bronchus arises from the right main bronchus before the hilum and, after entering the lung substance, divides into apical, anterior and posterior segmental bronchi (**Fig. 4.8**).

The middle lobe bronchus arises beyond this and divides into medial and lateral segmental bronchi. The continuation of the right main bronchus passes to the lower lobe and divides into apical, anterior, medial, lateral and posterior basal segmental bronchi. The left upper lobe bronchus arises from the main bronchus within the lung and divides into five segmental bronchi, the anterior and inferior passing to the lingula. The continuation of the left bronchus passes to the lower lobe and also, similar to the right side, divides into five segmental bronchi. Each segmental bronchus is divided into a functionally independent unit of lung tissue with its own vascular supply – a **bronchopulmonary segment** (**Figs. 4.8– 4.10**). The walls of the bronchi are lined with smooth muscle and hyaline cartilage, and lined by pseudostratified columnar epithelium and mucous glands. Their thin terminal branches, the bronchioles, contain no cartilage and are lined by non-ciliated columnar epithelium.

The comatose or anaesthetized patient is subject to a particular risk of aspiration, and such material will gravitate to the most dependent, posterior part of the lung. The apical segment of the lower lobe is supplied by the highest, most posterior of the segmental bronchi and it is, therefore, this segment (particularly on the right) that is the most common site for aspiration pneumonia in these patients.

Relations

The lung borders closely follow the lines of pleural reflection on the chest wall, except inferiorly, where the lower border

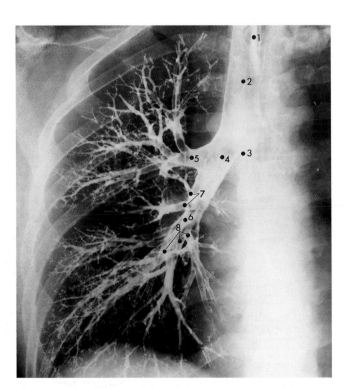

Figure 4.9 Bronchogram of the right lung, anteroposterior view: 1, intubation catheter; 2, trachea, 3, carina; 4, right main bronchus; 5, right upper lobe bronchus; 6, right middle lobe bronchus; 7, right apical lower lobe bronchi; 8, right basal lower lobe bronchi

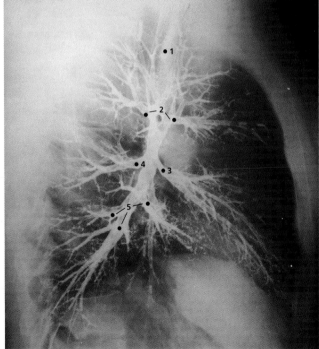

Figure 4.10 Bronchogram of the right lung, lateral view: 1, trachea; 2, right upper lobe bronchi; 3, right middle lobe bronchus; 4, right apical lower lobe bronchus; 5, right basal lower lobe bronchi

of the lung lies about two intercostal spaces above the pleural reflection (costodiaphragmatic recess), and in front, where, near to the cardiac notch, the anterior border of the left lung lies some 3 cm lateral to the pleural reflection (costomediastinal recess) (Figs. 4.1 and 4.2). The costal surfaces are related to the thoracic wall; the base is separated by the diaphragm from the right lobe of the liver on the right and the liver, stomach and spleen on the left. The apex, covered by the dome of the pleura, lies under the suprapleural membrane, a fibrous sheet extending from the transverse process of the 7th cervical vertebra to the inner border of the 1st rib. The subclavian vessels arch over the membrane. Posteriorly lie the anterior primary ramus of the first thoracic nerve, passing to the brachial plexus, and the sympathetic trunk, both lying on the neck of the 1st rib.

The **medial** relations differ on each side. On the left (Figs. 4.6b and 4.11), a large concavity for the left ventricle continues superiorly with a groove for the aortic arch, which passes in front of the hilum. Above the arch, the lung is in contact, from before backwards, with the left brachiocephalic vein, left common carotid artery, left subclavian artery and oesophagus. On the right (Figs. 4.7b and 4.12), a shallow concavity in front of the hilum for the right atrium is continuous above with a groove for the superior vena cava, and below with a shorter groove for the inferior vena cava. The azygos vein grooves the lung as it arches forwards above the hilum. The oesophagus is in contact throughout its length near to the posterior border, except where the azygos vein separates it from the lung. The oesophagus lies between the superior vena cava and the trachea.

Blood supply

Lung tissue is supplied by the bronchial arteries – branches of the descending aorta – and some of this blood returns to the heart via the pulmonary veins. Other bronchial veins drain to the azygos or hemiazygos veins. The pulmonary artery conveys poorly oxygenated blood to the alveoli by branches that accompany the bronchial tree. From the alveolar capillary network arise veins that accompany the bronchi to form the upper and lower pulmonary veins.

Pulmonary embolism may be a fatal condition. It is caused by large blood clots (thrombi) that originate in the deep veins of the legs or pelvis, becoming dislodged and then being conveyed through the right side of the heart to rest in and occlude large or segmental pulmonary arteries (Fig. 3.5, p. 56, and Fig. 4.13), or worse, the pulmonary trunk. The result is partial or complete obstruction of the arterial supply to a segment or lobe of the lung, which, although ventilated, is no longer perfused with blood. If the embolus blocks the main pulmonary artery, acute respiratory distress and cyanosis results and death often follows within a few minutes. Segmental emboli cause death of lung tissue, a pulmonary infarct that, if small, resolves over a few weeks.

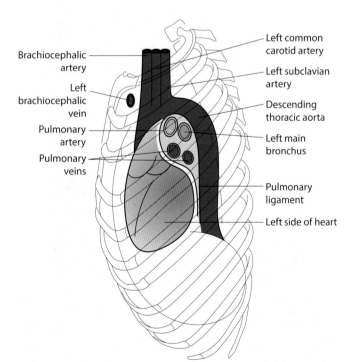

Figure 4.11 Medial relations of the left lung

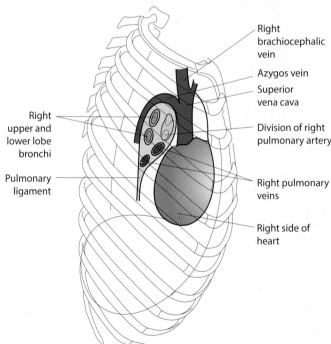

Figure 4.12 Medial relations of the right lung

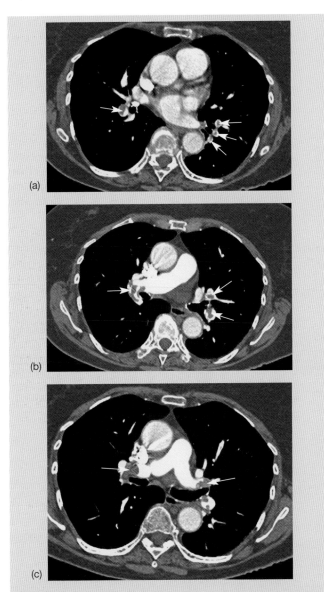

Figure 4.13 These three axial transverse CT images show various cases of pulmonary emboli (arrowed). This is when a blood clot, often from the lower leg or pelvis, detaches and rushes through the venous side of the heart before lodging within the lungs. If, as in (c), it is a recently dislodged 'saddle' embolus in both pulmonary arteries, it may be fatal. (a) Multiple emboli appear as darker areas within the small peripheral arteries (arrows); (b) bilateral clots in the main pulmonary arteries; (c) large bilateral clots in both right and left pulmonary arteries

Lymphatic drainage

This is by a superficial subpleural lymph plexus and by a deep plexus of vessels accompanying the bronchi. Both groups drain through hilar (bronchopulmonary) nodes to tracheo-bronchial nodes around the tracheal bifurcation (carina) and thence to mediastinal lymph trunks.

Nerve supply

The lungs are supplied by sympathetic (bronchodilator) fibres from the upper thoracic segments and parasympathetic (bronchoconstrictor) fibres from the vagus. The latter provide afferent fibres for the cough reflex, which is so important for clearing mucus and inhaled material. Both supply the lungs via the pulmonary plexuses (p. 71).

X-rays of the chest allow accurate localization of disease in the lung and may also define abnormal collections of air or fluid in the pleural space (Fig. 1.6, p. 24). CT and MRI scans can improve the definition of pulmonary lesions and can be used to guide fine biopsy needles inserted percutaneously towards suspect lesions (Fig. 4.14). Radiopaque contrast media can outline the bronchial tree (Figs. 4.9 and 4.10) and radioisotopes assist in the assessment of ventilation and perfusion of lung tissue. Excision of pulmonary segments for localized disease is directly assisted by knowledge of the anatomy of the bronchopulmonary segments. This knowledge is also used to employ effective physiotherapy for drainage of infected lung segments (Fig. 4.15).

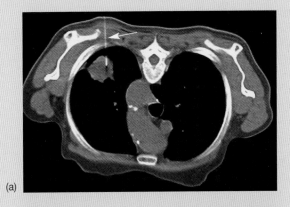

(a)

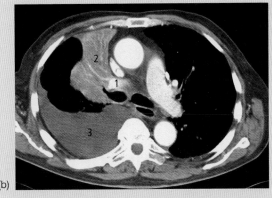

(b)

Figure 4.14 (a) Axial transverse CT of lung biopsy into a carcinoma in an apical segment of the lower lobe, patient lying prone (arrow indicates needle). (b) CT taken at the level of the pulmonary arteries, patient lying supine. The left lung field is normal but the right contains an upper lobe carcinoma (1) just posterior to the collapsed lung (2); the posterior part of the pleural cavity is filled with a large malignant pleural effusion (3)

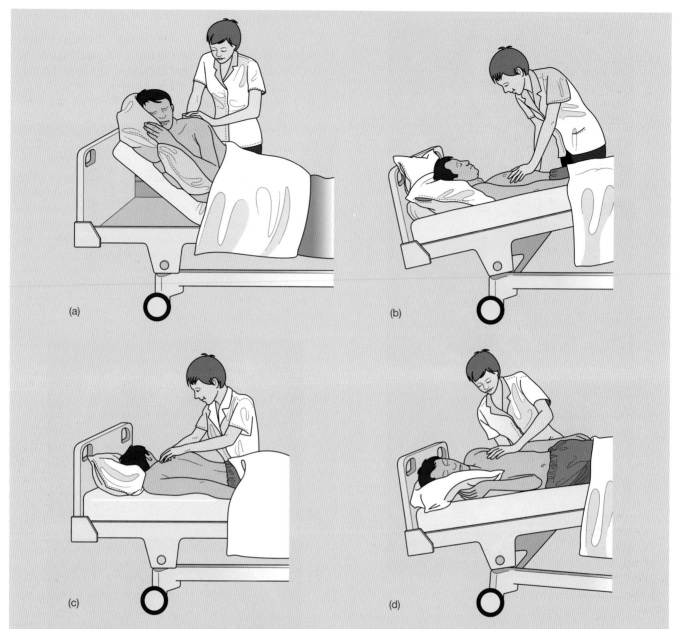

Figure 4.15 Postural drainage positions: (a) posterior segment, left upper lobe; (b) anterior basal segments, lower lobes; (c) posterior segment, right upper lobe; (d) lingula segment, left upper lobe

LYMPHATIC DRAINAGE OF THE THORAX

There are two groups of lymph vessels in the thorax: those draining the chest wall and those of the thoracic viscera (Fig. 4.16).

The **chest wall** drains by superficial and deep systems. The superficial vessels, like those of the breast, drain to the pectoral and central groups of axillary lymph nodes. There is some communication with vessels of the opposite side.

The vessels draining the deeper chest wall drain to the:

- **Parasternal nodes** alongside the internal thoracic artery, whose efferents drain to the bronchomediastinal lymph trunk.

- **Intercostal nodes** lying at the back of the intercostal spaces, whose efferents drain to the right lymph duct and the thoracic duct.

- **Diaphragmatic nodes** on the upper surface of the diaphragm, whose efferents drain to parasternal and posterior mediastinal nodes and, through the diaphragm, to communicate with those draining the upper surface of the liver.

The **thoracic viscera** drain to the:

- **Anterior mediastinal nodes** in front of the brachiocephalic veins and drain the anterior mediastinum. Their efferents join those of the tracheobronchial nodes.

- **Tracheobronchial nodes**, alongside the trachea and main bronchi, which drain the lungs, trachea and heart. Their

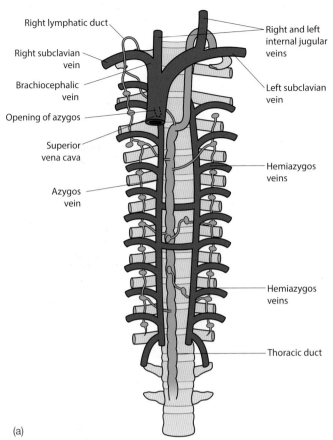

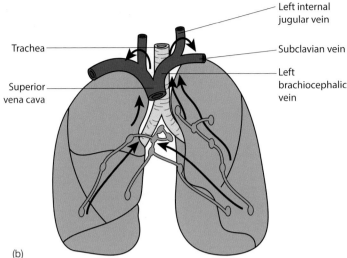

Figure 4.16 Lymphatic and venous drainage of the chest: (a) azygos system and thoracic lymphatics; (b) lymphatic and venous drainage of the lungs. Lymph nodes are situated along the course of the bronchial tree and drain to the hilar nodes and around the carina and tracheal bifurcation. Lymph from the right lung and the left lower lobe tends to follow the nodes on the right side of the trachea and from there passes in the right mediastinal lymph duct into the right subclavian vein. Lymph from the left upper lobe follows the left side of the trachea and passes into the thoracic duct, thence draining into the left subclavian vein as indicated by the arrows

A chylothorax is the abnormal collection of lymph within the pleural cavity. This is most commonly the result of surgical damage from either surgery at the root of the neck, a left-sided subclavian venous puncture, or extensive surgery in the posterior mediastinum. More rarely, a chylothorax may result from a malignant infiltration or a filarial parasitic infection blocking the thoracic duct.

efferents join those of the anterior mediastinal nodes to form the **bronchomediastinal trunk**, which, on the right side joins the right lymph duct and on the left the thoracic duct.

- **Posterior mediastinal nodes**, alongside the oesophagus. Their efferents pass into the thoracic duct.

The **thoracic duct** and the smaller right lymph duct return lymph to the bloodstream.

The thoracic duct, about 45 cm long, arises in the abdomen as a continuation of the cisterna chyli (Fig. 10.10a, p. 161) and enters the thorax on the right of the aorta through the aortic opening of the diaphragm. It ascends, behind and on the right of the oesophagus, with the azygos vein, passing to the left in front of the 5th thoracic vertebra. At the level of the 7th cervical vertebra, it arches laterally behind the carotid sheath and then forwards to enter the origin of the left brachiocephalic vein. It conveys lymph from below the diaphragm and the left half of the thorax, as well as from the head and neck, via the left jugular and subclavian lymph trunks and the left bronchomediastinal lymph trunk that joins it.

The **right lymph duct** is a short vessel, formed in the neck by the union of the right jugular, subclavian and bronchomediastinal lymph trunks. It enters the origin of the right brachiocephalic vein, conveying lymph from the right side of the head and neck and thorax.

AUTONOMIC NERVOUS SYSTEM

The autonomic nerve supply of the thoracic viscera is via the cardiac, pulmonary and oesophageal plexuses, which each receive sympathetic and parasympathetic contributions.

The **cardiac plexus** lies partly on the ligamentum arteriosum and partly on the tracheal bifurcation. The parts communicate and are a single functional unit. They receive branches from each of the cervical and upper thoracic sympathetic ganglia, and parasympathetic branches from both vagi. Branches of the plexus are distributed with the coronary arteries to the heart and its conducting system. The cardiac plexus also sends branches to the pulmonary plexus.

A **pulmonary plexus** lies around the root of each lung; it receives branches from the upper four cervical ganglia and from both vagi, and supplies the lung substance.

The **oesophageal plexus** is a network surrounding the lower oesophagus. It receives branches from the upper cervical ganglia and both vagi. It supplies the oesophagus, and over the lower oesophagus the right and left vagal trunks emerge from it and descend with the oesophagus to enter the abdomen as the anterior and posterior gastric nerves (Fig. 10.13, p. 163).

Each thoracic sympathetic trunk (Figs. 4.17a,b) lies alongside the vertebral column behind the parietal pleura. It is continuous above with the cervical trunk and below with the lumbar sympathetic trunk. It usually possesses 12 ganglia, each contributed by a thoracic nerve, but half of the first thoracic ganglion is fused to the 7th cervical to form a larger stellate ganglion on the neck of the 1st rib. Each ganglion receives preganglionic fibres in a white ramus communicans from its corresponding spinal nerve, and sends postganglionic fibres back to that nerve as a grey ramus communicans.

Sympathetic denervation (sympathectomy) of the upper limb is employed to dilate cutaneous blood vessels or inhibit sweating. It is achieved by surgically removing the 2nd and 3rd thoracic ganglia. The 1st ganglion is left intact to preserve sympathetic innervation to the head and neck and prevent the development of Horner's syndrome (Fig. 4.18). The features of the syndrome are unilateral ptosis, flushed and dry skin on the same side of the face, enophthalmos and a small pupil (meiosis). The syndrome is due to damage to the upper cervical trunk. It is often caused by cancerous infiltration from the apex of the lung (Fig. 4.19), but may also be caused by surgical removal of the stellate ganglion or a stellate ganglion block.

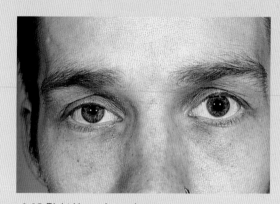

Figure 4.18 Right Horner's syndrome

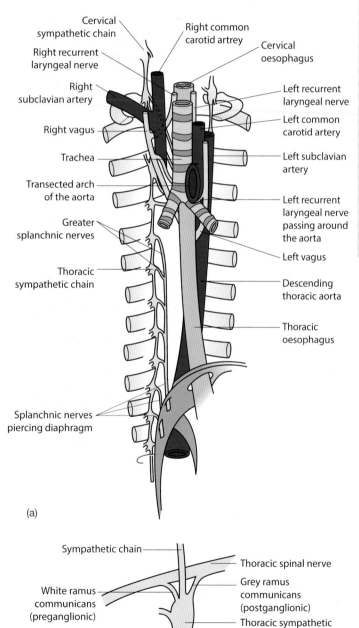

(a)

Cervical sympathetic chain
Right recurrent laryngeal nerve
Right subclavian artery
Right vagus
Trachea
Transected arch of the aorta
Greater splanchnic nerves
Thoracic sympathetic chain
Splanchnic nerves piercing diaphragm

Right common carotid artrey
Cervical oesophagus
Left recurrent laryngeal nerve
Left common carotid artery
Left subclavian artery
Left recurrent laryngeal nerve passing around the aorta
Left vagus
Descending thoracic aorta
Thoracic oesophagus

(b)

Sympathetic chain
White ramus communicans (preganglionic)

Thoracic spinal nerve
Grey ramus communicans (postganglionic)
Thoracic sympathetic ganglion

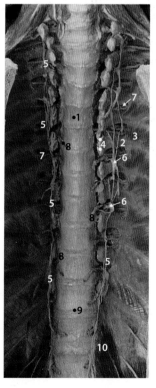

(c)

Figure 4.17 The sympathetic nervous system in the chest. (a) Sympathetic nerves in the thorax and root of neck. (b) Typical thoracic sympathetic ganglion. (c) Posterior thoracic wall dissection after removal of organs to show vertebral bodies and sympathetic chains: 1, vertebral bodies; 2, rib; 3, internal intercostal muscles; 4, disarticulated heads of ribs to show demi-facets; 5, sympathetic chain; 6, sympathetic ganglia; 7, intercostal, segmental neurovascular bundles; 8, posterior intercostal arteries; 9, intervertebral discs; 10, psoas major muscle

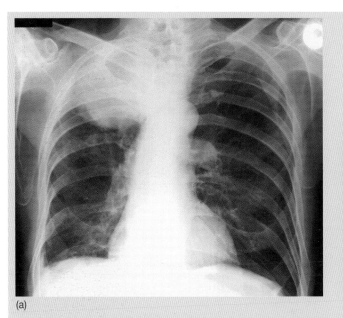

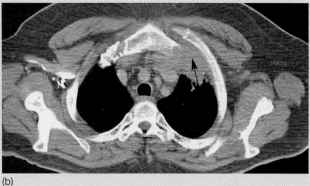

Figure 4.19 Apical cancer of the lung (Pancoast's syndrome): (a) chest X-ray, right-sided lesion; (b) CT scan, left-sided lesion (arrow)

The sympathetic trunk supplies:

- rami communicantes to each of its spinal nerves;
- branches to the cardiac, pulmonary and oesophageal plexuses from the upper four ganglia;

- branches to form the **greater, lesser and least splanchnic nerves** (Fig. 4.17a and Fig. 10.13, p. 163). These descend medial to the sympathetic chain and enter the abdomen by piercing the diaphragmatic crura. They contribute branches to the coeliac and other preaortic ganglia.

DEVELOPMENT OF THE TRACHEA, BRONCHI AND LUNGS

The lungs and tracheobronchial tree develop from the respiratory (laryngotracheal) diverticulum, an outgrowth of tissue that buds off the ventral aspect of the proximal foregut in the region of the 6th pharyngeal arch during week 4 of development (Figs. 4.20 and 22.13). The lining of the larynx and tracheobronchial tree is therefore derived from endoderm. The respiratory diverticulum grows caudally and gains a covering of splanchnic mesoderm, thus forming the respiratory bud. The respiratory bud subsequently branches into the left and right primary bronchial buds. (Fig. 4.22). The primary bronchial buds continue to subdivide, first into secondary bronchi (three on the right, and two on the left) followed by tertiary/segmental bronchi (ten on the right, and eight on the left), and continue to sequentially branch both *in utero* and postpartum

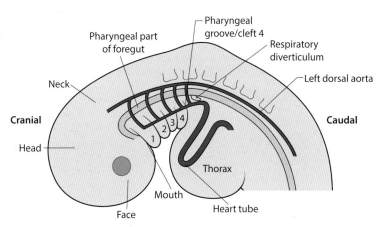

Figure 4.20 Early stage development of the tracheobronchial tree via branching of the respiratory diverticulum from the ventral surface of the proximal foregut (left lateral view)

to create the bronchial tree. The number of secondary and tertiary bronchi that develop reflects the number of lobes and bronchopulmonary segments present in the fully developed lung.

The longitudinal cavities either side of the pericardial sac become the pericardioperitoneal canals, from which the future pleural sacs develop. The primary bronchial buds grow into the pericardioperitoneal canals via the medial wall and in doing so acquire a covering of splanchnopleuric mesoderm; this develops into the connective tissue, smooth muscle and blood vessels of the adult organ (Figs. 4.22a–c). The innermost linings of the canals form the visceral and parietal pleural membranes.

The tracheal part of the respiratory diverticulum becomes separated from the foregut via the growth and union of the paired tracheo-oesophageal ridges (Fig. 4.21a,b). Fusion of the ridges forms the tracheo-oesophageal septum, which separates the oesophagus from the trachea. Abnormalities in the formation of the septum can lead to oesophageal atresia, which may be combined with a tracheo-oesophageal fistula (Fig. 4.23).

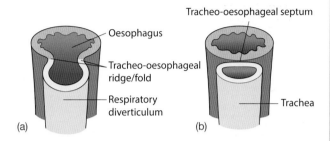

Figure 4.21 Separation of the respiratory diverticulum (tracheal part) from the oesophagus via the formation of the tracheooesophageal (a) ridges and (b) septum (anterior view)

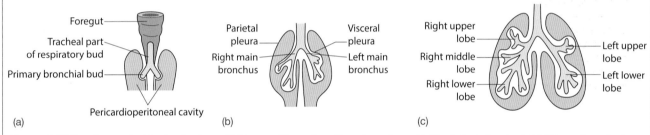

Figure 4.22 Development of the tracheobronchial tree and lungs from the primary bronchial buds (anterior view). (a) Primary bronchial bud growth into the pericardioperintoneal cavities. (b) and (c) Formation of the primary, secondary and tertiary bronchi, and lung lobes, via sequential branching of the bronchial buds

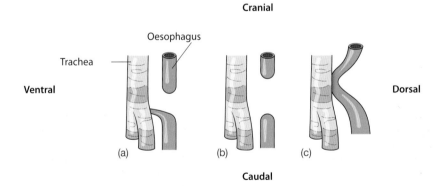

Figure 4.23 Tracheo-oesophageal defects (left lateral view) resulting from the malformation of the tracheo-oesophageal septum. (a) Upper oesophagus ends in blind pouch and the lower oesophagus forms a fistula with the trachea; (b) Oesophageal atresia, (c) Tracheo-oesophageal fistula (H-type)

MCQs

1. The surface markings of the pleural sacs: T/F
a do not extend above the clavicle   (___)
b meet anteriorly in the midline   (___)
c are similar on both sides   (___)
d extend to the 8th rib in the midaxillary line   (___)
e extend to the 12th rib in the paravertebral line   (___)

Answers
1.
a **F** – On both sides, the upper limit of the pleural sacs lies 3 cm above the mid-clavicle.
b **T** – The pleura meet in the midline at the level of the 2nd to 4th costal cartilages.
c **F** – At the 4th costal cartilage, the right pleura descends close to the midline, whereas the left pleura deviates laterally to accommodate the heart to descend to the 6th costal cartilage along the lateral border of the sternum.
d **F** – Both deviate laterally to reach the 8th rib in the midclavicular line and the 10th rib in the midaxillary line.
e **T** – The lower limit of the pleural reflection often descends to just below the 12th rib in the paravertebral line.

2. The right lung: T/F
a is smaller than the left   (___)
b is divided into upper and lower lobes and the lingula   (___)
c possesses 10 bronchopulmonary segments   (___)
d is related to the oesophagus only in the lower part of its medial surface   (___)
e is related to the liver   (___)

Answers
2.
a **F** – The right weighs about 620 g and the left about 560 g.
b **F** – Oblique and horizontal fissures divide it into upper, middle and lower lobes. The lingula exists only in the left lung and is the equivalent of the middle lobe on the right.
c **T** – Bronchopulmonary segments are functionally independent units of lung. In the right lung, there are three in the upper lobe, two in the middle and five in the lower lobe. In the left lung, there are five in the upper and four in the lower lobe, the medial segment being replaced by the left ventricle of the heart.
d **F** – The whole length of the thoracic oesophagus lies close to the medial surface of the right lung, separated only by the azygos vein crossing over the hilum of the lung.
e **T** – It is separated from the liver only by the diaphragm and the pleural and peritoneal coverings.

3. Lung tissue: T/F
a receives oxygenated arterial blood from branches of the aorta   (___)
b drains venous blood into the azygos veins   (___)
c has no lymph drainage   (___)
d is lined throughout by ciliated epithelium   (___)
e is supplied by the vagus nerve   (___)

Answers
3.
a **T** – It receives blood from small bronchial arteries arising from the descending thoracic aorta.
b **T** – Drainage is via bronchial veins draining into the azygos and hemiazygos veins.
c **F** – There is an extensive subpleural lymph plexus and a deep lymph plexus that accompanies the bronchi. These drain into hilar and tracheobronchial nodes and then into the mediastinal lymph trunks.
d **F** – Ciliated epithelium lines only the extra- and intrapulmonary bronchi. The distal bronchioles are lined by non-ciliated columnar epithelium and the alveoli by squamous epithelium.
e **T** – Innervation is via branches that pass through the pulmonary plexuses.

4. **The sympathetic chain:**   **T/F**
   a is formed by contributions from the ventral   (___)
      roots of T1–L2
   b carries parasympathetic fibres below L2   (___)
   c lies anterior to the common iliac vessels   (___)
   d lies anterior to the lumbar arteries and veins (___)
   e lies posterior to the psoas fascia   (___)

Answers

4.
a **T** – *The sympathetic chain extends from the base of the skull to the coccyx.*
b **F** – *It carries no parasympathetic fibres.*
c **F** – *It lies behind the iliac vessels.*
d **T** – *It lies anterior to segmental vessels such as the lumbar vessels.*
e **F** – *Inferiorly, it lies on the psoas fascia.*

5. **The thoracic duct:**   **T/F**
   a arises in the thorax   (___)
   b lies anterior to the vertebral column   (___)
   c drains into the left brachiocephalic vein   (___)
   d drains only thoracic structures   (___)
   e is joined by the right lymph duct   (___)

Answers

5.
a **F** – *It arises in the abdomen from the cisterna chyli, entering the thorax through the aortic opening of the diaphragm ...*
b **T** – *... alongside the azygos vein, behind the oesophagus.*
c **T** – *It arches forwards from behind the carotid sheath over the subclavian artery to enter the vein.*
d **F** – *It drains all structures below the diaphragm and the left half of the body and head and neck above it through the left superior mediastinal, jugular and subclavian lymph trunks.*
e **F** – *The right lymph duct is often absent but, when present, enters the right brachiocephalic vein separately, draining lymph from the right side of the head, neck and thorax.*

SBA

1. A comatose or anaesthetized patient is particularly at risk of aspiration, and this is frequently followed by development of right lower lobe pneumonia. Why is this?
   - a the right main bronchus is longer than the the left main bronchus
   - b the right main bronchus is narrower than the left main bronchus
   - c the right main bronchus is more vertical than the left main bronchus
   - d the right lung has a higher pulmonary vascular resistance than the left lung
   - e venous drainage is poorer from the right lower lobe than from other lobes

Answer

c *The right bronchus is more vertical, shorter and wider than the left, so aspirated material is more likely to pass into it and thence to the most dependent part of the right lobe. There are no differences in pulmonary vascular resistance or venous drainage between the right lower lobe and any other pulmonary lobe, and these play no part.*

2. A patient is admitted with a cough, fever and painful breathing. A pleural rub is heard on auscultation. Lobar pneumonia with pleurisy is diagnosed. In addition to respiratory support and antibiotics, the doctor has decided to give pain relief by injection of local anaesthetic into which nerve(s)?
   - a phrenic nerve
   - b intercostal nerves
   - c recurrent laryngeal nerves
   - d cardiopulmonary nerves
   - e vagus nerve

Answer

b *Pleuritic pain is the consequence of inflammation of the parietal pleural, which is supplied by the intercostal nerves. The phrenic nerve supplies only the diaphragmatic part of the visceral pleura and is not amenable to nerve blocks. None of the other nerves innervates the pleura.*

EMQs

Each question has an anatomical theme linked to the chapter, and a list of 10 related items (A–J) placed in alphabetical order: these are followed by five statements (1–5). Match **one or more** of the items A–J to each of the five statements.

Relationships of the lungs and bronchial tree
A. 8th costal cartilage
B. 8th rib
C. 4th costal cartilage
D. 4th rib
E. 2nd costal cartilage
F. 2nd rib
G. 6th costal cartilage
H. 6th rib
I. 10th rib
J. 12th rib

Answers
1 H; 2 C; 3 CD; 4 B; 5 I

Match the following statements with the appropriate item(s) from the above list.
1. Line of the oblique fissure of each lung
2. Surface marking of the cardiac notch
3. Surface marking of the horizontal fissure of the right lung
4. Surface marking of the parietal pleura in the mid-clavicular line
5. Surface marking of the parietal pleura in the mid-axillary line

APPLIED QUESTIONS

1. You are informed that a patient has a pleural effusion. Where is the fluid situated?

1. A pleural effusion is an abnormal collection of fluid in the pleural cavity, which normally contains only a thin film of fluid sufficient for lubrication of the opposing visceral and parietal layers of pleura. The exact position of any abnormal collection is influenced by gravity and the patient's posture. In bedridden patients, therefore, it tends to collect at the base of the pleural cavity posteriorly, where it will be detected by percussion and auscultation.

2. How would you drain the pleural cavity of air, and through which structures would your needle or catheter pass?

2. A pneumothorax is drained by a needle or, more commonly, a tube attached to an underwater seal apparatus inserted at one of two sites, either the 2nd intercostal space in the midclavicular line or the 7th intercostal space in the midaxillary line. With the upper approach, the needle or trocar and cannula pass through skin, superficial fascia and pectoralis major and minor, before the intercostal muscle fibres and, finally, the parietal pleura. The lower approach avoids penetration of the pectoral muscles and produces less discomfort for the patient.

3. Your patient has unwanted bronchial secretions in her posterior basal segments. Into which position should she be placed to maximize postural drainage?

3. Effective postural drainage is achieved by positioning the patient so that the lung secretions drain from the diseased segment with the aid of gravity. Basal segments therefore require the patient to be tipped head downwards and, for the posterior basal segment, into a prone position. A physiotherapist helps the drainage by chest wall percussion over the diseased segment.

4. Why may a misplaced central venous catheter cause a chylothorax?

4. It is prudent to avoid performing a left subclavian or brachiocephalic puncture because of the presence of the thoracic duct terminating in the angle between the internal jugular and subclavian veins. If the pleura is punctured at the same time as the duct is damaged, a chylothorax may result from leakage of lymph into the pleural cavity.

5. Why may an apical carcinoma of the lung cause pain in the little finger and a drooping upper eyelid on the same side?

5. An apical carcinoma often affects structures lying in contact with the suprapleural membrane (Sibson's fascia), namely the sympathetic trunk, the stellate ganglion and the 1st thoracic nerve root. Damage to the sympathetic nerves at this level may produce a Horner's syndrome – a constricted pupil (meiosis), flushed and dry skin on the side of the face, drooping of the upper eyelid (ptosis) and retraction of the eyeball (enophthalmos). The ptosis is caused by partial paralysis of levator palpebrae superioris, whose smooth muscle is innervated by sympathetic fibres. The finger pain may be caused by direct involvement of T1 nerve, whose dermatome lies along the medial border of the forearm and hand. This combination is known as Pancoast's syndrome.

6. A young boy throws a peanut in the air and, in attempting to catch it in his mouth, inhales it. Into which bronchus is it likely to pass?

6. It is most likely to be inhaled into the right main bronchus, which is shorter, wider and nearly in the same line as the trachea. Once inhaled, material such as peanuts, pins or even gastric contents tends to pass into the right middle or lower lobe. However, in the unconscious patient lying on the right side, inhaled material frequently collects in the posterior segment of the right upper lobe.

Bailey & Love · Essential Clinical Anatomy

Essential Clinical Anatomy · Bailey & Love

Bailey & Love · Essential Clinical Anatomy

PART **2**

The abdomen

Chapter **5**

The abdominal wall and peritoneum

THE ANTERIOR ABDOMINAL WALL

The anterior abdominal wall is divided, for descriptive and clinical purposes, into nine regions by two horizontal and two vertical planes: horizontal – the **subcostal** (lower costal margin and lower border of the 3rd lumbar vertebra) and the **transtubercular** plane (through the tubercles of the iliac crests); and vertical – the **right and left lateral** planes, which are extensions of the midclavicular line down to the mid-inguinal points. These define nine regions: centrally from above downwards, the epigastric, umbilical and supra-pubic, laterally on each side, the hypochondrial, lumbar (lateral) and iliac regions. The **transpyloric** plane, which passes through the first part of the duodenum, is midway between the xiphisternum and the umbilicus at the level of the body of the 1st lumbar vertebra posteriorly (**Figs. 5.1** and **5.2**).

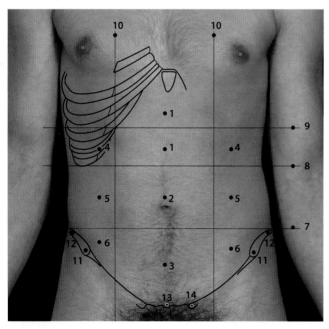

Figure 5.1 Surface anatomy of the abdominal wall, showing abdominal planes and regions. Regions: 1, epigastric; 2, umbilical; 3, suprapubic; 4, left and right hypochondrial; 5, lumbar; 6, iliac. Planes: 7, transtubercular; 8, subcostal; 9, transpyloric. 10, midclavicular line; 11, anterior superior iliac spine; 12, iliac tubercle; 13, symphysis pubis; 14, pubic tubercle

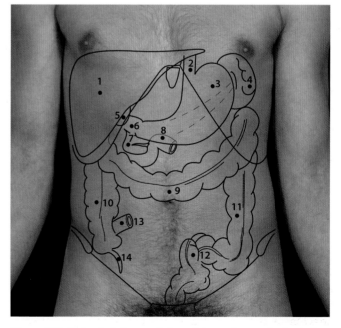

Figure 5.2 Abdominal viscera: 1, liver; 2, oesophagus; 3, stomach; 4, spleen; 5, gallbladder; 6, first part of duodenum; 7, head of pancreas; 8, duodenojejunal flexure; 9, transverse colon; 10, ascending colon; 11, descending colon; 12, sigmoid colon; 13, terminal ileum; 14, appendix

TABLE 5.1 Muscles of the abdominal wall

Muscles	Proximal attachment	Distal attachment	Nerve supply	Functions
External oblique	Outer surface of 5th–12th ribs	Linea alba, pubic tubercle, anterior half of iliac crest	T6–T12	Support and compression of abdominal contents. Flexion and rotation of trunk
Internal oblique	Thoracolumbar fascia, anterior iliac crest, lateral two-thirds of inguinal ligament	External surface of 10th–12th ribs, linea alba and pubic crest via conjoint tendon	T6–T12, L1	Support and compression of abdominal contents. Flexion and rotation of trunk
Transversus abdominis	Internal surface of 7th–12th costal cartilages, thoracolumbar fascia, iliac crest and lateral one-third of inguinal ligament	Jointly with internal oblique into linea alba and pubic crest via conjoint tendon	T7–T12, L1	Support and compression of abdominal contents
Rectus abdominis	Xiphoid process and 5th, 6th and 7th costal cartilages	Pubic symphysis and pubic crest	T7–T12	Flexion of trunk, compression of abdominal contents

The skin of the anterior abdominal wall is supplied by the 6th thoracic to 1st lumbar nerves in segmental overlapping dermatomes (Figs. 1.10 and 1.11, p. 26). T6 innervates the skin of the epigastric region, T10 the umbilical region and L1 the groin. The subcutaneous tissues are divided by fascia; the most superficial is fatty and continuous with that of the thorax and thigh; the deeper layer is membranous and thickened in the lower abdomen where it is attached to the iliac crests, the fascia lata of the thigh and the pubic tubercles. It continues between the tubercles to gain attachment inferiorly to the ischiopubic rami and the posterior border of the perineal membrane (Fig. 9.5a, p. 140).

Muscles

Laterally, the anterior abdominal wall contains three overlapping, flat sheet-like muscles: an outer external oblique, a middle internal oblique and an inner transversus abdominis. Anteriorly these become aponeurotic. The aponeuroses of each side fuse in the midline at the **linea alba** and form the **rectus sheath**. Their attachments, nerve supply and function are summarized in Table 5.1.

- **External oblique** lies superficially and its fibres descend inferomedially. Its origin interdigitates with serratus anterior.
- **Internal oblique** is deep to external oblique and its fibres are at right angles to it.
- **Transversus abdominis** is deep to internal oblique and its fibres, apart from its lowest, run horizontally.

The pubic crest forms the base of a triangular deficiency in the aponeurosis of the external oblique, the **superficial inguinal ring** (Fig. 5.3b). Between the **pubic tubercle** and the **anterior superior iliac spine** the thickened lower border of the aponeurosis is known as the **inguinal ligament** (Figs. 5.3b–d). Its free lower border is curved back on itself and gives attachment laterally to the internal oblique and transversus abdominis; its medial 2 cm, attached to the pectineal line on the pubis, forms the pectineal (lacunar) ligament, which, with the inguinal ligament proper, forms the gutter-like floor

of the inguinal canal (Fig. 5.5 below). Below the inguinal ligament the aponeurosis of the external oblique is continuous with the fascia lata of the thigh. The fibres of the internal oblique arising from the inguinal ligament arch medially over the spermatic cord and unite with the transverse abdominis aponeurosis to form the **conjoint tendon** (Figs. 5.3c,d), attached to the crest and pectineal line of the pubis.

Rectus abdominis, a strap-like muscle alongside the midline, is enclosed in a **rectus sheath** (Figs. 5.3a–f). It is attached to the sheath's anterior layer by three **tendinous intersections**, situated at the xiphoid process, the umbilicus, and midway between these two points (Fig. 5.3b). The anterior layer of the rectus sheath is formed of the fused aponeuroses of the external and internal oblique, while the posterior layer consists of the fused aponeuroses of the internal oblique and transversus abdominis. The lowest quarter of the sheath's posterior layer is deficient, revealing its lower crescentic border, the **arcuate line** (Fig. 5.3d). Here the aponeuroses of all three flat muscles pass into the anterior layer (Fig. 8.11, p. 128).

The rectus sheath contains the rectus muscle, the superior and inferior epigastric vessels and the anterior primary rami of T7–T12.

Function

The four muscles of the anterior abdominal wall usually act together and provide a flexible, strong, expandable support and protection for the abdominal contents. Contraction of the muscles moves the trunk, compresses the viscera, assists expiration by depressing the lower ribs and increases intra-abdominal pressure, thus assisting evacuation, i.e. defecation, micturition and childbirth. Rectus abdominis is the strongest flexor of the trunk.

Blood supply

This consists of the superior and inferior epigastric, intercostal and subcostal arteries, and branches of the femoral artery. Venous drainage follows the arterial supply.

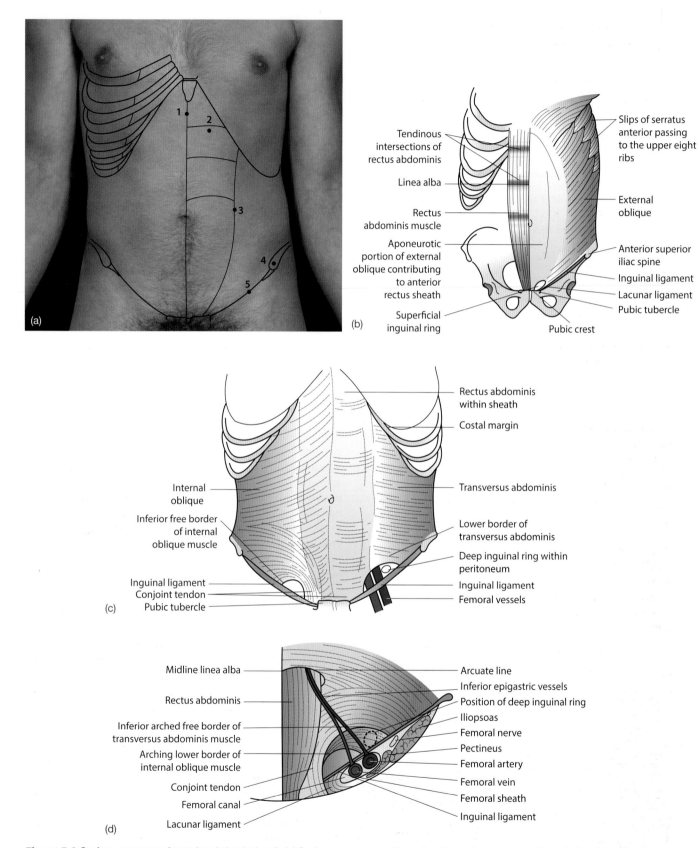

Figure 5.3 Surface anatomy of anterior abdominal wall. (a) Surface anatomy: 1, linea alba; 2, tendinous intersections; 3, linea semilunaris; 4, anterior superior iliac spine; 5, inguinal ligament. (b) Outer musculofascial layer, anterior rectus sheath removed on the right. (c) Deep layer (external oblique on right and internal oblique on left, muscles removed). (d) Inguinal region viewed from within the abdomen

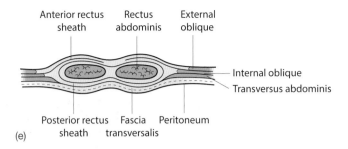

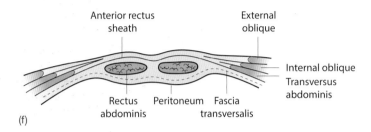

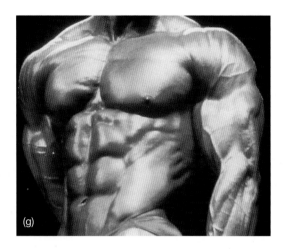

Figure 5.3 (*continued*) (e) Transverse section at the supraumbilical level. (f) Transverse section below the level of the arcuate line. (g) Contraction of rectus abdominis emphasizes the '6-pack' produced by the tendinous intersections

Surgical access to the abdomen can be gained by a variety of incisions. The nerve supply of the abdominal wall is a dense network of rich communications, so surgical division of a few of the terminal branches of the cutaneous nerves produces little or no consequence. Surgical exposure of the stomach, duodenum, transverse colon or aorta is frequently by a midline or paramedian incision (**Fig. 5.4**), and that of the gallbladder or spleen by a subcostal or transverse incision. A short oblique 'gridiron incision' in the right iliac fossa is usually sufficient for an appendectomy; longer ones allow access to the caecum and right colon and, on the left side, the sigmoid colon and rectum. Lower midline incisions may also be used. Pelvic organs and the uterus can be gained by low transverse incisions and lateral retraction of the recti.

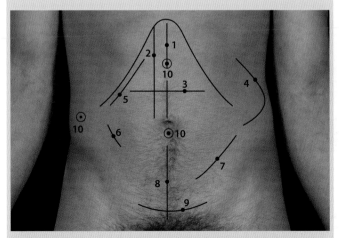

Figure 5.4 Abdominal incisions: 1, upper midline; 2, right paramedian; 3, transverse; 4, nephrectomy; 5, subcostal cholecystectomy; 6, appendectomy; 7, left iliac; 8, lower midline; 9, suprapubic; 10, laparoscopic ports

The inguinal canal

The **inguinal canal** (**Figs. 5.5a–e**) is an oblique pathway through the anterior abdominal wall extending from the deep (internal) inguinal ring, a deficiency in the transversalis fascia just above the midpoint of the inguinal ligament, to the superficial (external) inguinal ring, a deficiency in the external oblique aponeurosis above, medial to the pubic tubercle. The canal is about 4 cm long with a floor, roof and anterior and posterior walls:

- **Anterior wall** – formed throughout by the external oblique aponeurosis, reinforced laterally by internal oblique.
- **Posterior wall** – formed by transversalis fascia throughout, reinforced by the conjoint tendon medially. The inferior epigastric artery lies medial to the deep ring.
- The **floor** is the recurved edge of the inguinal ligament and its medial (pectineal) part.
- The **roof** is formed by the arching fibres of transversus abdominis and internal oblique, which become the conjoint tendon medially.

In the male the inguinal canal contains the spermatic cord; in the female it contains the round ligament of the uterus.

The **spermatic cord** (**Figs. 5.5b–d**) is formed when the testis, in late fetal life, descends the inguinal canal to reach the scrotum, carrying with it its ductus (vas) deferens, vessels and nerves. The **processus vaginalis**, a prolongation of peritoneum, connecting it with the tunica vaginalis of the testis, is usually obliterated at birth but, when patent, forms the sac of an indirect inguinal hernia (see below).

The cord gains three fascial coverings from the layers through which it passes and contains three nerves, three arteries, three other structures and lymph vessels:

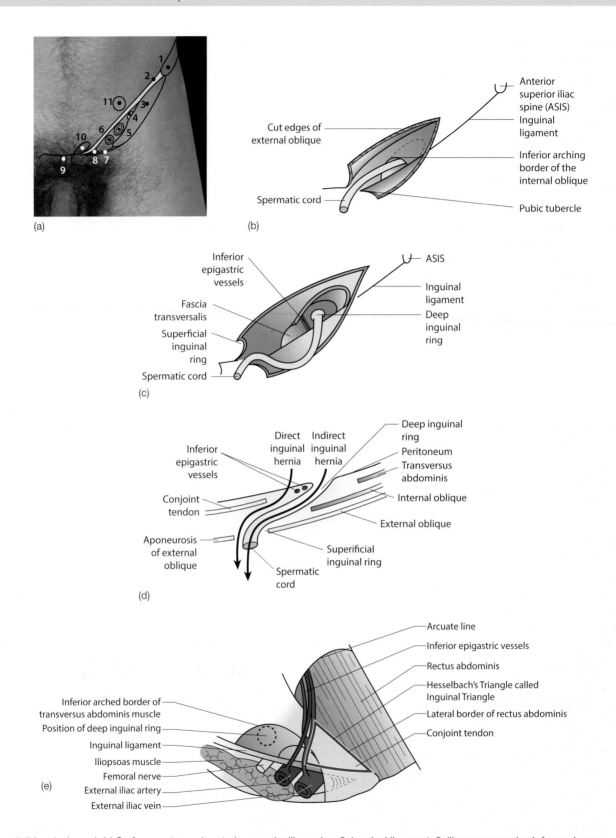

Figure 5.5 Inguinal canal. (a) Surface anatomy: 1, anterior superior iliac spine; 2, inguinal ligament; 3, iliopsoas muscle; 4, femoral nerve; 5, femoral artery passing beneath mid-inguinal point; 6, femoral vein; 7, origin of pectineus muscle; 8, reflected part of the inguinal ligament (pectineal [lacunar] ligament); 9, symphysis pubis; 10, superficial inguinal ring; 11, position of deep inguinal ring above midpoint of the inguinal ligament. (b) Anatomy of the inguinal region, external oblique being divided to demonstrate the course of the inguinal canal. (c) Deeper dissection through the internal oblique. (d) Diagram of horizontal section through the inguinal canal. (e) Posterior aspect, as viewed laparoscopically, of inguinal region showing inguinal (Hesselbach's) triangle (thick red lines)

Hernias, defined as protrusions of the contents of a body cavity through the wall of that cavity, are common in the inguinal region. They are especially common in males, because during development the testis carries with it, during its descent into the scrotum, a tongue of peritoneum, the processus vaginalis. Normally, part of the processus forms the tunica vaginalis of the testis and the remainder of the tube is obliterated at birth. When the processus stays patent there remains a hernial sac of peritoneum lying in the inguinal canal, a congenital defect that forms an **indirect inguinal hernia** (so-called because of its oblique emergence from the abdomen – see **Figs. 5.6** and **5.7**). This may appear at the superficial ring and become symptomatic at any age from birth onwards. It can be felt above and medial to the pubic tubercle. The superficial ring can be palpated superolateral to the pubic tubercle, and this is most easily done by invaginating the neck of the scrotum with the index finger and gently sliding the finger superiorly along the spermatic cord.

Middle-aged adults may develop a **direct inguinal hernia** due to a weakness in the posterior wall of the inguinal canal, the transversalis fascia. Such hernias are covered by the weakened conjoint tendon. **Femoral hernias**, which are less common, result from protrusions through the femoral ring. They can be palpated below the inguinal ligament (**Fig. 15.27**, p. 257).

Congenital **umbilical hernias** present in infants through a weakened umbilical scar. Adults are susceptible to hernias in this region, but these occur usually through a weakened linea alba, just above the umbilicus (**Fig. 5.8**) and, because of their situation, are known as paraumbilical hernias. Less frequently, adults present with small **epigastric hernias** in the midline through the linea alba, midway between the umbilicus and the xiphoid process (**Fig. 5.9**).

Surgical repair of hernias is advisable in young individuals because all hernias tend to enlarge as time passes, and the possibility of abdominal contents becoming trapped within the sac increases. Hernia repair usually involves the removal of the peritoneal sac together with repair of the abdominal wall defect.

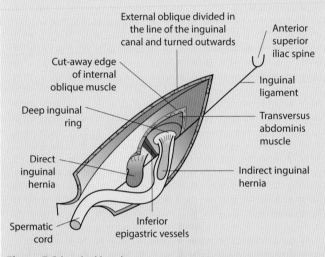

Figure 5.6 Inguinal hernia

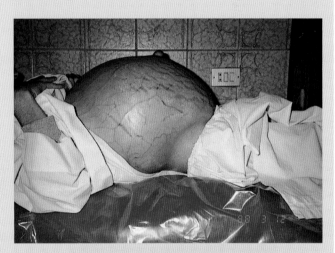

Figure 5.8 Umbilical hernia protruding from a grossly distended abdomen, due to ascites

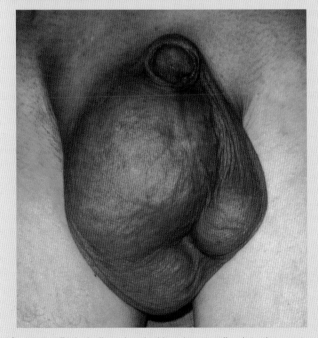

Figure 5.7 Right indirect inguinal hernia extending into the scrotum

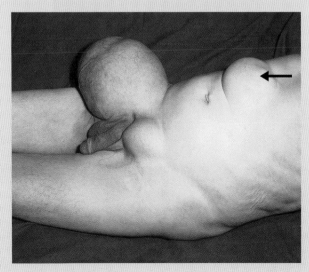

Figure 5.9 Epigastric hernia (arrow) accompanying bilateral direct inguinal hernias. These are recognized as direct inguinal hernias because they do not descend into the scrotum

- **Fascial coverings** – the innermost layer, the internal spermatic fascia, derived from transversalis fascia; the middle layer, the cremasteric muscle and fascia, derived from internal oblique and transversalis muscles; and the outer external spermatic fascia, derived from external oblique fascia as the cord passes through the external ring.
- **Nerves** – genital branch of the genitofemoral, ilioinguinal and autonomic nerves.
- **Arteries** – testicular (from the aorta), cremasteric and artery to the ductus deferens.
- **Structures** – the pampiniform plexus of veins, the ductus (vas) deferens and remains of the processus vaginalis.
- The **lymphatics** drain to the para-aortic nodes.

THE TESTIS AND EPIDIDYMIS

The two testes are oval, about 4 cm × 2.5 cm, and suspended in the scrotum by the spermatic cord (Fig. 5.10). Each is separated from its fellow by the midline scrotal septum. Vessels and nerves enter the testis at its lower pole (Fig. 5.11). The epididymis and ductus deferens lie posterolaterally and, with the testis, are covered by the inner layer of a closed serous sac, the **tunica vaginalis**. The testis, spermatic cord and epididymis are accessible to clinical examination, the epididymis being palpable posterior to the testis. The tunica and its contents are in turn covered with extensions of the coverings of the spermatic cord – the internal spermatic fascia, the cremaster muscle and fascia, external spermatic fascia, superficial fascia and dartos muscle, and scrotal skin.

The **epididymis**, a tightly coiled tube, about 6 cm long, applied to the posterolateral surface of the testis, consists of a widened head, a body and a thinner tail. The head, attached to the upper pole of the testis by the efferent ducts, connects via the body to the ductus deferens below.

Blood supply

This is by the testicular artery and, in part, the artery to the ductus deferens. Venous blood drains via a mass of veins, the pampiniform plexus, which forms around the spermatic cord to drain, asymmetrically, by the right testicular vein into the inferior vena cava and by the left testicular vein into the left renal vein.

Nerve supply

Sympathetic fibres, originating from T10, pass to the gland; afferent fibres are conveyed by the genitofemoral and ilioinguinal nerves to the spinal cord.

Lymphatic drainage

Vessels pass along the testicular arteries to para-aortic lymph nodes. There is no lymphatic drainage to the inguinal nodes.

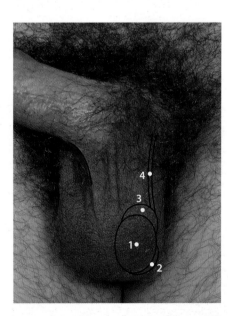

Figure 5.10 Surface anatomy of testis and spermatic cord: 1, testis; 2, inferior and 3, superior pole of the epididymis; 4, ductus deferens

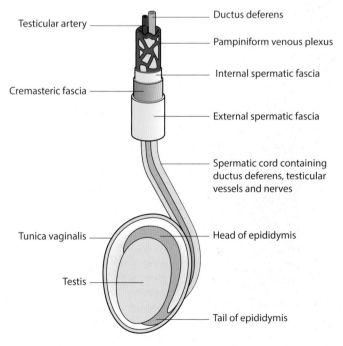

Figure 5.11 Testis, spermatic cord and their coverings

Testicular descent may occasionally be retarded or impeded (**cryptorchidism**; Fig. 5.12). It may descend through the inguinal canal but fail to enter the scrotum, remaining over the pubis in an ectopic position. Surgical correction of the abnormal position is desirable to ensure normal development of the testis and production of testicular hormones.

Fluid may accumulate within the tunica (**hydrocoele**) as the result of infection or trauma. A chronic hydrocoele (Fig. 5.13) may be drained by a needle, but this rarely produces a permanent cure. A surgical operation may be required to excise the parietal surface of the tunica. Cysts may develop in the epididymis. If this occurs once spermatogenesis has started, the cyst will contain sperm and is known as a spermatocoele. The pampiniform plexus of veins may distend and dilate to form a varicocoele; this is more common on the left side where the vein drains into the left renal vein (Fig. 5.14). The majority are left-sided and are idiopathic, but occasionally they may be a presenting sign of a left renal cancer that has blocked the left renal vein and, with it, the left testicular vein.

The testis is prone to **torsion** because of the nature of its suspension within the scrotum, and the twisting occludes the organ's arterial supply, rendering the ischaemic testis tender and painful (Fig. 5.15). This, however, rarely occurs outside the 10- to 20-year age group. Unless surgical correction of the torsion is achieved within 8–12 hours, the impairment of the blood supply results in death of the testis.

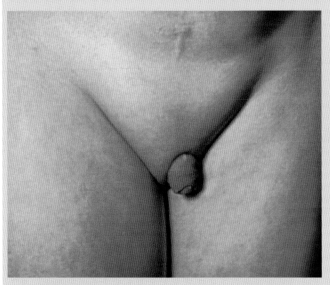

Figure 5.12 Left-sided cryptorchidism showing a poorly developed scrotum and swellings over the external inguinal rings

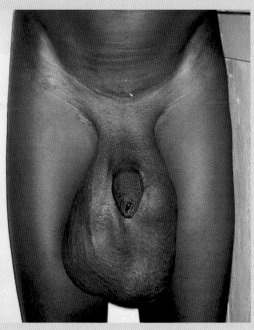

Figure 5.13 Chronic bilateral hydrocoele with scrotal enlargement

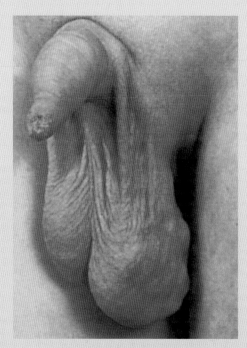

Figure 5.14 Left varicocoele revealing nodular soft swelling around the upper pole of the testis and spermatic cord

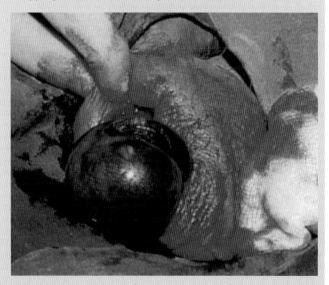

Figure 5.15 Surgical exposure shows torsion of the testis. The tense, dark vascular congestion probably indicates testicular death

THE PERITONEUM

The peritoneum lines the abdominal cavity. It is a thin membrane folded into a serous sac enclosing the peritoneal cavity. The part lining the abdominal wall is known as the **parietal layer** and this, in places, leaves the abdominal wall, the diaphragm or the pelvic floor to partially or completely invest the viscera. This layer is known as the **visceral layer**. The parietal and visceral peritoneum are separated by a small amount of serous fluid. Some of the viscera are almost completely invested by peritoneum and are attached to the abdominal wall or adjacent structures by double layers of peritoneum known variously as mesenteries, ligaments, folds or omenta (Figs. 5.16a–d). Others, incompletely invested, have bare areas in contact with the posterior abdominal wall and diaphragm (Fig. 5.17). This invagination increases the complexity of the peritoneal cavity.

To study the complexities of the peritoneum it is best to trace it from one point travelling around the abdominal cavity to return to that point. Beginning on the upper anterior abdominal wall and diaphragm: between the umbilicus and the liver there is a double layer of peritoneum, known as the falciform ligament, that passes back and separates to enclose the liver (Figs. 5.18 and 5.19). Superiorly, the right layer reflects from the diaphragm, forming the coronary and right triangular ligaments and enclosing the bare area of the liver (Fig. 7.2, p. 113). The left layer forms the left triangular ligament. On the undersurface of the liver the two layers reunite along the porta hepatitis (Fig. 7.2, p. 113) to form the **lesser omentum**, whose two layers descend to the oesophagus and stomach before separating again to enclose them. Rejoining along the greater curvature of the stomach, the two, often fat-laden, peritoneal layers descend in a lax fold, the **greater omentum**, before ascending anterior to the transverse colon and its mesentery.

The **mesocolon**, which suspends the transverse colon from the posterior abdominal wall, forms an attachment that runs across the anterior surface of the pancreas (Fig 5.17). The upper peritoneal layer covers the posterior wall of the abdomen and the undersurface of the diaphragm as far as the oesophageal opening. Over the anterior surface of the left kidney the two layers of the peritoneum split to enclose the spleen before joining again to extend to the stomach; the spleen is thus suspended by two peritoneal ligaments, the **gastrosplenic** and the **lienorenal**.

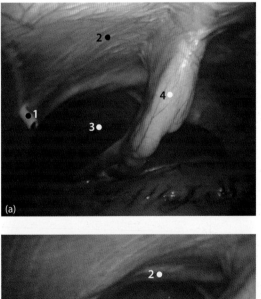
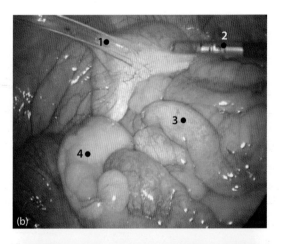
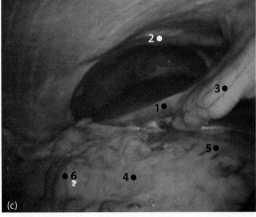
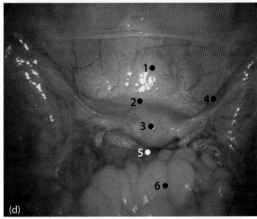

Figure 5.16 Laparoscopic views of intra-abdominal peritoneum. (a) Right upper quadrant: 1, porthole for instruments; 2, anterior abdominal wall; 3, liver; 4, falciform ligament covered in fat. (b) Intestinal folds covered in shiny visceral peritoneum: 1, bowel adhesion; 2, instrument; 3, small intestine; 4, fat overlying large intestine. (c) View from umbilicus on the right-hand side: 1, right lobe of liver; 2, diaphragm; 3, falciform ligament; 4, greater omentum; 5, greater curvature of stomach; 6, transverse colon. (d) Pelvic peritoneum: 1, bladder; 2, uterovesical pouch: 3, fundus of uterus; 4, round ligament of uterus covered in broad ligament peritoneum; 5, rectouterine pouch (Douglas); 6, loops of fat-covered bowel

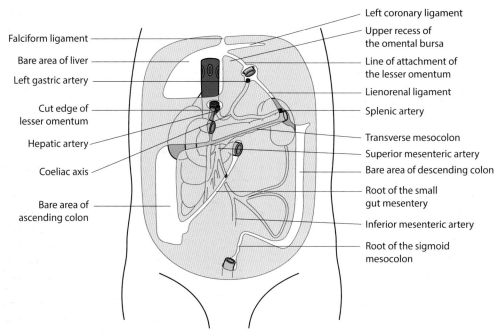

Figure 5.17 Posterior abdominal wall showing peritoneal reflections

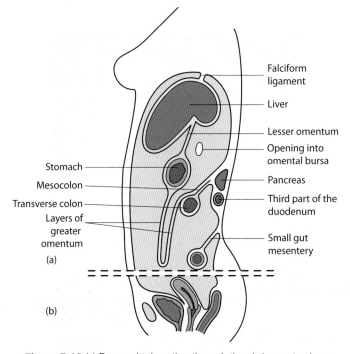

Figure 5.18 (a) Parasagittal section through the abdomen to show the peritoneal reflections. (b) Below the dotted line is a mid-sagittal section through the female pelvis

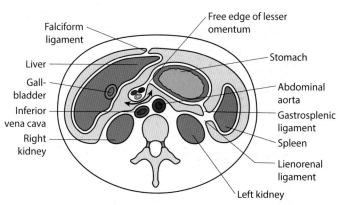

Figure 5.19 Transverse section through the abdomen showing peritoneal reflections, viewed from below. The arrow indicates the opening into the omental bursa (epiploic foraman), sited at this level

The peritoneum covering the posterior abdominal wall below the mesocolon descends, covering the third part of the duodenum and anterior surfaces of the ascending and descending colon, but it forms a mesentery for the sigmoid colon, which is attached along the inverted V-shaped line over the left sacroiliac joint (Fig. 5.17). The **small bowel mesentery** – the posterior parietal peritoneum – also forms a mesentery for the whole jejunum and ileum; this is attached along an oblique line (Fig. 5.17). The **lesser sac** (omental bursa) of peritoneum is a diverticulum of the peritoneal cavity lying between the stomach and the posterior abdominal wall, with its opening, the epiploic foramen, lying to the right bounded by the liver above, the inferior vena cava posteriorly, the duodenum inferiorly and the free edge of the omentum (Figs. 5.18 and 5.19). In the free edge of the lesser omentum lie the portal vein, the common bile duct and the hepatic artery.

Surgeons employ their knowledge of this anatomy to control haemorrhage from the liver or cystic artery by compressing the hepatic artery between a finger inserted into the epiploic foramen and a thumb applied to its anterior wall.

The anterior abdominal peritoneum descends into the pelvis to cover the pelvic walls and the upper surfaces of the pelvic viscera. In the male it spreads from the bladder to the seminal vesicles to descend into the rectovesical fossa before ascending to cover the front of the rectum. In the female it covers the body of the uterus and uterine tubes. Between the rectum and uterus there is a pouch of peritoneum known as the rectouterine **pouch of Douglas** (Fig. 5.16d). The peritoneal folds over each uterine tube extend to the lateral pelvic wall as the **broad ligament** of the uterus.

Nerve supply

The parietal peritoneum is supplied segmentally by the somatic nerves supplying the overlying muscles: the diaphragm in its central portion by the phrenic nerve; the peripheral part of the diaphragm and the parietal peritoneum of the abdominal wall by intercostal and lumbar nerves; and the pelvic peritoneum largely by the obturator nerve. The visceral peritoneum is innervated by autonomic nerves that are sensitive only to stretch and pressure, and produce only a dull and generalized abdominal ache. Parietal peritoneum is sensitive to pain and therefore, when it is inflamed, pain is felt over the area of the dermatome supplying the affected part. The central portion of the diaphragm supplied by the phrenic nerve, when inflamed, produces pain referred to the tip of the shoulder. The greater omentum has considerable mobility and the potential to wrap itself around any infected focus. Thus an inflamed appendix or small perforated duodenal ulcer is frequently found, at operation, to be 'walled off' and its infection partially localized.

Peritoneal anatomy and gravity ensure that fluid or pus tends to collect in certain locations. The right and left **subphrenic spaces** lie between the diaphragm and liver, separated by the falciform ligament. In each space infected peritoneal fluid can accumulate to form subphrenic abscesses. Below the liver is the **right subhepatic space** (the **hepatorenal pouch of Morison**), the most dependent part of the peritoneal cavity in a patient lying on their back, and hence this too is a frequent site for a peritoneal abscess. To the lateral side of the ascending colon is the **right paracolic gutter**, a potential route for transmission of infection from the pelvis or appendix to the subhepatic space. The **lesser sac** (omental bursa) may contain inflammatory fluid arising from pancreatitis or infection from a posterior perforation of the stomach. The **pouch of Douglas** (Fig. 5.16d), low in the pelvis, frequently contains localized peritoneal abscesses that have gravitated there from higher in the peritoneal cavity. They can be palpated by rectal or vaginal examination. Drainage of intra-abdominal abscesses can be achieved by ultrasonically guided needle aspiration or surgical procedures.

An abnormal collection of fluid in the peritoneum (**ascites**; Fig. 5.20) may be the result of heart, liver or renal failure, low-grade infection or malignancy. It can be drained from the abdomen or samples obtained for diagnostic purposes by inserting a cannula into the peritoneal cavity through the anterior abdominal wall below the umbilicus. In order to avoid puncturing the inferior epigastric vessels the puncture site should be in the midline or lateral to the rectus muscle. The same site may be used for peritoneal cavity lavage – the washing out of peritoneal fluid with saline – or for aspiration as a diagnostic test for the presence of intraperitoneal bleeding after abdominal trauma.

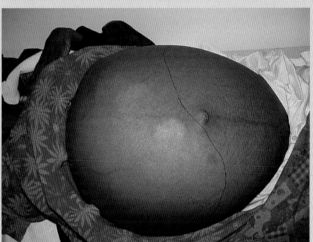

(a)

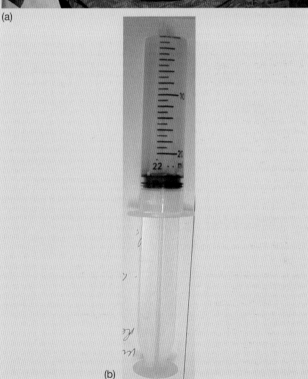

(b)

Figure 5.20 (a) Gross ascites due to haematoma, pre-paracentesis. The liver edge is marked with a line on the abdomen. (b) Ascites fluid from paracentesis showing the typical colour

MCQs

1. The inguinal canal: T/F
a transmits the ilioinguinal nerve in men only   (____)
b transmits the genital branch of the   (____)
   genitofemoral nerve in both sexes
c is more oblique in the newborn than in the   (____)
   adult
d has fascia transversalis and conjoint tendon   (____)
   along its posterior wall
e has the external oblique muscle as its roof   (____)

Answers
1.
a F – The ilioinguinal nerve (L1) is transmitted in both sexes. In the male the contents of the spermatic cord are also transmitted, whereas in the female the ilioinguinal nerve, the genital branch of the genitofemoral nerve and the round ligament of the uterus pass along the canal.

b T – In the male the genital branch of this nerve is involved in the cremasteric reflex. Although the female has no such muscle, the nerve passes along the canal to supply the labia majora.

c F – In the newborn infant the deep ring lies almost directly behind the superficial ring, so the canal is shorter and less oblique than in the adult.

d T – The inguinal canal has the fascia transversalis along its whole posterior wall and this is reinforced in its medial third by the conjoint tendon. This strong tendon attached to the pubic crest and pectineal line forms a tough posterior wall behind the superficial inguinal ring.

e F – The roof of the canal is formed by the arching fibres of internal oblique and transversus muscles. The external oblique aponeurosis forms the entire anterior wall.

2. The porta hepatis: T/F
a is enclosed by the lesser omentum   (____)
b contains the hepatic veins   (____)
c contains the portal vein anterior to the   (____)
   hepatic artery
d contains the whole of the cystic duct   (____)
e contains lymph nodes   (____)

Answers
2.
a T   Ascending from the anterior aspect of the epiplogic foramen

b F – The hepatic veins pass from the liver's posterior surface to drain to the inferior vena cava.

c F – The portal vein lies posterior to the hepatic artery and common bile duct.

d F – Only the distal end of the cystic duct lies in the porta hepatis.

e T – These drain the gallbladder and its bed.

3. The lesser omentum: T/F
a is attached superiorly to the porta hepatis   (____)
b extends inferiorly to the transverse colon   (____)
c separates the lesser and greater sacs of   (____)
   peritoneum
d forms part of the boundary of the foramen   (____)
   of the lesser omentum
e contains the portal vein   (____)

Answers
3.
a T – Its two layers are formed from the left and right sacs of peritoneum, which meet at this point.

b F – Inferiorly it meets to enclose the oesophagus and stomach.

c T – The lesser sac lies behind the stomach and lesser omentum and communicates with the greater sac only via the foramen of the lesser sac.

d T – The foramen is bounded by the free edge of the lesser omentum anteriorly, the liver superiorly, the inferior vena cava posteriorly and the duodenum inferiorly.

e T – The free edge of the lesser omentum contains the common bile duct, the hepatic artery and the portal vein.

SBA

1. An attack of acute pancreatitis most frequently results in fluid collecting in which peritioneal space?
a right paracolic gutter
b left paracolic gutter
c lesser sac (omental bursa)
d left subphrenic space
e pouch of Douglas

Answer
c *These patients are very unwell, lying supine for considerable periods of time. The peritoneal inflammatory exudate typically collects in the adjacent lesser sac.*

2. A 15-year-old boy presents with a reducible swelling in the groin that can be palpated above and medial to the pubic tubercle. His testes are of normal size. What is the likely diagnosis?
a hydrocoele
b direct inguinal hernia
c indirect inguinal hernia
d spermatocoele
e varicocoele

Answer
c *Indirect inguinal hernias are most common in males and are usually of congenital origin, although they often first appear during the teenage years. They are caused by the processus vaginalis remaining patent, and thus pursue an oblique course down the inguinal canal to present at the superficial inguinal ring, which lies medial and slightly superior to the pubic tubercle.*

EMQs

Each question has an anatomical theme linked to the chapter, and a list of 10 related items (A–J) placed in alphabetical order: these are followed by five statements (1–5). Match **one or more** of the items A–J to each of the five statements.

Inguinal region
A. Conjoint tendon
B. Deep inguinal ligament
C. External oblique muscle aponeurosis
D. Inferior epigastric artery
E. Inguinal ligament
F. Mid-inguinal point
G. Midpoint of the inguinal ligament
H. Reflected part of the inguinal ligament
I. Superficial inguinal ring
J. Transversalis fascia

Match the following statements with the appropriate item(s) from the above list.
1. Posterior relationship to the medial end of the inguinal canal
2. Forms the superficial inguinal ring
3. Forms the deep inguinal ring
4. Lies between the deep and superficial inguinal rings
5. Surface marking of the femoral artery

Answers
1 A; 2 C; 3 J; 4 D; 5 F

APPLIED QUESTIONS

1. Why might a patient, after an inguinal hernia repair, complain of a pain in his scrotum?

    1. The patient was unfortunate enough to have his ilioinguinal nerve trapped in the hernia repair and now suffers pain in the L1 dermatome, which includes the scrotum. There may also be haemorrhage from the surgical site, which has produced a haematoma in the scrotum.

2. Where does a kick in the testes produce pain?

    2. The testis is an internal organ innervated by the T10 dermatome. Therefore, pain arising in the testis is felt as dull pain in the umbilical region.

3. What structures develop from the gubernaculum in the female?

    3. The gubernaculum of the ovary becomes both the ligament of the ovary and the round ligament of the uterus in the adult. These are continuous and attached to the uterus just below the uterine tube, and take a course similar to that in the male, passing along the inguinal canal to end in the female scrotal homologue, the labia majora.

4. What are the subphrenic spaces and why are they important?

    4. The subphrenic spaces are potential spaces within the peritoneal cavity that may become filled with pus or fluid and form subphrenic abscesses. The right and left subphrenic spaces lie between the diaphragm and the liver but are separated by the falciform ligament. Both spaces are limited anteriorly by the anterior abdominal wall and superiorly by the diaphragm. The posterior border on the right is the coronary ligament, and on the left is the left triangular ligament. Abscesses more commonly accumulate in the right subphrenic space.

Chapter 6

The abdominal alimentary tract

Figure 6.1 shows the approximate surface markings of the major abdominal viscera.

THE OESOPHAGUS

The **abdominal oesophagus**, about 3 cm long, enters the abdomen to the left of the midline through the right crus of the diaphragm to join the stomach at the cardiac orifice (Fig. 6.2). The fibres of the right crus form a sling around the oesophagus. At the gastro-oesophageal junction (cardia), or just above it, the oesophageal lining of stratified squamous epithelium changes to columnar epithelium, and this lines the whole of the remainder of the gastrointestinal tract. The junction between the two different epithelial linings is normally 40 cm from the incisors and is readily recognizable endoscopically (Fig. 6.2). The oesophagus lies between the diaphragm posteriorly and the liver anteriorly, covered anterolaterally by peritoneum. Gastric vessels and nerves lie in its walls. Reflux of gastric contents is normally prevented by the lower oesophageal sphincter and the oblique angle of entry of the oesophagus into the stomach, as well as the positive abdominal pressure that compresses the walls of the intra-abdominal oesophagus.

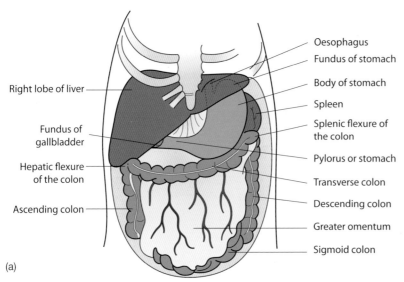

(a)

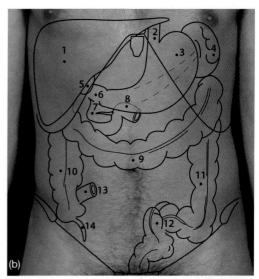

(b)

Figure 6.1 (a) Abdominal cavity showing the positions of the viscera. (b) Abdominal viscera: 1, liver; 2, oesophagus; 3, stomach; 4, spleen; 5, gallbladder; 6, first part of duodenum; 7, head of pancreas; 8, duodenojejunal flexure; 9, transverse colon; 10, ascending colon; 11, descending colon; 12, sigmoid colon; 13, terminal ileum; 14, appendix

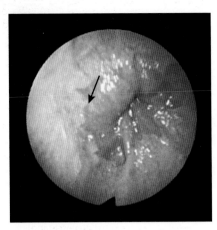

Figure 6.2 Endoscopic view of normal gastro-oesophageal junction: note the junction of the pale pink squamous epithelium of the oesophagus on the left with the redder stomach mucosa (arrow)

If reflux does occur, inflammation, spasm and stricture of the lower oesophagus may follow. In later life the oesophageal opening in the diaphragm may become more lax and allow part of the upper stomach to slide into the mediastinum. This condition (**hiatus hernia**) also predisposes to reflux of gastric contents.

THE STOMACH

The **stomach**, although variable in size, shape and position, is usually J-shaped. It is situated in the left hypochondrium and epigastrium, its lower part extending to the umbilicus.

The stomach is divided into a fundus, a body and a pyloric part (Figs. 6.3 and 6.4). It possesses anterior and posterior surfaces, both covered by peritoneum, and lesser (right) and greater (left) curvatures. The **fundus** is the part above the oesophageal opening; the **body** extends from the fundus to the **angular notch**, which is the most dependent part of the lesser curvature. The **pyloric portion** extends from the notch to the pyloric sphincter (pylorus), which separates the stomach and duodenum. The pyloric part possesses a proximal dilated **pyloric antrum** and a distal tubular **pyloric canal**. The pyloric sphincter, a thickening of the stomach's circular muscle, lies at the level of the 1st lumbar vertebra. It regulates the flow of stomach contents into the duodenum. The **lesser curvature** extends from the oesophagus to the pylorus; attached to it is the lesser omentum. The **greater curvature** extends from the left of the oesophagus, over the fundus to the pylorus, and gives attachment to the gastrosplenic ligament and the greater omentum.

Relations

Anterior are the left lobe of the liver, diaphragm and anterior abdominal wall. Posteriorly the lesser sac separates it from a group of structures known collectively as the stomach bed: the diaphragm above and the splenic vessels, pancreas, left kidney and suprarenal gland and spleen below. Below these are the transverse mesocolon and the splenic flexure of the colon (Fig. 6.4a).

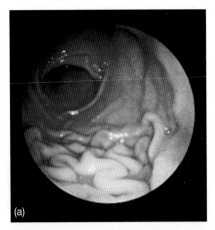

(a)

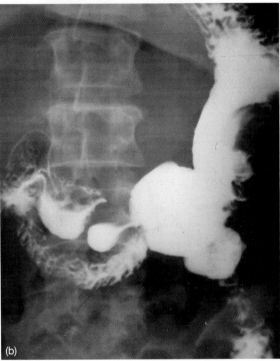

(b)

Figure 6.3 (a) Gastric body and antrum: endoscopic view showing normal rugal folds in the body of the stomach – the distal antrum is smooth. (b) Barium meal and follow through showing extensive carcinoma of the greater gastric curve with irregular mucosal thickening and penetrating ulceration

Blood supply

The left and right gastric arteries supply the lesser curvature and nearby gastric wall; the left and right gastroepiploic arteries supply the greater curvature and nearby tissue, and the short gastric branches of the splenic artery supply the gastric wall of the fundus (Fig. 6.4b). Veins from the stomach pass to the portal vein either directly or via the splenic or superior mesenteric veins (Fig. 6.4c).

Nerves

Anterior and posterior vagal trunks enter the abdomen through the oesophageal hiatus; the anterior trunk is in contact with the oesophagus; the posterior trunk lies in areolar

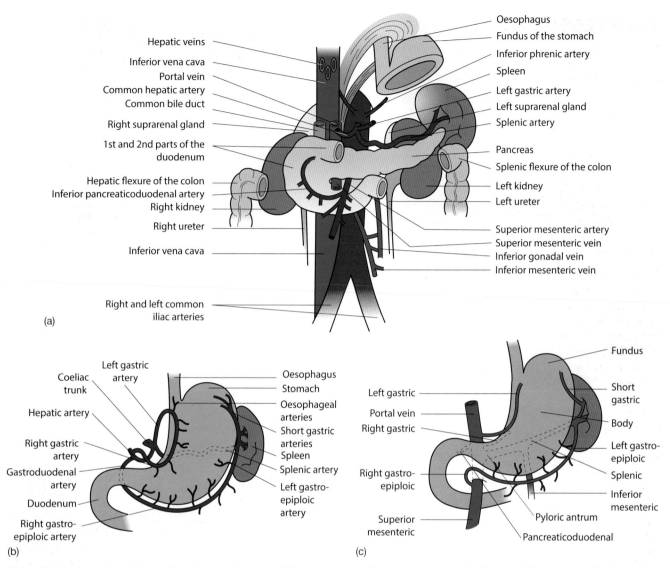

Figure 6.4 (a) Posterior relations of the stomach (shown with the major part of the stomach removed). (b) Arterial blood supply of the stomach. (c) Venous drainage of the stomach to the portal vein

tissue to the right of the oesophagus. The anterior trunk supplies a branch to the liver and each trunk supplies many branches to the stomach. The posterior trunk supplies the coeliac plexus and via that plexus, the pancreas, small intestine and right half of the colon. The vagi provide motor and secretomotor nerves to the stomach.

Differences in the size, shape, motility and rate of emptying of the stomach can be demonstrated by radiographs taken after a barium meal. The mucosal pattern and its irregularities can also be seen. The contours of the fundus can usually be seen outlined by air in a radiograph. Diagnosis of all gastric and duodenal disease is aided by barium meals and by fibreoptic **gastroduodenoscopy**. The oesophagus, stomach and duodenum can be directly inspected by a gastroscope and biopsies taken of suspected abnormalities. Benign gastric ulcers are usually situated along the lesser curvature, particularly near to the angular notch. Malignancies may be found in any part of the stomach. Gastrectomy (partial or total) may be indicated for malignancy.

Surgical vagotomy is occasionally employed in the treatment of duodenal ulceration. It abolishes gastric acid secretion but is always accompanied by gastric atony, with the result that the stomach empties with difficulty unless drainage is encouraged by widening the pylorus (pyloroplasty) or by a gastrojejunostomy (anastomosis of the stomach and proximal small intestine). It is performed less frequently since the development of effective drugs that block gastric acid output, such as proton pump inhibitors.

Lymph drainage

This is to the coeliac group of preaortic nodes, via nodes along the left gastric artery, nodes in the porta hepatis and nodes around the splenic artery and greater curvature.

Occasionally a gastric cancer (**Fig. 6.3b**) may spread via the left thoracic duct to involve and produce palpable enlargement of the left supraclavicular node (Troisier's sign).

THE DUODENUM

The **duodenum** lies on the posterior abdominal wall. About 25 cm long, it extends from the pylorus to the duodenojejunal flexure, embracing the head of the pancreas in a C-shaped curve open to the left. The duodenum is retroperitoneal apart from the first part of duodenum and duodojejunal flexure.

For descriptive purposes it is divided into four parts. The first part, 5 cm long, ascends to the right from the pylorus and turns down to form the second part (8 cm long), which descends to the right of the 3rd lumbar vertebra. The third part (10 cm long) passes left across the posterior abdominal wall to turn upwards as the fourth part on the left of the 2nd lumbar vertebra.

Relations

The **first part** is covered with peritoneum; posteriorly it lies on the portal vein, the common bile duct and the gastroduodenal artery (**Figs. 6.4a,b**); anteriorly it is in contact with the liver and gallbladder. The **second part** lies on the right kidney and ureter; it is crossed by the attachment of the transverse mesocolon, above which it is in contact with the liver and below which it is in contact with coils of small intestine. On its left lies the head of the pancreas, the common bile duct and the duodenal papilla; the common opening of the pancreatic and bile ducts opens into its lumen halfway down its posteromedial border (see **Figs. 7.9** and **7.10**, p. 116). The **third part** lies below the head and uncinate process of the pancreas and crosses, from the left, the right ureter, the inferior vena cava, the inferior mesenteric artery and the aorta. It is crossed anteriorly by the superior mesenteric vessels and the root of the small bowel mesentery. The **fourth part** lies on the left psoas muscle to the left of the vertebral column, with the inferior mesenteric vein, left ureter and left kidney on its left. The pancreas lies medial to it.

The **duodenojejunal flexure** lies to the left of the 2nd lumbar vertebra. A well-marked peritoneal fold, the suspensory ligament (ligament of Treitz), descends from the right crus of the diaphragm to the flexure. Small peritoneal recesses are occasionally found to the left of the flexure.

Blood supply

The superior pancreaticoduodenal artery, a branch of the gastroduodenal artery, anastomoses with the inferior pancreaticoduodenal artery from the superior mesenteric artery in the groove between the duodenum and pancreas to supply both structures. This is an anastomosis between foregut and midgut arteries.

Duodenal ulcers are common; the majority occur in the superior part of the first part of the duodenum. Posterior ulcers may penetrate and cause bleeding from the gastroduodenal artery or erosion into the pancreas, which results in severe back pain. Anterior ulcers may be complicated by perforation into the peritoneal cavity or sometimes by penetration into the adjacent gallbladder.

Gallstones may ulcerate through an infected gallbladder wall into the duodenum and then pass down the small intestine to impact and cause intestinal obstruction in the narrower ileum (gallstone ileus). Treatment of duodenal ulcers is aimed at reducing the stomach's acid output by pharmacological means, but removal of the acid-producing part of the stomach (partial gastrectomy) and denervation of the stomach and drainage (vagotomy and pyloroplasty) are employed in emergency situations.

THE SMALL INTESTINE

The **small intestine** comprises the jejunum and ileum, with a total length that varies between 4 and 7 m. It lies in the central abdomen, below the transverse colon, suspended from the posterior abdominal wall by a mesentery that conveys blood and lymph vessels and nerves to it. The **jejunum** is wider and thicker walled than the **ileum**; its mucous membrane is thrown into circular folds, which give it a characteristic appearance in radiographic contrast studies (**Fig. 6.5**), and it has less fat in its mesentery, which allows the surgeon to distinguish it from the ileum at operation.

Relations

The shorter jejunum lies above and to the left of the ileum. The root of the mesentery, some 15 cm long, passes obliquely down from the left of the 2nd lumbar vertebra to the right sacroiliac joint, crossing the left psoas, aorta, inferior vena cava and right psoas (**Fig. 5.17**, p. 89).

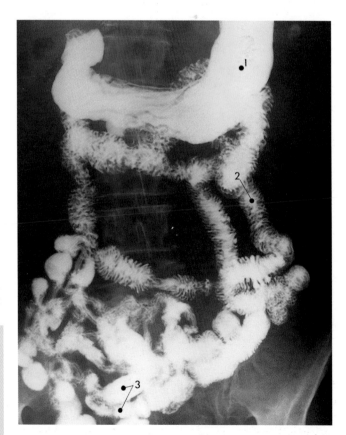

Figure 6.5 Barium meal and follow-through, demonstrating stomach and small intestine showing circular folds of duodenal mucosa and featureless ileum: 1, stomach; 2, jejunum; 3, loops of ileum

Blood and nerve supply

The superior mesenteric artery supplies almost the whole small intestine by numerous jejunal and ileal branches, anastomosing with the right colic artery in the terminal ileum. Its venous drainage is by branches of the superior mesenteric vein and thence to the portal vein. Vagal branches convey a parasympathetic supply and stimulate both motor and secretory activity; the sympathetic supply inhibits both motor and secretory activity. Pain is conveyed by afferents of the sympathetic system; these cells lie in the T9 and T10 segments. Hence pain arising from the small intestine is felt in the central paraumbilical region of the abdomen.

THE LARGE INTESTINE

This extends from the ileocaecal junction to the anus and is about 1.5 m long. It comprises the caecum, appendix, ascending, transverse, descending and sigmoid colon, rectum and anal canal. The longitudinal muscle of the colon, lying outside a continuous circular muscle coat, is confined to three bands, the **taeniae coli**, which are shorter than the rest of the colonic wall and cause it to be sacculated (**Fig. 6.6**). Fatty tags, the **appendices epiploicae**, project outwards from the wall. The large intestine is commonly investigated by radio-graphic contrast studies; barium and gas, injected per anum, are manipulated to coat the mucosa of the whole colon and rectum (**Fig. 6.6**).

The **caecum** is a blind sac, about 8 cm in diameter and invested in peritoneum, and is continuous with the ascending colon. It lies in the right iliac fossa on the iliacus and psoas muscles. Its taeniae coli converge on the appendix, attached to its posteromedial wall. The **ileocaecal orifice**, an oval slit on its medial wall, allows onward progression of small bowel contents into the caecum.

The **appendix**, a narrow diverticulum of variable length but usually about 8 cm long, arises from the posteromedial wall of the caecum below the ileocaecal orifice (**Fig. 6.7**). It is covered with peritoneum and connected to the terminal ileum by a mesentry, the mesoappendix, which contains the appendicular artery. Much lymphoid tissue is found in its wall. It is very mobile and therefore its relations are variable; most commonly it lies in a retrocaecal position, but not infrequently it is in the pelvis (**Fig. 6.8**).

Appendicitis – inflammation of the appendix – is usually a consequence of obstruction of its lumen by faeces. Because the lumen is wider in infancy and often non-existent in elderly individuals, appendicitis is uncommon in these age

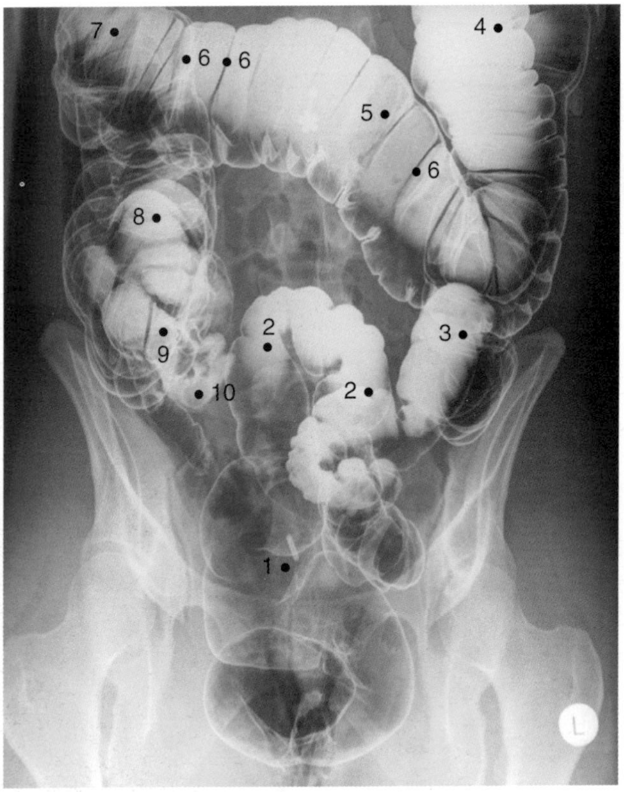

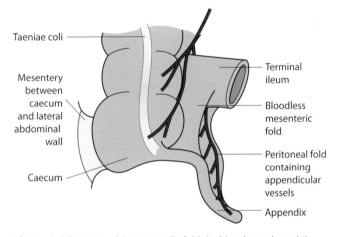

Figure 6.7 Diagram of the appendix fold, its blood supply and the ileocaecal junction

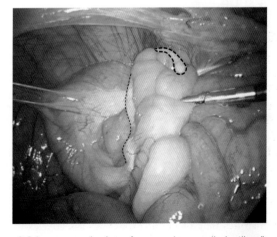

Figure 6.8 Laparoscopic view of a normal appendix (outlined), elevated from a pelvic position

Figure 6.6 Double-contrast enema of large bowel. The two contrast media used are barium and air, which are inserted in that order via the anus and the patient tilted so that all regions are outlined: 1, rectum; 2, sigmoid colon; 3, descending colon; 4, splenic flexure; 5, transverse colon; 6, haustrations; 7, hepatic flexure; 8, ascending colon; 9, caecum; 10, terminal ileum. Note the twisting, angulated sigmoid colon, which has a long mesentery

groups. Appendicitis causes tense swelling of the organ and this may be severe enough to impair flow in the appendicular artery, an end artery, which is followed by gangrene of the appendicular wall and perforation, with the development of generalized peritonitis. Distension of the organ in early appendicitis produces vague colicky pain in the central abdomen, but later, when local inflammation develops in the parietal peritoneum of the right iliac fossa, the pain changes in character, becoming localized to the right iliac fossa, continuous and exacerbated by movement.

The ascending colon

The **ascending colon** lies in the right lateral region, extending from the caecum to the **hepatic flexure** of the colon under the right lobe of the liver. It is about 15 cm long and peritoneum covers it anteriorly and on both sides, fixing it to the posterior abdominal wall. There is a **right paracolic gutter** of peritoneum along its right side, which leads to the right subphrenic space.

Relations

The ascending colon lies on the iliacus, the quadratus lumborum and the lower pole of the right kidney. It is covered anteriorly by coils of small intestine.

The transverse colon

The transverse colon extends from the hepatic flexure to the **splenic flexure** across the abdomen, suspended by the transverse mesocolon. It is about 50 cm long.

Relations

Initially it lies directly on the second part of the duodenum and the head of the pancreas, but subsequently it is attached by its long mesentery to the body of the pancreas. Above it is in contact with the liver, gallbladder, stomach, greater omentum and spleen; posteriorly it lies on the second part of the duodenum and head of the pancreas, the small intestine and the left kidney.

The descending colon

The descending colon, the narrowest part of the colon and about 30 cm long, lies in the left lateral region, extending from the left colic flexure to the brim of the pelvis, where it becomes the sigmoid colon. Peritoneum covers it anteriorly and on both sides, fixing it to the posterior abdominal wall; to its left lies the paracolic gutter (of peritoneum). The left colic flexure lies higher than the right and is attached to the diaphragm by a peritoneal fold, the phrenocolic ligament.

Relations

Posteriorly it lies on the lower pole of the left kidney, quadratus lumborum, iliacus and psoas. Anteriorly it is in contact with coils of small intestine.

The sigmoid colon

The sigmoid colon, about 40 cm long, lies in the left iliac region extending from the pelvic brim to the front of the 3rd sacral vertebra, where it becomes the rectum. It is attached to the pelvic wall by an inverted V-shaped mesentery, the sigmoid mesocolon (Fig. 5.17, p. 89). The apex of the inverted V-shaped mesentery overlies the left ureter, the bifurcation of the left common iliac artery and the left sacroiliac joint.

Relations

The sigmoid colon lies on the left ureter and common iliac vessels; above it is covered by coils of small intestine, and inferiorly lie the bladder and, in the female, the uterus.

Advances in fibreoptic technology over the last two decades have permitted **colonoscopy** – the passage of a flexible light and lens system – to become a most useful method of visualizing the whole of the large bowel (Fig. 6.9). It is particularly useful in looking for tumours and ulcerations. The bowel may be obstructed anywhere by narrowing due to inflammation or malignancy. **Chronic colonic obstruction** often presents with a change in bowel habit. More acute obstruction causes colicky lower abdominal pain, and swelling of the abdomen and high-pitched bowel sounds may be noted. **Cancer** of the large intestine (Fig. 6.10) arises from mucosal epithelial cells and spreads to invade the deeper layers of the wall and, eventually, the peritoneum. It may spread via the lymphatics to the nodes in the mesentery and para-aortic region, and by blood vessels to the liver. Peritoneal involvement may result in cancer seeding throughout the peritoneal cavity and lead to an increase in peritoneal fluid (ascites).

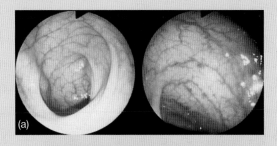

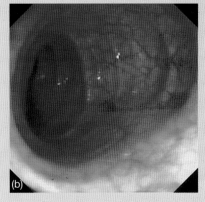

Figure 6.9 (a) and (b) Colonoscopic view of the left colon. The mucosa is indented by contracting circular muscle

Surgical resection of cancers in the left colon or rectum is frequently accompanied by the formation of a colostomy – the establishment of a temporary or permanent abdominal wall exit for the colon that allows faeces to be collected into a bag on the abdominal wall (Fig. 6.11). Colostomies are also used in the temporary surgical relief of large bowel obstruction.

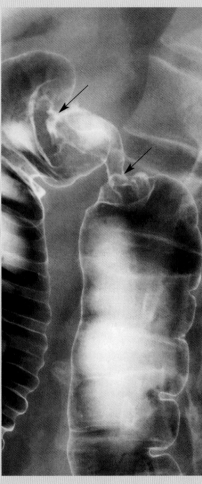

Figure 6.10 Barium enema showing carcinoma of the large bowel producing an 'apple core'-shaped narrowing of the colon (arrows)

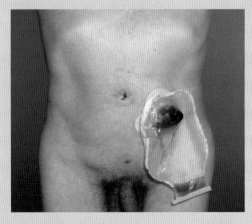

Figure 6.11 End colostomy

ARTERIAL SUPPLY OF THE GASTROINTESTINAL TRACT

Three arteries arising from the front of the aorta, the coeliac, superior and inferior mesenteric arteries, supply, respectively, the foregut, midgut, hindgut and their derivatives (Figs. 6.12–6.14).

The **coeliac artery** arises just above the pancreas and soon divides into the left gastric, common hepatic and splenic arteries (see also Figs. 6.4a and 7.17, p. 119). The **left gastric artery** passes upwards and left to the oesophagus, where it turns down into the lesser omentum. Branches anastomose with those of the right gastric artery, and it supplies the lower oesophagus and the stomach. The **common hepatic artery** passes above the first part of the duodenum to enter the lesser omentum, in whose free edge it ascends in front of the portal vein. It branches to form:

- The **right gastric artery**, which runs along the lesser curvature to anastomose with the left gastric artery in the lesser omentum.
- The **gastroduodenal artery**, which descends behind the duodenum to divide into the right gastroepiploic and superior pancreaticoduodenal arteries. The former passes along the greater curvature to anastomose with the left gastroepiploic artery; the latter descends between the duodenum and pancreas to supply both structures.
- The **right and left hepatic arteries**, which both ramify in the liver. The right gives a small cystic artery to the gallbladder. Knowledge of the variations in the pattern of these vessels is important in gallbladder surgery.

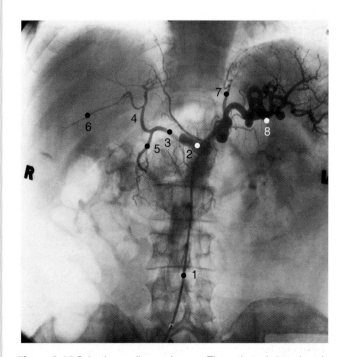

Figure 6.12 Selective coeliac angiogram. The catheter is introduced percutaneously via the femoral and iliac arteries and passes along the aorta to the coeliac trunk at the level of the 1st lumbar vertebra. The computer technique of subtraction 'removes' other tissues to highlight the arteries: 1, catheter in aorta; 2, coeliac trunk; 3, common hepatic artery; 4, proper hepatic artery; 5, gastroduodenal artery; 6, cystic artery; 7, left gastric artery; 8, splenic artery – note its convolutions

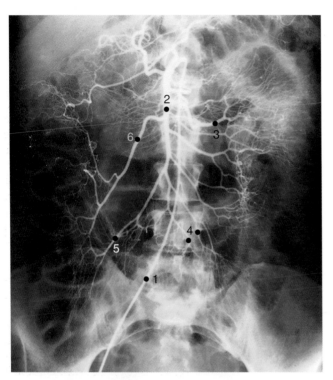

Figure 6.13 Selective superior mesenteric angiogram showing multiple jejunal, ileal, ileocolic and colic branches: 1, catheter; 2, superior mesenteric artery; 3, jejunal branches; 4, ileal branches; 5, ileocolic artery; 6, right colic artery

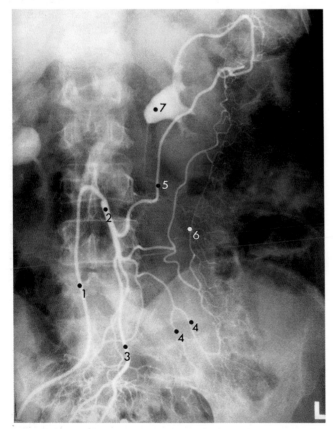

Figure 6.14 Selective inferior mesenteric angiogram: 1, catheter; 2, inferior mesenteric artery; 3, superior rectal artery; 4, sigmoid arteries; 5, left colic artery; 6, marginal artery; 7, left renal pelvis (outlined by contrast medium being excreted by the kidney)

The **splenic artery** runs a tortuous course to the left along the upper border of the pancreas and passes in the lienorenal ligament to the splenic hilum, before dividing into many terminal branches. It branches to form the:

- **Pancreatic vessels**, several.
- **Short gastric arteries**, several of which pass in the gastro-splenic ligament to the fundus of the stomach.
- **Left gastroepiploic artery**, which runs in the gastrosplenic ligament to the greater curvature, supplying the stomach and greater omentum to anastomose with the right gastro-epiploic artery.

The **superior mesenteric artery** (Fig. 6.13) arises below the coeliac artery, descends behind the body of the pancreas, anterior to its uncinate process and crosses the third part of the duodenum to enter the root of the mesentery of the small intestine. It supplies the small intestine and ends by dividing into the ileocolic, middle and right colic arteries (Fig. 6.15). Within the mesentery it is accompanied by veins, lymph vessels and nerves. It branches to form the:

- **Inferior pancreaticoduodenal artery** (see Fig. 6.4a) which runs between the pancreas and the duodenum to anastomose with the superior pancreaticoduodenal artery.
- **Right colic artery**, which descends to the right on the posterior abdominal wall to divide into ascending and descending branches. It supplies the ascending colon and anastomoses with the ileocolic and middle colic arteries.
- **Middle colic artery**, which passes upwards on the body of the pancreas to the mesocolon, within which its branches supply the right two-thirds of the transverse colon.
- **Jejunal and ileal arteries**, 15–20 in number, arising from the left of the artery within the small bowel mesentery. There are many side-to-side anastomoses between these branches, and tiers of arterial arcades are formed.
- **Ileocolic artery**, which descends to the right, dividing to supply the caecum, appendix and lower ascending colon.

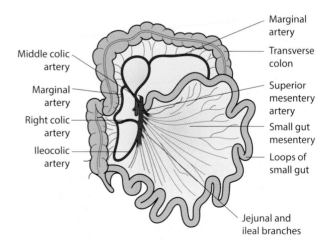

Figure 6.15 Superior mesenteric artery and its branches (large bowel fanned out and pulled to the right to reveal the blood supply of the small bowel)

The **inferior mesenteric artery** (Figs. 6.14 and 6.16) arises behind the duodenum and descends behind the peritoneum to the left, continuing beyond the pelvic brim as the superior rectal artery. Its branches form the:

- **Left colic artery**, which ascends to the left to the left colic flexure to supply the transverse and descending colon. It anastomoses with the middle colic and sigmoid arteries.
- **Sigmoid arteries**, which enter the sigmoid mesocolon and supply the sigmoid and lower descending colon.
- **Superior rectal artery**, which is the continuation of the inferior mesenteric artery, descends in the sigmoid mesocolon to reach the back of the rectum. It supplies the rectum and upper anal canal.

The terminal arteries supplying the gut form a continuous anastomotic arcade, known as the marginal artery, along the mesenteric border of the colon.

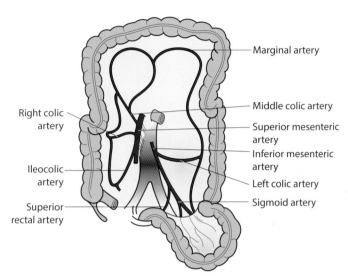

Figure 6.16 Superior and inferior mesenteric arterial supply of the large intestine (for clarity, small bowel removed and large colon lifted up)

Bowel ischaemia is most commonly the result of torsion (twisting) of the bowel or entrapment of the bowel in a hernial sac (Fig. 6.17). **Volvulus**, the twisting of the bowel on its mesentery, may occur in the sigmoid colon and the caecum. Bowel ischaemia in elderly individuals may also be the result of arterial disease and inadequate blood flow, which threatens the viability of the colon in the region where its blood supply is the lowest, the so-called 'marginal' area in the region of the splenic flexure.

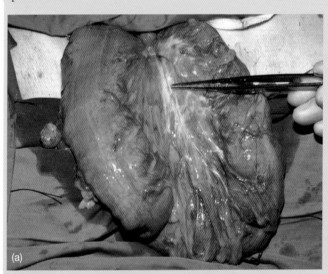
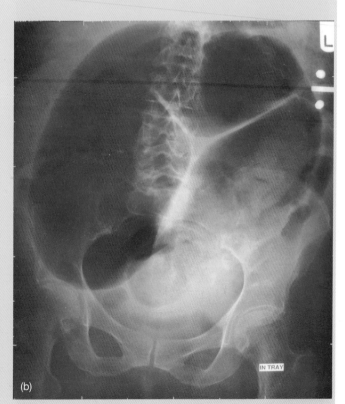

Figure 6.17 (a) Volvulus of the sigmoid colon caused by fibrosis. (b) Volvulus of the sigmoid colon before decompression (courtesy of Professor Paul Finan, Leeds University, UK)

VENOUS DRAINAGE OF THE GASTROINTESTINAL TRACT – THE PORTAL VENOUS SYSTEM

From the lower end of the oesophagus to the upper end of the anal canal, blood from the gastrointestinal tract drains into the liver (Fig. 6.18). The distal tributaries correspond to the arterial branches described above, but more proximally the venous anatomy differs: the superior mesenteric vein joins the splenic vein behind the pancreas to form the portal vein; the inferior mesenteric vein enters the splenic vein to the left of this (Fig. 6.18). The **portal vein** ascends behind the pancreas and first part of the duodenum to the free edge of the lesser omentum, and thence to the porta hepatis, where it divides into right and left branches. It is 8 cm long and receives branches from right and left gastric veins and the superior pancreaticoduodenal vein. This pattern, as with all veins, is variable. Injection of

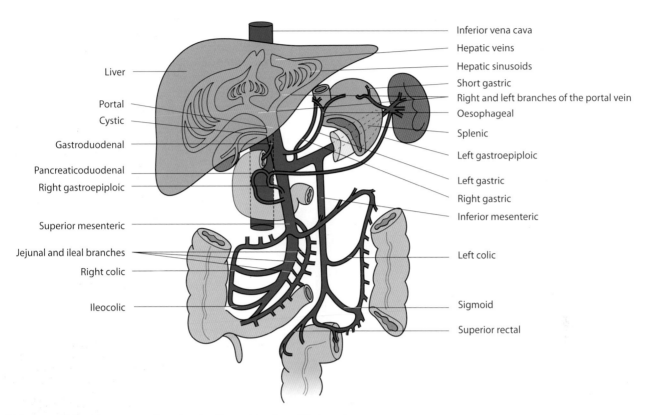

Liver
Portal
Cystic
Gastroduodenal
Pancreaticoduodenal
Right gastroepiploic
Superior mesenteric
Jejunal and ileal branches
Right colic
Ileocolic

Inferior vena cava
Hepatic veins
Hepatic sinusoids
Short gastric
Right and left branches of the portal vein
Oesophageal
Splenic
Left gastroepiploic
Left gastric
Right gastric
Inferior mesenteric
Left colic
Sigmoid
Superior rectal

Figure 6.18 Portal venous system showing the portal vein and its branches

contrast into the spleen permits radiological demonstration of the portal venous system (**Fig. 6.19**).

Relations

In the lesser omentum the portal vein lies behind the common hepatic artery and the common bile duct, and is separated from the inferior vena cava by the opening into the lesser sac (epiploic foramen).

Tributaries of the portal vein divide to supply all the liver cells, and from them blood is conveyed into the systemic venous system, i.e. the inferior vena cava, via the numerous hepatic veins.

Anastomoses between the portal and systemic system are only clinically important when there is a blockage in the portal system. It may be blocked by pathological processes or a congenital abnormality, e.g. portal vein thrombosis, cirrhosis or hepatic vein stenosis. If a block occurs, new anastomotic pathways develop between the portal and systemic venous systems, namely:

- In the submucosa of the lower end of the oesophagus between the left gastric and azygos veins, producing large oesophageal varices that are prone to haemorrhage.
- In the lower part of the anal canal between the superior and inferior rectal veins, resulting in rectal bleeding.
- In the umbilical region of the anterior abdominal wall between the anterior abdominal wall veins and the paraumbilical veins in the falciform ligament of the liver. This causes the development of a paraumbilical collection of dilated subcutaneous veins that look like the hair of the mythological Greek queen, the so-called 'caput Medusae'.

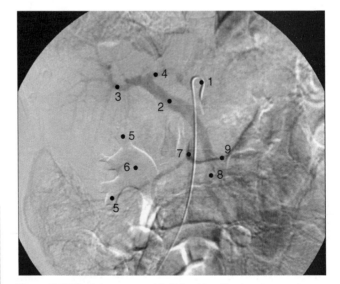

Figure 6.19 Portal venogram (digital subtraction has removed background tissues). A catheter is inserted via the femoral artery in the groin and passes up the aorta to the superior mesenteric artery where an iodine-based contrast is injected – this image has been taken as the contrast enters the veins: 1, catheter; 2, portal vein; 3, right portal branch within liver; 4, left portal vein branch in liver; 5, renal calyx; 6, renal pelvis; 7, gastroduodenal vein; 8, superior mesenteric vein; 9, gastroepiploic vein

- In the veins between the bare area of the liver and the diaphragm.

Portal hypertension may require surgery to reduce the pressure in the portal system, e.g. by anastomosing the portal vein directly into the inferior vena cava – a portocaval shunt.

LYMPHATIC DRAINAGE OF THE GASTROINTESTINAL TRACT

The intestinal mucosa is richly supplied with lymph vessels which drain, via submucosal and subserosal plexuses, to nodes alongside the viscus (Fig. 6.20). These drain to nodes in the mesentery or on the posterior abdominal wall, which in turn drain to one of three groups of **preaortic nodes** around the origins of the coeliac, superior and inferior mesenteric arteries. The **inferior mesenteric group** drains the distal transverse colon, sigmoid colon and upper rectum. The **superior mesenteric group** drains the distal duodenum, small intestine, and ascending and proximal transverse colon. The **coeliac group** drains the stomach, proximal duodenum, liver, spleen and pancreas, and also takes efferents from the superior and inferior mesenteric groups. Efferent vessels pass from it to the **cisterna chyli**, which drains into the thoracic duct (p. 71).

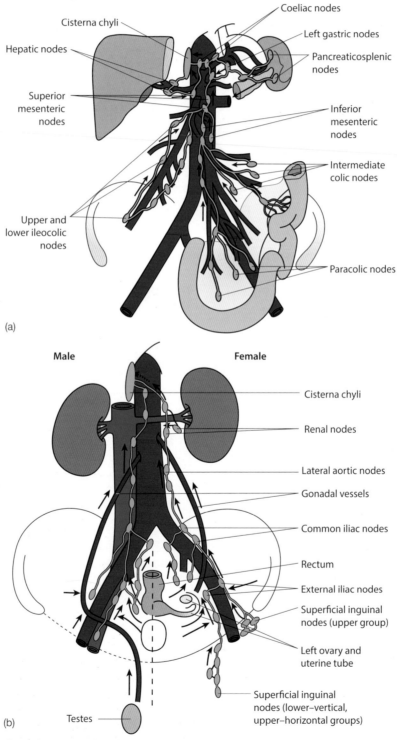

Figure 6.20 Lymphatic drainage and lymph nodes of: (a) the gut, and (b) the pelvis and abdomen (arrows show direction of lymph flow)

DEVELOPMENT OF THE GUT

Gut tube

The primordial gut tube is formed during folding of the embryonic disc. It extends from the oro/buccopharyngeal membrane to the cloacal membrane and is separated into three main parts: the foregut, midgut and hindgut (Fig. 6.21). The buccopharyngeal membrane breaks down in the 3rd week of intrauterine life; failure of this process is associated with choanal atresia. The embryonic endoderm forms the gut tube's epithelial lining, the hepatocytes and the exocrine and endocrine pancreatic cells. The muscle, vessels and visceral peritoneum associated with the gut tube are formed from splanchnic (visceral) mesoderm. The endodermal lining of many gut tube regions proliferates rapidly to occlude the lumen with a mass of cells, but subsequent recanalization restores a functional lumen (Fig. 6.22). Failure of recanalization

can result in stenosis (partial occlusion) or atresia (complete blockage) of a given part of the gut tube (e.g. oesophagus, duodenum, biliary tree or anorectal region), which may present before or after birth.

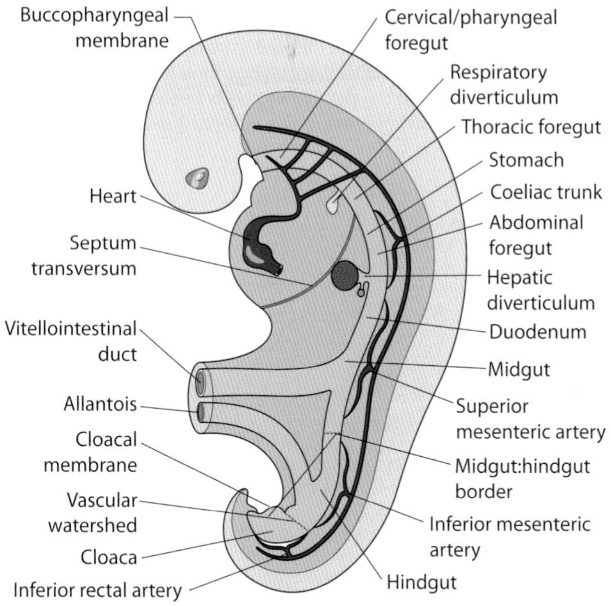

Blood supply to the gut tube and its watersheds

The intra-abdominal parts of the foregut, midgut and hindgut receive blood from one of three major vessels: the coeliac trunk, the superior mesenteric artery and the inferior mesenteric artery, respectively. Each artery supplies a specific territory of the gut tube, and it is this arterial supply that defines the three classic intra-abdominal gut tube regions. It also determines the location of the vascular watershed points of the gut tube which are located in the mid-to-distal transverse colon/splenic flexure (where the supplies from the superior and inferior mesenteric arteries meet; Griffith's point) and the rectum (where the inferior mesenteric artery supply meets branches of the internal iliac artery; Sudeck's point) (Fig. 6.21).

Mesenteries and intestinal fixation

The abdominal region of the gut tube initially has a dorsal mesentery along its length, through which travels all neurovasculature and lymphatics to and from the gut tube (Figs. 6.23a, 6.24). During development some sections of the dorsal mesentery persist (e.g. the mesentery of the small intestine) and some sections undergo mesenteric zygosis; in this process the mesentery fuses with the peritoneum of the posterior abdominal wall and disappears as regions of the gut tube move to contact the posterior abdominal wall (Figs. 6.23b,c). The process of mesenteric zygosis causes certain gut tube regions or organs to become secondarily retroperitoneal; this helps to fix the gut tube in position. Zygosis occurs in the mesentery of the caecum, ascending colon, descending colon, pancreas and duodenum. A knowledge of the planes of mesenteric zygosis enables avascular and aneural surgical planes to be defined for retroperitoneal organs, since the neurovascular supply to the gut or a particular organ will follow the direction and plane of the original dorsal mensentery (Fig. 6.23c). In general, incisions are made lateral to the section of gut tube requiring mobilization, e.g. the ascending colon, descending colon, second part of the duodenum or head of the pancreas.

The abdominal foregut also has a ventral mesentery, which attaches it to the midline of the anterior abdominal wall from the diaphragm to the umbilicus. The ventral mesentery contains the liver, ventral pancreatic bud and gallbladder and forms the lesser omentum and falciform ligament (Fig. 6.24). The lower free edge of the falciform ligament contains the

Figure 6.21 The embryonic gut tube passing from buccopharyngeal to cloacal membrane and showing the foregut, midgut and hindgut regions with their blood supplies. Regions of vascular watershed are shown using dashed red lines. The connections of the midgut to the yolk sac via the vitellointestinal duct and of the cloaca to umbilicus via the allantois are shown

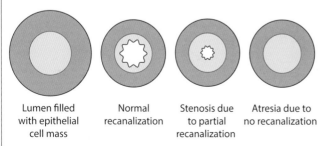

Figure 6.22 Normal process of gut tube lumen development and the outcomes of defective recanalization

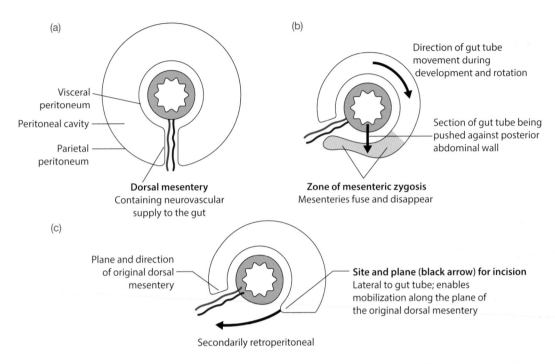

Figure 6.23 Mesenteric zygosis and the location of the avascular aneural plane for surgical mobilisation of secondarily retroperitoneal organs and/or access to the posterior abdominal wall. (a) An intraperitoneal section of gut tube with its neurovasculature contained within the dorsal mesentery. B) A section of gut tube being pushed against the posterior abdominal wall resulting in the loss of its dorsal mesentery via mesenteric zygosis. C) A secondarily retroperitoneal section of gut tube showing the positioning of its neurovasculature. Surgical incisions made lateral to the midline provide a safe route for mobilisation (black arrow) of secondarily retroperitoneal organs or regions of gut tube

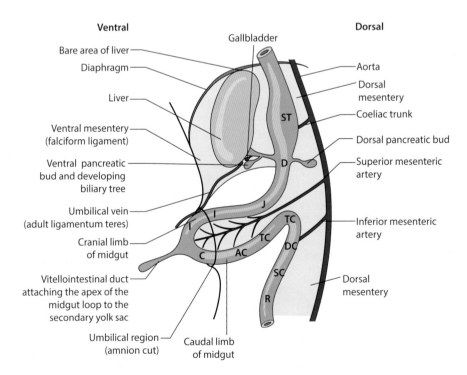

Figure 6.24 Formation and derivatives of the midgut loop and its herniation through the umbilicus (left lateral view). The liver, biliary tree and ventral pancreatic bud are developing in the ventral mesentery. ST stomach, D duodenum, J jejunum, I Ileum, C caecum, AC ascending colon, TC transverse colon, DC descending colon, SC sigmoid colon, R rectum

umbilical vein (which forms the ligamentum teres in the adult) and that of the lesser omentum contains the portal vein, hepatic artery and bile duct.

Foregut and lesser sac (omental bursa)

The foregut has cervical, intrathoracic and intra-abdominal regions (Fig. 6.21). It extends from the oropharyngeal membrane to the hepatic diverticulum, a point marked by the major duodenal papilla and the entrance of the hepatopancreatic duct. The foregut gives rise to the pharynx, oesophagus, stomach, duodenum, liver, biliary tree and pancreas, as well as the lower respiratory tract via the respiratory diverticulum (Fig. 4.20, p. 73). The pharynx develops in the region between the oropharyngeal membrane and the respiratory diverticulum. Below this the intrathoracic oesophageal part of the foregut passes through the thorax and septum transversum of the diaphragm, where it meets the stomach region of the intra-abdominal foregut. The oesophageal portion of the foregut normally lengthens rapidly and a failure to do so can pull the stomach superiorly, resulting in a congenital hiatus hernia. The oesophageal lumen is temporarily occluded by epithelial cell proliferation but soon reopens via recanalization. Oesophageal atresia, resulting from failure of recanalization or malformation of the tracheo-oesophageal septum (Figs. 4.21, 4.23, p. 74), prevents the normal swallowing of amniotic fluid, resulting in polyhydramnios. Incomplete recanalization can cause oesophageal stenosis.

During development the stomach region of the intra-abdominal foregut rotates to the right around a longitudinal axis (Fig. 6.25) such that the original right side of the stomach and right vagus nerve move to a posterior location, and vice versa. The duodenum and pancreas also rotate to the right and are pushed against the posterior abdominal wall by the colon, where both become secondarily retroperitoneal as a result of mesenteric zygosis. During rotation, the section of dorsal mesentery attached to the greater curvature of the stomach, the dorsal mesogastrium, grows rapidly and elongates to form the greater omentum. The dorsal mesentery also contains the spleen and the dorsal bud of the developing pancreas, which move to the left during rotation. The lesser omentum is formed by the ventral mesentery passing from the stomach and proximal duodenum to the liver.

The lesser sac is formed during foregut rotation and is mainly located posterior to the stomach and lesser omentum (Fig. 6.26). The left and inferior limits of the lesser sac are sealed off by the attachment of the dorsal mesogastrium and greater omentum to the posterior abdominal wall and by zygosis of the dorsal mensentery of the duodenum and pancreas. The right side of the lesser sac becomes sealed off by the hepatic veins entering the inferior vena cana and the liver

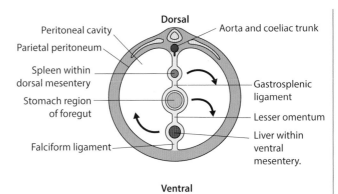

Figure 6.25 Axial section through the developing upper abdomen showing the rightwards rotation (arrows) of the intraabdominal foregut, associated organs and the ventral and dorsal mesenteries

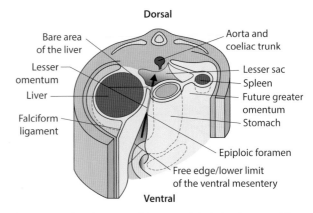

Figure 6.26 Development of foregut-related structures and the formation of the lesser sac in the region behind the stomach following the rightwards rotation of the foregut and associated mesenteries. The arrow indicates the route into the lesser sac (omental bursa) via the epiploic foramen

growing out of the ventral mesentery to produce the bare area. The only entrance or exit point (the epiploic foramen) is located between the liver and duodenum, posterior to the free edge of the lesser omentum.

Midgut

The midgut extends from the hepatic diverticulum of the duodenum to the middle/distal part of the transverse colon (Fig. 6.21). It is initially arranged in a U-shaped loop, with cranial and caudal limbs, and is supplied by the superior mesenteric artery (Fig. 6.24). The cranial limb undergoes significant growth to form much of the ileum and jejunum, whereas the caudal limb shows relatively little growth and forms the caecum, appendix and proximal parts of the colon. During week 5 of development the midgut grows quickly, and by week 6 it has outgrown the remaining space in the embryonic abdominal cavity and consequently herniates into the umbilicus. The vitellointestinal (omphaloenteric) duct connects the secondary yolk sac in the umbilicus to the apex of the midgut loop in the region of the future ileum. The duct normally fibroses and disappears

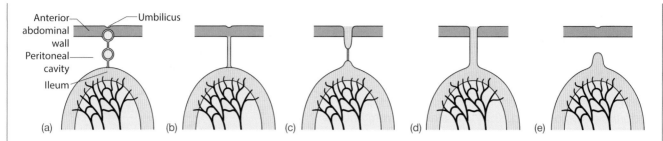

Figure 6.27 Developmental defects associated with the failure of degeneration or closure of the vitellointestinal/omphaloenteric duct. (a) omphaloenteric cysts. (b) fibrous cord. (c) umbilical sinus. (d) omphaloenteric fistula. (e) Ileal (Meckel's) diverticulum

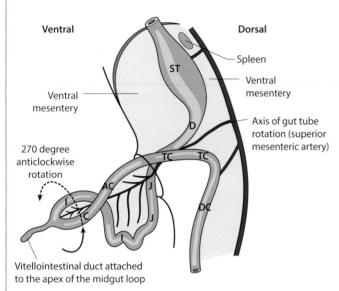

Figure 6.28 Left lateral view of the 270 degrees anticlockwise rotation of the midgut around the axis of the superior mesenteric artery. 90 degrees of rotation occurs within the umbilicus (solid curved black arrow), with the cranial limb moving to sit to the right of the caudal limb. A further 180 degrees of rotation occurs inside the abdominal cavity (dashed curved black arrow) to bring the gut tube into its near final disposition. ST stomach, D duodenum, J jejunum, I Ileum, C caecum, AC ascending colon, TC transverse colon, DC descending colon

during development; its persistence can result in a variety of conditions including cysts, sinuses or fistulae that pass from the gut tube to the umbilicus, or a blind-ended outpouching of the ileal wall known as an ileal (Meckel's) diverticulum (Figs. 6.27). Due to the midgut origin of the vitellointestinal duct, the symptoms of ileal diverticulitis can mimic those of appendicitis.

During development the midgut loop rotates a total of 270 degrees anticlockwise (when viewed from anteriorly) around the axis of the superior mesenteric artery, which runs to the apex of the loop (Fig. 6.28). Ninety degrees of rotation occurs while the gut tube is herniated in the umbilicus. The caudal limb, comprising parts of the large intestine, undergoes an additional 180 degrees of rotation during retraction of the herniated gut tube loop back into the abdominal cavity during week 10. This rotation forms the classic 'n'-shaped disposition of the large intestine and situates the transverse colon anterior to the mesentery of the small intestine. Absent rotation or malrotation results in abnormal positioning of the gut tube, which can be associated with volvulus or intestinal compression by, for example, the gut tube vasculature (Fig. 6.29). A congenital omphalocele is a herniation of the gut tube into the proximal umbilicus, with the hernial sac being covered in amniotic membrane (Fig. 6.30); it occurs in around 1:5000 births. The condition may be

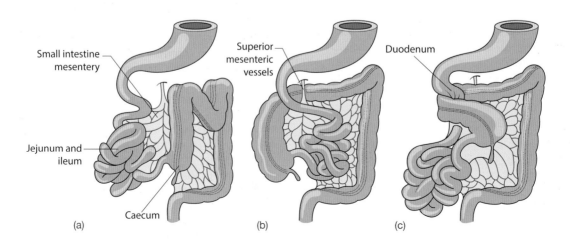

Figure 6.29 Anterior view of defects of gut tube rotation. (a) Absent/incomplete rotation. (b) Reversed rotation causing compression of the transverse colon by the superior mesenteric artery. (c) Malrotation causing large intestine volvulus and duodenal obstruction

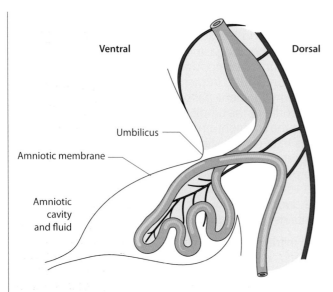

Figure 6.30 Congenital omphalocele; abdominal viscera herniate into the proximal umbilical cord and are covered by amniotic membrane

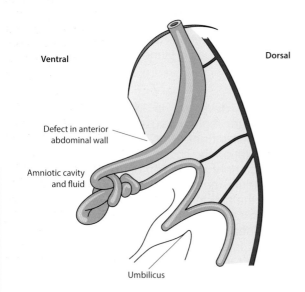

Figure 6.31 Gastroschisis; abdominal viscera pass through a defect in the anterior abdominal wall, just lateral to the midline, directly into the amniotic cavity and fluid

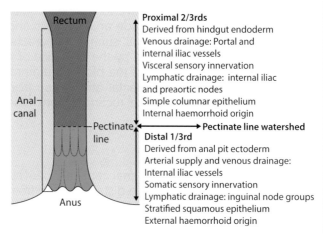

Figure 6.33 Division of the anal canal into proximal 2/3rds and distal 1/3rd and the functional significance of the pectinate line watershed

associated with an underdeveloped abdominal wall or cavity and other congenital defects. Gastroschisis (approximately 1:2000 births) looks similar to an omphalocele but is a defect in the anterior abdominal wall lateral to the midline that results in protrusion of the intestine directly into the amniotic cavity without an amniotic membrane covering (Fig. 6.31).

Hindgut, cloaca and urorectal septum

The hindgut extends from the distal one-half to one-third of the transverse colon to the anal membrane, approximately two-thirds of the way down the anal canal. It is supplied by the inferior mesenteric artery and its branches, and forms the distal part of the transverse colon, descending colon, sigmoid colon, rectum and upper anal canal.

The cloaca is the relatively dilated or expanded region of the terminal hindgut that communicates with both the hindgut and the allantois (Fig. 6.21). The distal cloaca is initially covered by the cloacal membrane, which later disappears. Growth of the urorectal septum divides the cloaca into the urogenital sinus, and the rectum and upper anal canal (Fig. 6.32). Malformation of the urorectal septum can lead to regional defects that are classified as low or high depending the

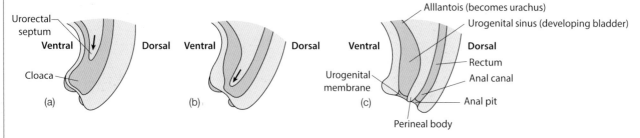

Figure 6.32 Left lateral views of the cloaca and its division into the bladder, rectum and anal canal by the urorectal septum. Arrow indicates the direction of growth of the urorectal septum

level of rectal termination relative to the pelvic floor musculature. Low defects include anal stenosis and imperforate anus; high defects such as anorectal agenesis may be accompanied by the presence of a fistula between the rectum and the bladder, urethra, vagina or vaginal vestibule. Rectal atresia can also occur and may result from absent recanalization of the rectal lumen.

Anal canal

The proximal two-thirds of the anal canal are derived from hindgut endoderm and the distal one-third from anal pit ectoderm (Fig. 6.33). The pectinate line marks the junction between these tissues of differing origin and represents the watershed point for the nervous and arterial supply and the lymphatic and venous drainage. Although the cloacal membrane covering the anal canal normally disappears, the lumen of the anorectal canal becomes occluded again by epithelial cell proliferation. Subsequent recanalization of the anal canal lumen by cellular apoptosis forms the externally visible anal pit (Fig. 6.32c). Incomplete recanalization can result in one form of imperforate anus, which requires operative correction.

Liver, falciform ligament and lesser omentum

The hepatic diverticulum grows from the ventral surface of the distal foregut into the ventral mesentery, about half way down the second part of the duodenum (Figs. 6.21, 6.24). It gives rise to the liver, gallbladder, biliary duct system and ventral pancreatic bud. The site of bile duct entry into the duodenum moves to the dorsal duodenal wall during foregut rotation and pancreatic development (Fig. 7.19, p. 120). The left and right lobes of the liver initially grow equally but the right lobe ends up larger than the left due to an unequal blood supply.

The liver eventually outgrows the ventral mesentery such that its superior part leaves its mesenteric covering to contact the diaphragm, thus creating the bare area of the liver (Figs. 6.24, 6.26). The peritoneal reflections around the margins of the bare area form the coronary and triangular hepatic ligaments. The section of ventral mesentery located between the liver and the anterior abdominal wall forms the falciform ligament, and the section between the liver and the stomach (hepatogastric ligament) and first part of the duodenum (hepatoduodenal ligament) is the future lesser omentum. *In utero* the free lower edge of the falciform ligament passing from the umbilicus to the liver contains the umbilical vein, whose fibrous remnant forms the ligamentum teres after birth. The ligamentum teres may recanalize in portal hypertension, resulting in portosystemic anastomoses at the umbilicus and the presence of a caput Medusae. The lowest part of the ventral mesentery passing between the liver and the duodenum, the free edge of the lesser omentum, contains the bile duct, hepatic artery and portal vein.

The extrahepatic bile duct system develops from the hepatic diverticulum and its branches. Surgically relevant developmental variations can occur within the bile duct system, e.g. accessory hepatic ducts passing directly into the gallbladder. As with other lumens within the developing gut tube (Fig. 6.22), the bile duct system is initially occluded by epithelial cell proliferation and later recanalizes. Extrahepatic biliary atresia may result from a failure of the duct system to recanalize or may be associated with disease-associated inflammation. The condition presents as a posthepatic obstructive jaundice.

Spleen

The spleen develops in the dorsal mesentery (mesogastrium region) and derives a blood supply from the coeliac trunk (Figs. 6.25, 6.26, 6.28). During gut tube rotation the spleen moves to the left, pulling the splenic artery with it. Part of the dorsal mesentery (mesogastrium region) containing the splenic artery fuses to the posterior body wall and undergoes mesenteric zygosis, thus explaining the mostly retroperitoneal disposition and course of the splenic artery. The spleen initially develops as a segmented or lobulated organ, the lobes later disappearing. Remnants of the lobes can be seen as notches on the anterior border of the spleen. Small islands of functional accessory splenic tissue may be present in or around the splenic mesenteries, e.g. within the gastrosplenic or splenorenal ligament or associated with the tail of the pancreas.

MCQs

1. The duodenum: **T/F**
  a is almost completely covered by peritoneum (___)
  b lies behind the portal vein   (___)
  c lies anterior to the hilum of the right kidney (___)
  d is crossed anteriorly by the superior mesen- (___)
     teric vessels
  e is about 25 cm long   (___)

Answers
1.
  a *F* – *Only its first and last centimetres are invested with peritoneum. The remainder lies retroperitoneally, with only its anterior surface and sides being covered.*
  b *F* – *The first part of the duodenum is anterior to the portal vein, common bile duct and gastroduodenal artery.*
  c *T* – *Its second part lies anterior to the hilum of the right kidney and the right psoas muscle.*
  d *T* – *The root of the mesentery and the superior mesenteric vessels cross anteriorly to the third part of the duodenum.*
  e *T* – *It comprises the first part (5 cm), the second part (8 cm) descending on the right of the vertebral column, the third part (10 cm) running horizontally, and the fourth part (3 cm), which ascends to the left of the 2nd lumbar vertebra.*

2. The ileum can be distinguished from the   **T/F**
jejunum because the ileum has:
  a thicker walls than the jejunum   (___)
  b fewer valvulae conniventes than the jejunum (___)
  c appendices epiploicae and, occasionally,   (___)
     taeniae coli
  d less fat in its mesentery   (___)
  e fewer arterial arcades   (___)

Answers
2.
  a *F* – *The jejunum is thicker walled because of the presence of larger circular muscle folds in the mucous ...*
  b *T* – *... membrane (valvulae conniventes).*
  c *F* – *These two features distinguish large bowel from small bowel. The appendices epiploicae are small numerous fat-laden peritoneal tags seen over most of the large bowel; the taeniae coli are flattened bands of longitudinal muscle that create the characteristic haustrations of the large bowel.*
  d *F* – *The mesentery carries more fat in the ileum.*
  e *F* – *The ileum has a greater number of arterial arcades.*

3. The structures on which the stomach lies   **T/F**
are often referred to as the stomach bed.
The immediate posterior relations of the
stomach include the:
  a lesser sac of peritoneum   (___)
  b pancreas   (___)
  c splenic artery   (___)
  d gastric surface of the spleen   (___)
  e duodenojejunal flexure   (___)

Answers
3.
  a *T* – *The lesser sac is the true immediate posterior relation of the stomach, separating it from all ...*
  b *F*   *... other structures: the pancreas, left kidney, adrenal gland, splenic artery, left colic flexure ...*
  c *F*   *... and the transverse mesocolon.*
  d *F* – *The gastric surface of the spleen is separated from the stomach by the greater sac of peritoneum.*
  e *F* – *The greater omentum and the transverse mesocolon separate the stomach from the duodenojejunal flexure and the small intestine.*

SBA

A 30-year-old woman presents with a 12-hour history of nausea and periumbilical pain, which has preceded the discomfort that she now feels in the lower abdomen. Examination reveals tenderness in the right iliac fossa. What is her most likely diagnosis?
  a ectopic pregnancy
  b appendicitis
  c cholecystitis
  d torsion of the right ovary
  e diverticulitis of the colon

Answer
  b *Appendicitis is usually caused by obstruction of the lumen appendix by faeces. This results in distension of the appendix and stimulates visceral pain afferents, which are carried by sympathetic nerves to the T10 spinal cord level. The patient feels a vague pain in the periumbilical region. Later, when the continuing obstruction causes local inflammation in the appendicular wall, the parietal peritoneum in the region becomes inflamed to produce tenderness and pain in the right iliac fossa.*

EMQs

Each question has an anatomical theme linked to the chapter, and a list of 10 related items (A–J) placed in alphabetical order: these are followed by five statements (1–5). Match **one or more** of the items A–J to each of the five statements.

Relationships of the abdominal viscera
A. Appendix
B. Duodenojejunal junction
C. Hepatic flexure of the colon
D. Ileocaecal valve
E. Ileum
F. Oesophagogastric junction
G. Pylorus
H. Second part of the duodenum
I. Sigmoid colon mesentery
J. Splenic flexure of the colon

Match the following statements with the appropriate item(s) from the above list.
1. Lies to the left of the xiphisternal joint
2. Lies to the right of the midline, at the level of the 1st lumbar vertebra
3. Overlies the left ureter
4. Overlies the hilum of the right kidney
5. Is in contact with the spleen

Answers
1 F; 2 G; 3 I; 4 H; 5 J

APPLIED QUESTIONS

1. Which artery and its branches supplies the foregut?

1. The artery of the foregut and its derivatives is the coeliac artery. The foregut extends as far as the point of entry of the ampulla of Vater into the second part of the duodenum and comprises the lower oesophagus, the stomach and the proximal duodenum, together with the liver, spleen and pancreas.

2. What radiological features distinguish large from small bowel?

2. Barium radiographs, small bowel enemas or barium meals and follow-throughs reveal that the small bowel is seen in the central abdomen with indentations of the circular folds of the mucosa, which commence in the second part of the duodenum but disappear by the mid-ileum. The large bowel is positioned more peripherally. A barium enema reveals sacculations or haustrations, especially in the transverse colon, and particularly if the radiographic examination is by the double-contrast technique, in which a mixture of gas and the contrast medium is used to emphasize the fine mucosal pattern. The pattern is caused by the relative shortness of the longitudinal muscle (taeniae coli) of the colon compared with that of the circular muscle it encloses. The sacculations are rather like the appearance of a piece of woven material in which a thread has been pulled.

Bailey & Love · Essential Clinical Anatomy · Bailey & Love · Essential Clinical Anatomy
Essential Clinical Anatomy · Bailey & Love · Essential Clinical Anatomy · Bailey & Love
ailey & Love · Essential Clinical Anatomy · Bailey & Love · Essential Clinical Anatomy

Chapter 7

The liver, spleen and pancreas

THE LIVER

The liver, the largest organ in the body, weighs about 1.5 kg in the adult. Wedge-shaped, it lies under the diaphragm, mainly in the right hypochondrium. It possesses two surfaces, a rounded diaphragmatic and an irregular visceral (inferior) surface. The **diaphragmatic surface** is rounded and convex, fitting closely to the diaphragm. Its sharp inferior border separates it from the visceral surface (**Figs. 7.1** and **7.2**).

The **visceral surface** (Fig. 7.3) is set obliquely, facing downwards, backwards and to the left. It is divided into a right and a smaller left lobe by the **interlobar fissure**, the ligamentum venosum superiorly and the ligamentum teres below. The ligamentum venosum is a remnant of the ductus venosus which, in the fetus, connects the umbilical vein and inferior vena cava and allows blood to bypass the liver. The ligamentum teres is the obliterated left umbilical vein. The right lobe contains the small **quadrate lobe** anteriorly between the interlobar fissure and the gallbladder, and the **caudate lobe** behind between the interlobar fissure and the inferior vena cava. These two lobes are separated by the **porta hepatis**, a transverse sulcus through which pass the portal vein, hepatic artery, common hepatic duct and lymph vessels (**Figs. 7.3** and **7.4**).

The liver is largely covered by peritoneum, folds of which are reflected onto the anterior abdominal wall, diaphragm and stomach (**Figs. 7.1–7.4**):

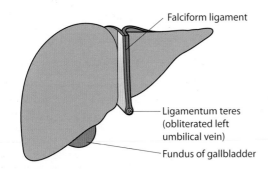

Figure 7.1 Liver, anterior surface

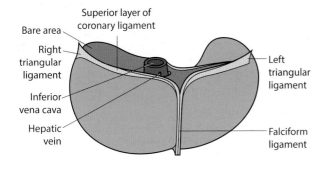

Figure 7.2 Liver, superior surface

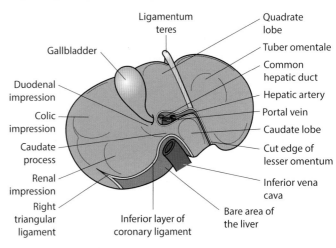

Figure 7.3 Liver, inferior (visceral) surface

- The sickle-shaped **falciform ligament** extends from the diaphragm and supraumbilical abdominal wall to the anterior and superior surfaces of the liver, where it defines the division of the right and left lobes and also separates the right and left subphrenic spaces. Its inferior free border contains the umbilical vein and the ligamentum teres.
- The **coronary ligament** has two layers connecting the back of the right lobe to the diaphragm. Between these layers the liver is in direct contact with the diaphragm (the bare area).
- The **right triangular ligament** is the right extremity of the coronary ligament, where its upper and lower layers are in continuity.
- The **left triangular ligament** connects the posterior surface of the left lobe to the diaphragm.

The peritoneal reflection onto the stomach, the two-layered lesser omentum, encloses the right and left hepatic ducts, the hepatic arteries and the right and left branches of the portal vein at the **porta hepatis**. The hepatic ducts are in front of the portal vein, which is to the right of the hepatic artery. The **gallbladder** lies in a shallow fossa to the right of the porta, its fundus usually projecting beyond the inferior border of the liver (**Figs. 7.3** and **7.4**).

The liver moves with the diaphragm during respiration because of the surface tension between the visceral and parietal layers of peritoneum. Its lower border may be felt, especially in thin individuals, descending just below the right subcostal margin during deep inspiration.

Relations

The diaphragm separates the liver from the heart and pericardium, lungs, pleura and chest wall. The inferior vena cava is closely applied to the posterior surface within the bare area. The abdominal relations of the visceral surface should be noted: the left lobe is in contact with the abdominal oesophagus, the fundus and body of the stomach, and the lesser omentum (**Fig. 7.3**), which separates it from the pancreas.

The gallbladder is in relation with the first part of the duodenum and the transverse colon. The upper recess of the lesser sac separates the caudate lobe from the diaphragm (**Fig. 7.4**). Adjacent to the right lobe inferiorly are the right colic flexure and right kidney (**Fig. 7.5**), but they are separated from it by a potential peritoneal space, the right subhepatic space,

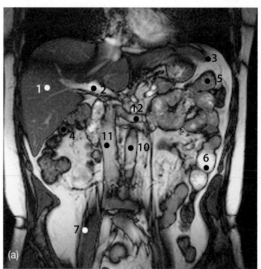

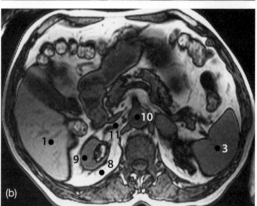

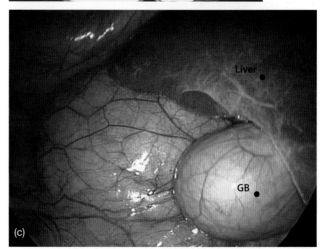

Figure 7.5 (a) Coronal MR image of abdomen and (b) axial MR image of upper abdomen: 1, liver; 2, portal vein; 3, spleen; 4, hepatic flexure of colon; 5, splenic flexure of colon; 6, descending colon; 7, psoas muscle; 8, perinephric fat; 9, right kidney; 10, aorta; 11, inferior vena cava; 12, left renal vein. (c) Laparoscopic cholecystectomy showing gallbladder (GB) and liver

Figure 7.4 Liver, posterior surface (the arrow is in the entry to the lesser sac of omentum)

which is continuous with the right paracolic gutter and the lesser sac.

Blood supply and lobular arrangement

The liver has two sources of blood: arterial from the hepatic artery and venous from the portal vein. Each divides at the porta hepatis into right and left lobar branches, from which interlobular branches ramify to supply the liver. Further branching of these vessels divides each lobe into four segments, each with a distinct arterial and venous supply that has only minor communications with neighbouring segments (Fig. 7.6). Blood drains by three major and numerous tiny hepatic veins into the inferior vena cava. Although the liver does possess two lobes, the traditional division into a right and a left lobe, divided by the line of attachment of the falciform ligament and the fissure for the ligamentum venosum, does not coincide with the anatomical arrangement of the finer terminal branches of the biliary ducts and blood vessels. The demarcation line between the portal and hepatic arterial branches to the right and left lobes lies along an imaginary line joining the inferior vena cava to the gallbladder bed, rather than, as one might expect, between the anatomical right and left lobes.

Nerve supply

The liver is supplied by both vagi via the anterior gastric nerve and by sympathetic fibres from the coeliac plexus.

Lymphatic drainage

The bare area of the diaphragmatic surface drains through the diaphragm to posterior mediastinal nodes. The remaining liver drains to nodes in the porta hepatis and thence to the coeliac nodes.

The fact that there is no major communication between the arteries, portal veins and bile ducts of the lobes of the liver makes surgical removal of the right or left lobe possible. An understanding of the segmentation of the liver also allows surgical removal of segments of the lobes. The liver is the most common site of secondary spread (**metastasis**; Fig. 7.7) of cancer cells, usually seen as nodular deposits just under the capsule; these are readily diagnosed by **ultrasound** scanning. Tissue samples, biopsies, can be obtained from the liver using a percutaneous needle. The site usually chosen for introduction of the needle is the 9th/10th intercostal space in the midaxillary line but, in choosing this site, one must be aware of the potential risk of accidentally entering the pleura and causing a pneumothorax. Thus the biopsy should be taken with the patient holding their breath in full expiration to reduce the size of the costodiaphragmatic recess. The regenerative properties are great and this permits resection of either lobe of the liver in some cases of trauma or localized malignancy.

Patients with oesophageal varices secondary to cirrhosis and portal hypertension may require a portosystemic shunt, in which the portal or splenic vein is anastomosed to the inferior vena cava or neighbouring large systemic vein. The aim of this is to reduce venous congestion and reduce pressure in the haemorrhage-prone oesophageal varices (Fig. 7.8).

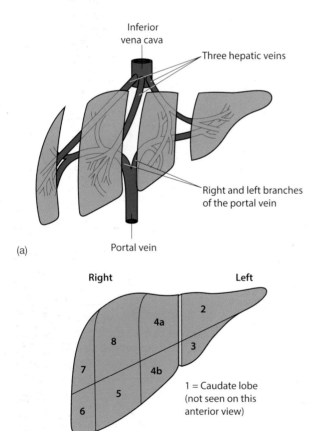

(a)

(b)

Figure 7.6 (a) Liver lobular arrangement. (b) Segmentation of the liver. This knowledge is useful in surgical removal of segments containing cancer metastases (partial hepatectomy). It is also essential in the area of transplant surgery where resected lobes or segments may be used so that a single donor liver can supply one or more recipients. Less commonly, a segment may be obtained from a living donor

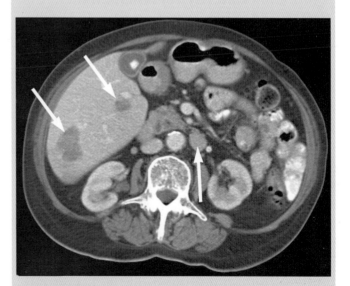

Figure 7.7 Axial CT scan showing secondary deposits in the liver (two arrows) and an enlarged para-aortic lymph node (single arrow)

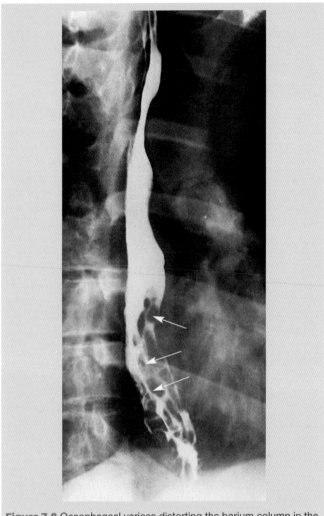

Figure 7.8 Oesophageal varices distorting the barium column in the lower oesophagus (arrows)

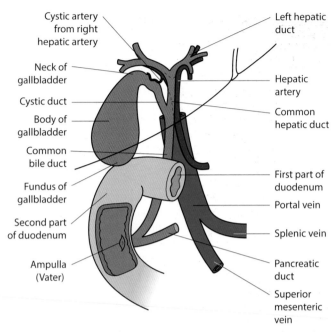

Figure 7.9 Extrahepatic biliary system

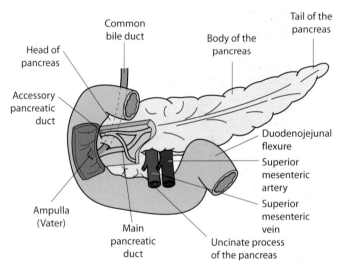

Figure 7.10 Pancreas: part of the head has been removed to show the duct system

THE EXTRAHEPATIC BILIARY SYSTEM

This comprises the right and left hepatic ducts, the common hepatic duct, the gallbladder and cystic duct and the common bile duct (Figs. 7.9–7.12). It conveys bile to the duodenum.

The **common hepatic duct**, formed by the union of the **right and left hepatic ducts** in the porta hepatis, descends in the free edge of the lesser omentum to be joined by the cystic duct from the gallbladder to form the bile duct.

The **bile duct**, 8 cm long, descends in the free edge of the lesser omentum behind the first part of the duodenum and the head of the pancreas to enter the duodenum at the duodenal papilla.

Relations

In the lesser omentum, the portal vein lies posterior to the bile duct; the hepatic artery lies to its left. Behind the duodenum, the bile duct is accompanied by the gastroduodenal artery; behind the head of the pancreas and anterior to the inferior vena cava it is joined by the main pancreatic duct,

and both open into the ampulla. The **ampulla** opens into the medial wall of the second part of the duodenum at the **duodenal papilla** (Fig. 7.10), 10 cm beyond the pylorus. The papilla contains a sphincter of smooth muscle. A postoperative cholangiogram gives an excellent *in-vivo* demonstration of the anatomy (Fig. 7.11).

The gallbladder

The gallbladder concentrates and stores bile. It is a pear-shaped sac lying in the right hypochondrium, firmly connected to the visceral surface of the right lobe of the liver by fibrous tissue. It has a fundus, body and neck. Its mucous membrane shows a honeycombed appearance and is thrown into numerous folds.

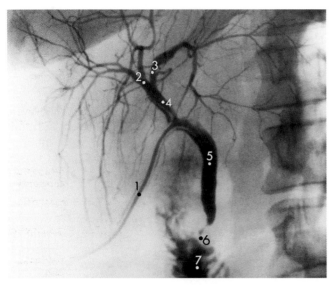

Figure 7.11 Biliary tree, contrast material having been introduced into the common bile duct by a T tube (the gallbladder has been removed): 1, T tube; 2, right hepatic duct; 3, left hepatic duct; 4, common hepatic duct; 5, common bile duct; 6, site of biliary ampulla; 7, duodenum

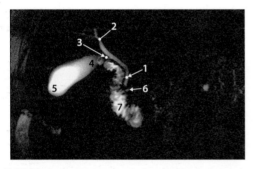

Figure 7.12 Magnetic resonance cholangiopancreatography. 1, common bile duct; 2, common hepatic duct; 3, cystic duct; 4, neck of gallbladder; 5, fundus of gallbladder; 6, pancreatic duct; 7, duodenum, second part

The neck of the gallbladder is sinuous, contains a constant spiral fold and is continuous with the cystic duct. The fundus and inferior surface of the body are covered with peritoneum.

Relations

The fundus lies just below the inferior border of the liver in contact with the anterior abdominal wall deep to the tip of the 9th costal cartilage; the transverse colon is adjacent. The body overlies the second part of the duodenum.

Vessels

The cystic artery, usually a branch of the right hepatic artery, supplies the gallbladder. Lymph drains via nodes in the porta hepatis to the coeliac group of nodes.

Some radiopaque media are excreted by the liver and concentrated by a normally functioning gallbladder, a feature that is exploited by **cholecystography**, and which can thus explore irregularities of function as well as potentially reveal the presence of gallstones (Fig. 7.13b). Stones formed in the gall-

bladder may pass into the common bile duct and occasionally cause obstructive jaundice. Their presence may be confirmed by endoscopic retrograde cholangiopancreatography (ERCP) via the ampulla of Vater and subsequent injection of contrast. Gallstones that impact in the gallbladder neck obstruct the gallbladder and cause painful biliary colic; this is typically felt in the epigastrium. If infection of the gallbladder (cholecystitis) follows, tenderness over the area of the 9th right costal cartilage is present and, if the inflammation spreads to the diaphragm, the pain may be referred to the right shoulder region.

Stones in the common bile duct may produce obstructive jaundice. They can usually be removed by opening the common bile duct, although a stone impacted in the ampulla requires an incision in the second part of the duodenum to gain access to the ampulla. Modern duodenoscopes equipped with diathermy allow this to be done endoscopically. Symptomatic gallstones are usually treated by surgical removal of the gallbladder (cholecystectomy; Fig. 7.13a) and exploration and removal of stones (if present) from the bile duct. The biliary tree may be visualized radiographically by cholangiography (Fig. 7.11) or by magnetic resonance cholangiopancreatography (Fig. 7.12).

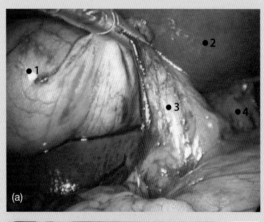

(a)

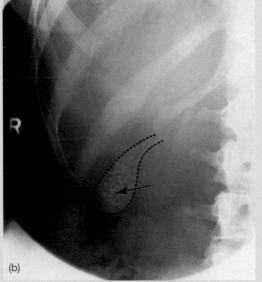

(b)

Figure 7.13 (a) Laparoscopic view of gallbladder during cholecystectomy: 1, gallbladder; 2, right lobe of liver; 3, free edge of lesser omentum; 4, lesser omentum. (b) Oral cholecystogram showing multiple gallstones in the gallbladder (arrow)

THE SPLEEN

This large lymphoid organ lies deep in the left hypochondrium, obliquely beneath the 9th, 10th and 11th ribs. In health it is approximately 3 cm thick, 8 cm wide and 13 cm long, and weighs about 200 g. It has anterior and posterior surfaces, inferior, posterior and superior (notched) borders, and a diaphragmatic and a visceral surface that bears the hilum containing the splenic vessels (Fig. 7.14).

Relations

The spleen is invested in peritoneum and suspended at its hilum by two peritoneal folds, the lienorenal and gastrosplenic ligaments, which form the lateral limit of the lesser sac (omental bursa) (Fig. 5.19, p. 89). The diaphragm separates the spleen from the left pleural sac, the left lung and the 9th, 10th and 11th ribs; the visceral surface is in contact with the stomach anteriorly, the left kidney posteriorly and the splenic flexure of the colon inferiorly. The tail of the pancreas, lying in the lienorenal ligament, is close to the hilum (Fig. 7.15). Anteriorly the normal spleen extends no further than the left midaxillary line and its tip may be palpated in the left hypochondrium during deep inspiration. If enlarged the spleen extends down towards the right iliac fossa and may be recognized by palpating the notch on its anterior border (Fig. 7.16).

Blood supply

This is by the splenic artery and vein.

Lymphatic drainage

This is to the suprapancreatic and coeliac nodes.

The chest wall gives protection to the spleen, but severe blows over the left lower chest may fracture the ribs and result in contusion or fracture of the splenic tissue. Severe intraperitoneal haemorrhage then usually results, and urgent surgery is required to remove the spleen unless the injury allows conservation of part of it. An enlarged spleen that extends beyond the costal margin is more susceptible to injury. When removing the spleen the close relation of the tail of the pancreas to the splenic hilum must be taken into account. A splenectomized patient has a reduced immunity to infection so prophylactic antibiotics and vaccination are advised, particularly against pneumococcal infections.

THE PANCREAS

The pancreas is both an endocrine and an exocrine gland. It is about 15 cm long and weighs about 80 g. It possesses a head with an uncinate process, a neck, a body and a tail, and lies obliquely across the posterior abdominal wall, crossing the 1st

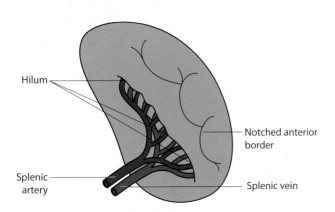

Figure 7.14 Hilum of the spleen

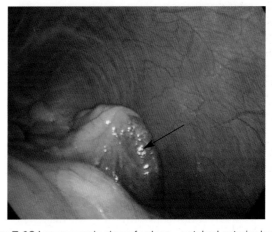

Figure 7.16 Laparoscopic view of spleen – notched anterior border arrowed

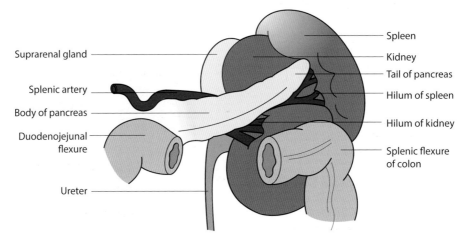

Figure 7.15 Anterior view and relations of the spleen, tail of the pancreas and left kidney

lumbar vertebra and the aorta and inferior vena cava. The head, the expanded right extremity of the gland, bears inferiorly the **uncinate process**. The body, triangular in section, has anterior, inferior and posterior surfaces; the tail is the narrow left extremity and lies in the lienorenal ligament.

Relations

The head lies within the curve of the duodenum (Fig. 7.17). Anteriorly it is covered, from above downwards, by the pylorus, the transverse colon and the small intestine; posteriorly it lies on the inferior vena cava, the right renal vessels and the bile duct. The **uncinate process** lies on the left renal vein and the aorta and is crossed by the superior mesenteric vessels. The **neck** overlies the portal vein and is behind the pylorus and the gastroduodenal artery. Above the **body** is the coeliac artery, and the common hepatic and splenic arteries run along its superior border. Anteriorly lie the stomach and lesser sac. Inferiorly its surface is covered by the peritoneum of the greater sac and it is related to coils of small intestine. The transverse mesocolon is attached by its mesentery to its anterior surface. The body, from right to left, lies on the aorta and superior mesenteric artery, the left crus of the diaphragm, the left renal vessels and the left kidney, and the splenic vein runs behind it throughout its length, being joined by the inferior mesenteric vein.

The **pancreatic duct** (Figs. 7.9 and 7.10) traverses the length of the gland to the head of the pancreas, where it joins the bile duct in the ampulla before opening into the second part of the duodenum. An accessory duct drains the uncinate process and usually drains into the ampulla, but it may open separately into the duodenum about 3 cm proximal to the main duct (Fig. 7.10).

Blood supply

This is from the splenic and superior and inferior pancreaticoduodenal arteries. The veins drain to the splenic vein and, via the pancreaticoduodenal veins, to the superior mesenteric vein.

Nerve supply

This is from the thoracic splanchnic nerves (p. 73) and the vagi via the coeliac plexus. Pain fibres, whose cell bodies are located in the 6th to 10th thoracic segments, are conveyed with the sympathetic nerves. Pancreatic pain is commonly referred to the back.

Lymphatic drainage

This is via suprapancreatic nodes to the preaortic coeliac nodes.

Rarely the two embryonic buds encircle the duodenum (see below) and may cause duodenal obstruction. **Pancreatitis** (inflammation of the gland) is often the result of gallstone impaction in the ampulla or reflux of bile into the pancreatic duct. It causes glandular secretions rich in proteolytic enzymes to escape into the surrounding tissues and produce severe abdominal and back pain, peritonitis and severe systemic upset. The inflammatory fluid produced may accumulate in the lesser sac to form a 'pseudocyst' of the pancreas.

The pancreas is rarely **injured** because of its deep-seated location, but severe crush injuries of the abdomen may result in the pancreas being crushed against the vertebral column, producing ductal tears and leakage of pancreatic secretions into the abdomen. **Cancer of the pancreas** (Fig. 7.18) is usually advanced at the time of diagnosis because of spread to the lymph nodes, and curative excision is rarely possible. If the cancer involves the head, obstructive jaundice secondary to bile duct or ampullary obstruction is a likely presentation; if it involves the body, unremitting back pain may result, owing to the invasion of the neighbouring neural plexuses.

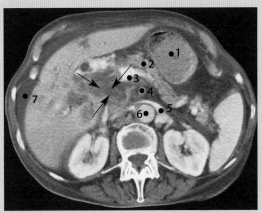

Figure 7.18 CT scan showing a malignant tumour in the head of the pancreas (arrows): 1, stomach; 2, pancreatic body; 3, origin of portal vein; 4, superior mesenteric artery; 5, left renal vein; 6, aorta; 7, ascites (viewed from below)

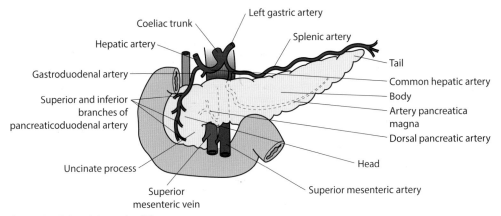

Figure 7.17 Arterial supply of the pancreas

Coeliac trunk

Left gastric artery

Hepatic artery

Splenic artery

Gastroduodenal artery

Tail

Common hepatic artery

Superior and inferior branches of pancreaticoduodenal artery

Body

Artery pancreatica magna

Dorsal pancreatic artery

Uncinate process

Head

Superior mesenteric vein

Superior mesenteric artery

DEVELOPMENT OF THE PANCREAS

The pancreas develops from two separate growths (buds) of tissue, both of which arise from the distal foregut and develop within the mesenteries (Figs. 7.19a–c). The small ventral pancreatic bud branches from the hepatic diverticulum in the ventral mesentery and therefore shares a duct drainage system with the liver. The larger dorsal pancreatic bud forms in the dorsal mesentery. Rotation of the foregut to the right causes the ventral pancreatic bud and bile duct to rotate to the original dorsal aspect (now on the left hand side) of the gut tube, where it joins and fuses with the dorsal bud. The ventral bud forms the pancreatic head and uncinate process whereas the dorsal bud forms the pancreatic neck, body and tail. The main pancreatic duct, which joins the common bile duct to drain into the second part of the duodenum via the major duodenal papilla, is formed by a union of the duct systems of the ventral bud and the distal part of the dorsal bud. The accessory pancreatic duct, which drains via the minor duodenal papilla, is formed from the duct system in the proximal part of the dorsal bud.

Pancreatic tissue can be located in numerous ectopic positions including within the stomach, duodenum or jejunum, or in an ileal diverticulum. Malformation of the ventral pancreatic bud, possibly as a result of its bifurcation, can lead to an annular pancreas where pancreatic tissue surrounds, and therefore obstructs, the second part of the duodenum (Fig. 7.20a,b).

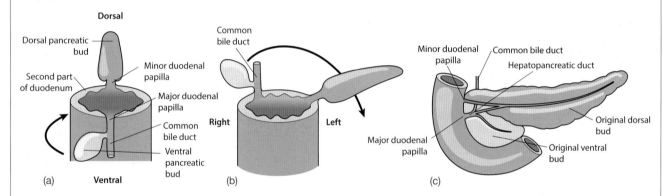

Figure 7.19 Development of the pancreas from ventral and dorsal pancreatic buds (anterior view). (a) The ventral and dorsal buds, and associated bile duct system, rotate during the rightward rotation of the foregut. (b) The ventral bud and associated bile duct system pass behind the gut tube to join the dorsal bud. (c) The ventral and dorsal buds and their duct systems join, fuse and remodel to form a single pancreas. The main pancreatic duct forms from the duct system of the ventral bud; the accessory pancreatic duct (green) forms within the proximal part of the dorsal bud

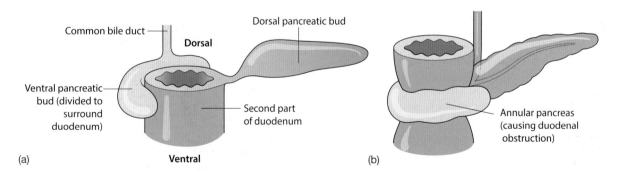

Figure 7.20 Development of an annular pancreas. (a) Malformation/division of the ventral pancreatic bud. (b) The ventral bud encircles the second part of the duodenum causing either partial or complete obstruction

MCQs

1. The pancreas: **T/F**
  a is an intraperitonal structure   (___)
  b usually has two major ducts   (___)
  c is related to the greater sac of peritoneum   (___)
  d lies anterior to the right and left renal veins   (___)
  e is closely related to the hepatic duct   (___)

Answers

1.

a **F** – *It is only covered by peritoneum anteriorly; the tail lies within the lienorenal ligament.*

b **T** – *The main pancreatic duct joins the bile duct in the ampulla and opens about the middle of the medial wall of the descending duodenum. The accessory duct draining the uncinate process may open separately into the duodenum proximal to the duodenal papilla, but frequently joins the main pancreatic duct.*

c **T** – *The transverse mesocolon, which is attached to the border between the anterior and inferior surfaces of the gland, separates these two peritoneal sacs.*

d **T** – *Both renal veins join the inferior vena cava behind the head of the pancreas.*

e **F** – *The hepatic duct lies superior to the duodenum and pancreas.*

2. The spleen: **T/F**
  a lies deep to the 9th, 10th and 11th ribs   (___)
  b is separated by the diaphragm from the   (___)
     chest wall
  c is closely related to the stomach   (___)
  d is separated by the stomach from the tail   (___)
     of the pancreas
  e is closely related to the left kidney   (___)

Answers

2.

a **T** – *It lies posterior to the midaxillary line deep to these ribs ...*

b **T** – *... being separated from them by the diaphragm and the left pleural sac.*

c **T** – *Its anterior surface is directly related to the greater curvature of the stomach.*

d **F** – *The tail of the pancreas extends in the lienorenal ligament to the hilum of the spleen.*

e **T** – *The posterior surface is closely related to the left kidney and suprarenal gland.*

SBA

1. A road traffic accident victim is admitted in shock with low blood pressure. A chest X-ray reveals fractures of the left 9th and 10th ribs, and aspiration of the peritoneum reveals heavily blood-stained fluid. What is the likely diagnosis?
  a liver trauma
  b pancreatic trauma
  c splenic trauma
  d trauma to the left kidney
  e rupture of the inferior vena cava

Answer

c *The chest wall gives protection to the underlying spleen, but the spleen may be injured by a fracture of the overlying ribs (9th, 10th and 11th) and then bleed rapidly into the peritoneal cavity. In such cases urgent laparotomy is indicated to either repair or remove the spleen.*

2. A patient is admitted with progressive jaundice that has been worsening over the past week. X-rays show gallstones. If gallstones are the cause of the jaundice, where are they likely to be lying?
  a cystic duct
  b common bile duct
  c gallbladder
  d hepatic ducts

Answer

b *The jaundice is worsening so the gallstones are obstructing the common bile duct. Cystic duct obstruction may be associated with mild, temporary jaundice; gallstone obstruction of a single hepatic duct is rare and will not cause jaundice. Stones with the gall bladder are usually assymtomatic and do not cuase obstruction.*

EMQs

Each question has an anatomical theme linked to the chapter, and a list of 10 related items (A–J) placed in alphabetical order: these are followed by five statements (1–5). Match **one or more** of the items A–J to each of the five statements.

Liver
A. Caudate lobe
B. Caudate process
C. Coronary ligament
D. Falciform ligament
E. Left lobe
F. Left triangular ligament
G. Lesser omentum
H. Porta hepatis
I. Quadrate lobe
J. Right triangular ligament

Answers
1 I; 2 H; 3 CJ; 4 E; 5 G

Match the following statements with the appropriate item(s) from the above list.
1. Lies to the left of the gallbladder
2. Site of exit of the common bile duct from the liver
3. Encloses the bare area of the liver
4. Related posteriorly to the oesophagus
5. An anterior relation to the opening of the lesser sac

APPLIED QUESTIONS

1. What may be the consequences of a boy falling from his bike on his left side? Why may the abdominal injury sustained cause left shoulder tip pain?

1. Severe blows to the left hypochondrium, especially when associated with rib fractures, can tear the splenic capsule and lacerate the soft, pulpy, friable parenchyma of the spleen. Splenectomy often has to be performed to arrest haemorrhage, but repair is preferable because of the spleen's importance in immunity. Left shoulder tip pain is due to irritation of the nearby diaphragm; pain is referred by its nerve supply, the phrenic nerve, to the supraclavicular C4 dermatome, which also supplies the skin of the shoulder region.

2. Why must the patient hold his breath during a liver biopsy?

2. When the biopsy needle is in the liver the diaphragm must remain stationary, otherwise the liver will move and can be lacerated by the needle. Diaphragmatic movement may also cause the pleura to be punctured and result in a pneumothorax.

Essential Clinical Anatomy · Bailey & Love · Essential Clinical Anatomy
sential Clinical Anatomy · Bailey & Love · Essential Clinical Anatomy · Bailey & Love
ley & Love · Essential Clinical Anatomy · Bailey & Love · Essential Clinical Anatomy

Chapter 8

The kidneys and posterior abdominal wall

THE KIDNEYS

The **kidneys** lie on the posterior abdominal wall on each side of the vertebral column, their hila at the level of L1, the transpyloric plane. Each is about 10 cm long, 5 cm wide and 3 cm thick and weighs about 100 g; they possess upper and lower poles, anterior and posterior surfaces, a lateral convex border, and a medial border whose concavity gives the organ its characteristic shape. Each lies obliquely, its upper pole nearer to the midline than its lower; the liver displaces the right kidney slightly lower than the left (Fig. 8.1).

The kidneys are embedded in and protected by perirenal fat enclosed by the perirenal fascia; each is capped by a tricorn hat – the suprarenal gland.

Relations

Posterior

The kidneys are similar on both sides. The diaphragm separates the upper pole from the costodiaphragmatic recess of the pleura and the 11th and 12th ribs (Figs. 8.1 and 8.2). Below

this the kidney lies, from medial to lateral, on psoas, quadratus lumborum (which is crossed by the subcostal, iliohypogastric and ilioinguinal nerves) and transversus abdominis.

Anterior

- **Left kidney** (Fig. 7.15, p. 118) – the suprarenal gland lies superomedially, the spleen on its upper lateral border and the stomach between the two. The body of the pancreas and the splenic vessels cross the hilum and middle part, and the lower pole is in contact with the jejunum and left colic flexure.
- **Right kidney** (Fig. 8.3) – the suprarenal gland lies superiorly. It and the upper anterior surface are covered by the liver anteriorly. The hilum is covered by the second part of the duodenum, and below that lie the right colic flexure and jejunum.

In the **hilum** of each kidney lie the renal vein, renal artery and pelvis of the ureter in that order, from in front backwards. Within the kidney the pelvis of the ureter is formed by the union of **major calyces**, each of which has been formed in turn by the union of three or four **minor calyces**, into which project pyramids of renal tissue, the **papillae** (Figs. 8.4 and 8.5).

Blood supply

Each renal artery arises horizontally from the aorta and divides near the hilum into smaller branches (Fig. 8.6) that supply the five segments of each kidney. The segments have no collateral circulation between them. Venous tributaries unite in the hilum to form the renal vein, each draining to the inferior vena cava (Fig. 8.7).

Nerve supply

From the coeliac plexuses emerge sympathetic (vasomotor) nerves originating in the 12th thoracic and 1st lumbar

Figure 8.1 Surface anatomy of posterior abdominal wall, showing the relations of the kidney: 1, 11th rib; 2, spine T12; 3, lower pole of right kidney; 4, iliac crest; 5, intercristal plane; 6, S2

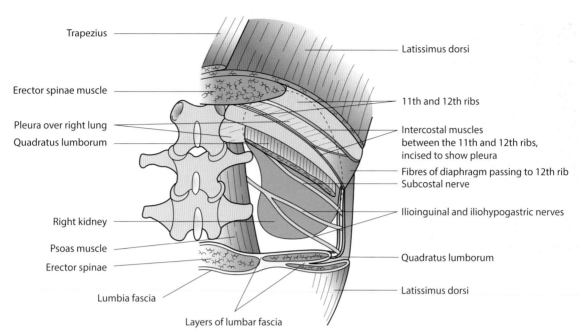

Figure 8.2 Muscle layers of the posterior abdominal wall encountered in the posterior approach to the right kidney (part of the superficial muscles and fascia removed)

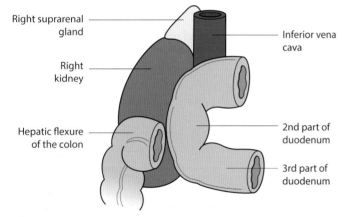

Figure 8.3 Anterior relations of the right kidney

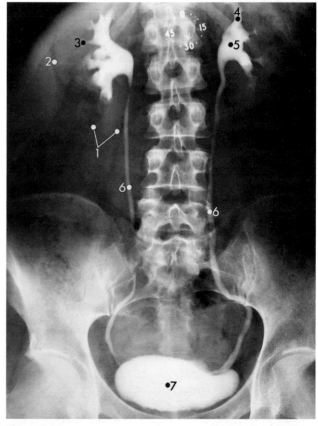

Figure 8.5 Intravenous urogram: 1, contour of lower pole of the right kidney; 2, lateral margin of the kidney; 3, minor calyx; 4, major calyx; 5, left renal pelvis; 6, left and right ureters; 7, urinary bladder

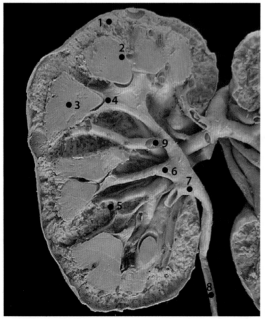

Figure 8.4 Dissection of right kidney to show the collecting system and arterial supply: 1, renal cortex; 2, renal medulla; 3, pyramid; 4, renal papilla; 5, minor calyx; 6, major calyx; 7, pelvis of ureter; 8, ureter; 9, branch of renal artery

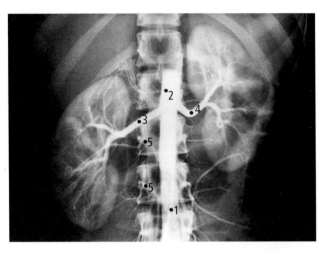

Figure 8.6 Angiogram showing both renal arteries: 1, catheter; 2, aorta; 3, right renal artery; 4, left renal artery; 5, lumbar arteries

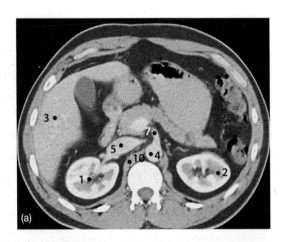

(a)

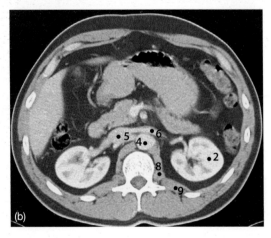

(b)

Figure 8.7 (a) and (b) Axial transverse CT scans at the L1/L2 level showing the hila of the kidneys: 1, right kidney; 2, left kidney; 3, liver; 4, aorta; 5, inferior vena cava; 6, left renal vein; 7, superior mesenteric artery; 8, psoas muscle; 9, quadratus lumborum muscle; 10, right crus of the diaphragm

segments. Pain fibres, conveyed with the sympathetic nerves, pass via the posterior roots to these spinal segments. Hence pain arising from the kidney is referred to the back and radiates to the lower anterior abdominal wall and genitalia. The parasympathetic supply is derived from the vagi.

Lymph drainage

This is into para-aortic nodes around the renal arteries.

Pus arising from infection in the renal parenchyma is usually retained within the perirenal fascia, leading to the formation of a **perinephric abscess**. **Cancer of the kidney** often invades and occludes the renal vein. An occasional consequence of this is the development of a left-sided varicocoele (distended veins around the testis), caused by occlusion of the junction of the left testicular vein with the left renal vein (Fig. 5.14, p. 87).

THE URETERS

The ureters are narrow muscular tubes about 25 cm long. Each has a dilated upper end, the pelvis. They are lined with transitional epithelium, as is the bladder. The upper half of each ureter lies on the posterior abdominal wall and the lower half is within the pelvis. There are three narrowings in the ureter: at the pelviureteric junction, at the brim of the pelvis and on entering the bladder. A stone or blood clot may impact at these sites, causing ureteric obstruction.

Relations

The abdominal course of the ureters is similar in both sexes but their relations differ on the right and the left sides, whereas in the pelvis, although their courses are different in the two sexes, their relations on both sides are the same.

- **Abdominal part** – the **right ureter** descends on the psoas muscle and is crossed by the second part of the duodenum and vessels supplying the right colon and small bowel. The **left ureter** also descends on psoas but is crossed by the root of the sigmoid colon. Both ureters are covered by and are adherent to the peritoneum.
- **Pelvic part** – in the **male**, in front of the sacroiliac joint it crosses the common iliac vessels and descends on the pelvic wall to the ischial spine, where it is crossed by the ductus deferens before turning medially above levator ani. In the **female** it similarly descends to the ischial spine and turns medially, passing under the root of the broad ligament, where it lies adjacent to the vaginal lateral fornix, and is there crossed superiorly by the uterine artery just before it enters the bladder.

Blood supply

This is via anastomoses between the renal, gonadal and inferior vesical arteries. Venous drainage is into renal, gonadal and internal iliac veins.

Lymphatic drainage

This is to the para-aortic and internal iliac nodes.

Radiology

The outline of the calyces, pelvis, ureter and bladder can be readily shown (Fig. 8.5) by injection of contrast material intravenously or by retrograde instillation into the ureter. Injection of contrast intra-arterially (Fig. 8.6) may reveal vascular abnormalities or abnormal vascular patterns characteristic of malignant change in the kidney. A plain X-ray of the abdomen may reveal radiopaque calculi along the course of the ureter, which lies, as seen radiographically, over the tips of the transverse processes of the lumbar vertebrae, in front of the sacroiliac joint, and over the ischial spine prior to passing medially to the bladder (Fig. 8.8b). Obstruction of the ureter by stone or clot produces sharp severe renal colic, felt in the lateral abdomen, the groin and, sometimes, the external genitalia (see 'Nerve supply', p. 125).

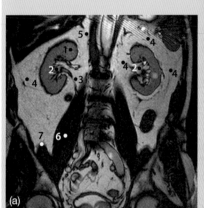
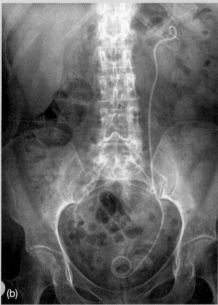
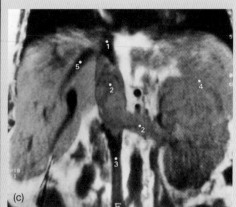

Figure 8.8 (a) Coronal MR image of normal kidneys: 1, upper pole of kidney; 2, hilum of kidney; 3, ureter; 4, perinephric fat (white region); 5, right crus of diaphragm; 6, psoas muscle; 7, quadratus lumborum muscle. (b) Plain X-ray of an abdomen showing a stent in the left ureter. (c) MR image of a coronal abdominal section illustrating left renal carcinoma with tumour extending along the renal vein into the inferior vena cava: 1, inferior vena cava above tumour mass; 2, tumour mass in inferior vena cava and left renal vein; 3, inferior vena cava below tumour mass; 4, renal carcinoma; 5, hepatic vein

THE SUPRARENALS

These lie on the upper pole of each kidney, enclosed in a sheath outside but adjacent to the perirenal fascia (Fig. 8.9). Each weighs about 5 g. The **right suprarenal** is pyramidal in shape (Fig. 8.10a) and lies on the right crus of the diaphragm behind the inferior vena cava. The **left suprarenal** is crescentic (Fig. 8.10b) and lies superomedially, its lower pole reaching the hilum of the kidney. It lies in front of the left crus, behind the pancreas and splenic vessels. Between the two glands is the coeliac plexus, with which they are intimately connected.

Blood supply

This is via suprarenal arteries arising on each side from the phrenic and renal arteries and the aorta. A large vein drains, on the right, to the inferior vena cava and, on the left, to the left renal vein.

Nerve supply

Preganglionic fibres from the thoracic splanchnic nerves, especially the greater splanchnic (Fig. 4.17, p. 72), pass via the coeliac plexus to end by synapsing with cells in the suprarenal medulla.

THE POSTERIOR ABDOMINAL WALL

The posterior abdominal wall is a series of layers starting with the lumbar vertebrae posteriorly, covered by the psoas and quadratus lumborum muscles. Lying over the muscles are the aorta and inferior vena cava and renal branches attached to the kidneys themselves. Next, moving anteriorly, are the gonadal vessels overlying the ureters and, most anteriorly, are the branches of the inferior mesenteric vessels, even more so on the left hand side. This arrangement leaves two deep channels known as the paravertebral gutters lateral to ascending and descending colons, which drain down towards the pelvis and crainally towards the diaphragm providing the potential of pelvic and subphrenic abscess.

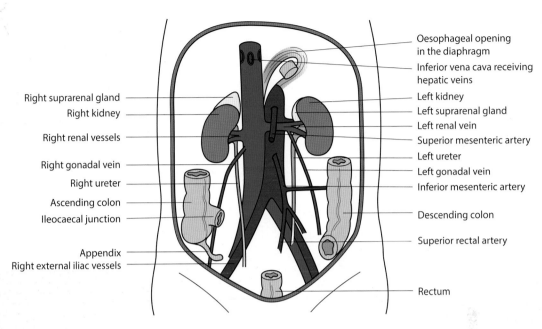

Figure 8.9 Posterior abdominal wall viscera

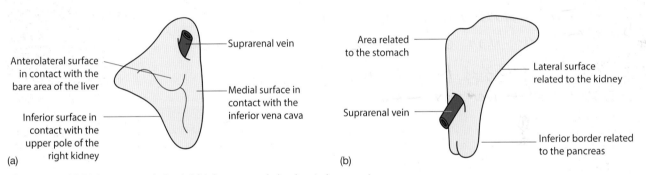

Figure 8.10 (a) Right suprarenal gland; (b) left suprarenal gland, anterior aspect

Psoas major

Its attachments are: *vertebral* – from the fibrous arches across the bodies of the lumbar vertebrae, intervertebral discs and transverse processes of the lumbar vertebrae; *femoral* – the lesser trochanter. It acts to flex and medially rotate the femur and, acting with its partner, flexes the trunk.

It is supplied by the 1st, 2nd and 3rd lumbar nerves.

Quadratus lumborum

This flat muscle lies between psoas major and transversus abdominis laterally. Its attachments are: *superior* – the lower border of the 12th rib; *inferior* – the iliolumbar ligament and the nearby iliac crest. Its action is to fix the 12th rib (which improves the effect of contraction of the diaphragm) and lateral flexion of the trunk.

It is supplied by the 12th thoracic and the upper four lumbar nerves.

The iliacus muscle is described on p. 140.

The **thoracolumbar fascia** (Fig. 8.11) encloses the muscles of the posterior abdominal wall and fuses laterally to give attachment to internal oblique and transversus abdominis muscles. It possesses three layers:

- The stronger posterior layer covers the erector spinae and is reinforced by the aponeurosis of latissimus dorsi. It is attached medially to the lumbar and sacral spines and continues superiorly to become the deep fascia of the back and neck.
- The middle layer lies between the erector spinae and quadratus lumborum; it is attached medially to the lumbar transverse processes and extends between the iliac crest and the 12th rib.
- The anterior layer is thin and covers quadratus lumborum, separating it from psoas. Superiorly it is thickened to form the lateral arcuate ligament, an origin for the diaphragm.

The **psoas fascia** forms a thick sheath over the muscle. It extends behind the inguinal ligament into the thigh to contribute to the femoral sheath. Superiorly it is thickened and forms the medial arcuate ligament of the diaphragm.

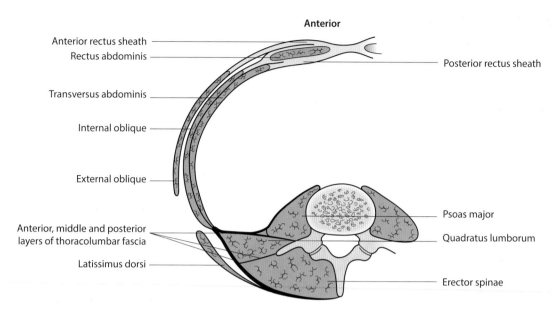

Figure 8.11 Transverse section through the abdomen showing abdominal muscles and thoracolumbar fascia

Tuberculosis arising in the lumbar spine may track down within the psoas sheath and present as a swelling in the groin below the inguinal ligament. Such **psoas abscesses** are always associated with spasm of the psoas muscle and a flexion deformity of the hip (Fig. 8.12). Infection or inflammation in any of the structures lying anterior to the psoas muscle, kidneys, ureters, appendix or sigmoid colon may produce some spasm and pain on contraction of the affected psoas muscle. The 'psoas' test involves lying the patient on the unaffected side and demonstrating painful and possibly limited extension of the hip.

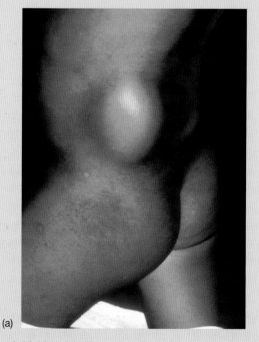

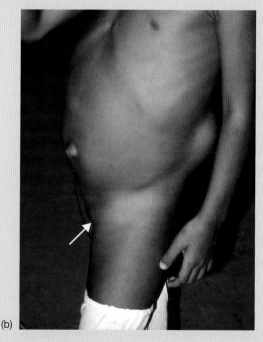

(a)

(b)

Figure 8.12 (a) and (b) This young girl has a tuberculous infection in the lower left lumbar vertebrae that has formed a large abscess in her back. The pus from this abscess has tracked down the sheath of the left psoas muscle from the posterior abdominal wall towards the lesser trochanter of the femur and has appeared as a soft swelling in the groin, easily mistaken for a hernia (arrow). It has also caused flexion of the left hip

Nerves of the posterior abdominal wall

These comprise the subcostal nerve and the upper branches of the lumbosacral plexus (Figs. 8.13 and 8.14).

The **subcostal nerve**, the ventral ramus of the 12th thoracic nerve, enters the abdomen under the lateral arcuate ligament on quadratus lumborum to cross the muscle obliquely. It supplies the posterior wall muscles and the skin and parietal peritoneum in the suprapubic region.

The **lumbar part of the lumbosacral plexus** forms in the substance of psoas from the ventral rami of the first four lumbar nerves.

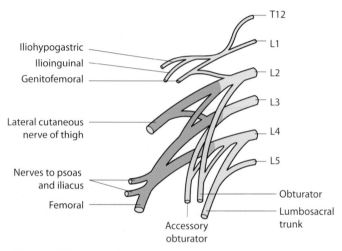

Figure 8.13 Lumbar plexus

Branches

The **iliohypogastric** and **ilioinguinal** nerves pass laterally around the posterior abdominal wall (Figs. 8.14a,b), the latter passing along the inguinal canal. They supply the anterior wall muscles and skin over the pubis and external genitalia. The genitofemoral nerve descends on the surface of psoas; the genital branch traverses the inguinal canal to supply the cremasteric muscle and the femoral branch, passing below the inguinal ligament to supply the skin of the femoral triangle. The **lateral femoral cutaneous nerve** descends on iliacus and enters the thigh under the lateral inguinal ligament just below the anterior superior iliac spine, to supply the skin over the upper lateral thigh. The **femoral nerve** (2nd, 3rd and 4th lumbar nerves) descends between iliacus and psoas, passing deep to the inguinal ligament on the lateral side of the femoral artery. In the abdomen it supplies iliacus. Its distribution in the thigh is described on p. 260. The **obturator nerve** (2nd, 3rd and 4th lumbar nerves) descends medial to psoas along the medial pelvic wall to the obturator foramen, through which it passes into the thigh. In the female it lies just lateral to the ovary. It has no branches in the pelvis; its branches in the thigh are described on p. 260. The **lumbosacral trunk** (4th and 5th lumbar nerves) descends medial to psoas over the lateral sacrum to join the sacral part of the lumbosacral plexus (p. 162). The autonomic nerves of the abdomen are described on p. 162.

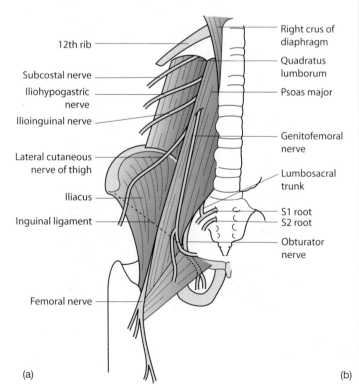

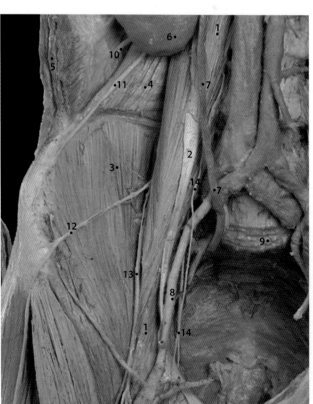

Figure 8.14 (a) Nerves of the lumbar plexus on the posterior abdominal wall and their relations to the psoas muscle. (b) Dissection of the posterior abdominal wall with lumbar plexus: 1, psoas major muscle; 2, psoas minor muscle; 3, iliacus muscle; 4, quadratus lumborum muscle; 5, lateral abdominal wall muscles (three layers); 6, kidney; 7, ureter; 8, external iliac artery; 9, sacral promontory; 10, iliohypogastric nerve; 11, ilioinguinal nerve; 12, lateral cutaneous nerve of the thigh; 13, femoral nerve; 14, genitofemoral nerve

Blood supply

1. Abdominal aorta

The abdominal aorta, the continuation of the thoracic aorta, enters the abdomen between the two crura of the diaphragm in front of the 12th thoracic vertebra. It descends on the posterior abdominal wall slightly to the left of the midline (Fig. 8.9), and ends on the body of the 4th lumbar vertebra by dividing into the two common iliac arteries (Fig. 8.15).

Relations

The abdominal aorta is surrounded by autonomic nerve plexuses and ganglia, lymph vessels and nodes. The cisterna chyli lies between it and the right crus. It lies on the bodies of the upper four lumbar vertebrae, and the lumbar veins traverse behind it. On its right is the inferior vena cava and cisterna chyli; on its left lie the left sympathetic trunk and, from above downwards, the left crus, the pancreas, the fourth part of the duodenum and the small intestine. Anteriorly, from above downwards, it is covered by the lesser sac, the pancreas and splenic vein, the left renal vein, the third part of the duodenum and coils of small intestine.

Branches

The abdominal aorta has unpaired and paired branches:

- **Unpaired** – these are the arteries supplying the abdominal alimentary tract, namely the **coeliac, superior and inferior mesenteric arteries** and the **median sacral**, descending to the pelvis to supply the lower rectum.
- **Paired** – the **inferior phrenic arteries** arise as the aorta enters the abdomen to supply the crura and the suprarenal arteries. The **suprarenal arteries** are two or three small short vessels to each gland; the **renal arteries** arise at the level of the 1st lumbar vertebra, pass laterally, and divide into terminal branches in the hilum of each kidney. The shorter left artery crosses the left crus and psoas behind the body of the pancreas; the right artery crosses the right crus and psoas behind the neck of the pancreas and the inferior vena cava. Each supplies the kidney, upper ureter and suprarenal gland.

The **testicular arteries** arise at the level of the 2nd lumbar vertebra, descend the posterior abdominal wall obliquely and pass around the pelvic brim to the deep inguinal ring, where each passes in the spermatic cord to supply the testis.

The **ovarian arteries** follow a course similar to the testicular arteries in the abdomen, but at the pelvic brim they cross the external iliac vessels to be conveyed in the suspensory ligaments of the ovary to supply that structure. Each anastomoses with the uterine artery in the broad ligament of the uterus.

There are four pairs of **lumbar arteries**, which each pass back, deep to psoas, to supply the vertebral column, spinal cord and posterior abdominal wall.

Atheroma, a degenerative arterial disease, produces several adverse effects: loss of elasticity of the walls of the larger vessels, luminal narrowing due to subintimal lipid deposits, and loss of smooth muscle of the arterial wall with thinning, loss of strength and consequent dilatation of the artery. The dilatation is known as an **aneurysm** and the abdominal aorta is the artery most commonly affected (Fig. 8.16).

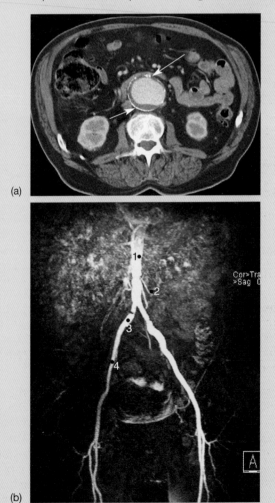

Figure 8.16 (a) Axial CT scan of the lumbar region showing an enlarged abdominal aortic aneurysm (arrows). Lying immediately anterior to the vertebral body it is about 4–5 cm in diameter and can be seen to have a double or false passage as well as calcification deposits along its outer edge; these are seen as white spots in the aortic wall (arrows). (b) Arteriogram showing arteries with atherosclerotic irregularity, the internal iliac arteries occluded: 1, aorta; 2, lumbar artery; 3, common iliac; 4, external iliac

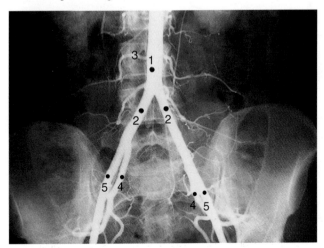

Figure 8.15 Abdominal aortogram: 1, aorta; 2, common iliac arteries; 3, lumbar artery; 4, internal iliac arteries; 5, external iliac arteries

2. Inferior vena cava

The inferior vena cava (Fig. 8.9) is formed in front of the body of the 5th lumbar vertebra by union of the two common iliac veins, and ascends the posterior abdominal wall covered by peritoneum to the right of the midline to the caval opening in the central tendon of the diaphragm. It traverses the diaphragm at the level of the 8th thoracic vertebra and, after a short thoracic course, opens into the right atrium.

Relations

The inferior vena cava lies on the right psoas, the sympathetic trunk, the lower two lumbar vertebrae and the right crus, from which it is separated by the right suprarenal gland and right renal artery. Anteriorly it is related, from below upwards, to the right common iliac artery, the root of the small bowel mesentery, the third part of the duodenum, the head of pancreas and common bile duct, the second part of the duodenum, the opening into the lesser sac and the visceral surface of the liver. The aorta is in contact with its left side and the right ureter lies to its right.

Tributaries

- The lower two **lumbar veins**.
- The right **gonadal vein** (the left gonadal vein drains into the left renal vein).
- The **renal veins**, formed in the hilum of the kidney, which lie anterior to the renal arteries. The right vein, 3 cm long, lies behind the second part of the duodenum; the left, about 8 cm long, lies behind the body of the pancreas and crosses anterior to the aorta.
- The right **suprarenal vein**.
- **Hepatic veins**, two or three large trunks and a variable number of smaller vessels conveying portal and systemic blood from the liver. They have no extrahepatic course.
- The **phrenic veins**.

If the inferior vena cava is obstructed by thrombus or tumour, collateral channels develop to return blood to the heart. For example:

- Within the rectus sheath of the anterior abdominal wall, the inferior epigastric veins, branches of the external iliac vein, anastomose with the superior epigastric vein, which passes via the internal thoracic veins to the superior vena cava.
- Branches of the saphenous vein, the circumflex iliac vein and the superficial epigastric vein anastomose in the lateral abdominal wall with branches of the axillary vein, such as the lateral thoracic vein, to carry blood to the superior vena cava. The collateral channels become dilated and tortuous and are visible in these circumstances.

Lymphatic drainage

See p. 104.

DEVELOPMENT OF THE KIDNEYS AND URETERS

During fetal development three different functional sets of kidneys form sequentially on the posterior body wall, from cranial to caudal, from three regions of intermediate mesoderm. The left and right pronephros (pronephric kidneys) appear first in a cranial position on the posterior abdominal wall. These degenerate to be replaced by the mesonephric kidneys, which themselves degenerate to be replaced by the metanephric kidneys, the final kidneys (Fig. 8.17). The metanephric kidneys form in the pelvic cavity from the ureteric bud and metanephric blastema.

Subsequent growth of the fetal body brings about a relative change in position of the metanephric kidneys such that they ascend the posterior abdominal wall to achieve their final position (Fig. 8.18d). Due to this movement the kidneys can be found in ectopic locations such as the pelvis or lower abdomen, or on the same side of the body (crossed renal ectopia), where they may also fuse together (Fig. 8.18). Fusion of the kidneys can also occur in other situations; pelvic kidneys may fuse to produce a discoid-shaped kidney, and fusion of the inferior poles of the kidneys while in the pelvic cavity can create a horseshoe kidney (Fig. 8.18c), the ascent of which is limited by the origin of the inferior mesenteric artery. Supernumerary kidneys (Fig. 8.18b) can be present along the route of ascent of the metanephric kidneys and may be due to the formation of duplicate ureteric buds.

During their ascent, the point of origin of the arterial supply to the kidneys changes regularly, with new

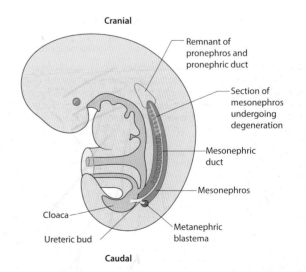

Cranial

Remnant of pronephros and pronephric duct

Section of mesonephros undergoing degeneration

Mesonephric duct

Mesonephros

Cloaca

Ureteric bud

Metanephric blastema

Caudal

Figure 8.17 Development of the kidneys (left lateral view) from the left pronephros, mesonephros and metanephros (ureteric bud and metanephric blastema) and the left mesonephric duct. Renal development occurs bilaterally. The final kidneys are the metanephric kidneys

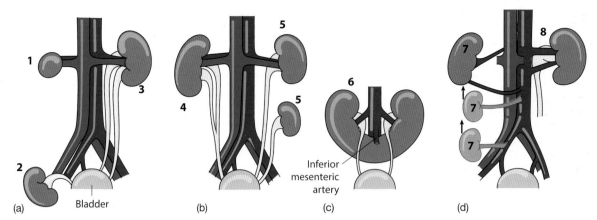

Figure 8.18 Abnormal renal development: 1, agenesis; 2, pelvic position; 3, duplicate ureter and renal pelvis; 4, bifid ureter; 5, multilpe/supernumerary kidneys; 6, horseshoe kidney; 7, route of ascent of the kidney (arrows) from the pelvic cavity to the posterior abdominal wall, and the changing origin of its blood supply – an additional polar artery remains in the final (superiormost) kidney; 8, aberrant renal artery obstructing the ureter leading to hydronephrosis

renal arteries arising from successively higher parts of the iliac and then abdominal aortic arterial system. Failure of regression of previous renal arteries can lead to accessory/multiple renal arteries or a polar renal artery that can obstruct the ureter, resulting in hydronephrosis (Fig. 8.18d).

The early stages of the developing kidneys drain urine to the cloaca via correspondingly named duct systems; for example this initially occurs via the the pronephric duct, a part of which subsequenlty becomes the mesonephric duct system. The ureteric bud of the metanephric kidney branches from the proximal mesonephric duct to form the ureter. The bud continues to sequentially branch to form the collecting duct system of kidney, including the glomerular capsule, nephron loop, convoluted tubules and calyces. The joining of some of the earlier branches of the collecting tubule system forms the major and minor renal calyces. Abnormalities in ureteric bud branching can lead to bifid or duplicate ureters (Fig. 8.18a,b).

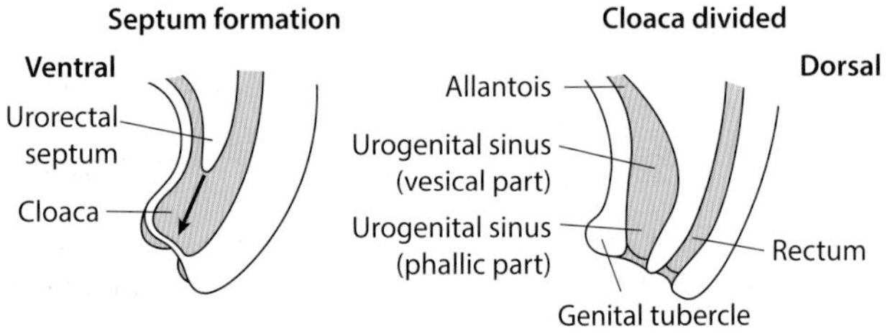

Bladder and urachus

The bladder epithelium forms from the vesical part of the urogenital sinus of the ventral cloaca. The cloaca is divided into ventral and dorsal parts by growth of the urorectal septum (Fig. 8.19). The ventral part is joined by the tube-like allantois, which projects into the umbilical region. The allantois normally fibroses to form the urachus, which can be seen in the adult as the median umbilical ligament. Defects of urachal development or remnants of urachal tissue can lead to the formation of cysts anywhere along the course of the urachus, or to sinuses that open to either the umbilicus or bladder (Fig. 8.20). A urachal sinus in the umbilical region may discharge into the umbilicus, become infected or lead to abscess formation. A urachal fistula may result in the discharge of urine from the umbilicus.

Figure 8.19 Division of the urorectal septum into the urogential sinus (ventral) and rectum (dorsal) via downgrowth of the urorectal septum (arrow). The vesical part of the urogenital sinus forms the bladder epithelium and receives the mesonephric ducts. The allantois passes from the anterior midline of the bladder to the umbilical cord

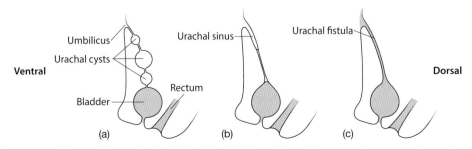

Figure 8.20 Developmental defects of the urachus (left lateral view). (a) Urachal cysts form anywhere along the urachus due to the persistence of part of its lining. (b) Urachal sinus opening into the umbilicus (can open into the bladder) due to persistence of a segment of the urachal lumen. (c) Urachal fistula due to failure of closure of the urachus, resulting in urine leaking from the umbilicus

MCQs

1. The inferior vena cava: **T/F**

a passes through the diaphragm at the level of the 8th thoracic vertebra   (___)

b lies in a deep groove on the posterior aspect of the liver   (___)

c is related to the fourth part of the duodenum   (___)

d in the abdomen, lies to the left of the aorta   (___)

e is formed by the union, in front of the right common iliac artery, of the two common iliac veins   (___)

Answers

1.

a **T** – *Accompanied by the right phrenic nerve.*

b **T** – *It is embedded in the posterior surface of the liver.*

c **F** – *It ascends the posterior abdominal wall, passing behind the third part of the duodenum.*

d **F** – *It lies to the right of the aorta throughout its abdominal course.*

e **F** – *Despite being formed by the two common iliac veins, their union lies posterior to the right common iliac artery.*

---

2. The psoas major muscle: **T/F**

a is attached to the middle of the sides of the lumbar vertebral bodies   (___)

b is attached to the lesser trochanter of the femur   (___)

c receives a nerve supply from all the lumbar nerves   (___)

d flexes both the hip joint and the trunk   (___)

e gains the thigh by passing below the pubic rami   (___)

Answers

2.

a **F** – *It is attached to fibrous arches that cross the concave sides of the vertebral bodies to the edge of the bodies, the intervertebral discs between them and the lumbar transverse processes.*

b **T** – *As it approaches the femur it is joined by the iliacus muscle on its lateral side.*

c **F** – *It is supplied by branches of the 1st and 2nd lumbar nerves.*

d **T** – *Contraction produces flexion and medial rotation at the hip joint or flexion of the lumbar trunk on the femur.*

e **F** – *It gains the thigh by passing posterior to the inguinal ligament above the superior pubic ramus.*

---

3. The ureter: **T/F**

a contains circular and longitudinal smooth muscle   (___)

b is lined by columnar epithelium   (___)

c is innervated by L2, L3 and L4   (___)

d develops from the mesonephric duct   (___)

e descends the posterior abdominal wall on a line joining the tips of the transverse processes of the lumbar vertebrae   (___)

Answers

3.

a **T** – *The ureter is a muscular structure and peristalsis occurs.*

b **F** – *It is lined, as is the bladder, with transitional epithelium.*

c **F** – *The sensory nerve supply is from the lower thoracic nerves, L1 and L2.*

d **T** – *The ureter develops from the mesonephric duct, the kidney from the metanephric cap.*

e **T** – *This radiologically defined relationship is of great clinical use. Radiopaque calculi within the ureter can be seen overlying this line.*

SBA

1. A young man is admitted with a 24-hour history of nausea, anorexia and vomiting. Examination reveals marked tenderness in the right iliac fossa and persistent flexion of the right thigh, which the patient finds painful to overcome. The likely diagnosis is appendicitis, but which muscle is in spasm?
a biceps femoris
b obturator externus
c psoas major
d adductor magnus
e gluteus maximus

Answer

1.
c *Psoas major is attached proximally to the lumbar vertebrae and distally to the lesser trochanter of the femur. In this case inflammation of the appendix, which often lies on the anterior surface of the psoas, has caused spasm of the muscle and thus flexion of the thigh on the trunk.*

2. During an operation for a bleeding duodenal ulcer the surgeon accidentally damages a structure posterior to the epiploic foramen, with the result that the operative field quickly fills with blood. What structure is likely to have been damaged?
a portal vein
b aorta
c inferior vena cava
d right renal artery
e superior mesenteric artery

Answer

2.
c *The inferior vena cava lies immediately behind the epiploic foramen, covered by the parietal peritoneum of the posterior abdominal wall.*

EMQs

Each question has an anatomical theme linked to the chapter, and a list of 10 related items (A–J) placed in alphabetical order: these are followed by five statements (1–5). Match **one or more** of the items A–J to each of the five statements.

Relationships of the kidney, ureter and adrenal glands
A. Female pelvic ureter
B. Left abdominal ureter
C. Left adrenal gland
D. Left kidney
E. Left renal pelvis
F. Male pelvic ureter
G. Right abdominal ureter
H. Right suprarenal gland
I. Right kidney
J. Right renal pelvis

Answers
1 B, 2 AF, 3 HI, 4 I, 5 E

Match the following statements with the appropriate item(s) from the above list.
1. Crossed by the root of the sigmoid mesentery
2. Turns medially near the spine of the ischium
3. Related to the bare area of the liver
4. Related to the proximal transverse colon
5. Related to the tail of the pancreas

APPLIED QUESTIONS

1. Describe the structures pierced by a needle in performing a percutaneous renal biopsy.

1. The needle pierces, in succession, the skin, the superficial fascia, the posterior layer of the lumbar fascia and, usually, the lateral part of quadratus lumborum. It passes through the anterior lumbar fascia and perinephric fascia and fat, and then, with the patient holding their breath in inspiration, it is advanced into the kidney. It is advisable to biopsy the lower pole, as parietal pleura covers the upper part of the kidney.

2. Discuss the clinical significance of the relations of the iliopsoas muscle.

2. The iliopsoas muscle has important relations to the kidney, ureter, caecum, appendix, sigmoid colon, pancreas and nerves of the posterior abdominal wall. When any of these structures are diseased, especially if they are the site of infection, the muscle goes into spasm – a protective reflex – and any movement of it causes pain. This physical sign often gives important diagnostic clues. A chronic tuberculous abscess in a lumbar vertebra may spread to the psoas and within its sheath, to track down within it and present as a fluctuant swelling in the femoral triangle of the thigh.

The pelvis

The bony pelvis comprises two hip (innominate) bones, the sacrum and the coccyx, which when articulated enclose the pelvic cavity. The hip bones articulate anteriorly with each other at the symphysis pubis and posteriorly with the sacrum at the sacroiliac joints.

THE HIP (INNOMINATE) BONE

This large irregularly shaped bone has three parts – the ilium above, the ischium below and the pubis in front. In the child they join in a Y-shaped epiphyseal cartilage in the **acetabulum**, a laterally placed cup-shaped fossa with which the femoral head articulates. The epiphyses close by late puberty. The ilium expands upwards as a fan-shaped bone and, below it, the pubis and ischium join to enclose the obturator foramen and form the anterolateral walls of the true pelvis (**Figs. 9.1a,b**).

The **ilium** forms the upper two-fifths of the acetabulum and expands superiorly into a flattened plate, the **ala**, which has lateral (gluteal) and medial (pelvic) surfaces surmounted by the **iliac crest** and separated by anterior and posterior borders. The gluteal surface gives attachment to the glutei: gluteus minimus, gluteus medius and gluteus maximus from anterior to posterior. The medial surface is divided into a posterior **auricular surface**, which articulates with the sacrum, and an anterior **iliac fossa** from whose upper two-thirds arises the iliacus muscle. Posteriorly it bears the roughened **iliac tuberosity** for the sacroiliac ligaments. The short **anterior border** bears two small projections, the subcutaneous **anterior superior iliac spine** to which the inguinal ligament is attached, and the **anterior inferior iliac spine**, an origin of rectus femoris. The posterior border gives attachment to the sacrotuberous ligament and also has two projections, the **posterior superior and posterior inferior iliac spines**. The

curved and palpable **iliac crest** extends from the anterior to the posterior superior iliac spines. It is thick and gives attachment to muscles of the lateral and posterior abdominal walls, tensor fascia lata anteriorly and gluteus maximus posteriorly.

The highest points of the two iliac crests (intercristal plane) are at the level of the 4th lumbar vertebra and mark the level of the preferred site for lumbar puncture (the L4–L5 intervertebral space is wide and allows access to the subarachnoid space below the termination of the spinal cord). The iliac crest is a common site for bone biopsy (see **Fig. 5.1**, p. 80 and **Fig. 8.1**, p. 123), using the posterior superior spine as a landmark (it lies under the skin dimple, the 'dimple of Venus') to the medial side of the upper buttock. It is more prominent in females and lies at the level of S2.

The **ischium**, an L-shaped bone, has a body and a ramus. The **body** forms two-fifths of the acetabulum and expands inferiorly to form the **ischial tuberosity**, which gives attachment to the hamstring muscles and the sacrotuberous ligament. To the femoral surface of the body is attached obturator externus. Above the tuberosity the body is crossed by the sciatic nerve, lying above a conical **ischial spine** that separates the **greater sciatic notch (foramen)** above from the **lesser sciatic notch (foramen)** below. To the spine are attached levator ani and the sacrospinous ligament, thus producing the lessor sciatic foramen (**Figs. 9.2a,b**). The pelvic surface of the body gives attachment to the obturator internus muscle, and levator ani and coccygeus are attached to the medial surface of the spine.

The **pubis** has a body and superior and inferior pubic rami, which join with the superior and inferior rami of the ischium to enclose the obturator foramen. The outer surface of the **body** gives attachment to adductor muscles, and the inner surface is related to the bladder and gives attachment to levator ani. The oval symphyseal surface is covered by hyaline

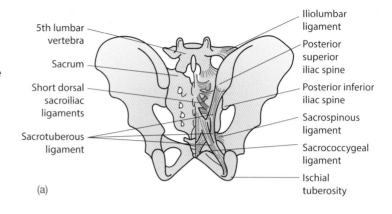

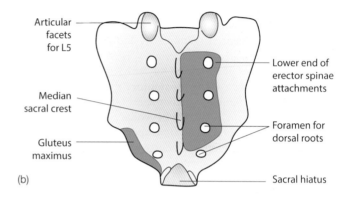

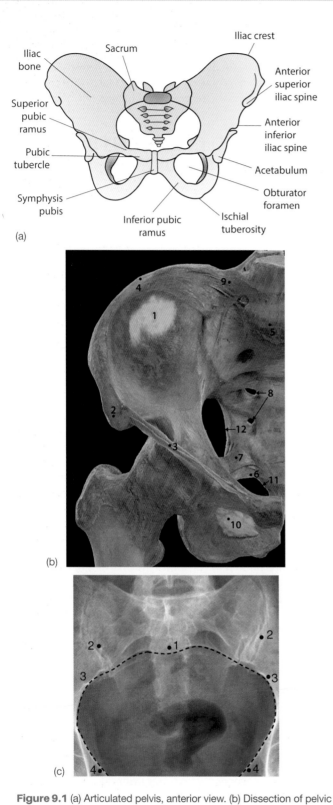

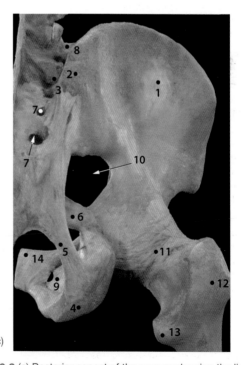

Figure 9.1 (a) Articulated pelvis, anterior view. (b) Dissection of pelvic bones and ligaments, anterior view: 1, iliac bone (thin); 2, anterior superior iliac spine; 3, inguinal ligament; 4, iliac crest; 5, sacral promontory; 6, sacrotuberous ligament; 7, sacrospinous ligament; 8, anterior sacral foramina; 9, iliolumbar ligaments; 10, obturator foramen covered by membrane; 11, lesser sciatic notch (foramen); 12, greater sciatic notch (foramen). (c) X-ray view: 1, sacrum; 2, sacroiliac joints; 3, arcuate line; 4, pectineal line. The pelvic inlet or brim, through which the fetal head must pass down into the true pelvis (dashed line), is bounded by these four structures above and the pubic symphysis anteriorly

Figure 9.2 (a) Posterior aspect of the sacrum showing the ligaments of the pelvis. (b) Muscle attachments. (c) Dissection of posterior view of the pelvic bones and ligaments: 1, iliac bone; 2, posterior superior iliac spine; 3, sacroiliac joint; 4, ischial tuberosity; 5, sacrotuberous ligament; 6, sacrospinous ligament; 7, posterior sacral foramina; 8, iliolumbar ligaments; 9, obturator foramen covered by membrane; 10, greater sciatic notch (foramen); 11, posterior hip joint capsule; 12, greater trochanter of femur; 13, lesser trochanter of femur, 14, pubic symphysis

cartilage and joined to its fellow by a fibrocartilaginous disc and ligaments. Its superior border, the **pubic crest**, is palpable and gives attachment to rectus abdominis, the conjoint tendon and the external oblique aponeurosis. The palpable **pubic tubercle**, at the lateral end of the crest, gives attachment to the inguinal ligament. The superior ramus bears a ridge diverging from the pubic tubercle; the **pectineal line** gives attachment to part of the inguinal ligament. In the midline the pubic bones articulate to form the **pubic arch**.

The **sacrum** is formed of five fused sacral vertebrae (Figs. 9.2b and 9.3a). Triangular in shape, it possesses a base superiorly, an apex inferiorly and a dorsal, a pelvic and two lateral surfaces. It is divided by four paired rows of sacral foramina into a median portion, corresponding to the fused vertebral bodies, and a pair of lateral masses, formed of the transverse processes. The pelvic and dorsal **sacral foramina** communicate with the central sacral canal and convey the sacral segmental nerves.

The **base** faces upwards and forwards; its projecting anterior margin is known as the **promontory**. It bears an articular facet for the 5th lumbar vertebra anterior to the opening of the sacral canal, on each side of which are two projecting **superior articular processes**. The **apex** articulates with the coccyx. The pelvic surface is concave; the alae give attachment to piriformis. The upper part of the surface is in contact with peritoneum and the lower part with the rectum. The dorsal surface is convex and irregular, giving attachment to erector spinae, the thoracolumbar fascia and gluteus maximus. In the midline it bears a **median sacral crest**. Inferiorly the posterior wall of the sacral canal is deficient between paired sacral cornua, forming the **sacral hiatus**, which is closed by fibrous tissue. The **sacral canal** contains, within the meninges, the end of the cauda equina and cerebrospinal fluid, and, extradurally, the external vertebral venous plexus and spinal nerves. The lateral surface bears a roughened **auricular sur-**face for articulation with the ilium and, posteriorly, a pitted area for attachment of the strong interosseous ligaments.

The **coccyx** is small and triangular and is formed by the fusion of four coccygeal vertebrae. It articulates with the apex of the sacrum and is the remnant of a human tail.

JOINTS AND LIGAMENTS OF THE PELVIC GIRDLE

Sacroiliac joint

The sacroiliac joint is a plane synovial joint between the irregular auricular surfaces of the sacrum and ilium; in older people it may become partly fibrous and may even fuse.

Ligaments

- **Capsular** – attached to the articular margins with capsular thickenings – the very strong ventral and dorsal sacroiliac ligaments.
- **Extracapsular** – the interosseous sacroiliac ligament is also very strong and unites the auricular surfaces of the two bones.
- **Accessory ligaments** – (i) the **sacrotuberous ligament** – a strong thick band from the ischial tuberosity to the coccyx, lateral crest of the sacrum and posterior iliac spines; (ii) the **sacrospinous ligament** – a triangular ligament that converges from the lateral margin of the sacrum and coccyx to the ischial spine (Fig. 9.2a); (iii) the **iliolumbar ligament** –which attaches the 5th lumbar transverse process to the posterior iliac crest.

Functional aspects

Movement is limited by the joint's irregularities to slight gliding and rotation; stability is maintained entirely by ligaments. Body weight is transmitted through the vertebral column and tends to rotate the sacrum forwards, but this is resisted by the sacrospinous and sacrotuberous ligaments.

The sacral hiatus is used to introduce anaesthetic solutions into the sacral canal and block the sacral nerve roots (**caudal epidural block**). Thus the birth canal, the pelvic floor and perineum can be anaesthetized, with the lower limbs being spared. A pudendal nerve block is often used during labour to block the pain of an episiotomy. The hormones of late pregnancy allow stretching of these ligaments and a slight increase in movement of the joint, all of which contribute to a 10 per cent increase in the transverse diameter of the female pelvis in late pregnancy, which in turn makes the passage of the fetus much easier.

Sacrococcygeal joint

The sacrococcygeal joint is a secondary cartilaginous joint whose stability is enhanced by a fibrocartilaginous intervertebral disc and a capsular ligament. In late pregnancy there is an increase in laxity of the ligaments and an increased range of movement, which may result in trauma during delivery.

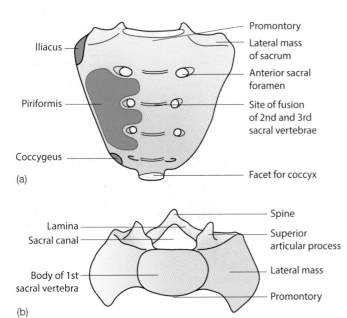

Iliacus

Promontory

Lateral mass of sacrum

Anterior sacral foramen

Piriformis

Site of fusion of 2nd and 3rd sacral vertebrae

Coccygeus

Facet for coccyx

(a)

Lamina
Sacral canal

Spine

Superior articular process

Lateral mass

Body of 1st sacral vertebra

Promontory

(b)

Figure 9.3 Disarticulated sacrum: (a) anterior view showing muscle attachments; (b) superior view

Symphysis pubis

The symphysis pubis (Fig. 9.1) is a secondary cartilaginous joint between the two pubic bones. Its articular surfaces are united by a fibrocartilaginous disc.

Little movement occurs except for a little separation of the pubic bones in late pregnancy. Splitting of this joint (symphysiotomy) is sometimes performed to enlarge the birth canal for delivery.

THE ARTICULATED PELVIS

In the erect posture the pelvis lies obliquely, with the anterior superior iliac spines and pubic symphysis in the same vertical plane; it is divided into greater and lesser parts by the pelvic brim, which runs between the arcuate lines and the promontory of the sacrum. The **greater (false) pelvis** is above the brim and bounds the lower abdominal cavity; the **lesser (true) pelvis** lies below the brim and, because it forms the birth canal, is a space of much obstetric importance. It has an inlet, a cavity and an outlet (Fig. 9.1c).

The **inlet** is the pelvic brim; the male's is heart-shaped but the female's is round or oval, with a transverse diameter (13 cm) usually greater than its anteroposterior diameter (11 cm). The **cavity** is a short curved canal whose posterior wall is three times longer than its anterior wall. It is bounded by the true pelvic surfaces of the hip bones, the sacrum and the sacrospinous and sacrotuberous ligaments. The outlet is diamond-shaped, bounded by the lower border of the pubic symphysis and ischiopubic rami, the sacrotuberous ligaments and the coccyx. In the female the anterior diameter (conjugate) is larger than the transverse diameter.

In the female, the maximum diameter of the pelvic inlet is transverse and that of the outlet is anteroposterior. Thus the larger diameter of the fetal head, the anteroposterior, normally lies along the wider diameter of that part of the pelvis containing it, and in normal labour the head undergoes partial rotation during descent.

Sex differences are more evident in the pelvis than in other bones. The male pelvis is rougher, thicker and heavier; its brim is heart-shaped rather than round/oval; its cavity is longer and the outlet narrower; its acetabulum is larger and the ischiopubic ramus is everted along the attachment of the crura of the penis; and the subpubic angle is less than 90 degrees, often as acute as 60 degrees, whereas the female's is 90 degrees or more (Fig. 9.4).

Pelvimetry

Obstetricians require measurements of the pregnant women's pelvis to assess whether problems may occur in childbirth. Previously done by X-ray, this is now achieved ultrasonically.

Fractures of the pelvis are commonly caused by crush injuries and frequently result in injuries to related soft tissues; i.e. bladder and urethral trauma is associated with fractures of the pubis and major vessel trauma (common and internal iliac) with sacroiliac fractures and dislocation.

MUSCLES AND FASCIAE OF THE PELVIS

The muscles lining the walls of the pelvis – iliacus, obturator internus and piriformis – are covered with pelvic fascia, which, where it overlies the obturator internus, gives attachment to levator ani.

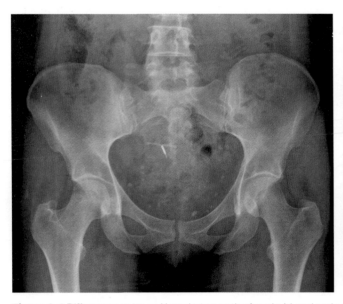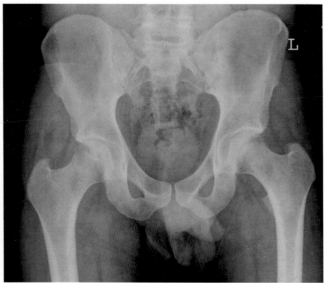

Figure 9.4 Differences seen on X-ray between the female (a) and male (b) pelvis

Note:
1. Female inlet is more circular, male more heart-shaped
2. Female subpubic angle is wide (90–120 degrees), male is narrower (60–90 degrees)
3. Female sacrum is wider and flatter
4. Female ischial spines are further apart (not shown)

Iliacus

Attachments

Pelvic – upper two-thirds of the iliac fossa and sacroiliac ligament; *distal* – the lesser trochanter of the femur.

Nerve supply

The femoral nerve.

Function

Flexion of the trunk on the thigh; flexion and medial rotation of the femur on the trunk.

Obturator internus

Attachments

Pelvic – pelvic surface of the obturator membrane and adjacent bone. It is covered with the strong obturator internus fascia; *femoral* – the fibres converge on the lesser sciatic notch (foramen) and turn laterally to its attachment on the greater trochanter of the femur.

Nerve supply

Nerve to obturator internus, a branch of the sacral plexus.

Function

Lateral rotation of the femur.

Piriformis

Attachments

Sacral – the lateral part of the pelvic surface of the sacrum; *femoral* – passes laterally through the greater sciatic notch (foramen) to the greater trochanter of the femur.

Nerve supply

Direct branches from the sacral plexus.

Function

Lateral rotation of the femur, but it is also an important landmark of the gluteal region.

THE PELVIC FLOOR

This fibromuscular diaphragm, separating the pelvic cavity from the perineum and ischioanal fossae below, is formed by the two levator ani and coccygeus muscles (Fig. 9.5). The **pelvic fascia** has parietal and visceral parts. The parietal part covers the walls and floor of the pelvic cavity. It is thick over obturator internus where levator ani is attached, and

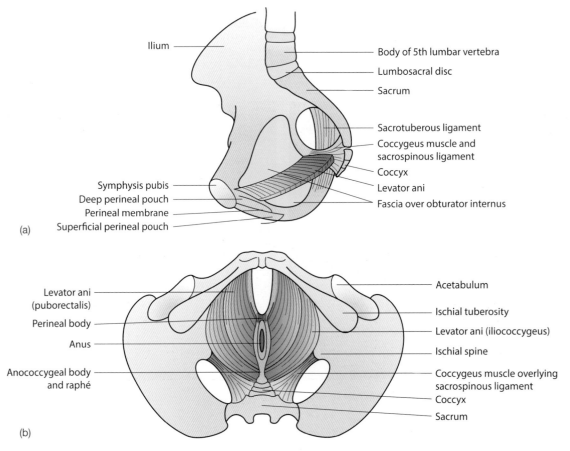

Figure 9.5 (a) Muscles and ligaments of lateral pelvis. (b) Pelvic floor showing parts of levator ani

continuous superiorly with iliacus and the transversalis fascia. It covers levator ani. The vessels of the pelvis lie internal to it and the spinal nerves external to it. The visceral fascia covers the bladder, uterus and rectum. It is thickened over the lower parts of these viscera, forming ligaments that attach and suspend them from the pelvic walls (p. 144).

Levator ani

This is a broad, flat, thin muscle (Fig. 9.5).

Attachments

Lateral – in a continuous line from the back of the body of the pubis, the ischial spine and fascia over obturator internus between the pubis and ischium. *Medial* – the muscle slopes downwards and backwards to the midline and there meets its fellow behind and below the rectum in the midline anococcygeal raphé, which forms a forward-facing gutter offering support to the pelvic viscera.

The anterior fibres pass backwards around the prostate or vagina to the fibrous perineal body or central tendon of the perineum; the middle fibres pass backwards and down around the rectum (puborectalis) to the fibrous anococcygeal body. Some of these fibres blend with the anal sphincter. The posterior fibres pass to the coccyx and the midline raphé lying behind the rectum between it and the anococcygeal body.

Coccygeus

This triangular muscle passes from the ischial spine to the sides of the lower sacrum and coccyx. It lies in the same plane as levator ani.

Functions

Both muscles form the pelvic floor and act together to provide muscular support for the pelvic viscera when intra-abdominal pressure rises during coughing or heavy lifting. The pelvic floor relaxes during the expulsive efforts of defecation and micturition and, by doing so, the floor descends to become more funnel-shaped. It rises again once defecation comes to an end and the anorectal angle is resumed (see p. 143). The muscles also reinforce the urethral sphincter during momentary increases in abdominal pressure such as occurs during coughing or lifting heavy weights. The gutter-like arrangement of the two muscles rotates the fetal head into the anteroposterior plane as it descends through the pelvis during birth.

Nerve supply

Both are supplied by the pudendal nerve and direct branches from S3 and S4.

THE RECTUM AND ANAL CANAL

The **rectum** extends from the sigmoid colon to the anal canal. It lies in the posterior pelvis, is about 12 cm long and begins in front of the 3rd sacral segment, curving forwards with a loop to the left to the tip of the coccyx. Inferiorly it widens – the **rectal ampulla**. It has no mesentery; its upper third is covered by peritoneum on its front and sides, the middle third is covered by peritoneum on its front only and its lower third lies extraperitoneally, embedded in pelvic fascia.

Relations

Its upper part is in contact laterally with coils of small intestine; below this it is related to levator ani and coccygeus. Posteriorly the superior rectal artery, the 3rd, 4th and 5th sacral nerves, the sympathetic plexus and the sacral vessels separate it from the lower sacrum and coccyx. Anteriorly in both sexes the upper two-thirds form the posterior wall of a peritoneal pouch, the rectovesical in the male and the rectouterine (pouch of Douglas) in the female. Below the pouch in the male, anterior to the rectum, lie the seminal vesicles, the ducta deferentia, the bladder and the prostate gland (Figs. 9.6 and 9.7); in the female the vagina and uterus lie anterior to the rectum.

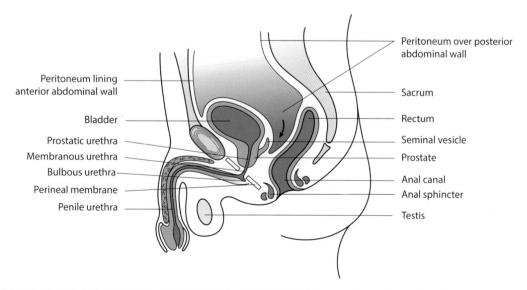

Figure 9.6 Mid-sagittal section of male pelvis showing peritoneal relations, The arrow indicates the peritoneal rectovesical pouch

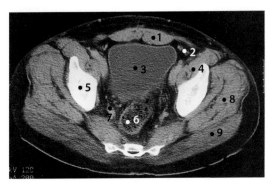

Figure 9.7 MR image of an axial (transverse) section through the male pelvis at the level of the upper bladder: 1, rectus abdominus; 2, external iliac vessels; 3, bladder; 4, iliopsoas; 5, hip bone; 6, rectum; 7, internal iliac vessels; 8, gluteus medius; 9, gluteus maximus

The rectovesical and rectouterine pouches form the lowest part of the peritoneal cavity and are palpable on rectal examination in both sexes. Inflammation of the peritoneum (peritonitis) from, for example, a perforated appendix may result in an abscess collecting in the pouch. Palpation will reveal a tender swelling anterior to the rectal wall. Infection may also be introduced into the pouch by a 'knitting needle' or 'back-street' abortion in which an unintentional perforation of the uterus or posterior vaginal fornix has occurred.

The anal canal

This, the terminal part of the alimentary tract, is 3–4 cm long (Figs. 9.8 and 9.9). It is surrounded by internal and external sphincters that hold it closed except for the occasional passage of flatus and faeces. It descends, turning posteriorly through the pelvic floor at 90 degrees to the rectum, to open externally at the anus. Posteriorly lies the anococcygeal body; laterally levator ani separates it from the ischioanal fossae, and anteriorly the perineal body separates it from, in the female, the lower vagina and, in the male, the bulb of the penis and prostate. The involuntary **internal sphincter**, a continuation of the circular muscle of the rectum, surrounds its upper two-

thirds. The voluntary **external sphincter** encircles the lower two-thirds of the anal canal and is arranged in deep, superficial and subcutaneous parts (Fig. 9.8):

- The deep part surrounds the middle anal canal and is reinforced by fibres of levator ani. Damage to this part of the muscle results in faecal incontinence.
- The superficial part surrounds the lower anal canal, and is attached to the anococcygeal body posteriorly and the perineal body anteriorly.
- The subcutaneous part is a thick ring of muscle surrounding the anal orifice.

The mucous membrane of the upper anal canal reveals 8–10 longitudinal ridges, the anal columns (Fig. 9.8), joined at their distal ends, at the **pectinate line**, by ridges or anal valves into which the anal glands open. Beneath the anal mucosa lie three **anal cushions**, one on the left and two on the right, which are composed of connective tissue and dilated venous tissue. They assist in maintaining continence and closure of the anal canal. The lowest few centimetres of the anal canal is lined by skin.

Blood supply

This is via the superior, middle and inferior rectal arteries. The veins form submucous plexuses that drain via the superior rectal vein to the portal system, and via middle and inferior rectal veins to the internal iliac vein.

Haemorrhoids are caused by congestion of the anal cushions, which is usually the result of straining at defecation. They result in prolapsed and congested anal mucosa that may bleed and, occasionally, strangulate. Haemorrhoids are best assessed with a proctoscope. **Perianal abscesses** originate in the anal glands that emerge in the anal valves. They may spread to form subcutaneous abscesses in the perineum or ischioanal space (clinically known as ischiorectal abscesses). Anal fistulae result from the rupture of abscesses through the skin and usually require surgical excision. Anal fissures – tears in the anal mucosa – are common and occur most frequently in the posterior midline.

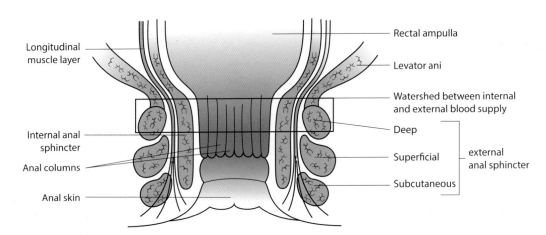

Figure 9.8 Anal sphincter – coronal section

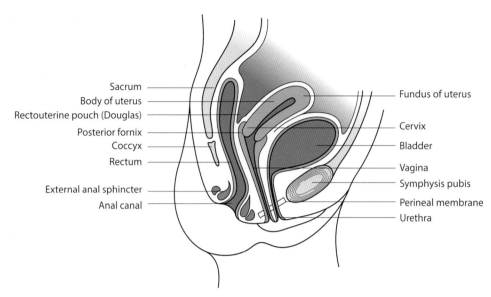

Figure 9.9 Mid-sagittal section of female pelvis showing peritoneal relationships

Labels (left): Sacrum; Body of uterus; Rectouterine pouch (Douglas); Posterior fornix; Coccyx; Rectum; External anal sphincter; Anal canal

Labels (right): Fundus of uterus; Cervix; Bladder; Vagina; Symphysis pubis; Perineal membrane; Urethra

Lymphatic drainage

The rectum and upper anal canal drain via the inferior mesenteric nodes to the para-aortic nodes and thence to preaortic nodes. The upper anal canal drains upwards with those lymphatics of the rectum; the lower anal canal drains to the superficial inguinal nodes.

Cancer of the rectum spreads via the lymph vessels, so surgical attempts at cure must include removal of these nodes. If the whole rectum and anal canal is removed, the cut end of the sigmoid colon is brought out and sutured to the anterior abdominal wall to form an artificial anus (colostomy) (see **Fig. 6.11**, p. 100). **Anal cancer** may present as an enlarged lymph gland in the groin. Its surgical treatment requires removal of the superficial inguinal lymph nodes, and radiotherapy, to which anal cancer is usually responsive, must include the groin nodes in the treatment fields.

Nerve supply

In the rectum and upper anal canal sympathetic nerves from the pelvic plexuses contract the circular muscle of the internal sphincter; parasympathetic nerves from the pelvic splanchnic nerves (S2, S3 and S4) relax the internal sphincter. The lower anal canal and the external sphincter are under voluntary control and are supplied by the inferior rectal nerves and the perineal branch of the 4th sacral nerve.

DEFECATION

Faeces entering the rectum give rise to the desire to defecate. Defecation begins with massive peristaltic waves passing through the colon, which advance more faeces into the rectum. The rectum then contracts to expel the faeces through a relaxed anal canal. Simultaneous contraction of the diaphragm and anterior abdominal wall helps this expulsion. The anal canal is emptied by levator ani pulling forwards the anorectal angle, squeezing its lumen flat while simultaneous relaxation of the voluntary external sphincter occurs. The anal canal is open only during the passage of faeces or flatus, and continence is maintained by these sphincter muscles.

Faecal continence is maintained by complex mechanisms that are not completely understood. It involves both internal and external anal sphincters, but possibly the most important is the anorectal angle maintained by the puborectalis fibres of levator ani. This is usually about 90 degrees, but if it is increased to more than 100 degrees incontinence is likely. Puborectalis, when functioning normally, is palpable rectally as a firm edge posteriorly just above the prostate (the anorectal ring).

On **digital examination** of the rectum, the tip of the coccyx and sacrum are felt posteriorly. Anteriorly, in the male, the prostate, and above it the ducta deferentia and seminal vesicles, may be palpable if diseased; in the female the cervix can be felt through the rectal and vaginal walls. This fact is used by midwives, who assess cervical dilatation during labour via a rectal examination. The anal canal and lower rectum are best examined by a **proctoscope**, but a **sigmoidoscope** is required to examine the whole rectum and lower sigmoid colon. Each gives an opportunity for biopsies to be taken.

THE BLADDER

The bladder is a hollow muscular organ lying extraperitoneally in the anterior pelvis, its lower part surrounded by fibrous tissue. Its wall is composed of smooth muscle, which is lined with transitional epithelium. Its size and shape vary with the amount of urine it contains: when empty it is pyramidal, with an apex behind the pubic symphysis, a posterior base and a superior and two lateral surfaces. When full it is ovoid and distends up behind the anterior abdominal wall. From the apex the median umbilical ligament, a remnant of the urachus, ascends to the umbilicus. The ureters enter the posterolateral angles of the base and the urethra leaves inferiorly at the narrow neck, surrounded by the bladder sphincter.

Peritoneum covers its superior surface and, in the female, passes backwards over the body of the uterus. Pelvic fascia surrounds the bladder base and is thickened to form ligaments, which attach at the back of the pubis (pubovesical and puboprostatic ligaments), the lateral walls of the pelvis (lateral ligaments of the bladder) and the rectum (posterior ligament). The mucosa of the bladder is thrown into many folds (trabeculations) except over a smooth triangular area, the trigone, between the two ureters and the internal urethral orifice inferiorly.

Relations

The inferolateral surfaces are separated by a fat-filled retropubic space from the pubic bones, levator ani and obturator internus; the superior surface is in contact with the small intestine and, in the female, the uterus. The base is in front of the rectum, separated from it in the female by the vagina and in the male by the seminal vesicles and ducta deferentia. Inferiorly the base overlies the prostate or, in the female, the urogenital diaphragm (Figs. 9.6, 9.9 and 9.15a,b below).

Blood supply

This is by superior and inferior vesical branches of the internal iliac arteries. Venous drainage is via the vesical venous plexus to the internal iliac veins.

Lymphatic drainage

This is to the internal and external iliac nodes.

Nerve supply

These are sympathetic fibres (motor to the vesical sphincter and inhibitory to bladder wall) from the 1st and 2nd lumbar segments via the pelvic plexuses. Parasympathetic fibres (motor to the bladder wall and inhibitory to the sphincter) are derived from the pelvic splanchnic nerves S2, S3 and S4. Bladder sensation is carried with the parasympathetic fibres.

MICTURITION

A bladder volume of more than about 300 mL in the adult usually provokes the desire to micturate. Micturition begins with slight relaxation of the vesical sphincter, which allows some urine to enter the urethra (or in the female the upper urethra). This initiates a reflex contraction of the bladder wall (detrusor muscle) and relaxation of the vesical and urethral sphincter muscles. Reflexes producing the desire to micturate can be voluntarily inhibited: the urethral sphincter is contracted, tone increases in the vesical sphincter and the detrusor relaxes. Once urine leaks into the urethra, however, micturition becomes inevitable.

The enlarged obstructed bladder, as it distends into the abdomen, strips off its peritoneal covering and hence it is a simple and safe procedure to introduce a needle/catheter in the midline suprapubically, without entering the peritoneum (suprapubic catheterization). The bladder is prone to injury in fractures involving the pubic and ischial rami. If the bladder is distended when this occurs, it is liable to rupture, with extravasation of urine intra- or extraperitoneally. Cystoscopy allows inspection of the bladder, biopsy of its mucosa and some treatments of small cancers. Advanced cancer of the bladder requires surgical excision.

THE FEMALE INTERNAL GENITAL ORGANS

These comprise the uterus and uterine tubes, the ovaries and the vagina (Figs. 9.9–9.11). All are related to the **broad ligament** of the uterus, a bilateral double layer of peritoneum containing fibrous tissue that extends from the lateral pelvic wall to the lateral margin of the uterus. The **uterine tubes** lie in the medial two-thirds of the ligament's free upper border; the suspensory ligament of the ovary, containing the ovarian vessels, forms in its lateral third. The ovary is attached to the posterior surface of the ligament by a peritoneal fold, the **mesovarium**; this contains the **ovarian ligament**, which is continuous with the **round ligament of the uterus**. Within the base of the broad ligament fibrous tissue, the **parametrium** contains ligaments that attach the uterus to pelvic structures. The uterine artery crosses over the ureter lateral to the cervix.

The uterus

The **uterus** is a pear-shaped, thick-walled, hollow muscular organ about 8 cm long, 5 cm wide and 3 cm thick, lying between the bladder and rectum. It provides protection and nourishment for the fetus. Contraction of its muscular walls propels the fetus through the birth canal. It opens into the vagina below and its long axis is usually directed forwards at right angles to the vagina (anteverted). The upper two-thirds, the **body**, meets the **cervix** at a slight angle, so that the body faces forwards (anteflexion) and overhangs the bladder. The uterine tubes join the body at its upper lateral angle. The part of the body above the tubes is known as the **fundus**.

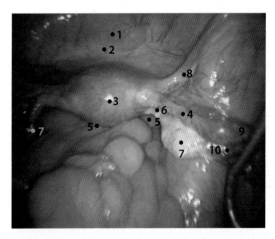

Figure 9.10 Laparoscopic view of the female pelvis: 1, bladder; 2, uterovesical pouch of peritoneum; 3, fundus of uterus; 4, uterine (Fallopian) tube; 5, rectouterine pouch (Douglas); 6, ligament of ovary; 7, ovary; 8, round ligament of uterus; 9, infundibulum of uterine tube; 10, suspensory ligament of ovary

The cylindrical cervix is, because of its attachments, the most fixed part of the uterus. It projects into the upper anterior vaginal wall and is surrounded by a sulcus, the **vaginal fornix**; on the apex of the cervix is the opening of the cervical canal. The larger supravaginal part of the cervix is surrounded by the parametrium and its ligamentous thickenings (see below).

Peritoneum covers much of the uterus posteriorly. It covers the fundus, body, supravaginal cervix and posterior wall (fornix) of the vagina, and anteriorly it covers the fundus and body, before passing on to the superior surface of the bladder (**Fig. 9.9**). From both anterior and posterior surfaces the peritoneum passes laterally as the broad ligament on to the lateral pelvic wall.

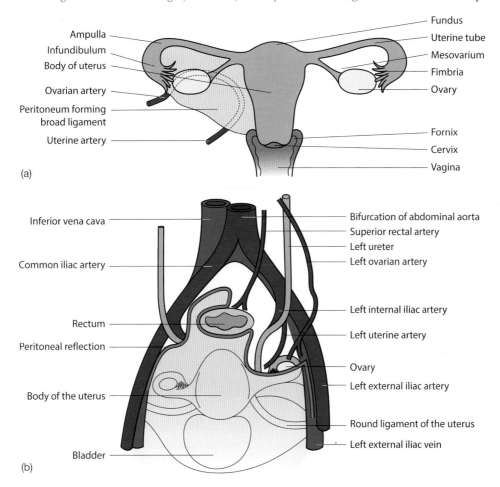

(a)

Ampulla
Infundibulum
Body of uterus
Ovarian artery
Peritoneum forming broad ligament
Uterine artery

Fundus
Uterine tube
Mesovarium
Fimbria
Ovary
Fornix
Cervix
Vagina

Inferior vena cava
Common iliac artery
Rectum
Peritoneal reflection
Body of the uterus
Bladder

Bifurcation of abdominal aorta
Superior rectal artery
Left ureter
Left ovarian artery
Left internal iliac artery
Left uterine artery
Ovary
Left external iliac artery
Round ligament of the uterus
Left external iliac vein

(b)

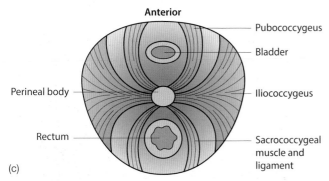

Anterior

Perineal body
Rectum

Pubococcygeus
Bladder
Iliococcygeus
Sacrococcygeal muscle and ligament

(c)

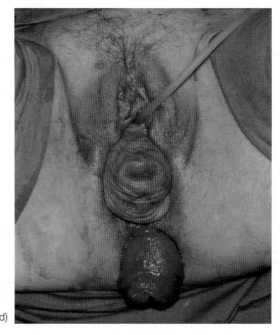

(d)

Figure 9.11 (a) Uterus, uterine tubes and ovaries, posterior view. (b) Pelvic viscera and peritoneum. (c) Perineal body and pelvic floor as seen from below. The perineal body, a tough knot of fibrous tissue, lies between the anal canal and the vagina or bulb of the penis, attached to the posterior border of the perineal membrane. It gives attachment to the external anal sphincter, bulbospongiosus, pubococcygeal and iliococcygeal fibres of levator ani and transverse perineal muscles. These attachments and its central position in the pelvis help stabilize pelvic structures. If torn during childbirth, the pelvic floor may be weakened and contribute to prolapse of the vagina and uterus. (d) Vaginal and rectal prolapse, with a urinary catheter *in situ*

An **intrauterine contraceptive device (IUCD)** is a small plastic device, often covered with copper, which, when placed inside the uterine cavity, reduces the chance of conception. **Dilatation and curettage (D&C)** is frequently employed in the diagnosis of irregular menstrual bleeding: the neck of the cervix is dilated and scrapings of the uterine mucosa are taken for microscopic study. **Cancer of the cervix** is common; it can be diagnosed at an early stage by vaginal examination, which should include obtaining a specimen of its superficial cells by gentle scraping of the cervix and examining the stained specimen microscopically (Papanicolaou smear). This is the basis of the screening programme for cervical cancer.

Ligaments of the uterus

The **round ligament** is a fibromuscular band passing from the upper lateral angle of the uterus through the broad ligament to the deep inguinal ring, and then through the inguinal canal to end in the labium majus (Figs. 9.11a,b). It is a remnant of the gubernaculum ovarii and carries lymph vessels from the uterus to the superficial inguinal lymph nodes.

The **parametrium** surrounds the supravaginal cervix. It is thickened to form three paired ligaments on the pelvic surface of levator ani:

- The **uterosacral ligaments** – pass posteriorly around the rectum to the sacrum.
- The **lateral cervical (cardinal) ligaments** – pass to the lateral pelvic wall.
- The **pubocervical ligaments** – pass forwards to the body of the pubis.

The uterus is supported and stabilized by these ligaments. The round ligaments may help to maintain the anteverted position. Major support is also given by levator ani. Stretching and tearing of levator ani during a difficult childbirth may prevent it from supporting and lifting the base of the bladder; the urethral sphincter then cannot prevent unintended loss of urine from the bladder (stress incontinence) when the intra-abdominal pressure is increased, e.g. during coughing or laughing.

Relations

Posterosuperiorly, coils of small intestine and sigmoid colon separate the uterus from the rectum; anteroinferiorly is the bladder and on each side are the broad ligaments. The vaginal cervix, surrounded by its fornix and vaginal walls, separates it from the rectum posteriorly and the ureter and uterine artery laterally.

This close relations of the ureter to the cervix and uterine artery means that it is at risk of injury when the artery is clamped during a hysterectomy. It also explains the frequent obstruction of the ureter in advanced cancer of the cervix or uterus.

Blood supply

This is from the uterine artery, a branch of the internal iliac. The veins drain via the uterine plexus in the lower broad ligament to the uterine and internal iliac veins.

Lymphatic drainage

Drainage is mainly to the external and common iliac nodes, but some drain along the round ligament to the superficial inguinal nodes in the groin.

Nerve supply

There are sympathetic and parasympathetic fibres from the pelvic plexus.

The uterine ligaments are stretched in pregnancy. Failure to regain their original tension may allow the uterus to descend into the vagina (uterine prolapse) and, if associated with laxity in the vaginal wall, would cause the bladder (cystocoele) or rectum (rectocoele) to bulge into the anterior vaginal wall and interfere with normal micturition and defecation. A difficult childbirth may result in partial tearing of levator ani and, thereafter, the support of the pelvic viscera is similarly weakened so that the uterus may descend (prolapse) and urinary incontinence result. Thus sudden increases in intra-abdominal pressure, which follow coughing for example, are followed by the involuntary expulsion of a small amount of urine (stress incontinence).

Age changes

Until puberty the cervix and body of the uterus are equal in size, but after puberty the body enlarges. Pregnancy produces a 30-fold increase in the uterine body due to muscle hypertrophy. Atrophy of muscle and endometrium occurs after the menopause.

The uterine tubes

The uterine tubes (Fig. 9.11a) are about 10 cm long and lie in the upper borders of the broad ligament. They open into the uterus at its superomedial angle. Each passes laterally to overlap the lateral surface of the ovary, and there opens into the peritoneal cavity. Their function is to convey ova to the uterus. They are described as having, from medial to lateral:

- A uterine part – within the wall of the uterus
- A narrow isthmus
- A dilated and convoluted ampulla
- A funnel-shaped infundibulum
- Several finger-like fimbriae, one of which is attached to the ovary.

Throughout its course the tube is related to coils of small intestine.

Blood supply

The uterine tubes are supplied by the uterine arteries; these anastomose with the ovarian vessels that arise directly from the aorta.

Nerve supply

There are sympathetic fibres from the pelvic plexuses.

Lymphatic drainage

Drainage is to para-aortic and iliac nodes.

Infection can spread directly to the uterine tubes from the vagina and uterus, causing **salpingitis** (infection of the tubes). This occasionally results in a tubal fibrosis and blockage and can be a cause of infertility. **Ectopic pregnancy** is a pregnancy that develops outside the uterine cavity, a consequence of implantation occurring in the uterine tubes and, rarely, in the peritoneum, rather than in the uterine body. In the uterine tubes these pregnancies usually develop for no longer than 6–8 weeks before the tube ruptures to cause an intraperitoneal bleed. The patency of the uterine tube may be assessed radiographically by hysterosalpingography, a procedure that employs the injection of radiopaque material into the uterine tubes (Fig. 9.12). Ligation of the uterine tubes is used as a method of birth control.

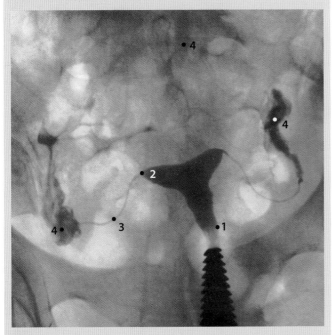

Figure 9.12 Hysterosalpingogram – contrast medium outlining: 1, body of uterus; 2, cornu; 3, uterine tube; 4, ampulla and intraperitoneal leakage (normal)

The ovary

The ovary is an almond-shaped organ about 3 cm long. Its position and mobility vary and it is displaced considerably during pregnancy. It lies on the back of the broad ligament, attached by a double fold of peritoneum, the mesovarium, which covers the ovary (Fig. 9.11a).

Relations

The lateral surface, adjacent to the pelvic wall, occupies the ovarian fossa. This is bounded by the obliterated umbilical ligament anteriorly, the internal iliac artery superiorly and the ureter posteriorly. Laterally the ovary is clasped by the infundibulum and the fimbriae of the tube; its medial surface lies close to the broad ligament. Its tubal end is attached to the

tube by one of the fimbriae and the suspensory ligament of the ovary, which conveys the ovarian vessels.

Blood supply

This is via the ovarian artery and branches of the uterine artery. Venous drainage is via an ovarian pampiniform plexus to the ovarian vein, which, on the left, drains to the left renal vein and on the right usually drains directly into the inferior vena cava.

Lymphatic drainage

Drainage is to para-aortic nodes.

Nerve supply

There are sympathetic fibres from the 10th thoracic segment via the aortic plexuses.

The ovary is subject to cyst formation and, occasionally, to malignant change. Surgical treatment of the latter requires excision of the ovary and associated lymph nodes. Some women feel their ovulation as pain referred to the para-umbilical region (T10). This occurs about halfway through the menstrual cycle and is known by the German term *mittelschmertz*.

THE MALE INTERNAL GENITAL ORGANS

The prostate

The prostate (Figs. 9.13 and 9.14) is a fibromuscular organ containing glandular tissue that lies below the bladder on the urogenital diaphragm (Fig. 9.5b). It resembles a truncated cone some 3 cm in diameter and possesses a base above, an apex below and anterior, posterior and two lateral surfaces. It is traversed by the urethra and, posteriorly, by the two ejaculatory ducts in its upper half. These, and fibrous septae, divide it into a median lobe and two lateral lobes: the **median lobe** lies between the urethra and the ejaculatory ducts; the **lateral lobes** lie below and lateral. Pelvic fascia – the prostatic sheath – invests the organ and its surrounding venous plexus; the fascia is continuous with that surrounding the bladder neck and covering the seminal vesicles; it separates the prostate from the rectum (rectovesical fascia).

Relations

Superiorly – the bladder neck; inferiorly – the urethral sphincter; anterolaterally – the levator ani; and posteriorly – the rectum and seminal vesicles (Figs. 9.6 and 9.15a).

Blood supply

This is by the inferior vesical and middle rectal branches of the internal iliac artery. Venous drainage is via the prostatic plexuses to the internal iliac veins and to vertebral venous plexus.

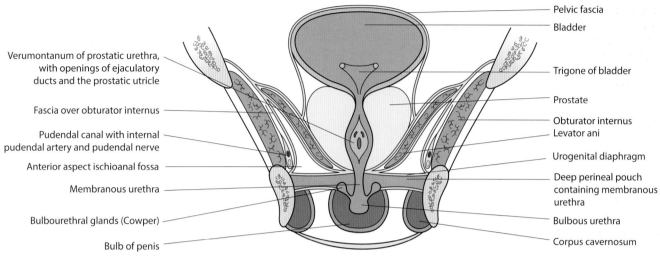

Pelvic fascia

Bladder

Trigone of bladder

Prostate

Obturator internus

Levator ani

Urogenital diaphragm

Deep perineal pouch containing membranous urethra

Bulbous urethra

Corpus cavernosum

Verumontanum of prostatic urethra, with openings of ejaculatory ducts and the prostatic utricle

Fascia over obturator internus

Pudendal canal with internal pudendal artery and pudendal nerve

Anterior aspect ischioanal fossa

Membranous urethra

Bulbourethral glands (Cowper)

Bulb of penis

Figure 9.13 Coronal section through the male pelvis and perineum, bladder and prostatic urethra

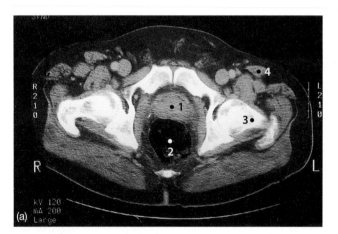

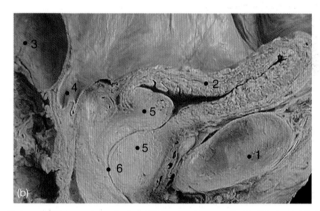

Figure 9.14 (a) Axial CT scan of low pelvis: 1, prostate gland; 2, rectum; 3, head of femur; 4, sartorius. (b) Sagittal dissection of male pelvis to show enlarged prostate: 1, pubic symphysis; 2, thickened bladder wall; 3, rectum; 4, rectovesical pouch; 5, enlarged prostate, part of which has enlarged into the bladder; 6, urethra trapped between swollen prostatic lobes

Lymphatic drainage

This is to the internal iliac nodes.

Nerve supply

There are sympathetic fibres (L1, L2) from the pelvic plexus and parasympathetic fibres from the pelvic splanchnics (S2, S3, S4).

The prostate is readily palpated by rectal examination; the normal gland is felt as a smooth firm mass, possessing a vertical sulcus, under the anterior rectal mucosa. In middle age there is often **hypertrophy** of the glandular tissue, especially that of the median lobe, which enlarges to project upwards, disturbing vesical sphincter action and rendering micturition difficult and incomplete (Fig. 9.14b). Surgical treatment is often employed, although pharmacological methods of reducing prostate size are now being used more frequently. Transurethral resection of the prostate (TURP) is carried out with an operating cystoscope and permits the 'coring out' of the median lobe. Infection in the prostate (**prostatitis**) is very difficult to eradicate because of the prostate's extremely coiled duct system. It is marked by vague perineal pain, and a swollen tender prostate may be felt rectally. **Cancer of the prostate** most commonly first affects the lateral lobes and may be diagnosed by a hard irregular mass on rectal examination. Secondary spread of the cancer is frequently to the vertebral column, the cancer cells being carried there in the vertebral venous plexus.

Ductus (vas) deferens

Each ductus is a narrow muscular tube about 45 cm long, a continuation of the canal of the epididymis. It extends from the tail of the epididymis through the scrotum, inguinal canal and pelvis to the ejaculatory duct.

Relations

It lies in the scrotum, where it is palpable as a firm 4 mm diameter cord, and the inguinal canal lies within the spermatic cord. It enters the pelvis at the deep inguinal ring, lateral to the inferior epigastric vessels, and then runs on the lateral pelvic wall covered by peritoneum across the external iliac vessels and ureter. At the ischial spine it descends behind the bladder, medial to the seminal vesicles. Here it is dilated and known as the ampulla. It ends by joining the duct of the seminal vesicles to form the common ejaculatory duct.

Seminal vesicles

Each is a coiled, sacculated diverticulum of the ductus deferens, about 5 cm long and lying obliquely above the prostate, behind the bladder base (Fig. 9.15). Each is separated from the rectum behind by the rectovesical fascia below and the rectovesical pouch of peritoneum above. The narrow lower end is rarely palpable on rectal examination, unless diseased.

Vasectomy is commonly performed for male sterilization: the vas is isolated from the spermatic cord in the upper part of the scrotum, a 1–2 cm section is removed and the divided ends are separated and tied. The patient does not become sterile for 3–6 months because of the sperm stored in the seminal vesicles.

Common ejaculatory ducts

About 2 cm long, each is formed behind the neck of the bladder by the union of the duct of the seminal vesicle and the terminal part of the ductus; it then traverses the upper prostate to open into the prostatic urethra (Fig. 9.13) just lateral to the posterior swelling the seminal colliculus (verumontanum).

Blood supply

All these structures are supplied by the inferior vesical and middle rectal arteries, and their venous drainage is via the vesical venous plexus to the internal iliac vein.

Lymphatic drainage

Drainage is to the internal iliac nodes.

Nerve supply

Sympathetic fibres from the pelvic plexuses (known as nervi erigentes) produce contraction of the muscles in the walls of the ducta and the seminal vesicles.

If the nervi erigentes are divided, as they may be during excision of the rectum, erection and ejaculation is not possible and impotence results.

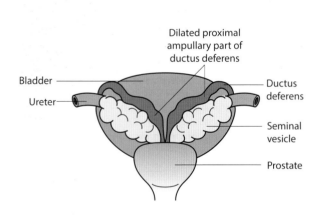

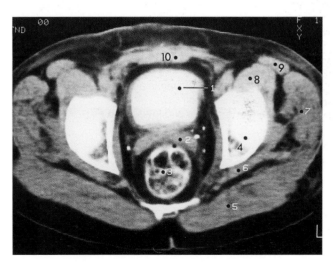

Figure 9.15 (a) Posterior aspect of the male bladder. (b) CT scan through the level of the seminal vesicles: 1, bladder containing contrast; 2, left seminal vesicle; 3, rectum; 4, roof of acetabulum; 5, gluteus maximus; 6, obturator internus; 7, gluteus medius and minimus; 8, iliopsoas; 9, sartorius; 10, rectus abdominis

MCQs

1. In the pelvis the: **T/F**
  a sacral hiatus permits injection into the   ( )
    epidural space
  b rectum follows the sacral concavity   ( )
  c sacral promontory is palpable on rectal   ( )
    examination
  d sacrotuberous ligament divides the greater   ( )
    from the lesser sciatic notch (foramen)
  e levator ani is attached to the pelvic fascia   ( )
    overlying obturator internus

Answers
1.
a **T** – *This is the site used for caudal epidural block, often performed in obstetrics.*
b **T** – *There is thus a sharp angle back into the anal canal.*
c **F** – *The sacral promontory lies high in the rectum and is not within reach of the examining finger.*
d **F** – *It is the sacrospinous ligament that separates the notches (foramina).*
e **T** – *Levator ani is attached to a tendinous arch over the obturator internus fascia.*

2. The prostate gland: **T/F**
  a is separated from the rectum by fascia   ( )
  b lies against the urogenital diaphragm   ( )
  c drains, with the dorsal vein of the penis, into   ( )
    the prostatic venous plexus
  d is traversed by the ducta deferentia   ( )
  e is supplied by the inferior vesical arteries   ( )

Answers
2.
a **T** – *Prostatic fascia invests the gland and, posteriorly, between the prostate and the rectum, the fascia is particularly well developed.*
b **T** – *The gland lies on the levator ani and its apex abuts against the urogenital diaphragm.*
c **T**
d **F** – *The ejaculatory ducts, formed by the union of the seminal vesicles and the ducta deferentia, traverse the gland. The ducts lie posterior to the prostate.*
e **T**

3. The rectum: **T/F**
  a has a short mesentery   ( )
  b is supplied mainly by the superior   ( )
    mesenteric artery
  c is the site of portosystemic anastomoses   ( )
  d has three taenia coli   ( )
  e has anteroposterior and lateral curves   ( )

Answers
3.
a **F** – *The rectum has no mesentery. Only the anterior and lateral surfaces of the upper third are covered by peritoneum.*
b **F** – *Its arterial supply is from the superior rectal branch of the inferior mesenteric artery.*
c **T** – *The superior and inferior rectal veins communicate in the mucosa of the lower rectum.*
d **F** – *The rectum has no taeniae coli. It is covered with a continuous tube of longitudinal muscle.*
e **T**

SBA

1. The intercristal plane is marked on a patient's back and the trainee clinician is asked to mark the spinous process below which it is recommended to perform a lumbar puncture. Where should he mark the skin?

a two spinous processes inferior to the line
b three spinous processes above the line
c the spinous process immediately above the line
d two spinous processes above the line
e three spinous processes below the line

Answer
c *The intercristal plane is a line joining the highest points of the two iliac crests, at the level of the 4th lumbar vertebra. This marks the level of the preferred site for lumbar puncture. Here the L4–L5 interspace is wide and allows safe access to the subarachnoid space below, where the spinal cord terminates.*

2. An anal carcinoma is found close to the anal verge. To which group of lymph nodes is it likely to spread to first?

a internal iliac
b middle rectal
c superficial inguinal
d deep inguinal
e external iliac

Answer
c *Anal carcinomas arising below the pectinate line drain primarily to the superficial inguinal nodes; those arising above the pectinate line drain to the internal iliac nodes.*

EMQs

Each question has an anatomical theme linked to the chapter, and a list of 10 related items (A–J) placed in alphabetical order: these are followed by five statements (1–5). Match **one or more** of the items A–J to each of the five statements.

Pelvic viscera
A. Broad ligament
B. Greater sciatic notch (foramen)
C. Lesser sciatic notch (foramen)
D. Membranous urethra
E. Obturator internus
F. Ovary
G. Penile urethra
H. Piriformis
I. Prostatic urethra
J. Vas deferens

Answers
1 B; 2 A; 3 F; 4 BC; 5 D

Match the following statements with the appropriate item(s) from the above list.
1. Transmits the inferior gluteal nerve
2. Contains the uterine tubes
3. Overlies the origin of the internal iliac artery
4. Transmits the internal pudendal nerve
5. Lies within the deep perineal pouch

APPLIED QUESTIONS

1. Discuss the functions of the pelvic diaphragm.

1. The pelvic diaphragm (levator ani and coccygeus) is the only striated muscle to possess resting tonus during sleep. It has an important role in support of the pelvic viscera, greatly aided by its attachment to the fibrous focal point of the perineum, the perineal body. It supports the prostate and indirectly the bladder and, in females, the vagina and uterus. It resists the downward displacement of the pelvic organs that accompanies increases in intra-abdominal pressure, e.g. in lifting, coughing, micturition and defecation. The anorectal angle, maintained by the puborectalis part of levator ani, plays a very important role in faecal continence.

2. What structures can one normally palpate during a bimanual pelvic examination in a female patient?

2. During a bimanual pelvic examination the clinician can feel the cervix and its external os and the vaginal fornices, as well as assessing the size and shape of the uterus. A normal ovary is often felt, but the uterine tubes are palpable only if enlarged. Examination of the posterior fornix may reveal abnormalities in the rectouterine pouch (Douglas) and, sometimes, a normal ovary. The size of the bony pelvis can also be assessed.

Bailey & Love · Essential Clinical Anatomy · Bailey & Love · Essential Clinical Anatomy
Essential Clinical Anatomy · Bailey & Love · Essential Clinical Anatomy · Bailey & Love · Essential Clinical Anatomy
Bailey & Love · Essential Clinical Anatomy · Bailey & Love · Essential Clinical Anatomy

Chapter 10

The perineum

The perineum lies below the pelvic diaphragm (levator ani and coccygeus). It is a diamond-shaped space between the pubic symphysis and the coccyx, bounded anterolaterally by the ischiopubic rami, posterolaterally by the sacrotuberous ligaments and laterally by the ischial tuberosities. A line joining the ischial tuberosities divides the space into a posterior anal triangle and an anterior urogenital triangle.

THE ANAL TRIANGLE

The anal triangle contains the anal canal in the midline and the two ischioanal fossae laterally.

The **ischioanal fossa** (Fig. 9.13, p. 148 and Fig. 10.1) is wedge-shaped, with its base lying inferiorly between the ischium and the anal canal. It is bounded superomedially by levator ani's attachment to the obturator fascia above and its junction with the external anal sphincter below, laterally by the fascia over obturator internus and inferiorly by perineal skin. Posteriorly it extends deep to gluteus maximus between the sacrotuberous and sacrospinous ligaments, and anteriorly it extends below levator ani, deep to the urogenital diaphragm. Its contents are identical in both sexes. The two fossae are separated by the anococcygeal body, the anal canal and the perineal body, but communicate behind the anal canal. Each fossa contains lobulated fat; the pudendal nerve and vessels lie on its lateral wall in a sheath of the fascia covering obturator internus (the **pudendal canal**), which lies about 3 cm above the ischial tuberosity. The perianal skin is supplied by the inferior rectal nerve, the perineal nerve and branches from the coccygeal plexus (S3, S4 and S5).

Infection of the glands of the anal canal frequently spreads through the anal wall into the ischioanal fossa (which clinicians still refer to as the ischiorectal fossa) to produce large abscesses. Should these discharge through the skin, a chronic fistula may develop between the anal canal and skin (fistula in ano).

THE UROGENITAL TRIANGLE

The urogenital triangle is divided by the inferior layer of the urogenital diaphragm – the perineal membrane – into superior and inferior compartments (pouches). The **urogenital diaphragm** is a triangular double layer of fascia (stronger in the male than the female) that stretches across the pubic arch between the ischiopubic rami. Its free posterior border is attached to a central subcutaneous fibrous mass, the **perineal body**. The diaphragm is pierced by the urethra and, in the female, the vagina. Its inferior fascial layer, the **perineal membrane**, gives attachment to the bulb and crura of the penis or clitoris. Its superior (deep) layer is continuous with the pelvic fascia where the viscera pass through between the two levatores ani. The deep layer fuses posteriorly with the posterior border of the perineal membrane to make a fascia-bound envelope, the deep perineal pouch (Fig. 9.13, p. 148). The superficial and deep perineal pouches differ markedly in males and females.

THE MALE UROGENITAL TRIANGLE

The **superficial perineal pouch** lies between the membranous layer of the superficial fascia and the urogenital diaphragm. The superficial fascia is attached to the posterior border of the diaphragm, and laterally to the ischiopubic rami, and anteriorly it is continuous with the superficial fascia of the anterior abdominal wall over the pubic symphysis (Fig. 9.5a, p. 140,

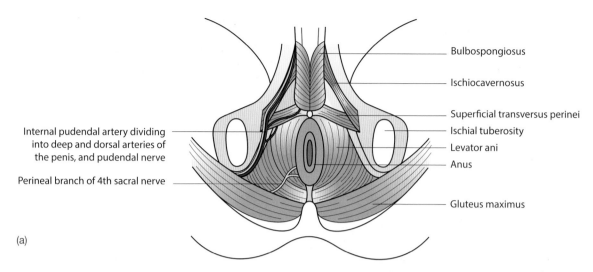

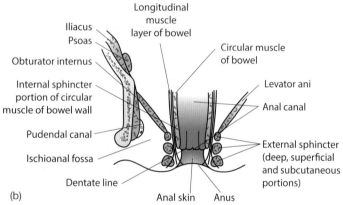

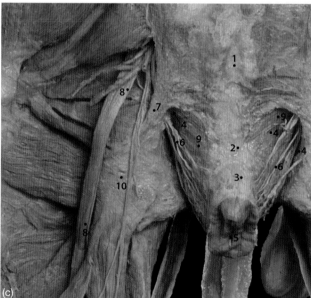

Figure 10.1 (a) Male perineum in the lithotomy position. (b) Anal canal – coronal section, showing the ischioanal fossa. (c) Dissection of the posterior view of the anal triangle and gluteal region with gluteus maximus removed: 1, sacrum; 2, coccyx; 3, anococcygeal body; 4, ischioanal fossa; 5, anus; 6, pudendal neurovascular bundle, 7, sacrotuberous ligament; 8, sciatic nerve; 9, levator ani muscle; 10, ischial tuberosity

and Fig. 9.6, p. 141). It provides a fascial sheath that contains the root and body of the penis and superficial perineal muscles (Fig. 10.1). The penis, testes and other scrotal contents lie in this fascial space, known as the superficial perineal pouch.

The penis

The **penis** comprises three longitudinal cylinders of erectile tissue: the central corpus spongiosum containing the urethra and the two lateral corpora cavernosa covered by fascia and skin (Fig. 10.2). It has a body and a root, and the root attaches it to the perineal membrane. The **corpus spongiosum** lies ventral and is expanded to form the bulb of the penis posteriorly and the glans penis anteriorly. The bulb, covered by the bulbospongiosus muscle, is attached to the perineal membrane. The urethra traverses the corpus and opens externally on the apex of the glans. The two **corpora cavernosa** unite dorsally and are embedded in the glans anteriorly. Posteriorly, beneath the symphysis, they diverge to form the two **crura** of the penis, which are covered by the ischiocavernosus muscles. The corpus spongiosum and the

corpora cavernosa are enclosed in a tough fibrous sheath, the tunica albuginea, which is itself enclosed by the deep fascia of the penis. This is attached dorsally by the suspensory ligament of the penis to the symphysis pubis. The skin of the penis forms a fold over the glans, the **prepuce or foreskin**, which is attached to the glans by a small skinfold, the frenulum.

Blood supply

This is by branches of the internal pudendal artery: the artery to the bulb supplies the bulb, the corpus spongiosum and glans; the deep artery of the penis supplies the corpora cavernosa; and the dorsal artery of the penis supplies the skin. Special attention must be paid to ligating the small frenular artery during circumcision, otherwise severe blood loss may occur.

Venous drainage is to the internal pudendal vein and, via the deep dorsal vein of the penis, to the prostatic plexus. Erection is achieved by engorgement of the cavernous spaces. The pelvic parasympathetic fibres cause dilation of the coiled penile arteries. The bulbospongiosus and ischiocavernosus muscles

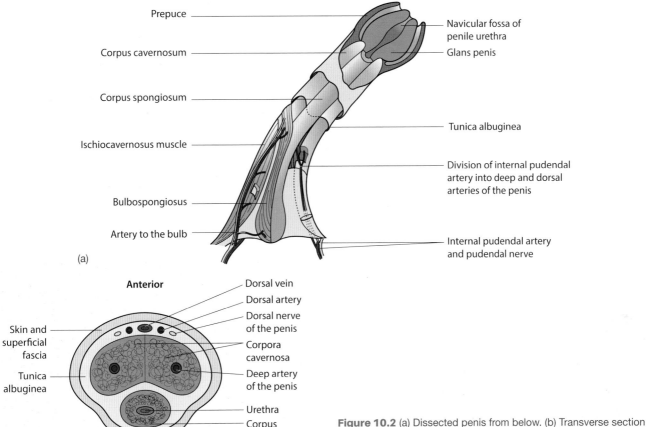

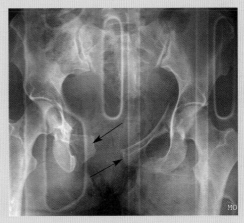

Figure 10.2 (a) Dissected penis from below. (b) Transverse section of the penis

compress the venous drainage from the cavernous spaces. Ejaculation is mediated by the sympathetic fibres – there is closure of the bladder neck and the sphincter urethrae, together with somatic contractions of the bulbospongiosus muscles.

Lymphatic drainage

This is to the superficial inguinal and iliac nodes.

Nerve supply

The somatic supply is by the ilioinguinal nerve and the dorsal nerve of the penis. Parasympathetic vasodilator fibres from the pelvic splanchnics (S2, S3 and S4) supply the erectile tissue.

The scrotum

The scrotum is a pouch of thin, rugose skin enclosing the two testes and spermatic cords, separated by a midline raphé and septum. Its walls contain smooth muscle fibres, the dartos muscle.

The superficial perineal pouch

The superficial perineal pouch contains the **superficial muscles of the perineum**, as well as the bulbospongiosus and ischiocavernosus muscles, both of which constrict the corpora and contribute to erection and ejaculation. There are also the paired **superficial transverse perineal muscles**, which lie in the posterior edge of the perineal membrane (Fig. 10.1a). All

are supplied by branches of the perineal branch of the pudendal nerve. The penis and penile urethra lie within the pouch.

Leakage of urine from a ruptured penile urethra, an injury that usually follows direct trauma to the perineum or is the result of a fractured pelvis (Fig. 10.3), spreads into the superficial perineal pouch. Its spread is confined by the attachments of the perineal fascia; initially the spread is into the subfascial tissues of the scrotum and penis, and then the **extravasation** ascends the anterior abdominal wall deep to its superficial fascia. It cannot spread into the thigh because of the attachments of the perineal fascia to the fascia lata.

Figure 10.3 Fractured pelvis showing gross disruption of the pubic symphysis and fracture of the pubic bones (arrows), with associated injury to the bladder

The deep perineal pouch

The **deep perineal pouch** is a closed space sandwiched between the two layers of the urogenital diaphragm. It contains the membranous urethra and the **sphincter urethrae muscle**, which surrounds the urethra. This voluntary muscle is attached on each side to the ischiopubic ramus and supplied by the pudendal nerves S2, S3 and S4 (Fig. 9.13, p. 148).

The urethra

The male urethra, about 20 cm long, runs from the internal urethral orifice in the bladder through the prostate, deep perineal pouch and corpus spongiosum to the external urethral orifice (Fig. 10.4). It is divided into prostatic, membranous and spongy parts:

- **The prostatic urethra**, about 3 cm long, is the widest part and descends through the gland. Its posterior wall possesses an elevation, the **urethral crest** (verumontanum), on whose summit is a small pit, the **prostatic utricle**, into which open the common ejaculatory ducts and numerous prostatic ducts.
- The **membranous urethra**, 1 cm long, is narrow. It descends through the deep perineal pouch surrounded by the sphincter urethrae muscle and the bulbourethral (Cowper's) glands.
- The **spongy urethra**, about 16 cm long, traverses the whole of the corpus spongiosum. Its slit-like lumen is dilated posteriorly in the bulb of the urethra (Fig. 10.4) and is narrowest at the external urethral meatus.

Blood supply

This is by the inferior vesical and branches of the internal pudendal artery. The veins drain to the prostatic venous plexus and internal pudendal vein.

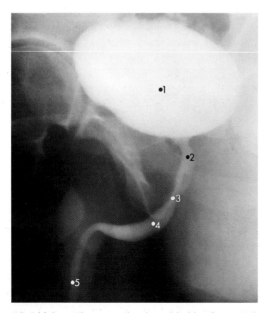

Figure 10.4 Male urethrogram: 1, urinary bladder; 2, prostatic urethra; 3, membranous urethra; 4, bulbous urethra; 5, spongy (penile) urethra

Nerve supply

The urethra is supplied by the pudendal nerve.

Lymphatic drainage

The prostatic and membranous parts drain to the internal iliac nodes and the spongy part to the superficial inguinal nodes.

Urethral catheterization is often required to relieve urinary obstruction, to monitor urine output or to provide a diagnostic sample.

In the male take care to avoid forcing the catheter onwards as the narrow, thin-walled membranous urethra is vulnerable to damage during this procedure. Obtain the patient's consent. The following equipment is required: 12–14 Fr gauge male Foley catheter, 25 mL antiseptic solution in a sterile pot, sterile gloves, a 25 mL tube of sterile lidocaine gel, a 10 mL syringe filled with sterile water, sterile swabs, paper towels and a bowl to receive the initial flow of urine. Obtain the patient's consent before the procedure. The patient should lie on his back with his legs slightly apart. Transfer the equipment to the sterile field, with the antiseptic solution poured into a receiver. Wash your hands and put on sterile gloves. Cleanse the penis with antiseptic solution, and then drape the area. Hold the penis with a sterile swab and cleanse it, paying particular attention to the glans. Squeeze some anaesthetic gel into the meatus, hold the meatus closed with a swab, and wait 5 minutes for the anaesthetic to work. Hold the penis vertically with the non-dominant hand and advance the catheter from its sterile sleeve into the urethra. Urine will flow once the catheter tip enters the bladder. Initially, direct the flow into the receiver; then attach the catheter bag and inflate the balloon with 10 mL of sterile water. Replace the foreskin if it has been retracted.

In the female the procedure uses the same equipment as for male patients except that the catheter should be a 12–14 Fr gauge female Foley catheter. First, obtain the patient's consent. The patient should lie on her back, with her heels together and her knees wide apart. Wash your hands, put sterile gloves on and lay the sterile equipment out. Cleanse the external genitalia with antiseptic solution, parting the labia with the non-dominant hand, and cleanse the urinary meatus. Insert the lidocaine gel syringe into the meatus and inject the contents. Wait for 5 minutes for the lidocaine to take effect. Insert the catheter from its sleeve until urine begins to flow into the receiver. Place the collecting receiver between the patient's legs, inflate the balloon to its capacity (10–25 mL) and connect the catheter bag.

The male urethra is susceptible to infection, subsequent ulceration and stricture. Urethral dilatation is achieved by the passage of fine, graduated urethral sounds.

THE FEMALE UROGENITAL TRIANGLE

The superficial and deep pouches of the female triangle are almost completely divided by the passage of the vagina through them. The **superficial pouch** contains the crura of

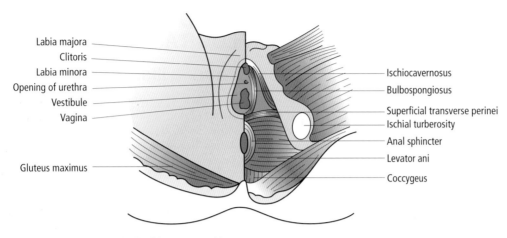

Figure 10.5 Female pelvic floor as seen in the lithotomy position

the clitoris, the bulb of the vestibule, the greater vestibular glands, the superficial perineal muscles and the terminal parts of the vagina and urethra (Fig. 10.5). The deep pouch is traversed by the vagina and membranous urethra and contains the sphincter urethrae and deep perineal muscles together with the pudendal nerve and internal pudendal vessels. The **female urethra** is about 3 cm long. From the bladder neck it descends through the deep perineal pouch, surrounded by its sphincter urethrae muscle, to open into the vestibule posterior to the clitoris. Also in the superficial pouch, alongside the vagina, are the bilateral **vestibular bulbs**, lying on the membrane covered by the bulbospongiosus muscles. Into this area drain the **greater vestibular glands** (Bartholin's).

Infection of the greater vestibular glands is not uncommon and produces a **Bartholin's abscess** at the side of the vaginal vestibule (Fig. 10.6). The perineum is most conveniently examined when the patient is lying in the 'lithotomy' position, i.e. supine with the hips flexed and abducted.

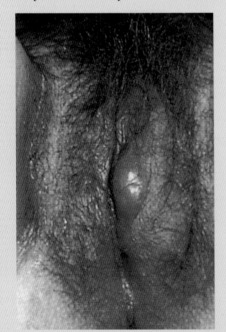

Figure 10.6 Bartholin's cyst (swollen greater vestibular gland) on the left vaginal wall

If a woman is having a prolonged labour and a perineal laceration looks likely, an episiotomy may be performed, with the assistance of a pudendal nerve block, to prevent damage to the anal sphincter or rectal wall. A mediolateral incision 3 cm in length is made, cutting through skin, posterior vaginal wall and bulbospongiosus muscle. After delivery it is sutured in layers. A pudendal nerve block is achieved by infiltration of local anaesthetic into the pudendal nerve, which can be located 3 cm deep to the ischial tuberosity, with a needle inserted into the vaginal wall and directed towards the ischial spine (palpable per vaginum). A pudendal block will anaesthetize the posterior vulva. The lateral walls, supplied by the ilioinguinal nerve, will require local infiltration to achieve anaesthesia of the whole vulva.

The female external genitalia

The **female external genitalia** comprise the mons pubis, two labia majora and two labia minora, clitoris and vestibule. The **mons pubis** is the mound of subcutaneous fat and hairy skin in front of the pubis. The **labia majora** are fatty folds of hairy skin forming the lateral boundaries of the vagina. The **labia minora** are thin cutaneous folds within the labia majora that unite anteriorly above the clitoris, a small, sensitive mass of erectile tissue, homologous with the penis, attached to the ischiopubic rami. The clitoris possesses two small corpora cavernosae and a diminutive glans. The **vestibule**, bounded by the labia minora, contains the external urethral meatus and the entrance of the vagina (Fig. 10.5).

The vagina

The vagina, a canal approximately 8 cm long, extends from the uterus to the pudendal cleft. It is supported by surrounding fascia and its supporting connections with the perineal body. It lies behind the bladder and urethra and in front of the rectum, its axis forming an angle of 90 degrees with the uterus. Its anterior and posterior walls are normally in contact, except at its upper end, into which projects the cervix, surrounded by a sulcus, the fornix. The lower end is partially occluded at birth by a perforated membrane, the hymen.

Relations

Anterior – the uterus, bladder and urethra; posterior – above, the peritoneum of the rectouterine pouch (Douglas), separating the vagina and rectum; below, the anal canal and perineal body and levator ani. The lowest part of the vagina lies in the perineum (Fig. 9.9, p. 143).

Blood supply

This is by internal iliac and uterine arteries. Venous drainage is via lateral plexuses to the internal iliac veins.

Lymphatic drainage

The upper two-thirds drain to internal and external iliac nodes, the lower third to superficial inguinal nodes.

A bimanual digital vaginal examination is usually performed with the patient in the lithotomy position, lying on her back with hips flexed. When combined with a hand on the lower abdominal wall, this examination allows bimanual assessment of the cervix, uterus and ovaries. The uterus is usually felt to be in an anteverted and anteflexed position, although 20 per cent of healthy women have a retroflexed or retroverted uterus. The non-pregnant cervix is firm and the pregnant cervix soft. The ovaries may be felt in the lateral fornices of the vagina and the size of the uterus can be assessed.

BLOOD SUPPLY OF THE PELVIC FLOOR AND PERINEUM

Common iliac arteries

The common iliac arteries arise at the aortic bifurcation on the front of the 4th lumbar vertebra slightly to the left of the midline. Each descends laterally to the front of the corresponding sacroiliac joint and ends by dividing into internal and external iliac arteries (Figs. 10.7 and 10.8).

Relations

Each artery is covered by peritoneum and surrounded by lymph nodes, sympathetic nerves and plexuses. It is crossed at its bifurcation by the ureter and, on the left, by the root of the sigmoid colon. Posteriorly it lies on the bodies of the 4th and 5th lumbar vertebrae and crosses over the psoas muscle and lumbosacral trunk. The common iliac veins lie behind the arteries.

Internal iliac artery

The internal iliac artery is a terminal branch of the common iliac. Arising anterior to the sacroiliac joint it descends on the posterior pelvic wall to the greater sciatic notch (foramen), where it divides into parietal and visceral branches.

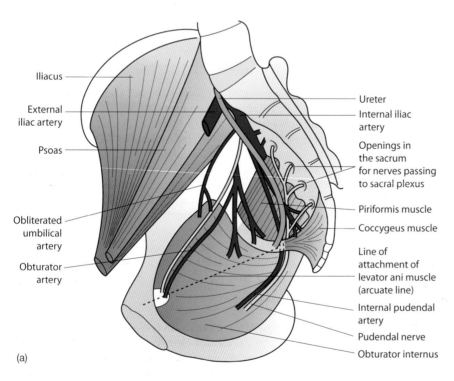

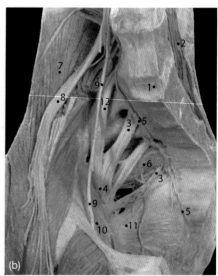

Figure 10.7 (a) Arteries of the lateral pelvic wall. (b) Dissection of the lateral pelvic wall with viscera removed to reveal neuronal components: 1, sacral promontory; 2, vertebral canal with cauda equina; 3, sacral spinal nerve roots; 4, formation of sacral plexus; 5, sympathetic chain terminating on coccyx; 6, piriformis muscle; 7, iliopsoas muscle; 8, femoral nerve; 9, obturator nerve, 10, obturator internus muscle; 11, levator ani muscle

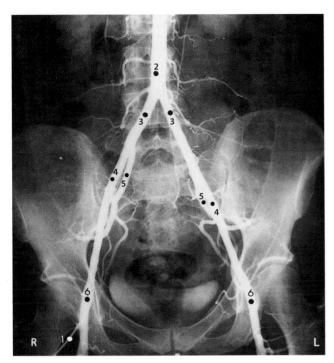

Figure 10.8 Angiogram showing iliac arteries: 1, fine plastic catheter that has been inserted percutaneously into the femoral artery and along which contrast media has been injected; 2, aorta; 3, common iliac arteries; 4, external iliac arteries; 5, internal iliac arteries; 6, femoral arteries

Relations

It is covered by peritoneum, surrounded by lymph nodes, and the ureter crosses its origin. Posteriorly lies the lumbosacral trunk and the sacroiliac joint, and laterally the external iliac vein and obturator nerve.

Visceral branches

The **superior vesical artery** is a branch of the patent remnant of the largely obliterated umbilical artery and supplies the bladder.

The **uterine artery** passes medially over the ureter alongside the lateral fornix of the vagina to gain the broad ligament, where it anastomoses with the ovarian artery. It supplies the vagina, uterus and uterine tubes.

The **middle rectal artery** supplies the seminal vesicles, prostate and lower rectum.

The **vaginal artery (inferior vesical artery in males)** supplies the vagina (vas deferens and seminal vesicles), bladder and ureter.

Parietal branches

The **umbilical artery** is obliterated soon after birth, but it remains as a fibrous cord between the pelvic wall and umbilicus, forming the medial umbilical ligament.

The **obturator artery** runs forwards on obturator internus, leaving the pelvis by passing above the obturator membrane to supply local muscles and, of importance in both children and adults, the hip joint.

The **internal pudendal artery** passes back to leave the pelvis through the greater sciatic notch (foramen). It enters the pudendal canal on obturator internus (Fig. 10.1) to give branches to the anal canal, scrotum (labia) and penis.

The **inferior gluteal artery** leaves the pelvis via the greater sciatic notch (foramen) below the piriformis to supply the gluteal muscles, the hip joint and the sciatic nerve.

The **superior gluteal artery** leaves the pelvis by the greater sciatic notch (foramen) above the piriformis and supplies the gluteal muscles and hip joint.

The **lateral sacral artery** supplies the contents of the sacral canal.

The **iliolumbar artery** ascends on the sacrum to supply the posterior abdominal wall muscles.

The external iliac artery

The external iliac artery, a terminal branch of the common iliac artery, begins over the sacroiliac joint and runs forwards around the pelvic brim. It enters the thigh below the midinguinal point to become the femoral artery.

Relations

It lies extraperitoneally, surrounded by lymph nodes on psoas, lateral to the external iliac vein. Anteriorly, in the male it is crossed by the ductus deferens and the testicular vessels, and in the female by ovarian vessels and the round ligament.

Branches (arising just above the inguinal ligament)

The **inferior epigastric artery** ascends medial to the deep inguinal ring behind the anterior abdominal wall to enter the posterior rectus sheath, whose contents it supplies.

The **deep circumflex iliac artery** also supplies the abdominal wall.

Veins

These drain mainly to the internal iliac vein via tributaries corresponding to the branches of its artery. The viscera drain via the venous plexuses surrounding them; the intercommunicating prostatic, vesical, uterine, vaginal and rectal plexuses also communicate with the vertebral venous plexuses (Fig. 10.9).

This accounts for the frequency with which some of the cancers affecting the pelvic organs, especially the prostate, spread to the vertebrae and the bones of the skull.

The **internal and external iliac veins** unite to form the common iliac vein anterior to the sacroiliac joint, and lie posterior to the accompanying arteries. The **common iliac vein** ascends obliquely to meet its fellow to the right of the midline on the 5th lumbar vertebra to form the inferior vena cava (p. 130). The left vein is longer than the right and is crossed by the right common iliac artery. The ovaries and testes drain via gonadal veins, which form pampiniform plexuses and drain into, on the right, the inferior vena cava, and on the left the left renal vein.

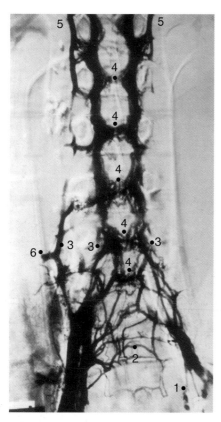

Figure 10.9 Subtracted lumbar venogram. Since the advent of CT and MR scanning these images are rarely performed, but they do illustrate the anatomy optimally. The drainage of the spinal cord, vertebrae and spinal musculature is via this complex internal and external venous plexus: 1, pelvic veins draining via the internal iliac veins to connections in the vertebral venous plexus; 2, pelvic bilateral venous drainage; 3, vertebral channels – up to six – alongside the vertebral column: these are valveless and connect to 4; 4, basivertebral segmental veins draining each vertebral body – direct from the bone marrow; 5, venous channels passing up to the thoracic and cervical region; 6, segmental intervertebral veins connecting to the posterior lumbar and intercostal systems

LYMPHATIC DRAINAGE OF THE PELVIS AND PERINEUM

Pelvis and perineum

The **internal iliac nodes** drain all of the pelvic viscera apart from the ovaries and testes, together with all of the perineum and the gluteal region. Lymph drains from the gonads directly to the para-aortic nodes around the renal vessels. The **external iliac nodes** receive vessels from the lower limb, the lower abdominal wall and also the bladder, prostate, uterus and cervix. Lymph drains from the perineum, the lower anal canal, the vagina and the perineal skin to the **superficial inguinal nodes**. Efferent vessels from the iliac nodes pass to the common iliac and para-aortic nodes (**Fig. 10.10** shows the general arrangement of the pelvic and abdominal lymph nodes).

Abdomen

The lymph vessels of the anterior abdominal wall pass to axillary, anterior mediastinal (p. 70) and superficial inguinal nodes (**Fig. 10.10b**). The abdominal viscera and posterior abdominal wall drain to **para-aortic nodes**, which lie alongside the aorta around the paired lateral arteries. They drain the posterior abdominal wall, kidneys, suprarenals and gonads and, through the common iliac nodes, the pelvic viscera and lower limbs. Their efferents unite and form the right and left lumbar lymph trunks. **Preaortic nodes** are arranged around the origins of the three arteries supplying the alimentary tract, the coeliac, superior and inferior mesenteric arteries, and drain the intestinal tract supplied by the arteries. Their efferents unite to form the **intestinal lymph trunk**, which enters the cisterna chyli. The **cisterna chyli** is a thin-walled slender sac, 5–7 cm long, that lies between the aorta and the right crus of the diaphragm in front of the upper two lumbar vertebrae. It receives the right and left lumbar lymph trunks and the intestinal lymph trunk, and leads directly to the thoracic duct (p. 71).

NERVES OF THE POSTERIOR ABDOMINAL WALL AND PELVIS

These comprise the lumbar and sacral plexuses, and the abdominal autonomic nervous system.

The **lumbar plexus** is formed from the ventral primary rami of L1–L4 on the surface of psoas (**Fig. 8.13**, p. 129). Its principal branches are the femoral nerve (pp. 129 and 260) and the obturator nerve; these also give **muscular** branches to the thigh and leg (quadriceps, sartorius and pectineus) and cutaneous branches (**medial and intermediate cutaneous nerves of the thigh, saphenous nerve**). The **obturator nerve** descends close to the medial border of psoas deep to the internal iliac vessels, and enters the thigh by passing through the obturator foramen. It supplies obturator internus, the adductor muscles of the thigh and cutaneous branches to the medial thigh as well as the joints of the thigh.

The **sacral plexus** is formed from the ventral primary rami of L4–L5 and S1–S4 on the surface of piriformis in the pelvis. Note that L4 contributes to both the lumbar and sacral (**Figs. 10.11** and **10.12**) plexuses, and that the contribution to the sacral plexus is by a branch that joins the L5 ramus to form the **lumbosacral trunk**. Branches from the plexus supply pelvic and hip muscles (p. 141), with cutaneous branches to the buttock and thigh, but its two major branches are the sciatic nerve (p. 255) and the **pudendal nerve**. The latter passes from the pelvis below piriformis and crosses the ischial spine to enter the perineum, where it lies in the pudendal canal (p. 153 and **Fig. 10.7**) on the lateral wall of the ischioanal fossa, giving branches to the external anal sphincter, the superficial muscles of the perineum, the penis (clitoris) and the scrotal (vulval) skin.

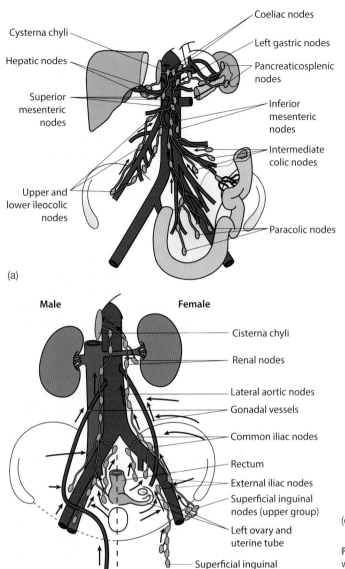

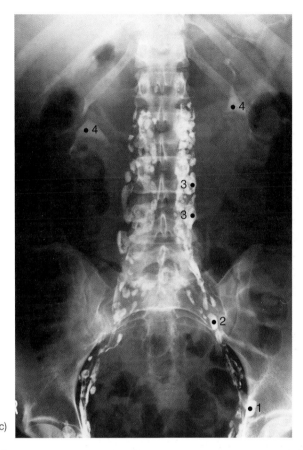

Figure 10.10 Lymph nodes of the pelvis and posterior abdominal wall: (a) preaortic nodes; (b) para-aortic nodes; (c) lymphangiogram: 1, external iliac nodes; 2, common iliac nodes; 3, para-aortic nodes; 4, renal pelvis (outlined by excreted contrast material)

THE AUTONOMIC NERVOUS SYSTEM OF THE ABDOMEN AND PELVIS

The **autonomic nervous system of the abdomen and pelvis** comprises the lumbar sympathetic trunk, the coeliac, aortic, hypogastric and pelvic plexuses, and the parasympathetic contribution, the vagi and the pelvic splanchnic nerves (S2, S3 and S4) (**Fig. 10.13**).

The **lumbar sympathetic trunk** commences deep to the medial arcuate ligament of the diaphragm as a continuation of the thoracic trunk (p. 72), and descends on each side of the lumbar vertebral bodies, behind the inferior vena cava and the aorta. It continues distally, deep to the iliac vessels, as the **sacral trunk** on the anterior sacrum. The lumbar trunk usually has four ganglia, all sending grey rami communicantes to

their spinal nerves and visceral branches to the **aortic plexus**, in front of the abdominal aorta and the **hypogastric plexus** on the common iliac arteries. The sacral plexus similarly sends branches to its spinal nerves and, via the **pelvic plexuses** on the internal iliac arteries, to the pelvic viscera.

Lumbar sympathectomy, i.e. surgical removal of the lower lumbar ganglia, is sometimes employed to reduce the excessive sweating of hyperhidrosis and, occasionally, to increase the distal cutaneous blood supply in arterial disease.

The **coeliac plexus** is formed of two communicating coeliac ganglia lying around the origin of the coeliac artery. Each ganglion receives greater, a lesser and sometimes the least splanchnic nerves (pp. 68 and 69) from the thoracic sympathetic trunk, and each gives branches that pass down the aorta to the aortic plexuses. From both plexuses fibres pass to the upper alimentary tract and its derivatives, e.g. liver,

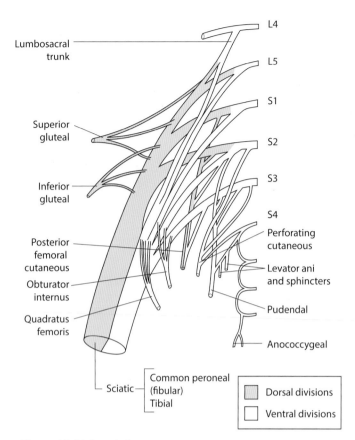

Figure 10.11 Sacral plexus

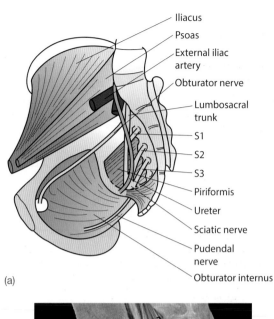

(a)

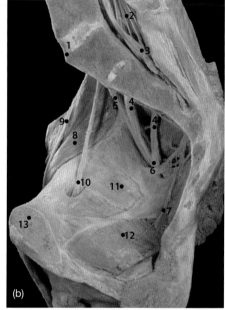

(b)

Figure 10.12 (a) Lateral pelvic wall demonstrating the position of the sacral plexus. (b) Dissection of the lateral pelvis with viscera removed to reveal the pelvic nerves and muscles: 1, sacral promontory; 2, vertebral canal with cauda equina; 3, terminal dural sac at S2; 4, sacral spinal nerve roots; 5, lumbosacral trunk; 6, formation of sacral plexus; 7, pudendal nerve; 8, iliacus muscle; 9, femoral nerve; 10, obturator nerve entering the obturator foramen; 11, obturator internus muscle; 12, levator ani muscle; 13, pubis

pancreas, and to the kidneys and gonads. There is a large communication between the coeliac plexus and the medulla of the suprarenal glands.

The **aortic plexus** lies on the lower aorta and receives branches from the coeliac plexus and the sympathetic trunk. Its postsynaptic fibres pass along the inferior mesenteric artery to the lower gastrointestinal tract, and it gives branches to the **hypogastric plexus**, which lies immediately below the aortic bifurcation formed of the above-mentioned branches from the aortic plexus and the sympathetic trunk. Its postsynaptic fibres supply the pelvic viscera.

Parasympathetic

Anterior and posterior vagal trunks

These receive contributions from both right and left vagi and are distributed to the coeliac plexus and then along the branches of the aorta to the alimentary tract as far distally as the splenic flexure.

Pelvic splanchnic nerves

The anterior primary rami of S2, S3 and sometimes S4 give off parasympathetic nerve fibres, the pelvic splanchnic, which join the sympathetic fibres within the inferior hypogastric plexus for distribution to the distal colon, and to the pelvic plexus for distribution to the pelvic viscera and perineal structures. Functionally they are responsible for 'emptying' the rectum (defecation) and bladder (micturition), and erection, supplying motor fibres to the walls of the viscus and inhibitory fibres to the internal anal and vesical sphincters.

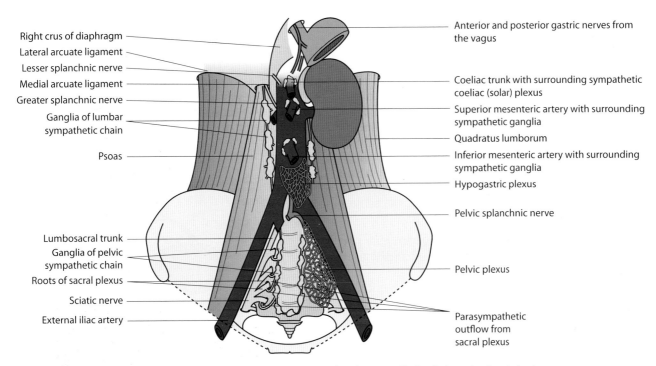

Figure 10.13 Autonomic nerves in the abdomen and pelvis demonstrating the sympathetic chain and autonomic plexuses

DEVELOPMENT OF THE REPRODUCTIVE SYSTEM

Development of the genital ducts

The internal genital duct systems of the male and female develop from parts of the paired mesonephric and paramesonephric duct systems, respectively (Fig. 10.14). During early development the undifferentiated duct system of the male and female are the same and are classed as 'indifferent'. In the male the mesonephric duct system persists and develops whereas the paramesonephric duct system degenerates, and vice versa in the female.

Development in males

In males the production of antimüllerian hormone causes regression of the paramesonephric (Müllerian) duct system and the production of testosterone drives the development of the mesonephric (Wolffian) duct system, which forms the epididymis, ductus deferens, ejaculatory duct and seminal vesicles (Fig. 10.15). A small remnant of the paramesonephric duct forms the appendix of the testicle, which is located by the superior pole of the testicle and is often visible on ultrasound imaging. The urethra develops mainly from the distal part of the urogenital sinus. The glandular parts of the prostate develop from numerous outgrowths of the prostatic part of the urethra, and the bulbourethral glands develop as outgrowths of the spongy urethra.

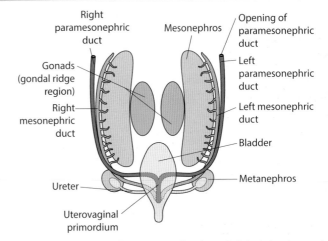

Figure 10.14 The indifferent stage of early genital duct development before sexual differentiation (anterior view). The paired mesonephric (purple) and paramesonephric duct (blue) systems are located close to the developing kidney on the posterior abdominal wall and pass from this region, and the developing gonad (green), toward the cloacal region

Development in females

In females a lack of testosterone results in a spontaneous degeneration of the gonad-associated part of the mesonephric duct system whereas the paramesonephric duct system persists to form the uterine tubes, uterus and proximal vagina (Figs. 10.16 and 10.17). The paramesonephric ducts form by an invagination of the coelomic epithelium (future parietal peritoneum) and their proximal ends remain open; hence the uterine tube ostium opens into the peritoneal cavity. The distal (caudal) ends of the paramesonephric ducts join to form the uterus and proximal vagina, and during this process each duct pulls a double-layered fold of peritoneum towards the midline to form the broad ligament (Fig. 10.16). Partial or complete failure of fusion, recanalization or development of the paramesonephric ducts can lead to a range of uterine and/or vaginal defects including a double uterus with a single or double vagina, septate uterus, arcuate uterus or atresia (Fig. 10.18).

Remnants of the mesonephric duct system may persist as an appendix vesiculosa (located proximal to the ovary), an epoophoron (located close to the ovary) or as Gartner's duct (located lateral to the uterus and vagina) (Figs. 10.16 and 10.17). Cysts may form in these remnants. The cranial part of the paramesonephric duct also usually degenerates; its persistence forms a hydatid (vesicular appendage) that is attached to the uterine tube infundibulum and may develop a cyst (Morgagni) in later life (Fig. 10.17).

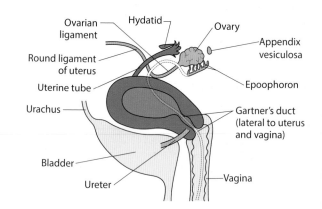

Figure 10.17 Development of the female reproductive tract, bladder and urinary tract from the urogenital sinus (yellow) and the mesonephric (purple) and paramesonephric (blue) ducts (left lateral view). Mesonephric duct remnants can be seen by the ovary (appendix vesiculosa and epoophoron) and lateral uterus/vagina (Gartner's duct). A small remnant of the cranial/proximal part of the paramesonephric duct, a hydatid, may remain connected to the uterine tube infundibulum

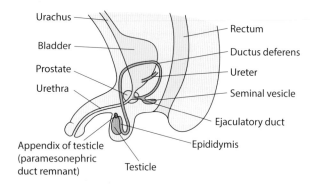

Figure 10.15 Development of the male reproductive tract, bladder and urinary tract from the urogenital sinus (yellow) and the mesonephric (purple) and paramesonephric (blue) ducts (left lateral view). The majority of the paramesonephric duct degenerates, although a small proximal segment can persist as the appendix of the testicle

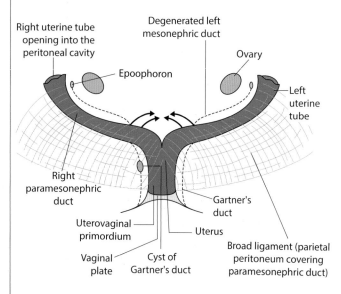

Figure 10.16 Formation of the uterus, uterine tubes and proximal vagina via the joining of the left and right paramesonephric ducts (anterior view). Note the basic shape of the uterus and uterine tubes. The course of the degenerated part of the mesonephric duct and the location of possible remnants are shown

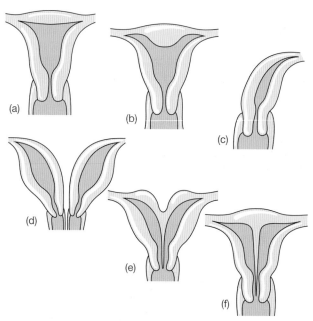

Figure 10.18 Developmental defects of the uterus and vagina. (a) Normal uterus. (b) Arcuate uterus, most likely due to the persistence of a small portion of the uterine septum. (c) Unicorn uterus, due to a failure of development of the contralateral paramesonephric duct. (d) Double uterus (didelphic) with double vagina. (e) Bicornuate uterus. (f) Septate uterus, due to persistence of the septum between the fused paramesonephric ducts

The meeting of the distal fused ends of the paramesonephric ducts (the uterovaginal primordium) and the distal part of the urogenital sinus promotes the formation of the paired sinovaginal bulbs, which join to form the vaginal plate (Fig. 10.19). Canalization of the vaginal plate forms the vaginal lumen, and varying degrees of failure of this process can cause vaginal atresia or the presence of vaginal septa (Fig. 10.20). The lumens of the vagina and urogenital sinus are separated by the hymen, a thin sheet of tissue that normally ruptures in early life (Fig. 10.19). The hymen can show varying patterns of rupture/perforation (Fig. 10.23) and a failure to rupture can present as primary amenorrhoea in early puberty.

Development of the external genitalia

During early development the external genitalia of the male and female are the same ('indifferent') (Fig. 20.21). Specifically, a pair of genital/labioscrotal swellings flank a pair of urogenital/urethral folds. The genital tubercle is located at the anterior midline apex of the urethral folds and will form the clitoris or penile glans and corpus cavernosum. The default state for development of the external genitalia is female, with relatively little remodelling required (Fig. 10.22a). The expression of testosterone leads to the development of male external genitalia in which the urethral and labioscrotal folds fuse in the midline with their contralateral partner, forming the spongy urethra and scrotum, respectively (Figs. 10.22b,c). Hypospadias (Fig. 10.24), the opening of the urethra onto the ventral surface of the penile glans, is a relatively common defect, while rarer forms involve the urethra opening onto the ventral penis, the scrotum or the perineum (Fig. 10.24). Both epispadias, the opening of the urethra onto the dorsal penis, and agenesis of the external genitalia are rare. Androgen insensitivity syndrome can result in a genetic male (46 XY) with normal external female genitalia and sexual characteristics that further develop during puberty; however, the vagina and uterus are underdeveloped or absent and the testicles are present but often undescended.

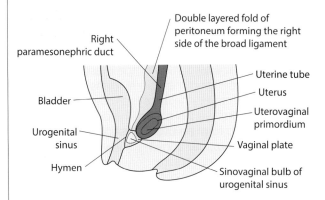

Figure 10.19 Development of the vagina from the sinovaginal bulb, uterovaginal primordium and vaginal plate (left lateral view). The hymen is located between the vaginal lumen and distal urogenital sinus

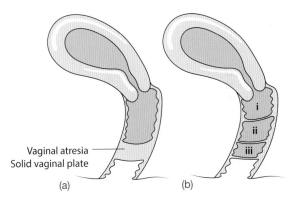

Figure 10.20 Vaginal atresia and septa. (a) Vaginal atresia caused by a failure of canalisation of the vaginal plate. (b) (i) High, (ii) middle and (iii) low vaginal septum caused by failure of complete canalisation of the vaginal plate or the uterovaginal primordium/duct

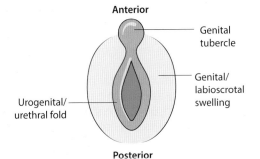

Embryological feature	Male	Female
Urogenital/urethral fold	Spongy urethra	Labia minora
Labioscrotal swelling	Scrotum	Labia majora
Genital tubercle	Penile glans and erectile tissue	Clitoris

Figure 10.21 External genitalia development. The indifferent stage of development of the male and female external genitalia. Male and female derivatives of each indifferent tissue type/structure are detailed in the table

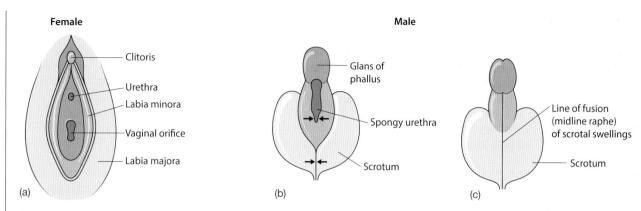

Figure 10.22 Differentiation of the external genitalia (complete around week 12) (a) Female external genitalia. (b) and (c) Male external genitalia. Note the urethral and labioscrotal swellings join in the midline (black arrows); a midline raphe can be seen on the scrotum and ventral penis

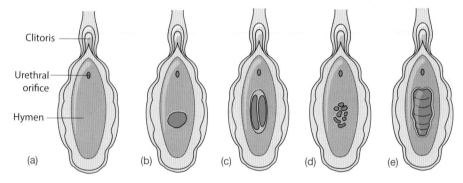

Figure 10.23 Varying patterns of hymen perforation: (a) imperforate; (b) annular; (c) septate; (d) cribriform; (e) parous

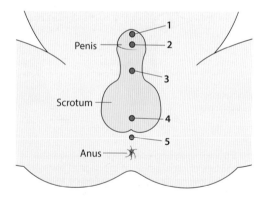

Figure 10.24 Hypospadias in the male. The urethra normally opens onto the tip of the glans (1), but in hypospadias can open onto the ventral glans (2) (a common penile defect), the ventral penis (3), the scrotum (4) or the perineum (5)

Development and descent of the testicles and ovaries

The ovaries and testicles both develop from the indifferent gonad, which is formed from three embryological tissues: the intermediate mesoderm medial to the mesonephros on the posterior abdominal wall (Fig. 10.14); the mesodermal epithelium covering this region; and primordial germ cells that migrate from the from the yolk sac (umbilical vesicle) into the interme-

diate mesoderm. Proliferation of the mesodermal epithelium and underlying mesoderm forms the gonadal ridges. Mesodermal epithelial cells penetrate the mesoderm to form primitive sex cords. The default developmental state is to form an ovary. Testicles only form in the XY chromosomal arrangement via the expression of testicular determining factor genes on the Y chromosome and the production of testosterone.

The downward movement of the testicles and ovaries to their final positions is guided by the gubernaculum, a fibrous cord attaching the caudal pole of a gonad to the ipsilateral labioscrotal fold (the future scrotum or labia majora) (Fig. 10.25). The gubernaculum also creates a pathway for the processus vaginalis (a loop of parietal peritoneum) to follow through the anterior abdominal wall. In both sexes the processus vaginalis pulls muscular and membranous layers of the abdominal wall with it to form the inguinal canal. The majority of the processus vaginalis usually disappears soon after birth, with only the distal part in contact with the testicle persisting as the tunica vaginalis. Persistence of the connection of the processus vaginalis to the peritoneal cavity in males can permit peritoneal fluid to pass into the tunica vaginalis, causing a scrotal hydrocele, which is often accompanied by swelling of the spermatic cord. Both swellings appear and disappear in a gravity-dependent manner.

In females, the ovary descends into the pelvic cavity and stops (Fig. 10.25b). The female gubernaculum attaches to the lateral uterus, therefore the gubernacular remnant passing from the ovary to the uterus forms the ovarian ligament, and the remnant passing from the uterus to the labia majora via the inguinal canal forms the round ligament of the uterus. The processus vaginalis in the female is small and quickly disappears. Its persistence, known as a processus vaginalis of the peritoneum or canal of Nuck, is rare and may present as swelling in the inguinal canal or proximal/anterior labia majora.

Maldescent of the testicle in the male can result in cryptorchidism or an ectopic testicle (Fig. 10.26). Cryptorchidism is a common congenital defect in males and represents a testicle that has not fully descended into the scrotum via the inguinal canal and is sitting somewhere along the normal route of testicular descent, most commonly in the inguinal canal. In contrast an ectopic testicle descends through the inguinal canal and subsequently to a non-scrotal location, e.g. the anterior abdominal wall, the upper medial or anterior thigh, the perineum or the opposite side of the scrotum or groin region.

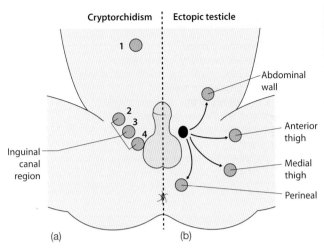

Figure 10.26 Maldescent of the testicle. (a) In cryptorchidism the testicle does not descend fully into the scrotum and can be located anywhere along the normal route of descent: 1, intra-abdominal; 2, deep inguinal ring; 3, inguinal canal (most common); 4, superficial inguinal ring. (b) An ectopic testicle descends through the inguinal canal as normal but then deviates to reside in one of a number of non-scrotal locations

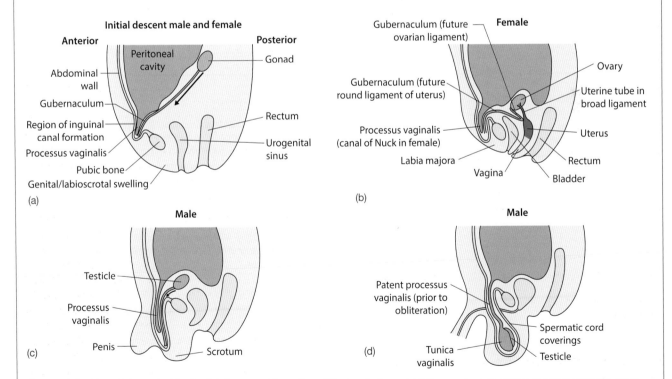

Figure 10.25 Normal descent of the testicle/ovary and formation of the inguinal canal. (a) The ovaries or testicles descend along the route of the fibrous gubernaculum, which passes into the ipsilateral labioscrotal fold. (b) In females ovarian descent stops in the pelvic cavity and remnants of the gubernaculum form the ovarian ligament and the round ligament of the uterus. (c) The processus vaginalis, a loop of parietal peritoneum, follows the gubernaculum through the anterior abdominal wall, pulling layers of the anterior abdominal wall with it, thus forming the inguinal canal (also occurs in females, forming the canal of Nuck [b]). The testicle passes through the inguinal canal and (d) into the scrotum where it sits adjacent to the distal part of the processus vaginalis, the stalk of which should obliterate leaving only the tunica vaginalis in contact with the testicle

MCQs

1. The ischioanal fossa: T/F
a is bounded medially by the rectum   (____)
b is bounded laterally by the fascia of the   (____)
   obturator internus muscle
c extends deep to the perineal membrane   (____)
d contains structures that have emerged   (____)
   from the pelvis via the lesser sciatic notch
   (foramen)
e is roofed by the fascia of levator ani muscle (____)

Answers

1.

a **F** – The ischioanal fossae are bordered by the anal canal
        and not by the rectum.
b **T** – Laterally the fascia over obturator internus forms a
        boundary.
c **T** – These fossae communicate with each other posterior
        to the anus, so infection in one may spread to the
        other.
d **F** – The structures that leave the lesser sciatic notch
        (foramen) are the obturator internus and gemelli
        muscles. The pudendal vessels and nerve that enter
        the perineum via the lesser sciatic notch (foramen)
        leave the pelvis via the greater sciatic notch (foramen).
e **T**

2. The deep perineal pouch: T/F
a is limited by the superficial perineal fascia   (____)
   and the perineal membrane
b contains the bulbourethral glands and the   (____)
   openings of their ducts
c contains the membranous urethra   (____)
d contains the sphincter urethrae and deep   (____)
   transverse perineal muscle
e transmits the dorsal nerve of the penis   (____)

Answers

2.

a **F** – These are the boundaries of the superficial perineal
        pouch. The deep pouch is bounded by the perineal
        membrane inferiorly and the urogenital diaphragm
        superiorly.
b **F** – The two small glands lie alongside the membranous
        urethra in the deep ...
c **T** – ... pouch, but their ducts open into the spongy urethra
        outside the deep pouch.
d **T** – Both muscles lie within the pouch.
e **T** – Branches of the internal pudendal vessels and
        pudendal nerve, among them the dorsal nerve of the
        penis, pass through the pouch.

3. The pelvic splanchnic nerve: T/F
a crosses the ischial spine medial to the   (____)
   pudendal artery
b contains postganglionic parasympathetic   (____)
   visceral motor fibres
c arises from the posterior primary rami of   (____)
   S2, S3 and S4
d supplies motor fibres to the sigmoid colon   (____)
e produces erection of the penis   (____)

Answers

3.

a **F** – The pelvic splanchnic nerve, carrying preganglionic
        parasympathetic fibres from ...
b **F** – ... S2, S3 and S4, to the hypogastric plexus below the
        aortic bifurcation, and its branches ...
c **F** – ... arise from ventral (anterior) rami.
d **T** – Its branches supply the pelvic viscera, including the
        sigmoid colon.
e **T** – The nerves (nervi erigentes) cause relaxation of
        the arteries supplying the pudendal erectile tissue,
        producing erection of the penis and clitoris.

SBA

1. A woman is admitted in an advanced stage of labour, the cervix is dilated and contractions are occurring every 5 minutes. The doctor administers a pudendal block to decrease the pain of what will be a vaginal delivery. Where should he aim to place the local anaesthetic?
a onto the ischial tuberosities
b to the medial side of the anterior superior iliac spines
c into the lateral vaginal wall pointing towards the ischial spines
d at the superiomedial corner of the obturator foramina
e in the sacral hiatus

Answer
c *The pudendal nerve (S2–S4) innervates the lower vagina and all of the perineum apart from the anterior labia majora. It enters the perineum curling around the sacrospinous ligament at its attachment to the ischial spine. Pudendal nerve blocks remove much of the discomfort of the third stage of labour.*

2. A young man is admitted the day after falling off his bicycle at speed. The next day he is found to have passed no urine and examination reveals an oedematous scrotum and tender swelling of the lower abdominal wall. He is thought to have extravasated urine following urethral trauma. Which part of his urethra is most likely to have been damaged?
a the prostatic urethra
b the pre-prostatic urethra
c the spongy urethra
d the urinary bladder
e the ureter

Answer
c *Rupture of the spongy urethra leads to extravasation of urine into the superficial perineal pouch. The superficial membranous layer of the perineal fascia (Colles' fascia) is continuous with the abdominal wall fascia (Scarpa's fascia) and this contains the leaking urine within the scrotum and subcutaneous tissues of the abdominal wall, first extravasating into the lower abdominal wall and thereafter ascending.*

EMQs

Each question has an anatomical theme linked to the chapter, and a list of 10 related items (A–J) placed in alphabetical order: these are followed by five statements (1–5). Match **one or more** of the items A–J to each of the five statements.

Vessels of the abdomen and pelvis
A. Abdominal aorta
B. Coeliac trunk
C. Inferior mesenteric artery
D. Internal pudendal artery
E. Left external iliac artery
F. Right common iliac artery
G. Right internal iliac artery
H. Right renal artery
I. Superior mesenteric artery
J. Uterine artery

Answers
1 G; *2* D; *3* AB; *4* I; *5* F

Match the following statements with the appropriate item(s) from the above list.
1. Supplies the bladder
2. Lies in a fascial tunnel on the obturator internus
3. Closely related to the fibres of the greater splanchnic nerve
4. Passes anterior to the uncinate process of the pancreas
5. Anterior relation of the left common iliac vein

APPLIED QUESTIONS

1. What structures are cut in a mediolateral episiotomy?

1. During a mediolateral episiotomy the perineal skin, posterior vaginal wall and bulbospongiosus muscle are cut. It is performed to ease the delivery of a fetus when a perineal laceration seems inevitable. If a tear is allowed to occur spontaneously in any direction, it may damage the perineal body (affecting pelvic visceral support), the external anal sphincter and the rectal wall (affecting anal continence). Episiotomy thus makes a clean cut away from important structures.

2. What anatomical knowledge is essential before male urethral instrumentation is performed?

2. When inserting urinary catheters and sounds, the course of the urethra must be considered. The spongy urethra is well covered inferolaterally by the erectile tissue of the penile bulb, but a short segment just inferior to the perineal membrane is relatively unprotected posteriorly – its thin, distensible wall here is vulnerable to injury during instrumentation, especially as a near right-angled bend occurs during entry into the deep perineal pouch through the perineal membrane. Hence at this junction the penis must be pulled down between the thighs. The instrument must never be forced, otherwise a false channel may be created. The gentle anteroinferior downwards curve of the prostatic urethra must also be considered.

3. What is the lithotomy position? Describe the boundaries of the anal triangle as seen in this position.

3. The lithotomy position is literally that used by surgeons in the middle ages for 'cutting for stone'. The patient lies supine with the legs abducted and raised in stirrups for easy access to the perineum. It is used mainly for gynaecological and anal procedures. In this rather undignified position the boundaries of the anal triangle are the coccyx and the two ischial tuberosities. The base of this triangle lies across the perineum between the tuberosities and the apex is the coccyx.

PART **3**

The back

Chapter **11**

The vertebral column and spinal cord

The curved, flexible column that forms the central axis of the skeleton supports the weight of the head, trunk and upper limbs and transmits it through the pelvic girdle to the lower limbs. Its great strength derives from the size and articulation of its bones, the vertebrae, and the strength of the ligaments and muscles that are attached to them. There are 33 vertebrae, united by cartilaginous discs (which contribute about one-quarter of its length) and ligaments. The column is about 70 cm long and within its canal contains and protects the spinal cord. There are five groups of vertebrae, each with specific characteristics: cervical (7), thoracic (12), lumbar (5), sacral (5) and coccygeal (4).

A **typical vertebra** (Fig. 11.1) has an anterior body with a vertebral arch behind enclosing the vertebral foramen. The arch consists of paired anterior pedicles and posterior flattened laminae; it bears two transverse processes arising near the junction of the pedicles and laminae, and a spinous process posteriorly. There are two superior and two inferior articular processes.

The **body** is short and cylindrical, with flat upper and lower articular surfaces. The **pedicles** are short and rounded, extending backwards from the posterolateral part of the body. Adjacent pedicles bound intervertebral foramina, which are traversed by spinal nerves. The **laminae** are flat and fuse posteriorly to form a projecting **spinous process**. Adjacent laminae overlap each other like tiles on a roof. The tips of the spinous process may be palpable posteriorly in the midline. Superior and inferior pairs of **articular processes** lie near the junction of the pedicles and laminae and bear articular facets covered with hyaline cartilage, which

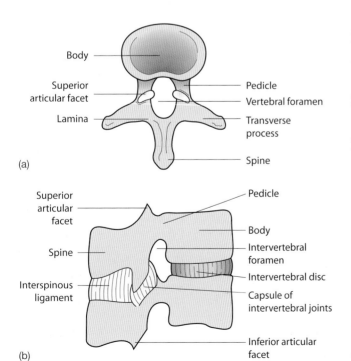

(a)

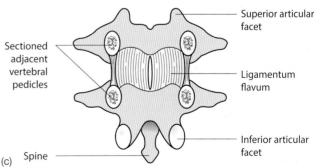

(b)

(c)

Figure 11.1 (a) Typical vertebra. (b) Intervertebral joints. (c) Ligamentum flavum viewed from within the vertebral canal – vertebral bodies removed

articulate in synovial joints between adjacent vertebral arches. The stout **transverse processes** project laterally, giving attachment to muscles and, in the thorax, articulation with the ribs.

REGIONAL VARIATIONS

Cervical

The typical cervical vertebra (Fig. 11.2) has a small oval body and a relatively large vertebral foramen. Each short, but wide, transverse process encloses a **foramen transversarium** containing vertebral vessels, and bears anterior and posterior tubercles. The surface of the superior articular facet faces backwards and upwards, and the inferior in the opposite direction. The spine is bifid. The 1st, 2nd and 7th cervical vertebrae show variations from this pattern.

The **atlas** (first cervical) is modified to allow free movement of the head (Fig. 11.3). It is a ring of bone with neither body nor spine, but bearing two bulky articular **lateral masses**. The kidney-shaped upper articular facets articulate with the occipital condyles. The lower circular articular facets articulate with the 2nd cervical vertebra. The transverse ligament of the atlas is attached to the medial aspect of the lateral masses. The **anterior arch** has a facet posteriorly for articulation with the dens of the axis. The **posterior arch** is grooved on each side superiorly by the vertebral artery. Its transverse processes are long and its tips, which are crossed by the spinal accessory nerve, are palpable behind the angle of the mandible.

The **axis** (second cervical) bears a conical projection, the dens, or odontoid peg, on the upper surface of its body (Figs.

11.4 and 11.5). The dens articulates with the back of the anterior arch of the atlas, where it is held in position by the transverse ligament of the atlas. The alar ligaments connect its apex to the occiput. The superior articular facets are almost horizontal and face upwards.

The 7th cervical vertebra (**the vertebra prominens**) has a long non-bifid spine, easily palpable and often visible in the midline at the level of the shirt collar on the back of the neck (Fig. 11.6).

Thoracic

A thoracic vertebra (Fig. 11.7) has a wedge-shaped body which is deeper posteriorly. The sides of each body articulate with paired ribs at **superior and inferior costal facets**. The transverse processes are directed backwards and laterally, and their ends bear a facet for articulation with the tubercle of the corresponding rib. The superior facets face backwards and laterally. The broad laminae and downward-projecting spines overlap with those below.

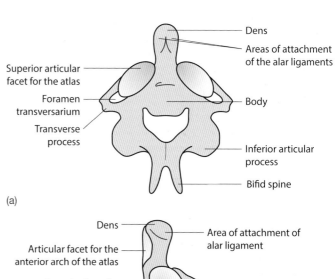

(a)

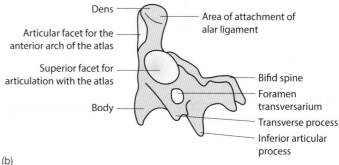

(b)

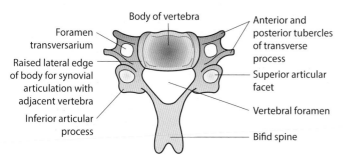

Figure 11.2 Typical cervical vertebra

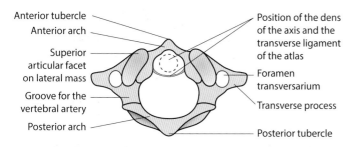

Figure 11.3 Superior surface of the atlas vertebra

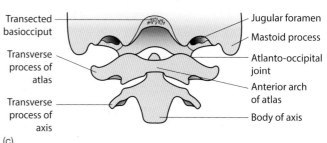

(c)

Figure 11.4 Axis and atlas: (a) posterosuperior view; (b) lateral view; (c) anterior view of atlantoaxial joint (*continued*)

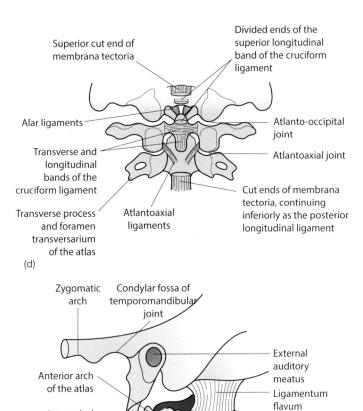

Superior cut end of membrana tectoria

Divided ends of the superior longitudinal band of the cruciform ligament

Alar ligaments

Atlanto-occipital joint

Transverse and longitudinal bands of the cruciform ligament

Atlantoaxial joint

Transverse process and foramen transversarium of the atlas

Atlantoaxial ligaments

Cut ends of membrana tectoria, continuing inferiorly as the posterior longitudinal ligament

(d)

Zygomatic arch

Condylar fossa of temporomandibular joint

Anterior arch of the atlas

External auditory meatus

1st cervical nerve

Ligamentum flavum

Styloid process

Posterior arch of atlas

Vertebral artery

Bifid spine of the axis

(e)

Figure 11.4 (*continued*) Axis and atlas: (d) posterior view; (e) lateral view

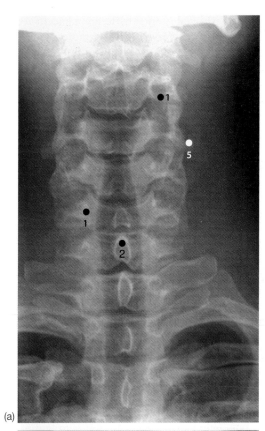

(a)

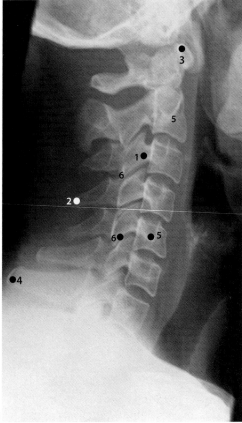

(b)

Figure 11.6 (a) Anteroposterior and (b) lateral X-ray views of cervical spine: 1, pedicle; 2, spinous process; 3, anterior arch of the atlas; 4, tip of the spinous process of the vertebra prominens; 5, transverse process; 6, facet joint

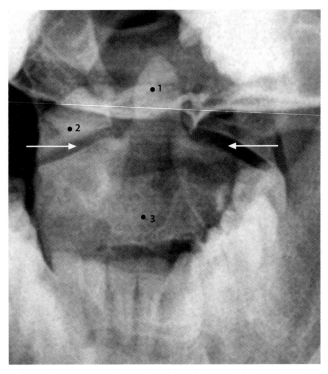

Figure 11.5 Transoral 'open-mouth' X-ray view of atlantoaxial joints (arrows): 1, dens; 2, lateral mass of C1; 3, body of C2

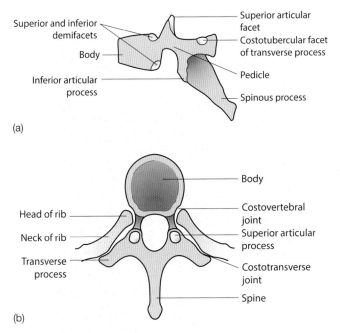

Figure 11.7 (a) Typical thoracic vertebra, lateral view. (b) Costovertebral articulation, superior view

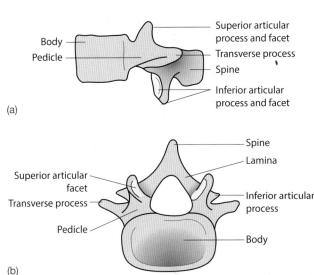

Figure 11.8 (a) Typical lumbar vertebra, lateral view. (b) 5th lumbar vertebra, superior view

The bodies of the upper vertebrae are small, whereas those of the lower ones are larger and their spines more horizontal. The costal facets on the bodies of the 10th, 11th and 12th vertebrae are usually single and complete.

Lumbar

A lumbar vertebra (Fig. 11.8) has a large kidney-shaped body, wider from side to side. Its bulky transverse processes project laterally and its superior articular facets face backwards and medially. The broad rectangular spinous process projects horizontally backwards. The **5th lumbar vertebra** is atypical – its body, being thicker anteriorly, is wedge-shaped and its transverse process is small and conical. Its forward-facing inferior articular facet prevents it sliding anteriorly over the top of the sacrum.

Spina bifida occulta is a common congenital abnormality in which the laminae of L5 or S1 fail to develop. The bony defect usually causes no problems and only comes to a physician's attention when the mother seeks advice for the cutaneous stigmata such as tufts of hair or a dimple found over the lumbar spine. In rare cases the defect is larger and the meninges and sometimes the spinal cord herniate (spina bifida cystica), with associated neurological symptoms such as lower limb paralysis.

The cervical, thoracic and lumbar vertebrae can be readily distinguished from each other: all cervical vertebrae have a foramen in the transverse process, all thoracic vertebrae have costal facets on each side of the body, whereas lumbar vertebrae have neither a foramen in their transverse process nor costal facets.

Sacrum and coccyx

The sacrum and coccyx are described on p. 138.

JOINTS AND LIGAMENTS

The articular surfaces of the bodies of adjacent vertebrae are covered by hyaline cartilage and united by a thick fibrocartilaginous **intervertebral disc**. The centre of the disc (**nucleus pulposus**) is gelatinous, with the consistency of toothpaste, and surrounded by a fibrous part, **the annulus fibrosus**. The disc is a shock absorber (Fig. 11.16).

Occasionally the semisolid nucleus protrudes through a defect in the annulus (**prolapsed disc**) and then may press on the spinal cord or a spinal nerve, to produce symptoms and signs of nerve compression (Fig. 11.9d). The majority of symptomatic disc protrusions occur at the L4/L5 or L5/S1 levels where the intervertebral foramina are small and the spinal nerve roots are relatively large.

The vertebral bodies are also united by **anterior and posterior longitudinal ligaments**. The anterior ligament extends from the occiput to the sacrum, and the posterior from the axis to the sacrum (Fig. 11.4d), and each is attached to each vertebral body and disc. Adjacent vertebrae articulate by two synovial joints between the paired articular processes. Additional support to the vertebral column is provided by:

- The **ligamenta flava** (Fig. 11.1c), which unite adjacent laminae. These ligaments contain a large amount of yellow elastic tissue and are strong. They maintain the curvatures of the spinal column and support it when it is flexed.
- The **supraspinous, interspinous** and **intertransverse ligaments**, which help unite adjacent vertebrae.

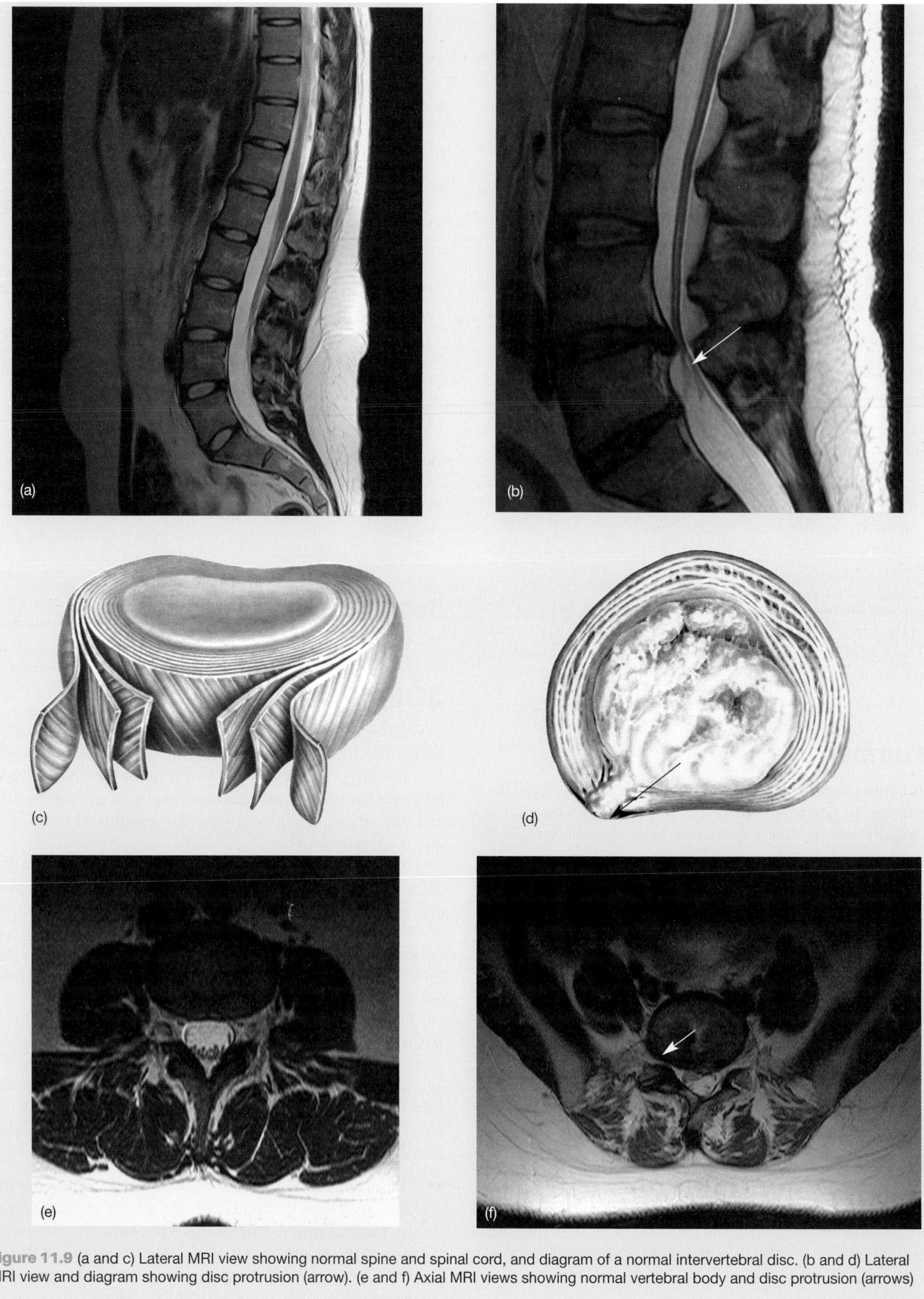

Figure 11.9 (a and c) Lateral MRI view showing normal spine and spinal cord, and diagram of a normal intervertebral disc. (b and d) Lateral MRI view and diagram showing disc protrusion (arrow). (e and f) Axial MRI views showing normal vertebral body and disc protrusion (arrows)

Variations

The atlanto-occipital and atlantoaxial joints are modified to allow free movement of the head.

X-rays taken through the wide-open mouth are used to demonstrate these joints (Fig. 11.5).

The **atlanto-occipital joints** are condyloid synovial joints between the convex occipital condyles and the concave upper articular surfaces of the atlas. They are strengthened by anterior and posterior atlanto-occipital membranes. The atlantoaxial joints comprise two lateral synovial plane joints between the lateral mass of the atlas and the pedicle of the axis, and a midline synovial pivot between the dens and a ring formed by the anterior arch and the transverse ligament of the atlas. The joint is strengthened by accessory ligaments, the **membrana tectoria**, which connect the back of the axis and the occiput and the adjacent **cruciate (cruciform) ligament** (Fig. 11.4d).

FUNCTIONAL ASPECTS

Curvatures and mobility

In fetal life the vertebral column is flexed – its primary curvature. After birth two secondary curvatures develop: extension of the cervical region by the muscles that raise the head, and extension of the lumbar region after adoption of the erect posture. The primary curvature is retained in the thoracic and sacral regions. These curves and the intervertebral discs give some resilience and spring to the column (Figs. 11.10 and 11.11).

Abnormalities in the curvature of the vertebral column occur. **Lordosis** gives an excessive hollowness to the back; an exaggerated lumbar curvature may be caused by weakened trunk muscles and is often present temporarily in late pregnancy. **Scoliosis**, an excessive lateral curvature, is always associated with rotation of the vertebral bodies so that the spinous processes point toward the concavity of the curve. It is often the result of weak back muscles or associated with failed growth of a vertebra (hemivertebra). **Kyphosis**, an exaggeration of the thoracic curvature, is usually the result of osteoporosis, a generalized bone atrophy, which causes erosion and collapse of several neighbouring vertebrae. The collapse of a single vertebra from tuberculous infection or fracture produces a localized kyphosis (kyphus).

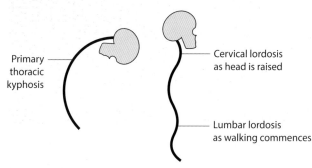

Primary thoracic kyphosis

Cervical lordosis as head is raised

Lumbar lordosis as walking commences

Figure 11.10 Primary and secondary vertebral curves

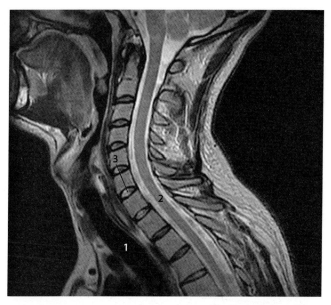

Figure 11.11 MR image of the mid-sagittal section of the cervical spine showing a normal cervical lordosis: 1, trachea; 2, spinal cord; 3, intervertebral disc

MUSCLES

The extensor muscles of the back and neck extend the head and vertebral column. They form a large composite mass lying deep to trapezius and girdle muscles, and extend from the sacrum to the occiput. The largest and most powerful are the erector spinae, but these are supported by shorter muscles attached to adjacent vertebrae and to nearby ribs (Fig. 11.12). These muscles play a large part in maintaining posture and are in constant action when standing at rest, as the centre of gravity lies anterior to the vertebral column. The muscles attached to the skull produce extension, lateral flexion and rotation of the head.

Movements

Only limited movements are possible between adjacent vertebrae, but because these can augment each other it is possible to produce extensive movement of the whole vertebral column. Flexion is most marked in the cervical region, rotation in the thoracic region, and rotation and lateral flexion in the lumbar region:

- **Flexion** – rectus abdominis and prevertebral muscles.
- **Lateral flexion** – in the neck by sternocleidomastoid and trapezius; in the trunk by the oblique abdominal muscles and quadratus lumborum.
- **Rotation** – sternocleidomastoid and oblique abdominal muscles.
- **Extension** – erector spinae muscles of the back.

Movements of the head

Rotation occurs at the atlantoaxial joints and all other movements, flexion, extension and lateral flexion, at the atlanto-occipital joint:

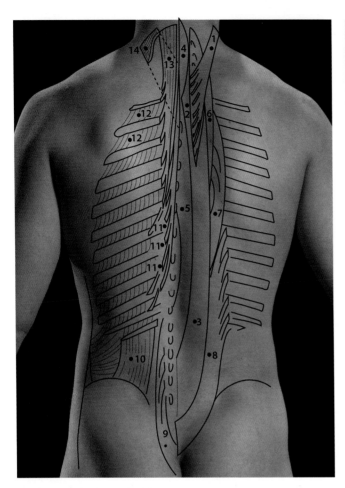

Figure 11.12 Surface anatomy of the back muscles: **Longissimus**:
1, capitis; 2, cervicis cord; 3, thoracis; **Spinalis**: 4, cervicis;
5, thoracis; **Iliocostalis**; 6, cervicis; 7, thoracis; 8, lumborum;
9, multifidus; 10, quadratus lumborum; 11, levator costae;
12, intercostals; 13, semispinalis capitis; 14, splenius capitis

- **Rotation** – sternocleidomastoid, trapezius.
- **Flexion** – longus capitis and the muscles depressing the fixed mandible.
- **Extension** – postvertebral muscles.
- **Lateral flexion** – sternocleidomastoid and trapezius aided and supported by stout muscles joining the atlas and axis to each other and to the base of the skull.

Stability

This depends almost entirely on the pre- and postvertebral muscles, helped by the ligamenta flava; neither the bones nor the ligaments alone could withstand the large forces that occasionally act on the vertebral column.

The commonest cause of vertebral fracture is a flexion-compression injury and this most commonly occurs at the thoracolumbar junction involving T12 and/or L1; it causes 'wedging' of the affected vertebrae. In the majority of such fractures the posterior longitudinal ligament remains intact

and there is no instability of the vertebral column (Fig. 11.14a). If, however, severe flexion is accompanied by forcible rotation of the vertebral column, the ligamenta flava (Fig. 11.1c) and interspinous ligaments are ruptured, and the vertebral column becomes unstable. Subsequent displacement may produce compression of the spinal cord and irreversible nerve damage.

Fracture–dislocation of a cervical vertebra may have serious consequences, especially if the transverse ligament of the atlas ruptures to cause atlantoaxial subluxation (incomplete dislocation) or complete dislocation. There is a risk of the dens impacting onto the spinal cord and paralysis of all four limbs (quadriplegia) – and the injury may be fatal. **Fractures of the vertebral bodies** (Fig. 11.14) are usually the result of forcible flexion of the vertebral column and may occur in any part of the column, but often occur at the thoracolumbar junction where the inflexible thoracic region meets the more mobile lumbar spine. A common genetic defect is a gap in the pars interarticularis of the pedicle of a lumbar vertebra (spondylolisthesis); this may give rise to slipping of the vertebrae. It is seen in an oblique X-ray of the lumbar spine. Disc prolapse posterolaterally (the most common type) often causes compression of a nerve root. The rarer posterocentral protrusion may produce pressure on the spinal cord. The diagnosis of disc prolapse has been made much easier by the use of MRI scans (Figs. 11.11 and 11.13). Prolapse of the L4/5 disc presses on the 5th lumbar nerve, and that of the disc below on the 1st sacral nerve.

Either of these events produces pain along the posterior thigh and leg. The diagnosis may be confirmed clinically by the 'straight leg raising' test (Fig. 15.27, p. 257); this produces pain along the irritated nerve root.

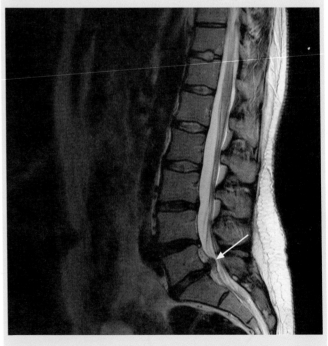

Figure 11.13 MR image showing lumbar disc protrusion (arrow)

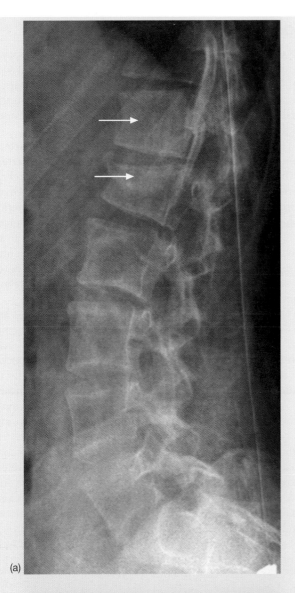

(a)

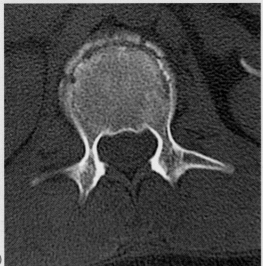

(b)

Figure 11.14 Lumbar crush fracture: (a) lateral X-ray (fracture arrowed); (b) axial CT scan showing fragmented rim of vertebral body

Management of a suspected spinal injury

Anyone who may have sustained a spinal injury, particularly one in the cervical region, should be handled with great care to protect the spinal cord from further damage. Until the extent of the injury is known all spinal injuries should be treated as unstable.

Do not move the patient; hold the head and neck in the position in which it was found. Do not help the patient to rise. Prevent further movement by placing rolled-up towels on each side of the head.

Check the circulation and breathing. If cardiopulmonary resuscitation (CPR) is required then do chest compression only. Do not roll the patient over unless there is a risk to the airway because of vomiting or bleeding. If you need to roll the patient over get someone to help you: one of you positioned at the patient's head, the other at the patient's side. Keep the patient's head, neck and back in line while you roll them to one side.

Remember, DO NOT:

- Bend, twist or flex the patient's head
- Move the patient until support is available in the form of a stiff sheet on to which the patient can be rolled and then carried safely
- Attempt removal of a motorcyclist's helmet.

Back pain is a common but poorly understood condition. Acute cases frequently follow extreme movements of the vertebral column or unaccustomed physical activity involving bending and/or lifting. It is likely that the cause in these cases is minor tearing of muscle fibres or ligaments. Long-standing cases of back pain are common; they are often caused by poor stance, as the body weight is not well balanced on the vertebral column and unequal strain is placed on part of the erector spinae muscles. In both types of back pain there is associated protective muscle spasm in the extensor muscles of the spine.

THE VERTEBRAL CANAL AND SPINAL CORD

The bony-ligamentous vertebral canal is formed by the series of vertebral foramina and the ligaments joining them. It extends from the foramen magnum to the sacral hiatus, becoming continuous below with the sacral canal. It contains the spinal meninges, the spinal cord and nerve roots. The bony wall of the canal is separated from the meninges by the epidural (extradural) space that contains the emerging spinal nerves, fat and internal vertebral venous plexus (Fig. 11.15). The spinal cord ends at the 2nd lumbar vertebra, and the **dural sac** at the 2nd sacral. The latter is separated from the walls of the vertebral canal by extradural fat and the internal vertebral venous plexus (Fig. 11.15 and p. 159), but is pierced by the ventral and dorsal nerve roots of the spinal nerves. It ensheathes the nerves as far as the intervertebral foramina. The spinal subarachnoid space communicates above the foramen magnum with the subarachnoid space of the posterior cranial fossa. Below the termination of the spinal cord at the level of L2 the space contains only the cauda equina.

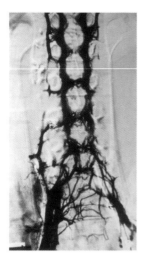

Figure 11.15 Vertebral venous plexus ascending from pelvis throughout the vertebral column

When performing **lumbar puncture** a needle is inserted just below the fourth lumbar spine in the midline (this level is found on the intercristal plane, which lies between the highest points of the iliac crests (Fig. 8.1, p. 123, and Fig. 25.3, p. 431). The needle is passed through the interspinous ligament to enter first the epidural space, and then it pierces the dura to enter the spinal canal, from which cerebrospinal fluid can be drawn off for examination. This site is used also for the injection of local anaesthetic solution into the epidural (extradural) space (epidural anaesthesia) or into the spinal canal (spinal anaesthesia) (Figs. 11.16 and 25.3, p. 431).

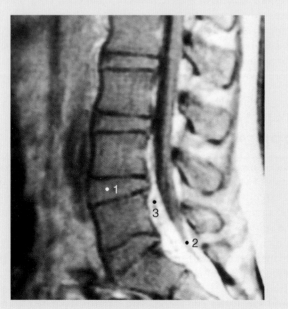

Figure 11.16 MR image, mid-sagittal view showing: 1, L4/5 intervertebral disc; 2, cauda equina; 3, epidural space

Blood supply

The **vertebral column** is supplied by small segmental spinal arteries. The veins drain into the external and internal vertebral venous plexuses, which in turn drain into the internal iliac, lumbar, azygos and basivertebral veins, which drain the vertebrae and communicate with both the pelvic plexuses and the intracranial sinuses.

The arterial supply is from a single **anterior spinal artery** (from both vertebral arteries) and two **posterior spinal arteries** (branches of the posterior inferior cerebellar or vertebral arteries). The anterior artery descends in the anterior median fissure of the cord, and each posterior artery descends posterior to the nerve rootlets. These three arteries receive reinforcement in the lower parts of the spinal cord by branches from the vertebral, deep cervical, posterior intercostal, lumbar and lateral sacral arteries. Venous drainage is by midline anterior and posterior spinal veins, which drain to the **vertebral venous plexus**.

The segmental additions to the longitudinal arteries are a most important contribution to the cord's blood supply. Thus spinal trauma, fractures and fracture–dislocations may each be attended by **spinal cord ischaemia**. Similarly, occlusive arterial disease in these small vessels, and especially in the important segmental vessel, the **great radicular artery (of Adamkiewicz)**, which contributes to the blood supply of the lower half of the spinal cord, may contribute to spinal cord ischaemia, muscle weakness and paralysis. If the aorta is clamped during surgery there is a risk of spinal cord ischaemia. The **vertebral venous plexus** (Batson's valveless plexus) (Fig. 11.15) has up to six longitudinal channels and numerous connections to each vertebral body via the basivertebral veins, which drain the newly formed cells from the vertebral marrow. It interconnects both outside and inside the spinal canal from pelvis to skull, and serves as an easy transport system for metastases, especially those of the prostate, ovary and breast, to both the vertebral column and the cranial cavity.

MCQs

1. In the vertebral column: T/F

a the individual vertebrae are all separately (___)
identifiable in the adult

b cervical vertebrae all have bifid spines (___)

c all thoracic vertebrae have articular surfaces (___)
for articulation with ribs

d the vertebral bodies bear articular (___)
processes arising near the base of their
pedicles

e in the adult the primary fetal curvatures (___)
are retained in the thoracic and sacral
regions

Answers

1.

a **F** – Five vertebrae fuse to form the sacrum and several to
form the coccyx.

b **F** – C1 has no spine, and that of C7 is not usually bifid.

c **T** – This is an identifying feature of thoracic vertebrae.

d **F** – The articular processes arise near the junction of the
pedicles and laminae ...

e **T** – ... and secondary curvatures develop after birth in
the cervical and lumbar regions (these are the most
mobile regions and most liable to injury).

**2. In the cervical region of the vertebral
column:**   T/F

a the atlas has no body (___)

b the superior articular facets of the atlas face (___)
anterolaterally

c the sixth cervical spine is the most (___)
prominent and palpable

d atlantoaxial dislocation is prevented by the (___)
alar and apical ligaments

e the upper vertebrae are related to the (___)
oropharynx

Answers

2.

a **T** – In early fetal life the body of the atlas is attached to
the axis to form the dens.

b **F** – The facets face upwards.

c **F** – C7 is known as the vertebra prominens.

d **F** – The cruciate (cruciform) ligament stabilizes the joint.

e **T** – X-rays of the atlanto-occipital and atlantoaxial joints
are best taken through the open mouth.

---

3. In the vertebral canal: T/F

a the dural covering of the spinal cord fuses (___)
with the periosteum of adjacent
vertebrae

b the adult spinal cord ends at about the level (___)
of the second lumbar vertebrae

c internal vertebral veins have large branches (___)
(basivertebral veins) draining the
vertebral bodies

d spinal nerve roots fuse in the intervertebral (___)
foramina

e the spinal cord cannot be damaged by a (___)
lumbar puncture performed between the
first and second lumbar spines

Answers

3.

a **F** – The bony-ligamentous wall of the canal is separated
from the dura by a fat-filled epidural space containing
emerging spinal nerves and the internal vertebral
venous plexus ...

b **T** – ... and in a child it ends somewhat lower.

c **T** – The bone marrow of the vertebral bodies is
haemopoietic throughout life.

d **T** – The dorsal root ganglion is situated near the point of
fusion.

e **F** – The spinal cord is still present at this level. The site of
election for a lumbar puncture is above or below the
spine of the 4th lumbar vertebra (interspace).

SBA

1. A young child is brought to the clinic for a routine check. All appears normal apart from dimpling of the skin with an associated tuft of hair found in the lumbar region. What is the likely cause of this?
a   Spina bifida cystica
b   Spina bifida occulta
c   Meningomyelocoele
d   Meningocoele
e   Congenital absence of 1st sacral vertebra

Answer

b   Spina bifida, a developmental condition resulting from incomplete fusion of the lumbar vertebral arches, presents most commonly without symptoms in its spina bifida occulta form. It usually causes parental concern because of its frequent association with the harmless cutaneous stigmata such as a tuft of hair or dimpling in the region. Its 'cystica' form is more severe and presents with associated protrusion of meninges and neurological deficits.

2. After an operation for ruptured aortic aneurysm the patient showed widespread paralysis of his lower limbs. What is the likely cause of this?
a   A cerebral thrombosis
b   Accidental ligation of the posterior spinal artery
c   Transection of the conal part of the spinal cord
d   Injury to the (great radicular) artery of Adamkiewicz
e   Accidental division of the thoracic sympathetic chain

Answer

d   The artery of Adamkiewicz gives rise to both the anterior and posterior spinal arteries and care should be taken to avoid its injury or ligation during aortic surgery or paraplegia will be likely to follow.

EMQs

Each question has an anatomical theme linked to the chapter, and a list of 10 related items (A–J) placed in alphabetical order: these are followed by five statements (1–5). Match **one or more** of the items A–J to each of the five statements.

Vertebrae
A. 1st lumbar
B. 1st thoracic
C. 3rd lumbar
D. 4th cervical
E. 5th lumbar
F. 7th cervical
G. 7th thoracic
H. 12th thoracic
I. Atlas
J. Axis

Answers
1 DJ; 2 I; 3 C; 4 BGH; 5 ACEH

Match the following statements with the appropriate vertebra(e) in the above list.
1. Has a bifid spine
2. Has no vertebral body
3. Has the longest transverse process
4. Has a costovertebral joint
5. Gives attachment to psoas major muscle

APPLIED QUESTIONS

1. Why should the cervical vertebrae be prone to dislocation in whiplash injuries?

1. *Because of the almost horizontal alignment of their articular facets.*

2. What might be an immediate consequence of a fracture–dislocation of the dens?

2. *Death, which is caused by the fractured dens being driven into the cervical spinal cord. Judicial hanging produces this effect. One of the most essential ligaments in the body is the transverse part of the cruciate ligament, which stabilizes the dens against the anterior arch of the atlas and prevents it from compressing the spinal cord.*

Bailey & Love · Essential Clinical Anatomy
Essential Clinical Anatomy · Bailey & Love
Bailey & Love · Essential Clinical Anatomy

PART 4

The upper limb

Bailey & Love · Essential Clinical Anatomy · Bailey & Love · Essential Clinical Anatom
Essential Clinical Anatomy · Bailey & Love · Essential Clinical Anatomy · Bailey & Lo
Bailey & Love · Essential Clinical Anatomy · Bailey & Love · Essential Clinical Anaton

Chapter 12

The shoulder region

The human upper limbs are specialized for prehension, sensation and grasping. They show little of their primitive functions of locomotion and support. Their ability to perform finely controlled movements is due to a well-developed sensory nerve supply, a large cerebral representation and a great mobility; pronation of the forearm and opposition of the thumb each contribute to this.

THE SHOULDER (PECTORAL) GIRDLE

This consists of the scapula (with which the humerus articulates), the clavicle and its articulation with the sternum, and the 1st costal cartilage. The shoulder girdle provides a very mobile connection of the upper limb with the axial skeleton, with two small joints, the sternoclavicular and the acromioclavicular, each with strong ligaments, and with a large muscular element.

The clavicle

The **clavicle** (Fig. 12.1) is a long bone but atypical in that it lacks a medullary cavity. Its expanded medial end articulates with the manubrium sterni and the 1st costal cartilage at the sternoclavicular joint (Fig. 12.2). It is subcutaneous throughout its length. The body is convex anteriorly in its medial two-thirds and concave in its lateral third. The flattened lateral end articulates with the acromion at the acromioclavicular joint. On the inferior surface of its medial end is attached the costoclavicular ligament, and on the inferior surface of its lateral end the strong coracoclavicular ligament. Four powerful muscles gain attachment: pectoralis major anteromedially, deltoid anterolaterally, sternocleidomastoid superomedially and trapezius posterolaterally.

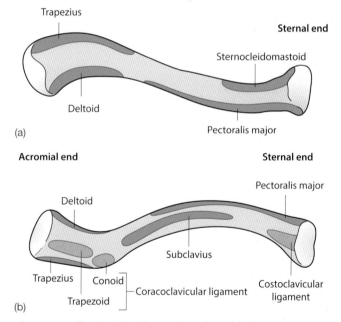

Figure 12.1 The clavicle: (a) superior surface; (b) inferior surface

Functions

The clavicle transmits part of the weight of the limb to the trunk and also allows it to swing clear of the trunk. It transmits shocks – commonly sustained by falling on to the outstretched hand – from the upper limb to the trunk, and thus is one of the most commonly fractured bones.

The scapula

The **scapula** (Fig. 12.3) is a flat triangular bone situated on the posterolateral part of the chest wall over the 2nd to

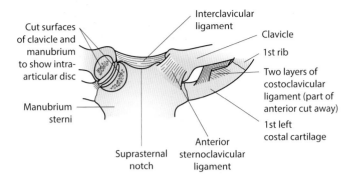

Figure 12.2 Sternoclavicular joint

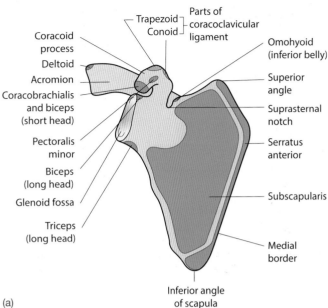

(a)

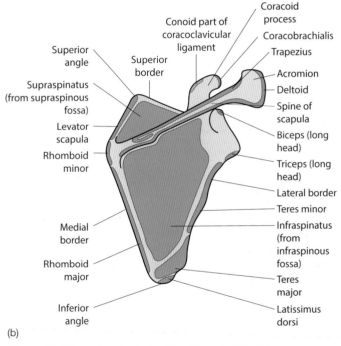

(b)

Figure 12.3 Scapula: (a) anterior view; (b) posterior view

7th ribs. Its costal surface gives attachment to subscapularis; its dorsal surface, divided by the projecting spine, gives attachment to the supraspinatus and infraspinatus muscles. The spine is expanded laterally into a flattened acromion, which articulates with the clavicle. The acromion and spine give attachment to trapezius and deltoid muscles. Near the lateral end of the superior border the beak-like coracoid process projects upwards and then forwards; it gives attachment to coracobrachialis, the short head of biceps and pectoralis minor muscles, and the coracoclavicular ligament.

The lateral angle is expanded to form the glenoid fossa for articulation with the humerus. Tubercles above and below it give attachment to the long heads of biceps and triceps, respectively. Latissimus dorsi, teres major and serratus anterior are attached to the stout inferior angle. Strong thick muscles cover much of the bone. Only the spine, acromion, coracoid process and inferior angle are palpable. The inferior angle overlies the 7th rib in the resting position and is an important surface landmark.

The humerus

The **humerus** is a long bone possessing an upper end, a shaft and a lower end (Fig. 12.4). The upper end has a humeral head and greater and lesser tubercles (tuberosities). The head articulates with the glenoid cavity of the scapula; it is bounded by the anatomical neck. The greater tubercle lies laterally behind the lesser tuberosity, separated from it by the bicipital (intertubercular) groove. To the greater tubercle are attached some of the muscles of the rotator cuff: supraspinatus, infraspinatus and teres minor. Subscapularis is attached to the lesser tubercle; the long head of biceps lies in the bicipital groove. The narrow junction between the upper end and the shaft of the humerus, its weakest part because of its propensity for fracture, is known as the surgical neck. The axillary nerve is in close relation to the bone at this point. The deltoid muscle gains attachment to a tuberosity halfway down its lateral border. Posteriorly, the oblique radial (spiral) groove, along which runs the nerve of the same name, separates the attachments of the lateral head of triceps above from the medial head below. The lower end of the shaft bears prominent lateral and medial supracondylar ridges; to the

lateral ridge are attached brachioradialis and extensor carpi radialis longus. Brachialis is attached to the anterior surface of the body.

The supracondylar ridges lead into the lateral and medial epicondyles, from which the common extensor and flexor origins, respectively, gain attachment. On the distal articular surface are a rounded capitulum laterally and a pulley-shaped trochlea medially; these articulate with the radius and ulna, respectively. Fossae, or concavities, are present anteriorly to accommodate the head of the radius and the coronoid process of the ulna during flexion, and posteriorly to accommodate the olecranon during extension.

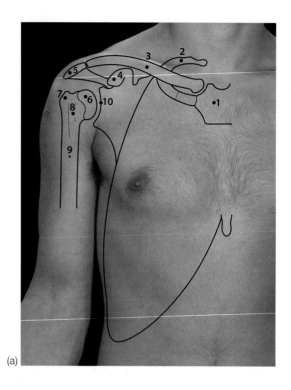

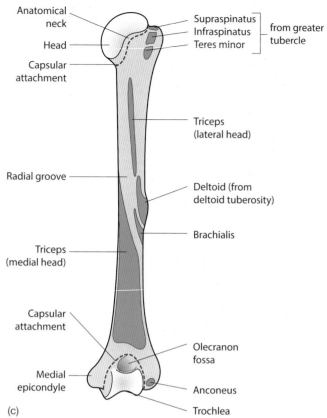

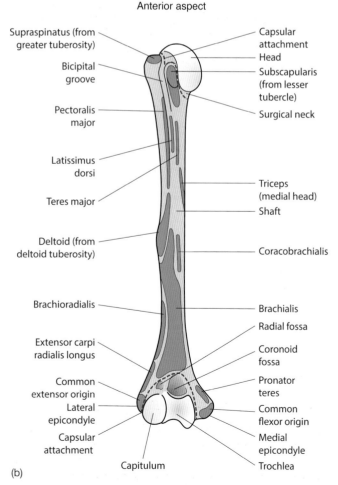

Anterior aspect

(b)

Figure 12.4 Bones of the shoulder joint. (a) Surface anatomy: 1, manubrium sterni; 2, 1st rib; 3, clavicle; 4, coracoid process; 5, acromion; 6, head of humerus; 7, greater tuberosity; 8, intertubercular groove; 9, shaft of humerus; 10, glenoid fossa. (b) Humerus anterior view and (c) humerus posterior view, each showing features, muscle attachments and capsular attachments (dotted red lines)

Fractures of the neck of the humerus (Fig. 12.5a), which usually follow a fall on the outstretched arm, may be complicated by injury to closely related nerves and vessels. The axillary nerve, lying close to the surgical neck, may be injured by a fracture at this level, as it may be following dislocation of the shoulder joint (Fig. 12.5b) and result in paralysis of the deltoid and inability to abduct the arm. There is associated sensory loss over the lateral upper arm. If the axillary nerve is severely injured then the normal rounded contour of the shoulder is lost because of the atrophy of the deltoid muscle. The radial nerve in the radial groove may be injured by fractures of the mid-shaft (Fig. 12.5d). A more common injury to the radial nerve is that of 'Saturday night palsy', wherein prolonged pressure to the radial nerve in the axilla after a drunken sleep resting with the arm thrown over a chairback results in prolonged paralysis of elbow and wrist extension. The ulnar nerve, lying subcutaneously behind the medial epicondyle, is often injured after trauma to the elbow region. The supracondylar region in children is a relatively weak spot and is often fractured (Fig. 13.4g, p. 212). In these cases the brachial artery may be occluded. Urgent attention is then required to prevent ischaemic contracture of the forearm muscles (Volkmann's contracture) (Fig. 12.6).

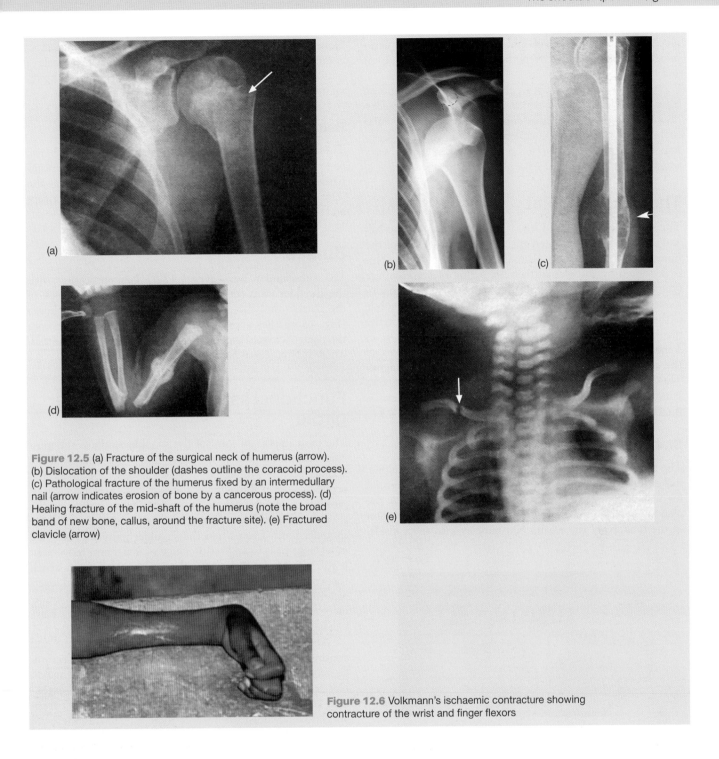

Figure 12.5 (a) Fracture of the surgical neck of humerus (arrow). (b) Dislocation of the shoulder (dashes outline the coracoid process). (c) Pathological fracture of the humerus fixed by an intermedullary nail (arrow indicates erosion of bone by a cancerous process). (d) Healing fracture of the mid-shaft of the humerus (note the broad band of new bone, callus, around the fracture site). (e) Fractured clavicle (arrow)

Figure 12.6 Volkmann's ischaemic contracture showing contracture of the wrist and finger flexors

The sternoclavicular joint

The **sternoclavicular joint** (Fig. 12.2) comprises the shallow concavity formed by the manubrium sterni and the 1st costal cartilage articulating with the medial end of the clavicle. It is lined by fibrocartilage and its capsule is strengthened by anterior and posterior sternoclavicular ligaments. The joint's stability is due to the strong accessory ligament, the **costoclavicular ligament**, and its fibrocartilaginous articular disc, which prevent the clavicle overriding the sternum.

The costoclavicular ligament acts as a fulcrum around which clavicular movements occur.

The acromioclavicular joint

The **acromioclavicular joint** lies subcutaneously (Fig. 12.7a). It permits a slight degree of gliding movement. It is a synovial joint with weak capsular ligaments and strong accessory ligaments. The **coracoclavicular ligament** provides a strong union between the scapula and the clavicle, and conveys much of the upper limb's weight to the clavicle. The **acromioclavicular ligament** covers the upper aspect of the joint and lends strength to it.

Acromioclavicular joint separation, a rather uncommon injury, can follow severe downward blows to the shoulder. Usually the coracoclavicular ligament remains intact and subluxation rather than complete dislocation occurs. Confirmation is easier to obtain if the X-ray is taken with a heavy weight in the hand (Fig. 12.7).

The shoulder joint

The **shoulder joint** (Fig. 12.8) is a synovial joint of the ball and socket variety, between the hemispherical head of the humerus and the shallow glenoid fossa of the scapula. This is deepened by the glenoid labrum, a ring of fibrocartilage attached to its rim. The capsule is strengthened by glenohumeral ligaments but it is lax, a necessity for a joint as mobile as the shoulder; it extends onto the diaphysis inferiorly on the medial side of the neck. The **coracohumeral ligament** gives some support. This is a broad band passing from the base of the coracoid process to the greater tubercle of the humerus. The synovial membrane communicates with the subscapular bursa and encloses the tendon of the long head of biceps as it crosses the joint in the intertubercular groove (Fig. 12.8).

Stability

The lax capsule and the shallow glenoid cavity would, alone, make the shoulder joint very unstable, but its potential for instability is reduced by strong contributions from the glenohumeral and coracohumeral ligaments and the fusion of the tendons of the rotator cuff muscles with the capsule.

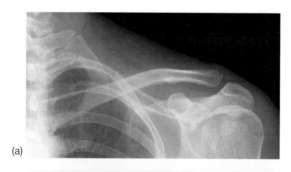

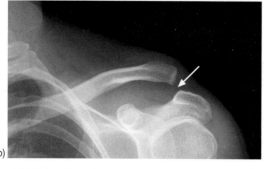

Figure 12.7 Acromioclavicular joint: (a) normal; (b) traumatic separation: weight distraction (arrow) – the scapula is dragged away from the acromion

Nonetheless, the shoulder joint is frequently dislocated, most commonly in a downwards direction because of the lack of muscles and tendons inferiorly. The coracoacromial arch prevents upward dislocation occurring very frequently.

Relations

These are seen in Fig. 12.9; *anterior* – subscapularis and bursa; *posterior* – infraspinatus and teres minor; *superior* – supraspinatus, subacromial bursa and coracoacromial arch; inside the joint is the long head of biceps; *inferior* – long head of triceps and the axillary nerve. The deltoid muscle embraces the joint.

Bursae

The **subscapular bursa** (Fig. 12.9) communicating with the shoulder joint separates subscapularis from the neck of the scapula and shoulder joint; a large **subacromial bursa** (Fig. 12.9b) lies above supraspinatus and separates it from the coracoacromial arch and the deep surface of the deltoid, where it often extends as the subdeltoid bursa.

Functional aspects of the shoulder girdle

The most important joint of the shoulder girdle is the muscular **scapulothoracic joint**, which allows movements of the scapula on the posterolateral thoracic wall: elevation and depression, as in shrugging of the shoulder, protraction, as in pushing or opening a door, and retraction, as in bracing the shoulders, are each usually combined with movements of the shoulder joint. Even when the shoulder joint has restricted movement or is fused, a wide range of upper arm movement is still possible by this scapulothoracic movement, in which the scapula pivots on the costoclavicular ligament and levers against the sternoclavicular joint (note that in forward movement and retraction of the scapula the medial end of the clavicle moves in the opposite direction).

Abduction of the arm is begun by supraspinatus and continued by deltoid (Fig. 12.10); **adduction** is by pectoralis major and latissimus dorsi; **flexion** is by pectoralis major, biceps brachii and the anterior fibres of deltoid; and **extension** is by the posterior fibres of deltoid, long head of triceps and latissimus dorsi. In most of these movements there are associated movements of the shoulder girdle. The scapula moves easily over the thoracic wall, elevated by trapezius, depressed by serratus anterior and the lower fibres of trapezius, and it moves forward as in punching by the action of serratus anterior and pectoralis minor, with latissimus dorsi holding the inferior angle to the chest wall. Retraction, as in bracing the shoulders, is effected by trapezius. Fixation of the humerus and shoulder girdle, achieved by placing the elbows on a table, or hands on the thighs, allows some of these muscles to act as accessory muscles of respiration during forced respiration. Their attachments to the ribs are then approximated to the now fixed humerus or scapula, and the chest wall is pulled up to increase the capacity of the thoracic cavity.

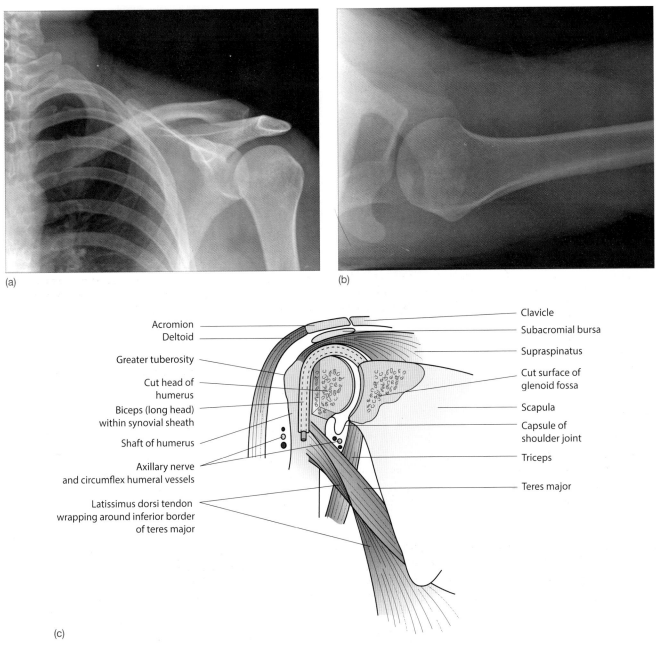

(a)

(b)

Clavicle

Subacromial bursa

Supraspinatus

Cut surface of glenoid fossa

Scapula

Capsule of shoulder joint

Triceps

Teres major

Acromion
Deltoid

Greater tuberosity

Cut head of humerus

Biceps (long head) within synovial sheath

Shaft of humerus

Axillary nerve and circumflex humeral vessels

Latissimus dorsi tendon wrapping around inferior border of teres major

(c)

Figure 12.8 Shoulder: (a) X-ray, anteroposterior view; (b) X-ray, axial view; (c) shoulder joint anterior view, with some bone removed from humerus and scapula

Dislocation of the shoulder (Fig. 12.5b) is a relatively common injury, usually caused by a blow on to the fully abducted arm – for example a backstroke swimmer colliding with the end of the pool. The dislocation is usually through the inferior capsule with the head of the humerus coming to lie anterior to the glenoid cavity. Such a dislocation frequently recurs due to tearing of the shoulder capsule and the rotator cuff muscles. The dislocation can be reduced by gentle traction on the hand, which is met by counterforce provided by a bare foot in the patient's axilla (Hippocratic method) or by Kocher's method, in which, while the operator grips and pulls on the epicondyles, the externally rotated arm is first adducted across the body and then internally rotated. Check for axillary nerve damage before and after reduction – it lies directly below the joint capsule and is thus subject to damage with this injury. The **rotator cuff syndrome** is painful and arises from impingement or injury of the tendons, particularly that of supraspinatus, under the coracoacromial arch (see below).

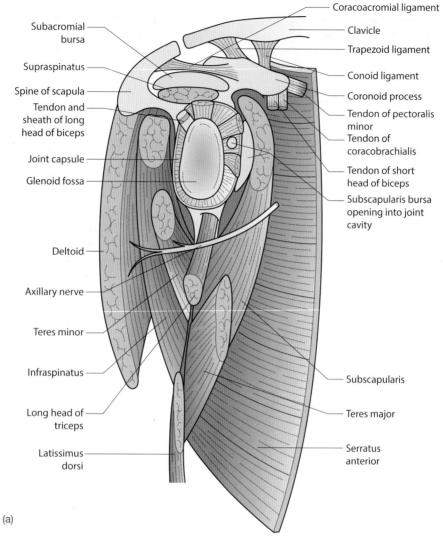

(a)

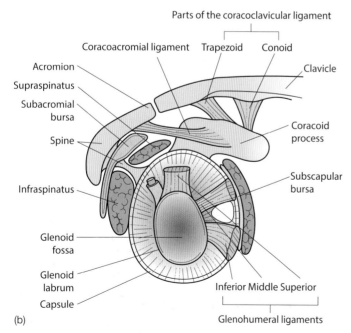

(b)

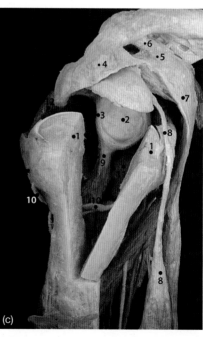

(c)

Figure 12.9 (a) Lateral view of right shoulder joint (humerus removed) showing the rotator cuff muscles. (b) Lateral view of right shoulder joint (humerus removed) showing bursae and ligaments. (c) Dissection of shoulder with division of the humeral head to reveal the glenoid fossa: 1, humeral head (split); 2, glenoid fossa; 3, glenoid labrum; 4, acromion; 5, coracoid process, 6, coracoclavicular ligament; 7, short head of biceps muscle; 8, long head of biceps tendon; 9, long head of triceps muscle; 10, axillary nerve; 11, subscapularis muscle; 12, deltoid muscle

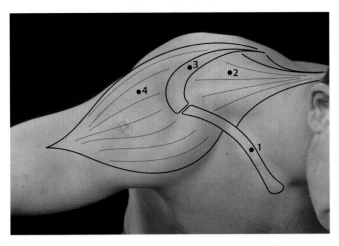

Figure 12.10 Deltoid muscle, superior view: 1, clavicle; 2, trapezius; 3, spine and acromion of scapula; 4, deltoid

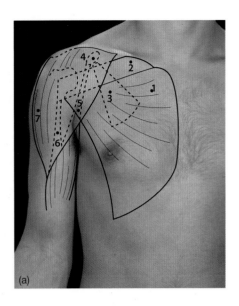

(a)

MUSCLES CONNECTING THE UPPER LIMB TO THE TRUNK

Anterior group

Four pectoral muscles move the shoulder girdle and attach it to the thoracic wall (Table 12.1 and Fig. 12.11). Pectoralis major covers the upper chest and its lower border forms the anterior wall of the axilla. Superiorly it is separated from deltoid muscle along the clavicle by the **deltopectoral triangle** (Fig. 12.11b). Pectoralis minor lies covered by pectoralis major in the anterior axillary wall. Serratus anterior lies on the lateral thoracic wall, forming the medial wall of the axilla. Subclavius lies below the clavicle and has no significant function.

Posterior group

These four muscles, trapezius, latissimus dorsi, levator scapulae and the rhomboids, attach the upper limb to the vertebral column (Table 12.2 and Fig. 12.12). Trapezius, levator scapulae and the rhomboids are attached to the shoulder girdle; only latissimus dorsi is attached to the humerus.

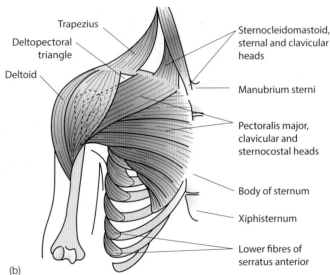

(b)

Figure 12.11 Shoulder. (a) Surface anatomy: 1 and 2, sternocostal and clavicular heads of pectoralis major; 3, underlying pectoralis minor; 4, coracoid process; 5 short and 6 long heads of biceps; 7 deltoid; (b) muscles, anterior view

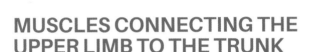

TABLE 12.1 Shoulder girdle muscles				
Muscle	Proximal attachment	Distal attachment	Nerve supply	Function
Pectoralis major	By two heads: Clavicular: medial half of clavicle. Sternocostal: anterior sternum, upper six costal cartilages and external oblique aponeurosis	Intertubercular groove of the humerus	Medial and lateral pectoral nerves (C5, C6, C7)	Adduction and medial rotation of humerus, pulls scapula anteriorly; anterior fibres flex shoulder, posterior fibres extend shoulder
Pectoralis minor	Anterior surfaces of 3rd–5th ribs	Coracoid process of scapula	Medial pectoral nerve (C8, T1)	Stabilization of scapula
Serratus anterior	External surface of lateral surface of 1st–8th ribs	Medial border of scapula	Long thoracic nerve (C5, C6, C7)	Protraction of scapula, holds scapula against chest wall

TABLE 12.2 Muscles of the shoulder girdle

Muscle	Proximal attachment	Distal attachment	Nerve supply	Function
Trapezius	Occipital bone, ligamentum nuchae, all the thoracic spines and supraspinous ligaments	Lateral third of clavicle, acromion, spine of scapula	Spinal accessory nerve, cervical nerves (C3, C4)	Elevates, retracts and rotates the scapula; upper fibres elevate, middle retract and lower depress. Both act to extend the head and neck
Latissimus dorsi	Spinous processes of lower six thoracic vertebrae, thoracolumbar fascia, posterior iliac crest and lower four ribs	Intertubercular groove of humerus	Thoracodorsal nerve (C6, C7, C8)	Adduction, extension and medial rotation of humerus; in climbing it raises the body on the arms
Levator scapulae	Transverse processes of first four cervical vertebrae	Medial border of scapula	Dorsal scapular nerve (C5)	Elevation of scapula
Rhomboids	Spinous processes of cervical and upper thoracic vertebrae	Medial border of scapula	Dorsal scapular nerve (C4, C5)	Retraction of scapula

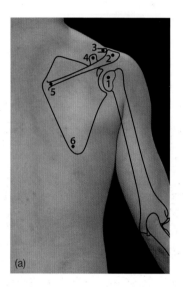

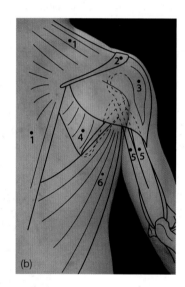

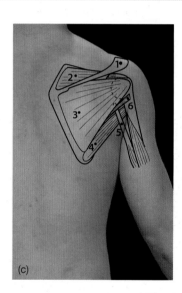

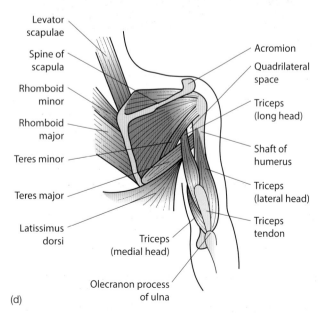

Figure 12.12 Shoulder, posterior view. (a) Bones, surface anatomy: 1, head of humerus; 2, acromion; 3, clavicle; 4, coracoid process; 5, spine of scapula; 6, inferior angle of scapula. (b) Superficial muscles, surface anatomy: 1, trapezius; 2, acromion; 3, deltoid; 4, infraspinatus; 5, long and lateral heads of triceps; 6, latissimus dorsi. (c) Deep muscles, surface anatomy: 1, acromion; 2, supraspinatus; 3, infraspinatus; 4, teres major; 5, long head of triceps; 6, teres minor. (d) Diagram of deep posterior muscles of shoulder joint

MUSCLES OF THE SHOULDER REGION

Deltoid (Fig. 12.10) forms the contour of the shoulder and is functionally divided into anterior, middle and posterior parts. Teres major, with the tendon of latissimus dorsi, forms the posterior axillary fold. Deep to deltoid are the four rotator cuff muscles: supraspinatus, teres minor, infraspinatus (all rotators of the humerus) and subscapularis (Table 12.3). Their tendons blend to form the **rotator cuff**, which gives stability to the shoulder joint.

Intramuscular injections, when necessary, can be made into deltoid's anterior fibres. Avoidance of the posterior part of the muscle prevents accidental injury to the axillary nerve.

Intraosseous infusion

The intraosseus route is indicated any time vascular accesss is difficult to obtain in emergency situations in both children and adult patients. It is contraindicated in those with clotting disorders, a fractured target bone, osteoporosis, local skin sepsis or skin ulcer. In children the preferred insertion site is the proximal tibia; in adults the preferred site is the proximal humerus.

The point of insertion is located just 1–2 cm proximal to the surgical neck of the humerus where the most prominent aspect of the greater tubercle of the humerus is found. Wear sterile gloves and 'prep' the skin with antiseptic solution. Drill downwards at an angle of 45 degrees to the horizontal, and confirm placement in the marrow by aspiration of blood or marrow. Secure the trochar/needle with tape and begin the infusion. The route should not be used for longer than 48 hours or infection may occur.

If the **supraspinatus tendon** is torn after injury then initiation of abduction is difficult without the trick manoeuvre of dipping the shoulder towards the injured side so that gravity can assist abduction of the arm away from the trunk. Repetitive injury may occur in sportsmen using a strong throwing action, and can result in inflammation of the supraspinatus tendon and associated inflammation of the underlying subacromial bursa (**rotator cuff syndrome**). This causes abduction to be painful, particularly during the middle range of this movement. This 'painful arc' of abduction, usually from 45 to 100 degrees, is diagnostic of this inflammatory condition. Rotator cuff tears are nowadays commonly diagnosed on MRI scans (Fig. 12.13).

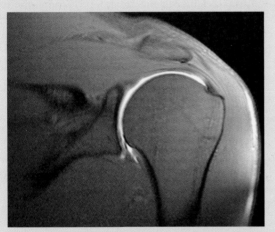 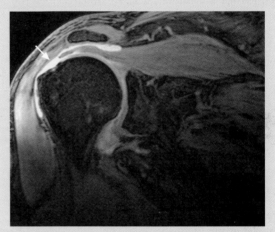

Figure 12.13 MR arthrogram of shoulder joint. (a) Normal; (b) tear in the supraspinatus tendon – the arrow shows the gap in the tendon

TABLE 12.3 Muscles of the shoulder joint

Muscle	Proximal attachment	Distal attachment	Nerve supply	Function
Deltoid	Lateral third of clavicle, acromion and scapular spine	Deltoid tuberosity of humerus	Axillary nerve (C5, C6)	Anterior – flexion, medial rotation of arm. Middle – abduction of arm. Posterior – extension and lateral rotation of arm
Supraspinatus	Supraspinous fossa of scapula	Greater tuberosity of humerus	Suprascapular nerve (C5)	Initiate abduction
Infraspinatus	Infraspinous fossa of scapula	Greater tuberosity of humerus	Suprascapular nerve (C5)	Adduction and lateral rotation of arm
Teres minor	Lateral border of scapula	Greater tuberosity of humerus	Axillary nerve (C5)	Adduction and lateral rotation of arm
Subscapularis	Subscapular fossa of scapula	Lesser tuberosity of humerus	Subscapular nerve (C6)	Adduction and lateral rotation of arm
Teres major	Inferior angle of scapula	Intertubercular groove of humerus	Subscapular nerve (C6)	Adduction, medial rotation of arm

THE AXILLA AND UPPER ARM

The **axilla** is a fat-filled pyramidal space between the lateral thoracic wall and the upper arm (Fig. 12.14). Its apex, which allows the axillary vessels, brachial plexus and lymphatics to pass from the neck to the axilla via the cervicoaxillary canal, is bounded by the 1st rib, scapula and middle third of the clavicle. Its base is formed by hairy axillary skin. Its anterior wall comprises pectoralis major and minor (Fig. 12.11); its posterior wall, lower than the anterior, comprises subscapularis, latissimus dorsi and teres major, which cover the scapula (Fig. 12.12). The medial wall is formed by the upper four ribs, their intercostal muscles and the overlying serratus anterior, and the narrow lateral wall is the intertubercular groove of the humerus, whose lips give attachment to the muscles of the anterior and posterior axillary walls. It contains the axillary artery and vein, the cords and branches of the brachial plexus, coracobrachialis and biceps, axillary lymph vessels, lymph nodes and fat.

Deep fascia

Around the shoulder region the deep fascia invests all the muscles and is drawn out as a tubular prolongation over the arm. Proximally it encloses pectoralis minor and extends above the clavicle as the clavipectoral fascia. Around the elbow the fascia ensheathes the muscles and gives attachment to some of their fibres; in the cubital fossa it is reinforced by the bicipital aponeurosis. In the forearm the fascia is attached to the posterior border of the ulna along its subcutaneous border; at the wrist it forms the flexor and extensor retinacula, and in the hand the palmar aponeurosis and fibrous flexor sheaths. Both the arm and forearm are divided into fascial compartments by strong fascial sheaths, each of which contain a nerve and blood vessels.

Clinically their importance is that if bleeding occurs during trauma, this can then cause compression within a compartment.

Lymphatic drainage

There are two groups of vessels, superficial and deep. The **superficial group** drain the skin. The medial vessels lie with the basilic vein and drain to axillary nodes; the lateral vessels lie with the cephalic vein and drain into infraclavicular nodes

and thence to the apical group of axillary nodes. The **deep group** drain bone and muscle and run with the deep veins to drain into the lateral group of axillary nodes.

The axillary nodes are arranged in five groups (Fig. 1.17, p. 28):

- **Pectoral** – deep to pectoralis major; drain the lateral and anterior chest wall, the breast and the upper anterior abdominal wall
- **Lateral** – on the lateral axillary wall; drain the efferents of the upper limb
- **Posterior** (subscapular) – on the posterior axillary wall; drain the back of the upper trunk
- **Central** – lie around the axillary vessels
- **Apical** – at the axillary apex; drain from all the preceding groups. They are continuous with the inferior deep cervical nodes.

Infection in the superficial tissues of the upper limb results in tender enlargement of the axillary nodes. Skin malignancies arising in the upper limb or anterolateral chest wall may spread lymphatically to produce enlarged axillary nodes. Blockage of the axillary nodes after, for example, radiotherapy treatment, may lead to lymphatic swelling of the limb (lymphoedema) (Fig. 1.20b, p. 29).

The **infraclavicular group** are grouped around the termination of the cephalic vein and drain to the apical nodes. Efferent vessels from the apical nodes form the **subclavian lymph trunk**, which, on the left, joins the thoracic duct and, on the right, opens into the right lymphatic duct, or the internal jugular or subclavian vein.

Blood supply

The **axillary artery** (Figs. 12.15 and 12.16) commences at the lateral border of the 1st rib as the continuation of the third part of the subclavian artery and ends at the lower border of teres major, where it becomes the **brachial artery.**

Dilatation of the axillary artery may occur beyond a stenosis due to an abnormal band of tissue or a cervical rib. Thrombus building up in the dilatation can break off and cause distal arterial ischemia. Axillary artery aneurysms are rare, but compress the surrounding part of the brachial plexus and adjacent axillary vein, causing nerve damage and arm swelling

Pectoralis minor divides the artery into three parts, the first above, the second behind and the third below the muscle. It is enclosed in the axilla by the axillary sheath, a continuation of the prevertebral fascia and surrounded by the cords and branches of the brachial plexus (p. 199). The **axillary vein** (Fig. 12.16) lies medial to this neurovascular bundle; coracobrachialis and the short head of biceps are lateral. The brachial plexus lies above and behind the first part of the artery, but below this its cords surround it closely in relationships according to their names, i.e. posterior, medial and lateral.

Branches

The first part has one branch, the superior thoracic artery. The second part has two branches, the thoracoacromial artery and the lateral thoracic artery, which supply the anterolateral

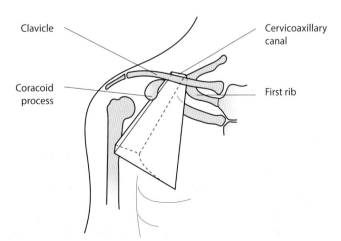

Figure 12.14 Pyramidal shape of the axilla

Clavicle

Cervicoaxillary canal

Coracoid process

First rib

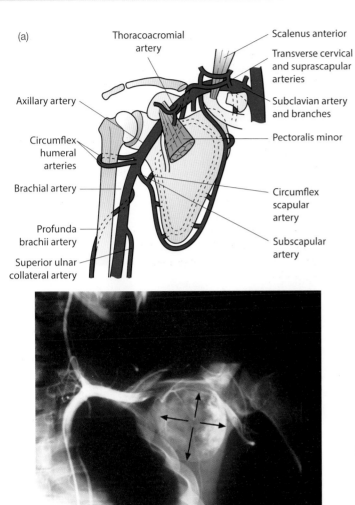

(a)

Thoracoacromial artery

Scalenus anterior

Transverse cervical and suprascapular arteries

Axillary artery

Subclavian artery and branches

Circumflex humeral arteries

Pectoralis minor

Brachial artery

Circumflex scapular artery

Profunda brachii artery

Subscapular artery

Superior ulnar collateral artery

(b)

Figure 12.15 (a) Axillary artery and shoulder girdle anastomoses. (b) Angiogram showing an aneurysm of the axillary artery (arrows)

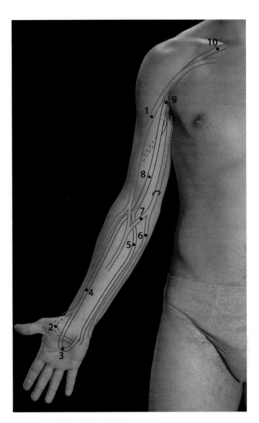

Figure 12.16 Upper limb arteries and veins: 1, cephalic vein; 2, deep palmar arch; 3, superficial palmar arch; 4, radial artery; 5, ulnar artery; 6, basilic vein; 7, medial cubital vein; 8, brachial artery; 9, axillary artery; 10, subclavian artery

aspects of the upper thoracic wall. The third part has three branches, the subscapular artery, which follows the lower border of subscapularis and gives a circumflex scapular branch to supply the infraspinous fossa, and the anterior and posterior circumflex humeral arteries which supply the shoulder region and anastomose around the surgical neck of the humerus. The **scapular anastomosis** acquires importance if the upper parts of the axillary artery are occluded. It comprises anastomoses between the **subclavian artery** via its thyrocervical trunk and the **third part of the axillary artery** via its subscapular and circumflex scapular branches.

Venous drainage

The veins are divided into superficial and deep groups that communicate via perforating veins, which under normal circumstances drain from superficial to deep systems.

Superficial group

The digital veins drain into a **dorsal venous arch** on the back of the hand. From its lateral side arises the cephalic vein, and

from its medial the basilic vein. The **cephalic vein** ascends the radial side of the forearm, crossing the cubital fossa to lie lateral to biceps in the upper arm. In the deltopectoral groove it pierces the clavipectoral fascia to join the axillary vein. The **basilic vein** ascends the ulnar side of the forearm, crosses the cubital fossa and lies medial to biceps. In the upper arm it pierces the deep fascia to join the brachial veins. The **median cubital vein**, frequently chosen for venepuncture, unites the cephalic and basilic veins superficial to the bicipital aponeurosis in the roof of the cubital fossa (Fig. 12.16).

The veins of the forearm and hand are most frequently chosen for intravenous infusions; patient comfort is more easily obtained when the puncture site is not too close to the wrist or elbow joint. The cephalic vein just proximal to the wrist is a popular site.

Deep group

The radial and ulnar veins accompany the arteries and join in the floor of the cubital fossa to form the brachial vein, which forms the axillary vein at the lower border of teres major.

The **axillary vein** is the continuation of the **basilic** and **brachial veins** above the lower border of teres major; it ascends medial to the axillary artery to the outer border of the 1st rib, where it becomes the subclavian vein. It gains tributaries that correspond to the branches of the axillary artery and the **cephalic vein**, which enters through the fascia in the deltopectoral groove.

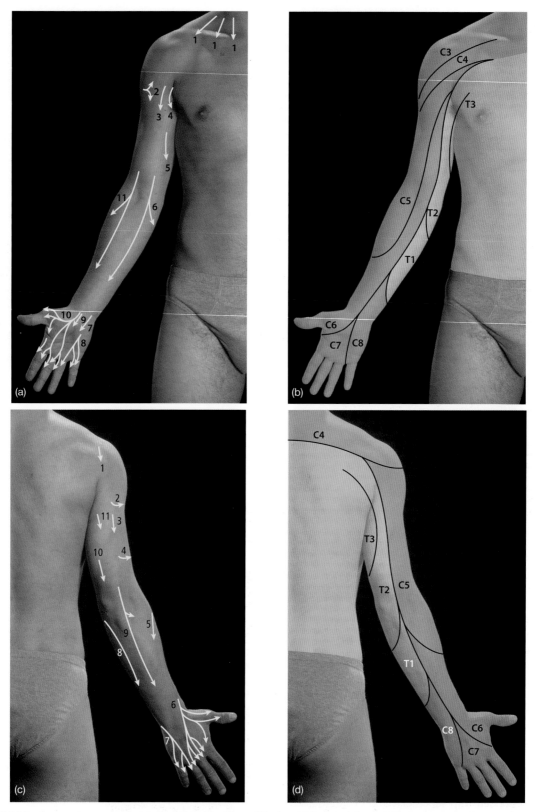

Figure 12.17 (a) Surface anatomy of anterior cutaneous branches of the brachial plexus: 1, supraclavicular nerve; 2, upper lateral cutaneous nerve of arm; 3, intermediate cutaneous nerve of arm; 4, intercostobrachial nerve; 5, medial cutaneous nerve of arm; 6, medial cutaneous nerve of forearm; 7, palmar branch of ulnar nerve; 8, ulnar nerve; 9, palmar branch of median nerve; 10, median nerve and its cutaneous branches to the lateral three and a half digits; 11, lateral cutaneous nerve of forearm. (b) Dermatomes of the upper limb, anterior view: the numbers denote the dermatomes of the brachial plexus and their distribution. (c) Posterior view, cutaneous nerves: 1, supraclavicular nerve; 2, axillary nerve; 3, posterior cutaneous nerve of arm; 4, lower lateral cutaneous nerve of arm; 5, lateral cutaneous nerve of forearm; 6, superficial radial nerve; 7, dorsal branch of ulnar nerve; 8, medial cutaneous nerve of forearm; 9, posterior cutaneous nerve of forearm; 10, posterior cutaneous nerve of arm; 11, intercostobrachial nerve. (d) Posterior view: dermatomes. C = cervical, T = thoracic

NERVES

The brachial plexus

The **brachial plexus** (Fig. 12.17) supplies the upper limb. It is formed from the anterior primary rami of the lower four cervical and the first thoracic nerves. These **five roots** of the plexus appear between the middle and anterior scalene muscles and unite to form three **trunks** in the posterior triangle of the neck. The upper two roots (C5, C6) form at the apex of the axilla. Each trunk divides into **anterior** and **posterior divisions**. The three posterior divisions join to form the posterior cord, the anterior divisions of the upper and middle trunks form the lateral cord and the anterior division of the lower trunk continues as the medial cord.

The cords lie close to the axillary artery, disposed around it according to their names. The posterior cord and its branches supply structures on the dorsal surface of the limb and end by dividing into axillary and radial nerves. The medial and lateral cords and their branches supply structures on the flexor surface of the limb; the lateral cord ends by dividing into the musculocutaneous nerve and the lateral head of the median nerve, while the medial cord ends as the ulnar nerve and the medial head of the median nerve.

The plexus and its branches can be best understood by study of Fig. 12.18b.

From the **roots**: small branches to the back muscles; C5 contributes to the phrenic nerve, and the long thoracic nerve passes behind the vessels to the medial wall of the axilla to supply serratus anterior.

Segmental nerve supply

Although the course of the nerve roots in the brachial plexus is complex, the skin of the upper limb has perfectly regular dermatomes (Figs. 12.17b,d). They originate from segments C4 to T2 (Fig. 12.18).

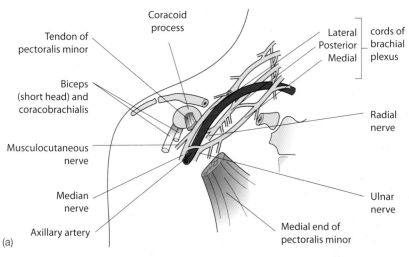

(a)

Figure 12.18 (a) Diagram of the brachial plexus showing the relationship of the cords to the axillary artery with a segment of clavicle and pectoralis minor removed. (b) Brachial plexus – diagram showing its roots, trunks, cords and branches

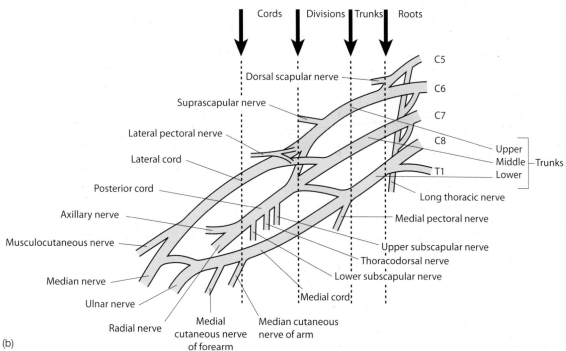

(b)

It is worth noting that the segmental innervation of the skin over the deltoid muscle, C4, is identical to that segment supplying the diaphragm, which explains the referral of pain originating in the diaphragm to the shoulder region.

C5 supplies the upper outer arm, C6 the radial side of the forearm and thumb, C7 the palm of the hand and first three fingers, C8 the ulnar forearm, T1 the ulnar upper arm and T2 the axillary skin (dermatomal patterns are subject to variation and overlap). Autonomic sympathetic nerves are carried in the branches of the brachial plexus and supply blood vessels, sweat glands and arrector pili muscles throughout the upper limb.

Injuries to the brachial plexus

Brachial plexus injuries, which are usually the result of forceful stretching or direct wounding, will produce signs of a segmental nature. **Upper trunk injury** is usually the result of forceful and excessive separation of the neck and shoulder, such as may happen when a motorcyclist is thrown forwards at high speed on to his shoulder, or following a difficult birth delivery which has been associated with excessive traction on the baby's head. Upper trunk damage produces sensory loss on the radial side of the arm and forearm (C5, C6) and paralysis of deltoid, biceps and brachialis. The limb hangs limply, medially rotated and fully pronated (the 'waiter's tip' position) (Erb's palsy; Fig. 12.19a). **Lower trunk injuries** are uncommon but may occur when the upper limb is pulled forcibly upwards. This may result from pulling too hard on an infant's arm during a difficult delivery. Injury to C8 and

THE UPPER ARM MUSCLES

In the anterior compartment of the arm there are three flexor muscles: biceps, brachialis and coracobrachialis (Table 12.4 and Fig. 12.20). The tendon of the long head of biceps lies in the shoulder joint, retained in the intertubercular groove by the transverse humeral ligament, surrounded by a synovial sheath. It unites with the short head in the lower arm. One extensor, triceps, occupies the posterior compartment. Anconeus lies close to triceps, but the bulk of it lies in the forearm.

T1 results in paralysis of the small muscles of the hand, and the unopposed action of the long flexors (flexing the interphalangeal joints) and the long extensors (extension of the metacarpophalangeal joints) produces the typical 'claw-hand' deformity (Klumpke's paralysis; Fig. 12.19b).

Non-traumatic causes of brachial plexus pathology occur: a cervical rib (Fig. 12.19c) may put undue pressure on the lower cord, as may direct invasion of an apical lung cancer to result in similar paralysis.

When viewed pushing against a wall, the patient in Fig. 12.19e is seen to have an obvious 'winging' of his scapula due to damage to the long thoracic nerve (C5, C6, C7) which arises from the roots of the brachial plexus and supplies serratus anterior muscle. This muscle, which normally holds the scapula against the chest wall when pushing, is here paralysed.

Peripheral nerve injuries are described on p. 236.

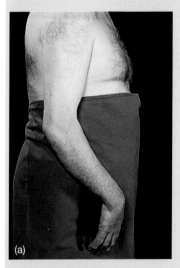

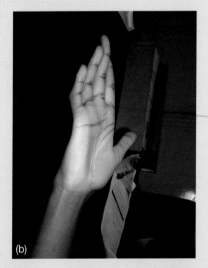

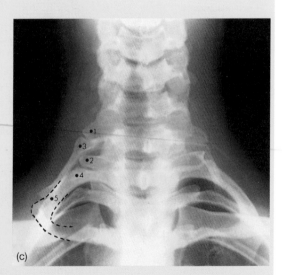

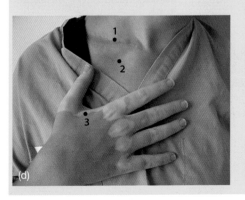

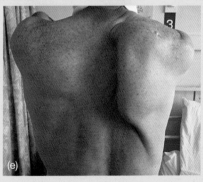

Figure 12.19 (a) Erb's palsy. (b) Injury to T1 producing a claw hand. (c) Cervical rib X-ray: 1, transverse process of 7th cervical vertebra; 2, transverse process of 1st thoracic vertebra; 3, abnormal cervical rib; 4, 1st rib; 5, prominent articulation between cervical and 1st rib. (d) This patient has: 1, a cervical rib scar; 2, hollow where 1st rib has been removed; 3, wasting of 1st dorsal interosseous muscle due to cervical rib pressure on the T1 nerve root, 'Klumpke's palsy'. (e) 'Winging' of the scapula

TABLE 12.4 Muscles of the arm

Muscle	Proximal attachment	Distal attachment	Nerve supply	Function
Biceps brachii	By two heads: Short head: coracoid process of scapula. Long head: supraglenoid tubercle of scapula	Radial tuberosity and by bicipital aponeurosis to deep fascia of forearm	Musculocutaneous nerve (C6)	Flexion of forearm, supinator
Brachialis	Distal half of anterior humerus	Coronoid process of ulna	Musculocutaneous nerve (C6)	Flexion of forearm
Coracobrachialis	Coracoid process of scapula	Medial side of mid-humerus	Musculocutaneous nerve (C6)	Adduction and flexion of humerus (the newspaper under the arm when running for a bus)
Triceps	By three heads: Long head: infraglenoid tubercle of scapula. Lateral head: posterior upper humerus. Medial head: posterior humerus below radial groove	Olecranon of ulna	Radial nerve (C7, C8)	Chief extensor of forearm
Anconeus	Lateral epicondyle of humerus	Olecranon and upper part of posterior surface of ulna	Radial nerve (C8, T1)	Weak extensor of forearm; abducts the ulna during pronation

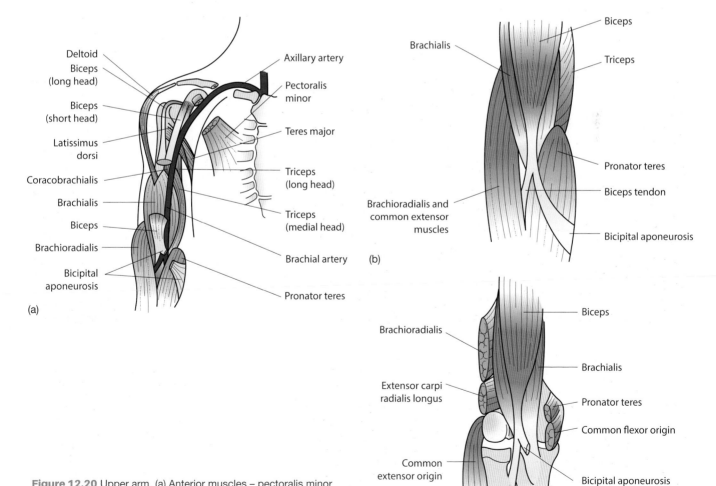

Figure 12.20 Upper arm. (a) Anterior muscles – pectoralis minor and biceps divided to reveal the artery. (b) Anterior elbow – bicipital aponeurosis. (c) Deep dissection of the elbow – attachment of biceps in the cubital fossa

Biceps

Biceps arises proximally by two heads: the **short head** from the coracoid process and the **long head** from the supraglenoid tubercle of the humerus.

Degenerative disease around the shoulder joint may cause the long head of biceps to fray and weaken, sometimes resulting in rupture. A noticeable bulge appears low on the anterior surface of the arm (Fig. 12.21) when the elbow is flexed, and supination against resistance is painful. Peripheral reflexes can be tested around the elbow joint: the biceps reflex (C5, C6) by tapping the thumb held against the biceps tendon in front of the elbow, and the triceps reflex by tapping the triceps tendon just above the olecranon (C6, C7).

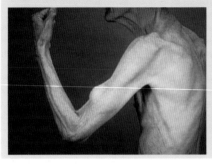

Figure 12.21 Rupture of the long head of biceps

The brachial artery

The **brachial artery** (Figs. 12.15, 12.20 and 12.22), the continuation of the axillary artery, begins at the lower border of teres major and descends subcutaneously on the medial side of the upper arm within the anterior compartment. Throughout its course it lies medial to biceps and its tendon. It is accompanied by veins and is crossed by the **median nerve** from lateral to medial halfway down the arm. It ends in the cubital fossa by dividing into the radial and ulnar arteries, and is here crossed by the **medial cubital vein** and separated from it by only the bicipital aponeurosis (Fig. 12.23).

Because the vein is frequently used for venepuncture this close relationship should be noted. Technique of venepuncture:

Prepare a tray of equipment – non-sterile gloves, tourniquet, butterfly needle and barrel, blood specimen bottles, sharps container and alcohol swab.

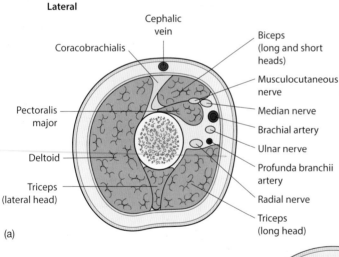

(a)

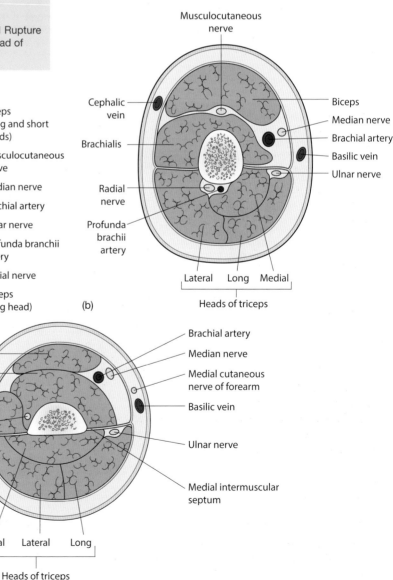

(b)

(c)

Figure 12.22 Transverse sections of the upper limb: (a) upper third; (b) middle third; (c) lower third

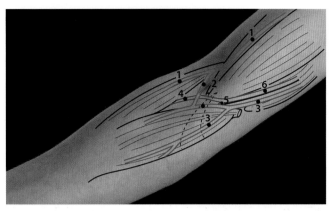

Figure 12.23 Surface marking of vessels and nerves in the cubital fossa (dotted lines show the bicipital aponeurosis separating the median cubital vein from the median nerve below): 1, cephalic vein; 2, median cubital vein; 3, basilic vein; 4, radial artery; 5, ulnar artery; 6, brachial artery

Wash your hands in alcohol gel. Confirm the patient's identity and position their arm comfortably extended; inspect the cubital fossa for a suitable vein. Apply the tourniquet about 10 cm proximal to the vein. Palpate the vein (it will feel 'springy').

Don non-sterile gloves, clean the chosen site with an alcohol swab for 20–30 seconds and allow it to dry.

Attach a needle to the barrel, warn the patient of 'a sharp scratch', insert the needle at about 30 degrees to the skin, and advance the needle 5 mm after blood is seen. Fill the sample bottle(s). Withdraw the needle and ask the patient to hold a cotton wool swab over the puncture site. Dispose of 'sharps' and apply an adhesive dressing to the puncture site. Complete the patient details on the sample bottles and laboratory request form and send both to the laboratory.

The artery provides branches to the muscles, the elbow joint and humerus and the **profunda brachii artery**, which runs with the radial nerve in the radial groove.

The brachial artery is palpable through most of its course on the medial side of the arm and in the cubital fossa medial to the bicipital tendon under the aponeurosis. In the latter situation it is usually palpated and auscultated when taking the blood pressure. The sphygmomanometer cuff is inflated until the arterial pulse can no longer be palpated, the stethoscope placed over the artery and the cuff slowly deflated. The pressure at which the arterial pressure waves are first heard is the systolic pressure and the pressure at which they disappear is the diastolic pressure. Laceration of the brachial artery or occlusion due to, for instance, displacement of an elbow fracture, is a surgical emergency because ischaemia and paralysis of the forearm muscles follows within a few hours. Subsequent fibrosis of the muscles results in contracture of the long forearm extensor and flexor muscles (Fig. 12.6).

Technique for measuring pulse rate
Extend the patient's elbow and place the tip of your index finger on the palpable brachial artery. Note the volume and regularity of the pulse, count the pulse beats for 30 seconds

measured by a watch and multiply this by 2 to obtain the pulse rate.

Technique for measuring blood pressure
Wash your hands, confirm the patient's name and apply the sphygmomanometer cuff to the upper arm. Place the your index finger of dominant hand on the radial artery and inflate the cuff until a palpable pulse disappears. Note the pressure reading. Now apply a stethoscope to the brachial artery position as previously felt in the cubital fossa and inflate the cuff to about 30 mmHg above the value noted. Begin a previously gradual release of air from the sphygmomanometer cuff until a pulsatile whooshing noise appears – this is the **systolic pressure**; continue deflating the cuff until the last sound disappears – this is the **diastolic pressure.**

The musculocutaneous nerve

The **musculocutaneous nerve** is a terminal branch of the lateral cord of the brachial plexus. Initially it lies lateral to the axillary artery and then it pierces coracobrachialis to descend between biceps and brachialis. It finally emerges lateral to these muscles to end, after piercing the deep fascia, as the **lateral cutaneous nerve of the forearm**. It supplies muscular branches to coracobrachialis, biceps and brachialis, and articular branches to the elbow joint. The lateral cutaneous nerve of the forearm supplies the flexor and extensor surfaces of the radial side of the forearm.

The nerve is rarely injured, but this occasionally occurs after a dislocation of the shoulder, producing paralysis of coracobrachialis, biceps and brachialis and a resultant weakness in elbow flexion and supination, together with loss of sensation on the lateral side of the forearm.

The radial nerve

The **radial nerve** (Figs. 12.22a–c), a terminal branch of the posterior cord of the brachial plexus, arises on the posterior wall of the axilla and descends between the long head of triceps and the shaft of the humerus to reach the posterior compartment of the arm. Here it descends with the profunda brachii artery between the medial and lateral heads of triceps in the radial groove of the humerus.

At this site it is susceptible to injury in mid-shaft fractures of the humerus.

It divides anterior to the elbow joint between brachioradialis and brachialis.

In the axilla it gives branches to triceps and the posterior cutaneous nerve of the arm, which supplies the skin of the posteromedial aspect of the upper arm.

In the posterior compartment of the arm it supplies triceps, brachioradialis and extensor carpi radialis longus, and gives off two sensory branches, the lower lateral cutaneous nerve of the arm, supplying the skin of the lower lateral aspect of the arm, and the posterior cutaneous nerve of the forearm, before piercing the lateral intermuscular septum.

The median nerve

The **median nerve** (Figs. 12.22a–c) in the upper arm arises by the union of its medial and lateral heads, both terminal branches of the brachial plexus. It descends through the upper arm, at first lateral to the axillary and brachial arteries, and then, halfway down the limb, it crosses the latter to the medial side. It has no branches above the elbow.

The ulnar nerve

The **ulnar nerve** (Figs. 12.22a–c) in the upper arm arises as the continuation of the medial cord of the brachial plexus. It descends medial to the axillary and brachial arteries and, halfway down the arm, pierces the medial intermuscular septum to continue its descent on the medial head of triceps to enter the forearm by passing behind the medial epicondyle. It has no branches in the upper arm above the elbow.

MCQs

1. The shoulder joint: **T/F**
  a has a scapular articular surface less than   (____)
    one-third that of the diameter of the
    humeral head
  b is surrounded by a tight capsular ligament   (____)
  c usually communicates with the subacromial   (____)
    bursa
  d depends for most of its stability on the   (____)
    capsular and accessory ligaments
  e is closely related inferiorly to the axillary   (____)
    nerve

Answers

1.
a **T** – *Even though the scapular articular surface includes the ring of fibrocartilage, the glenoid labrum, around its margin.*
b **F** – *The capsule is lax, particularly inferiorly, and allows for a wide range of movement in this joint.*
c **F** – *The subscapular bursa communicates with the joint, not the subacromial bursa.*
d **F** – *The lax capsule is of little support and the shallow glenoid cavity affords almost none. The tendons of the short articular (rotator cuff) muscles, subscapularis, supraspinatus, infraspinatus and teres minor, by their close fusion with the capsule, are the major stabilizing factors.*
e **T** – *Which is thus easily damaged in downward dislocations of the joint.*

2. Branches of the posterior cord of the   **T/F**
brachial plexus include the:
  a axillary nerve   (____)
  b lateral pectoral nerve   (____)
  c long thoracic nerve   (____)
  d nerve to the rhomboids   (____)
  e nerve to teres major   (____)

Answers

2.
a **T** – *The branches of the posterior cord are the axillary, radial, thoracodorsal and upper and lower subscapular nerves.*
b **F** – *The lateral pectoral nerve is a branch of the lateral cord.*
c **F** – *The long thoracic nerve to serratus anterior is a branch from the roots C5, C6 and C7.*
d **F** – *The nerve to the rhomboids is a branch from the root of C5.*
e **T** – *The nerve to teres major is a branch of the subscapular nerves, which are branches of the posterior cord.*

3. The axilla contains: **T/F**
  a the trunks of the brachial plexus   (____)
  b the superior thoracic artery   (____)
  c latissimus dorsi muscle   (____)
  d the dorsal scapular nerve   (____)
  e the long thoracic nerve   (____)

Answers

3.
a **F** – *The axilla contains the cords of the brachial plexus; the trunks lie in the posterior triangle of the neck.*
b **T** – *It arises in the upper axilla and supplies the upper thoracic wall.*
c **F** – *It is the tendon of latissimus dorsi, rather than the muscle, that is in the axilla.*
d **F** – *The dorsal scapular nerve (nerve to the rhomboids) lies posterior to the axilla.*
e **T** – *The long thoracic nerve (nerve to serratus anterior) lies on serratus anterior on the medial wall of the axilla.*

SBA

1. A patient is admitted after falling from a ladder complaining of shoulder pain in the shoulder region. He is unable to fully abduct the arm or rotate the arm laterally and has numbness over the shoulder area. What is his likely injury?

a   Fracture of the medial humeral epicondyle
b   Fracture of the surgical neck of the humerus
c   Fracture of the glenoid fossa
d   Fracture of the anatomical neck of the humerus
e   Fracture of the shaft of the humerus

Answer

b   Fracture of the surgical neck of the humerus frequently damages the axillary nerve, which supplies the deltoid and teres minor muscles. Abduction of the shoulder beyond 15 degrees is performed by the deltoid muscle, and lateral rotation largely by the deltoid and teres minor muscles.

2. During arthroscopy of the shoulder, erosion of a tendon crossing the joint is seen. Which tendon is this?

a   Long head of triceps brachii
b   Long head of biceps brachii
c   Coracobrachialis
d   Infraspinatus
e   Glenohumeral

Answer

b   The tendon of the long head of biceps passes through the shoulder joint enveloped in synovial membrane, to gain attachment to the glenoid tubercle of the scapula.

EMQs

Each question has an anatomical theme linked to the chapter, and a list of 10 related items (A–J) placed in alphabetical order: these are followed by five statements (1–5). Match **one or more** of the items A–J to each of the five statements.

Muscles of the shoulder and upper arm
A. Biceps
B. Brachialis
C. Deltoid
D. Latissimus dorsi
E. Pectoralis major
F. Serratus anterior
G. Subscapularis
H. Supraspinatus
I. Trapezius
J. Triceps

Match the following attachments to the appropriate muscle(s) in the above list.
1. Coronoid process of the ulna
2. Olecranon process of the ulna
3. Clavicle
4. Superior nuchal line of the skull
5. Infraglenoid tubercle of the scapula

Answers
1 B; 2 J; 3 CEI; 4 I; 5 J

Nerves of the shoulder and upper arm
A. Biceps
B. Brachialis
C. Deltoid
D. Latissimus dorsi
E. Pectoralis major
F. Serratus anterior
G. Subscapularis
H. Supraspinatus
I. Trapezius
J. Triceps

Match the following nerves to the appropriate muscle(s) in the above list.
1. Posterior cord of the brachial plexus
2. Axillary
3. Long thoracic
4. Thoracodorsal
5. Musculocutaneous

Answers
1 CDGJ; 2 C; 3 F; 4 D; 5 AB

APPLIED QUESTIONS

1. Where can the axillary artery be surgically ligated without compromise to the blood supply of the upper limb?

1. The scapular anastomosis, connecting the first part of the subclavian artery (via the thyrocervical trunk) with the third part of the axillary artery (via the subscapular artery), enables the blood supply to the upper limb to remain uncompromised in all positions of the shoulder joint. Accurate identification of the subscapular artery is therefore needed, as the axillary artery must be ligated above it to ensure a continued blood supply to the upper limb.

2. A patient complained that after she had had a radical mastectomy her scapula stuck out like a wing when she pushed open a door. She also now found difficulty reaching the top shelves in her kitchen. Why is this?

2. A 'winged' scapula is seen in some thin women, but following a radical mastectomy one must immediately think of a weak serratus anterior muscle. The most likely cause is trauma to the long thoracic nerve (Bell), which lies along the medial axillary wall, sending twigs to each of the eight slips of the muscle. It is here that breast surgeons may traumatize the nerve while clearing lymph nodes from the axillary fat. The resulting paralysis makes the patient unable to abduct the arm further than the horizontal, as the scapula cannot be rotated to raise the glenoid cavity.

3. Why is an intramuscular injection into the posterior part of the deltoid potentially dangerous?

3. The axillary nerve arises from the posterior cord of the brachial plexus. The anterior branch, accompanied by the posterior circumflex humeral vessels, winds posteriorly through the quadrangular (quadrilateral) space and round the surgical neck of the humerus to supply deltoid from its deep surface. This is usually some 6–8 cm inferior to the bony prominence of the acromion. Any injections below and posterior to the midpoint of the acromion endangers the axillary nerve. Muscular (and financial!) incapacity may result.

Chapter **13**

Bailey & Love · Essential Clinical Anatomy · Bailey & Love · Essential Clinical Anatomy
Essential Clinical Anatomy · Bailey & Love · Essential Clinical Anatomy · Bailey & Love
ey & Love · Essential Clinical Anatomy · Bailey & Love · Essential Clinical Anatomy

The elbow and forearm

THE RADIUS AND ULNA

The radius

The radius, the lateral bone of the forearm, has a head, a body and a lower end (Fig. 13.1). The **head** is a cupped circular disc which articulates with the capitulum of the humerus and the radial notch of the ulna (Fig. 13.2). It can be palpated in the depression behind the lateral side of the elbow in extension. Just below the head is the radial tuberosity, which gives attachment to the biceps tendon. The **body** has a slight lateral convexity and expands in its lower part for muscle attachments (Fig. 13.1). Its medial side bears a ridge for the attachments of the interosseous membrane. The **lower end** extends into a palpable styloid process laterally; posteriorly lie a dorsal tubercle, which guides the tendon of extensor pollicis longus, and ridges to which septa from the extensor retinaculum are attached. Its medial surface articulates with the head of the ulna and its inferior surface has facets for the carpal bones, and it gives attachment to a fibrocartilaginous articular disc.

A fall on the outstretched hand causes the body weight to be transmitted via the thenar eminence onto the lower end of the radius and occasionally causes a Colles' fracture, the distal fragment being impacted and characteristically displaced laterally and posteriorly (see Fig. 14.4b, p. 229).

The ulna

The ulna (Fig. 13.1), the medial forearm bone, has an upper end, a body and a lower end. The **upper end** has a deep trochlear notch bounded by two projections, the olecranon, giving attachment to the triceps, and the coronoid process to which brachialis is attached. The notch articulates with the trochlear notch of the humerus. On the lateral side of the coronoid process is an articular radial notch for the head of the radius; its borders give attachment to the annular ligament. Below the notch the anterior surface gives attachment to the supinator muscle. The medial side of the body and upper end have sites of attachment for flexor digitorum profundus. The **body** has anterior, medial and posterior surfaces, but towards the lower end it becomes cylindrical. The middle of the lateral border is prominently marked by the attachment of the interosseous membrane. The **lower end** possesses a rounded head and a prominent styloid process, between which lies the tendon of extensor carpi ulnaris; the head articulates with the lower end of the radius and with the articular disc attached to the base of the styloid process. The olecranon, the posterior border of the shaft, the lower medial surface and the styloid process are subcutaneous and palpable.

The cubital fossa

The cubital fossa (Fig. 12.23, p. 203) lies anterior to the elbow joint (Fig. 13.2). It is triangular, bounded by a line joining the humeral epicondyles, medially by pronator teres, and laterally by brachioradialis. It is roofed by deep fascia, here strengthened by the bicipital aponeurosis, across which the often-visible median cubital vein runs. The fossa contains, from medial to lateral, the median nerve, the brachial artery and its terminal branches, the radial and ulnar arteries and the biceps tendon. The radial and posterior interosseous nerves, lateral to the tendon, usually lie deep to brachioradialis. The brachial artery is palpable here lying medial to the tendon of biceps, a point taken advantage of when taking the blood pressure.

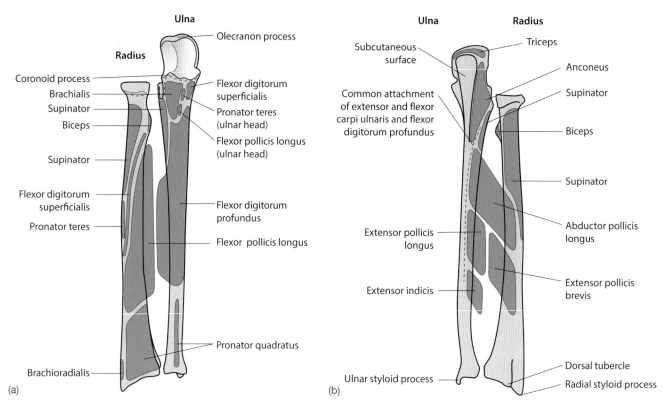

Figure 13.1 The right radius and ulna with muscle attachments: (a) anterior view (dotted red lines show capsular attachments); (b) posterior view

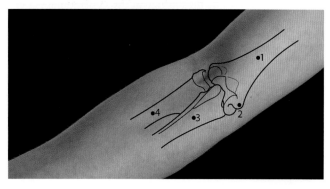

Figure 13.2 Bones of the elbow: 1, humerus; 2, medial epicondyle; 3, ulnar; 4, radius

THE ELBOW JOINT

The elbow joint (Fig. 13.3) is a synovial hinge joint between the lower end of the humerus and the upper ends of the radius and ulna. The humerus presents a rounded capitulum and a saddle-shaped trochlea for articulation with the cupped head of the radius and the trochlear notch of the ulna, respectively. In the anatomical position the forearm deviates laterally from the arm (carrying angle). The **capsular ligament** is attached to the humerus around the upper margins of its olecranon, coronoid and radial fossae, and inferiorly to the medial border of the trochlear notch and the annular ligament of the proximal radioulnar joint (Fig. 13.1). The capsule is thickened by strong **radial** and **ulnar collateral ligaments** (Fig. 13.4).

Functional aspects

The only movement permitted at the elbow is flexion and extension, but, in addition, the humeroradial articulation permits pronation and supination (Fig. 13.7 below).

- **Flexion** – brachialis and biceps are assisted by brachioradialis and the common flexor muscles.
- **Extension** – triceps.

The shapes of the bones, the strong capsule and the close envelope of brachialis and triceps contribute to the joint's sound stability.

The interosseous membrane

The radius and ulna are joined by the **interosseous membrane** (Figs. 13.4 and 13.5) and the radioulnar joints. The interosseous membrane is a strong fibrous sheet joining the adjacent interosseous borders of the two bones and giving attachment to the deep flexor and deep extensor muscles. The membrane's fibres are directed downwards and medially, hence a force passing from the hand to the radius, such as would occur in punching, is transmitted to the elbow by the ulna as well as through the head of the radius.

THE RADIOULNAR JOINTS

There are two radioulnar joints. The **proximal radioulnar joint** is a synovial joint of the pivot variety; the side of the disc-shaped radial head articulates within the osseoligamentous ring formed by the radial notch of the ulna and the annular

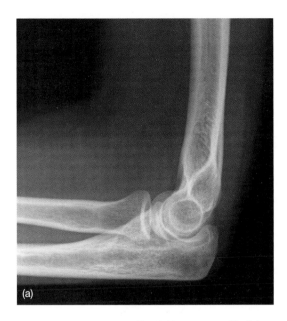

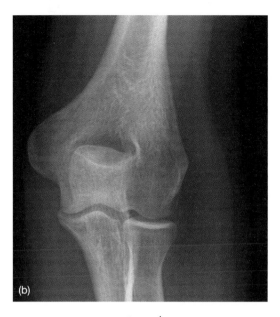

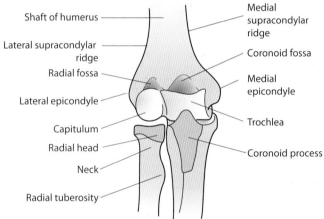

Shaft of humerus

Lateral supracondylar ridge

Radial fossa

Lateral epicondyle

Capitulum

Radial head

Neck

Radial tuberosity

Medial supracondylar ridge

Coronoid fossa

Medial epicondyle

Trochlea

Coronoid process

(c)

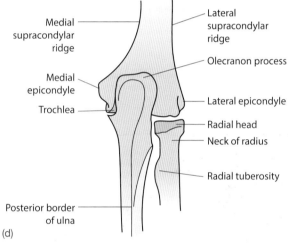

Medial supracondylar ridge

Medial epicondyle

Trochlea

Posterior border of ulna

Lateral supracondylar ridge

Olecranon process

Lateral epicondyle

Radial head

Neck of radius

Radial tuberosity

(d)

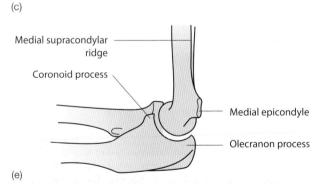

Medial supracondylar ridge

Coronoid process

Medial epicondyle

Olecranon process

(e)

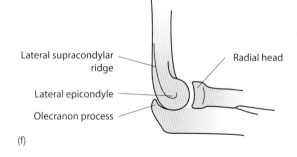

Lateral supracondylar ridge

Lateral epicondyle

Olecranon process

Radial head

(f)

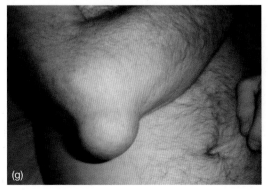

Figure 13.3 The right elbow joint: (a) X-ray, lateral view; (b) X-ray, anteroposterior view; (c–f) diagrams showing the bony features of the right elbow; (g) Olecranon bursitis

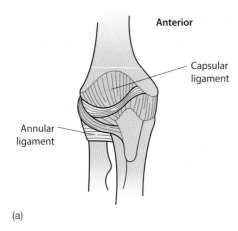

(a)

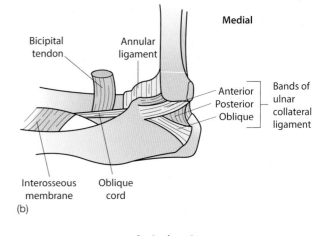

(b)

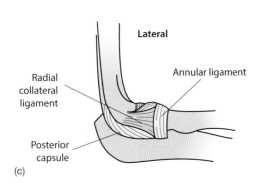

(c)

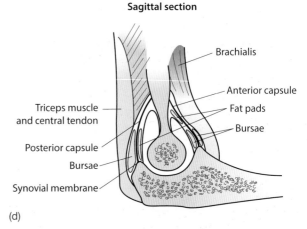

(d)

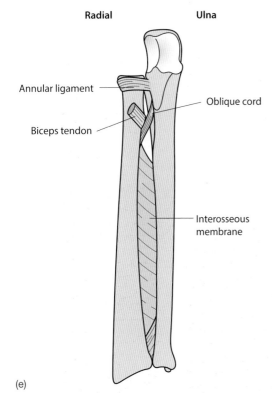

(e)

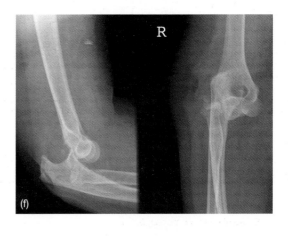

(f)

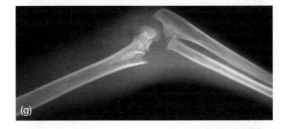

(g)

Figure 13.4 (a–c) Right elbow joint ligaments. (d) Sagittal section showing relations of tendons and bursae to the joint. (e) Forearm bones and ligaments of the superior radioulnar joint. (f) X-ray showing dislocation of the elbow – lateral and anteroposterior views. (g) Supracondylar fracture of the humerus in a child

ligament which encircles the radial head and is attached to the margins of the ulna's radial notch. Its synovial membrane is continuous with that of the elbow joint. It is a stable joint; the annular ligament, narrower below than above, holds the adult radial head firmly.

In the child, the radial head is less conical and therefore less firmly held by the annular ligament. A sharp tug on a child's arm can cause a dislocation (pulled elbow).

The **distal radioulnar joint** is also a synovial joint of the pivot variety, the head of the ulna articulating with the ulnar notch on the radius. A triangular fibrocartilaginous **articular disc** lies distal to the ulna and contributes to the articular surface of the wrist joint (Fig. 13.6). The weak capsular ligament is attached to the articular margin and the articular disc. The synovial membrane is not usually continuous with that of the wrist joint. Joint stability is dependent on the strength of the articular disc's attachments.

Functional aspects

Supination and pronation (Fig. 13.7) occur about an axis joining the centre of the radial head to the styloid process of the ulna. In the anatomical position the forearm is fully supinated. Pronation is produced by the radial head rotating within the annular ligament so that the lower end of the radius, tethered

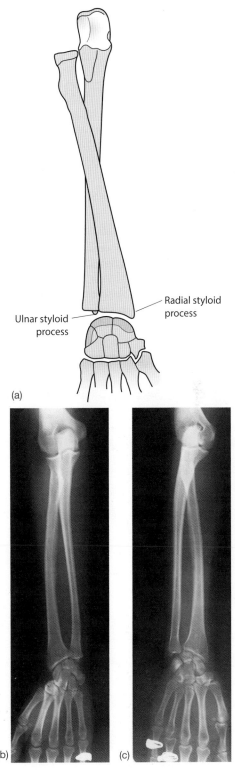

Figure 13.7 Right arm. (a) Position of the radius and ulna in pronation. (b) X-ray in supination. (c) X-ray in pronation

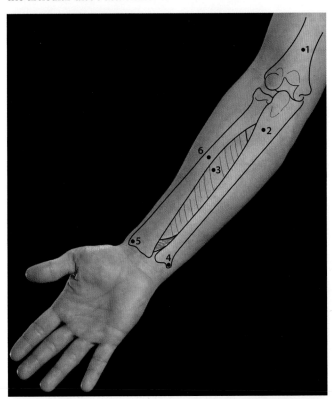

Figure 13.5 Surface anatomy of the interosseous membrane: 1, humerus; 2, ulna; 3, interosseous membrane; 4, ulnar styloid process; 5, radial styloid process; 6, radius

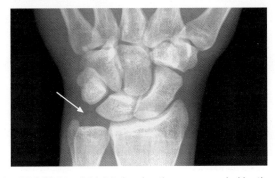

Figure 13.6 Right wrist joint showing the gap occupied by the articular disc (arrow)

by the articular disc, moves ventrally around the head of the ulna. The palm of the hand then faces dorsally. The range of these movements is high – more than 180 degrees – but can be increased further by simultaneous rotation of the humerus (provided the elbow joint is fully extended). Both supination and pronation are stronger when the elbow is flexed. Supination, produced by biceps and supinator, is stronger than pronation, which is produced by pronator teres and pronator quadratus. The power of supination is taken advantage of in the design of most screws, which are tightened by the action of supination in right-handed individuals.

MUSCLES OF THE FOREARM

These muscles act variously on several joints: the elbow, wrist and the joints of the fingers. The anterior (flexor) group, which includes pronator teres, arises from the common flexor attachment, the medial epicondyle of the humerus. The extensor group, which includes supinator, arises from the common extensor attachment, the lateral epicondyle of the humerus.

Flexor muscles

These are divided into the **superficial group** (Fig. 13.8a) comprising pronator teres, brachioradialis, flexor carpi radialis (FCR), palmaris longus and flexor carpi ulnaris (FCU); an **intermediate group** (Fig. 13.8b) comprising flexor digitorum superficialis (FDS); and a **deep group** (Fig. 13.8c) comprising flexor digitorum profundus (FDP), flexor pollicis longus

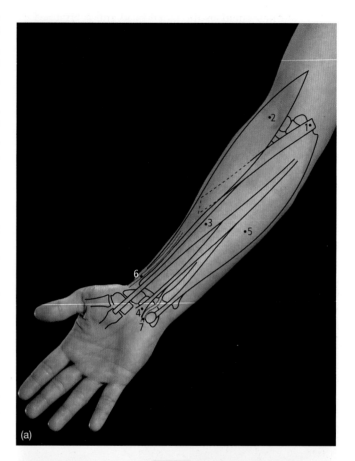

(a)

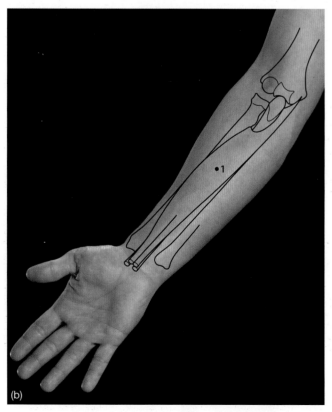

(b)

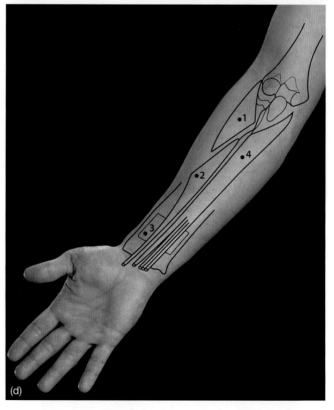

(d)

Figure 13.8 Surface anatomy of the forearm. (a) Superficial muscles: 1, pronator teres; 2, brachioradialis; 3, flexor carpi radialis; 4, palmaris longus; 5, flexor carpi ulnaris; 6, radial artery; 7, ulnar artery. (b) Intermediate muscles: 1, flexor digitorum superficialis. (c) Deep muscles: 1, supinator; 2, flexor pollicis longus; 3, pronator quadratus; 4, flexor digitorum profundus

(FPL) and pronator quadratus. The tendons of all but the two pronators pass over the anterior aspect of the wrist and are retained there by the flexor retinaculum, a thickening of the deep fascia of the forearm (Fig. 13.10).

The four tendons of FDS diverge in the palm, one passing to each finger. The tendon splits over the proximal phalanx to encircle the tendon of FDP and is attached to the sides of the middle phalanx (Fig. 13.9).

All these forearm flexor muscles are supplied by the median or ulnar nerves. The long flexors of the fingers (FDS and FDP) flex the wrist and the metacarpal and interphalangeal joints. Their attachments, nerve supply and functions are summarized below.

Brachioradialis is attached proximally to the lateral supracondylar ridge of the humerus and distally to the lower radius. It is a powerful flexor of the elbow, particularly when the forearm is in the midprone position, and it contributes to both pronation and supination, depending on the position of the forearm. It is supplied by the radial nerve.

Superficial group

All arise from the common flexor origin and all are supplied by the median nerve, apart from FCU, which is supplied by the ulnar nerve, and brachioradialis, which is supplied by the radial nerve (Table 13.1).

Deep group

All are supplied by the median nerve, but the ulnar half of FDP is also supplied by the ulnar nerve (Table 13.2).

Flexor synovial sheaths

The long flexor tendons are invested with synovial sheaths at points of maximum friction beneath the flexor retinaculum (Fig. 13.10 and p. 231) and within the digital fibrous flexor sheaths (Fig. 13.9 and p. 233). Deep to the retinaculum the tendons of FDS and FDP have a common sheath, the **ulnar bursa**. The tendon of FPL has its own sheath, the **radial bursa**. Each begins 2–3 cm above the wrist joint and they occasionally communicate with each other. The ulnar bursa ends in the palm, apart from a prolongation around the tendons of the little finger that extends to the distal phalanx. The radial bursa also continues to the distal phalanx of the thumb. There are separate digital synovial sheaths around the tendons to the index, middle and ring fingers. The tendons are nourished via membranous attachments called the vincula (Fig. 14.7b, p. 232).

Penetrating wounds of the palm may cause infection of the digital synovial sheaths, tenosynovitis. Localized swelling of the fingers and painful limitation of finger movement soon follow. Infections of the sheaths of the index, middle and ring fingers are confined to those fingers but infection of the little finger's sheath, which is in continuity with the common synovial sheath in the palm, may spread through the palm and through the carpal tunnel to the forearm. Tenosynovitis of the thumb may similarly spread to infect the whole of the radial bursa.

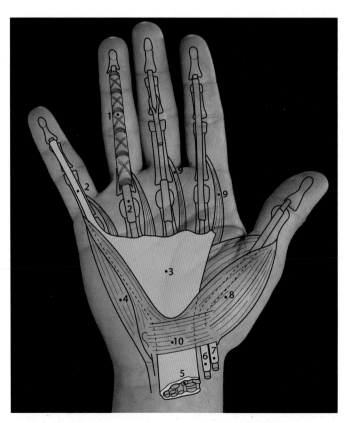

Figure 13.10 Surface anatomy of the flexor synovial sheaths and flexor retinaculum: 1, fibrous flexor digital sheath; 2, synovial digital sheath, sheath of the little finger being continuous with the ulnar bursa; 3, ulnar bursa; 4, hypothenar muscles; 5, tendons of flexor digitorum superficialis and profundus within ulnar bursa; 6, synovial sheath round flexor pollicis longus; 7, sheath of flexor carpi radialis; 8, thenar muscles; 9, lateral two lumbricals; 10, flexor retinaculum

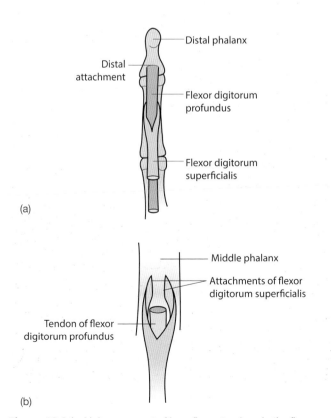

Figure 13.9 (a, b) Arrangement of long flexor tendons in the finger

TABLE 13.1 Superficial muscles of the forearm

Muscle	Proximal attachment	Distal attachment	Nerve supply	Function
Brachioradialis	Flexor origin of humerus	Styloid process of radius	Radial nerve (C5, C6)	Elbow flexion
Pronator teres	Flexor origin of humerus, coronoid process of ulna	Distal surface of radius	Median nerve (C6, C7)	Pronation
Flexor carpi ulnaris	Flexor origin of humerus, anterior surface of ulna	Pisiform, hamate and base of 5th metacarpal	Ulnar nerve (C8, T1)	Flexion and adduction of wrist
Flexor carpi radialis	Flexor origin of humerus	Bases of 2nd and 3rd metacarpals	Median nerve (C6, C7)	Flexion and abduction of wrist
Palmaris longus	Flexor origin of humerus	Palmar aponeurosis and flexor retinaculum	Median nerve (C6, C7)	Flexion of wrist
Flexor digitorum superficialis (intermediate group)	Flexor origin of humerus, neighbouring anterior surfaces of radius and ulna	Lateral surfaces of middle phalanges of fingers 2–5	Median nerve (C7, T1)	Flexion of proximal interphalangeal, metacarpophalangeal and wrist joints

TABLE 13.2 Deep muscles of the forearm

Muscle	Proximal attachment	Distal attachment	Nerve supply	Function
Flexor pollicis longus	Anterior shaft of radius, interosseous membrane	Base of distal phalanx of thumb	Median nerve (C8, T1)	Flexion of joints of thumb
Flexor digitorum profundus	Posterior surface of ulna, coronoid process and interosseous membrane	Bases of distal phalanges 2–5	Anterior interosseous branch of median nerve and ulnar nerve (C8, T1)	Flexion of distal interphalangeal joints and, to a lesser extent, the wrist
Pronator quadratus	Medial surface of distal ulna	Lateral surface of distal radius	Median nerve (C8, T1)	Pronation

Extensor muscles

The extensor (posterior) muscles of the forearm (Figs. 13.11 and 13.12, Table 13.3) can be functionally described as of three groups:

- Muscles that act on the wrist joint – extensor carpi radialis longus, extensor carpi radialis brevis (ECRB) and extensor carpi ulnaris (ECU)
- Extensor muscles of the fingers – extensor digitorum (ED), extensor indicis (EI) and extensor digiti minimi (EDM)
- Muscles extending/abducting the thumb (Fig. 13.13) – abductor pollicis longus (APL), extensor pollicis brevis (EPB) and extensor pollicis longus (EPL).

In addition to these muscles the posterior compartment of the forearm contains the supinator muscle. All are supplied by the radial nerve or its posterior interosseous branch.

The extensor muscle tendons pass under the **extensor retinaculum** (Figs. 13.14 and 13.15) as they pass over the wrist joint, and are retained so that 'bowstringing' does not occur during wrist extension. Here, closely contained between bones of the wrist joint and the retinaculum, they are covered by synovial sheaths, reducing the effects of friction. EI lies deeper. On the heads of the metacarpals and over the proximal phalanges the extensor tendons expand to form flat extensor expansions (Figs. 13.15 and 13.16), which wrap around the dorsum and sides of these bones. They help to retain the tendon in line with the finger and give attachment to the interossei and lumbrical muscles (Fig. 13.16 and p. 232). The tendon divides over the proximal interphalangeal joint into three slips: the middle is attached to the base of the middle phalanx and the outer two to the base of the terminal phalanx. The extensor muscles of the forearm may also be divided into superficial and deep groups. The superficial extensors (ECRB, ECU, ED, EDM) are all attached to the common extensor origin of the humerus, the lateral epicondyle, and are supplied by the posterior interosseous nerve. The deep extensors of the forearm, APL, EPL and EPB, act on the thumb and EI acts as a strong extensor on the forefinger. They lie deep to the superficial extensors and are all supplied by the posterior interosseous branch of the radial nerve (Fig. 13.17).

Tennis elbow – a common painful condition – is the result of repetitive flexion and extension of the wrist which, by putting strain on the common extensor origin, causes inflammation in the muscles' attachment to the lateral epicondyle. 'Mallet finger' is the name given to the deformity resulting from an unguarded forceful flexion of a finger's terminal interphalangeal joint, which avulses the attachment of the long extensor to the base of the terminal phalanx. It most commonly follows a failed attempt to catch a cricket- or baseball.

Extensor pollicis longus is attached proximally to the posterior surface of the ulna distal to abductor pollicis; distally the tendon descends under the extensor retinaculum on the medial side of the dorsal tubercle of the radius in its own synovial sheath. Here it forms the posterior margin of the 'snuffbox' as it crosses over the two radial extensors and the radial artery, before becoming attached to the base of the thumb's distal phalanx. It extends all the joints of the thumb.

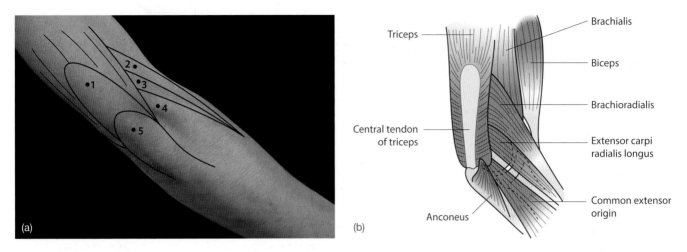

Figure 13.11 Extensor muscles of the forearm. (a) Surface anatomy at the elbow: 1, common extensor tendon of triceps muscle; 2, brachioradialis; 3, extensor carpi radialis longus; 4, common extensor origin; 5, olecranon process. (b) Diagram of the posterior aspect of the elbow showing brachioradialis and extensor carpi radialis longus

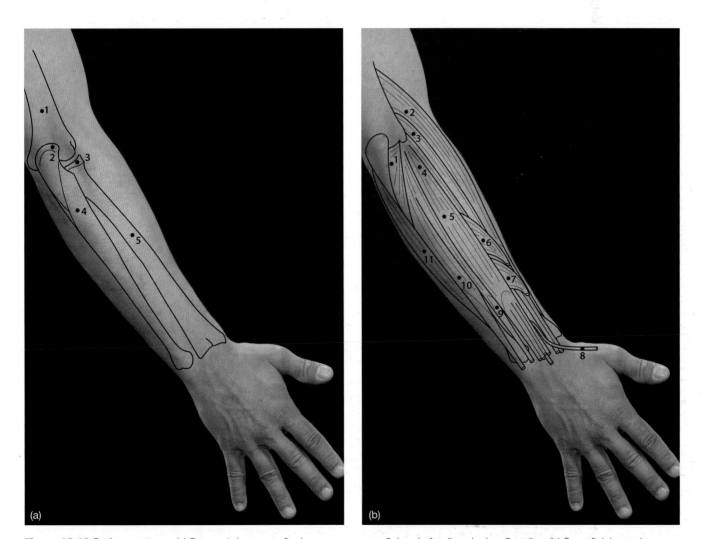

Figure 13.12 Surface anatomy. (a) Bones: 1, humerus; 2, olecranon process; 3, head of radius; 4, ulna; 5, radius. (b) Superficial muscles: 1, anconeus; 2, brachioradialis; 3, extensor carpi radialis longus; 4, common extensor origin; 5, extensor digitorum; 6, abductor pollicis longus; 7, extensor pollicis brevis; 8, tendon of extensor pollicis longus; 9, extensor digiti minimi; 10, extensor carpi ulnaris; 11, flexor carpi ulnaris

TABLE 13.3 Extensor muscles of the forearm

Muscle	Proximal attachment	Distal attachment	Nerve supply	Function
Extensor carpi radialis longus	Extensor origin of humerus	Base of 2nd metacarpal	Radial nerve (C6, C7)	Extension and abduction of wrist
Extensor carpi radialis brevis	Extensor origin of humerus	Base of 3rd metacarpal	Radial nerve (C6, C7)	Extension and abduction of wrist
Extensor carpi ulnaris	Extensor origin of humerus	Base of 5th metacarpal	Radial nerve (C6, C7, C8)	Extension and adduction of wrist
Extensor digitorum	Extensor origin of humerus	Posterior surfaces of phalanges, fingers 2–5	Radial nerve (C6, C7, C8)	Extension of finger joints and wrist
Abductor pollicis	Proximal extensor surfaces of radius and ulna	Lateral aspect of 1st metacarpal	Radial nerve (C6, C7)	Abduction of thumb and wrist
Extensor pollicis brevis	Distal shaft of radius	Base of proximal phalanx of thumb	Radial nerve (C6, C7)	Extension of thumb, abduction of wrist
Extensor pollicis longus	Posterior shaft of ulna and interosseous membrane	Base of distal phalanx of thumb	Radial nerve (C6, C7, C8)	Extension of thumb, abduction of wrist
Extensor indicis	Posterior surface of ulna and interosseous membrane	With tendon of ED into posterior surface of phalanges of index finger	Radial nerve (C6, C7, C8)	Extension of joints of index finger
Extensor digiti minimi	Extensor origin of humerus	Posterior surface of prox. phalanx of little finger	Radial nerve (C6, C7, C8)	Extension of joints of little finger
Supinator	Extensor origin of humerus and proximal ulna	Anterolateral surface of radius	Radial nerve (C6, C7, C8)	Supination (Fig. 13.17)

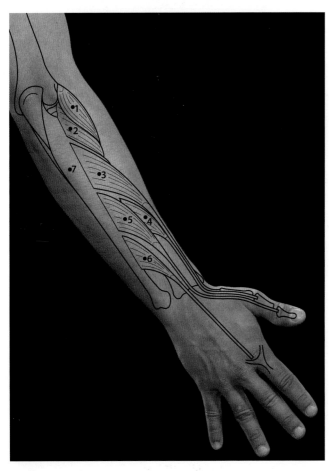

Figure 13.13 Surface anatomy of the deep extensor muscles of the forearm: 1, supinator (humeral head); 2 supinator (ulnar head); 3, abductor pollicis longus; 4, extensor pollicis brevis; 5, extensor pollicis longus; 6, extensor indicis; 7, ulna

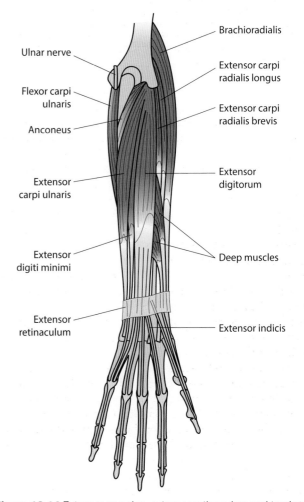

Figure 13.14 Extensor muscles, extensor retinaculum and tendons

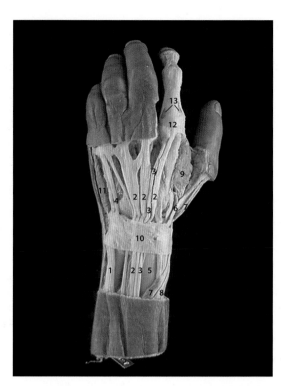

Figure 13.15 Dissection of extensor tendons and retinaculum: 1, extensor carpi ulnaris; 2, extensor digitorum tendons; 3, extensor indicis; 4, extensor digiti minimi; 5, radius; 6, extensor pollicis longus; 7, extensor pollicis brevis; 8, abductor pollicis longus; 9, first dorsal interosseous muscle; 10, extensor retinaculum; 11, abductor digiti minimi; 12, dorsal digital extensor expansion, 13, lateral 'wing' of extensor tendon expansion

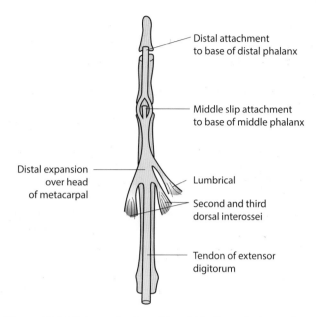

Figure 13.16 Extensor tendon of the middle finger, its expansion and attachments of the lumbricals and interossei

Tenosynovitis, an inflammatory thickening of the common sheath surrounding these two tendons, occurs sometimes after prolonged repetitive movements of the thumb. There is pain and swelling on movement of the thumb. It is given the name de Quervain's disease and usually responds to rest.

The **anatomical snuffbox** is the term applied to the depression formed on the lateral side of the wrist when the thumb is extended (Figs. 13.18 and 13.19). Its boundaries are: *anterior* – tendons of APL and EPB; *posterior* – tendon of EPL. In its base are the wrist joint, the radial styloid process, the scaphoid bone and the base of the first metacarpal; crossing its floor are the tendons of the two radial extensors of the wrist and the radial artery. Superficially are the cephalic vein and cutaneous branches of the radial nerve; the latter can be palpated crossing over the tendons – they feel like threads of cotton over the tendon of brachioradialis.

The **extensor retinaculum** is a band of deep fascia 2–3 cm wide passing obliquely over the back of the wrist from the distal end of the radius to the medial side of the carpus. It is attached by fibrous septae to the radius and ulna, forming fibro-osseous tunnels for the passage of the tendons (Fig. 13.20). The tendons' synovial sheaths commence at the retinaculum's proximal border. Those of abductor pollicis and both radial extensors reach the tendons' distal attachments, but all others end in the middle of the dorsum of the hand.

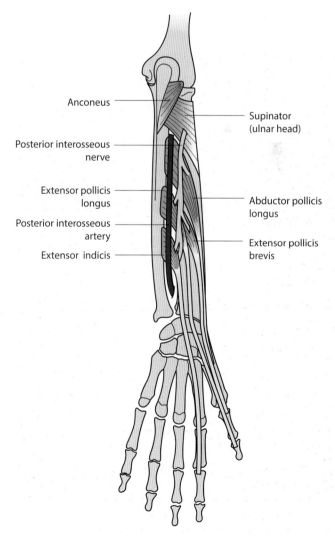

Figure 13.17 Deep extensors demonstrating the supinator muscle and course of the posterior interosseous nerve and artery

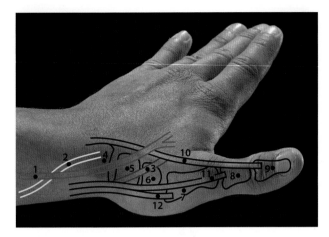

Figure 13.18 Surface anatomy of the anatomical snuffbox:
1, cephalic vein (blue); 2, radial nerve (yellow); 3, radial artery (red);
4, lower end of radius; 5, scaphoid; 6, trapezium; 7, first metacarpal;
8, proximal phalanx; 9, distal phalanx; 10, extensor pollicis longus;
11, extensor pollicis brevis; 12, abductor pollicis longus

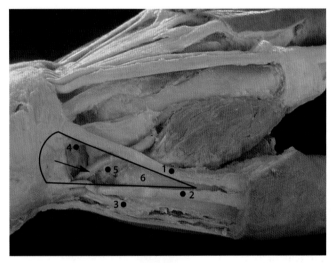

Figure 13.19 Snuffbox dissection, left hand: 1, extensor pollicis
longus; 2, extensor pollicis brevis; 3, abductor pollicis longus;
4, scaphoid; 5, trapezium; 6, first metacarpal; arrow = radial artery

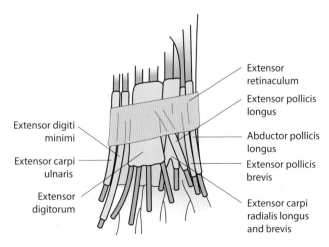

Figure 13.20 Extensor retinaculum and tendon sheaths across the
dorsum of the wrist

BLOOD SUPPLY

The radial artery

The radial artery (Fig. 13.21), a terminal branch of the brachial artery, arises in the cubital fossa. It descends the anterior forearm, passes over the lateral side of the wrist to the dorsum of the hand and ends in the palm.

Relations

Leaving the cubital fossa deep to brachioradialis it descends close to the radius, with the radial nerve on its lateral side. At the wrist it is palpable on the front of the radius, but then it crosses lateral to the wrist joint deep to the tendons bounding the 'snuffbox', to reach the dorsum of the hand by passing through the first dorsal interosseous and adductor pollicis muscles.

The radial pulsation can be felt against the lower radius and against the scaphoid in the floor of the snuffbox (Fig. 13.19). Arterial blood samples can be obtained at the wrist because here the artery is easily palpable. It is very important, though, before taking the sample, to establish that there is a pulse in the ulnar artery, which would provide an anastomotic blood supply should any damage or spasm follow the radial puncture (Allen's test: occlude both arteries, ask the patient to make a fist and then open the hand; release the arteries individually to see the return of blood flow).

The radial artery supplies the forearm muscles, contributes to anastomoses around the elbow and wrist joints (Fig. 13.21b) and supplies the elbow and wrist joints; it also contributes to the deep palmar arch and has a minor contribution to the superficial palmar arch (Fig. 13.22). It may be palpated in the floor of the anatomical snuffbox.

The ulnar artery

The ulnar artery (Fig. 13.21), also a terminal branch of the brachial artery, arises in the cubital fossa, descends in the anterior forearm, passes anterior to the flexor retinaculum near the wrist and ends mainly in the superficial palmar arch; a minor branch contributes to the deep palmar arch.

Relations

Leaving the cubital fossa it lies on FDP, deep to the muscles arising from the common flexor origin. In the lower forearm, under FCU, the ulnar nerve is medial to the ulnar artery. It crosses the wrist superficial to the flexor retinaculum and ends by continuing as the superficial palmar arch lateral to the pisiform bone. It supplies forearm muscles and the elbow and wrist joints. Its largest branch, the common interosseous artery, arises in the cubital fossa and then descends close to the interosseous membrane. It contributes to both the superficial and deep palmar arches.

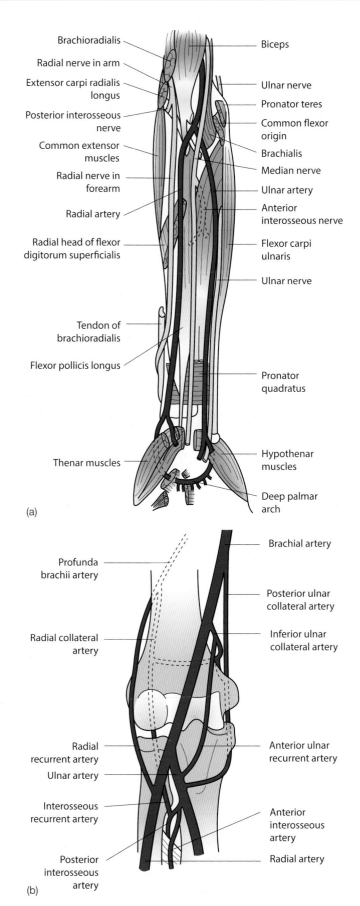

(a)

(b)

Figure 13.21 (a) Vessels and nerves of the forearm. (b) Arterial anastomoses around the right elbow joint

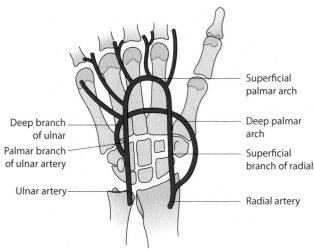

Figure 13.22 Palmar arterial arches of the right hand

NERVES

The radial nerve

The radial nerve lies on the anterolateral aspect of the forearm under brachioradialis (Fig. 13.23), lateral to the radial artery. Its largest branch, the **posterior interosseous nerve**, arises in the cubital fossa and passes posteriorly through the supinator muscle to gain the posterior compartment of the forearm, where it descends on the interosseous membrane supplying adjacent extensor muscles. Proximal to the wrist the superficial radial nerve turns posteriorly under the tendon of brachioradialis and superficial to the tendons bounding the 'snuffbox', to end on the dorsum of the hand as digital branches. It and its posterior interosseous branch supply brachioradialis, all the extensor muscles, the elbow, wrist and intercarpal joints and, by cutaneous branches, the lateral side of the dorsum of the hand and posterior aspects of the lateral 2½ digits, usually as far as the distal interphalangeal joints.

The median nerve

The median nerve descends in the anterior compartment of the forearm. In the cubital fossa it is medial to the brachial artery (Fig. 13.24a). Its largest branch, the **anterior interosseous nerve**, descends deep and close to the interosseous membrane, supplying most of the deep flexors and pronator quadratus. The median nerve then descends between the superficial and deep flexors to emerge, at the wrist, between the tendons of the FDS and the FCR, deep to palmaris longus. It enters the hand deep to the flexor retinaculum (Fig. 13.24b). It and its anterior interosseous branch supply all the forearm flexor muscles except the ulnar half of FDP and the FCU; in the hand it supplies abductor pollicis brevis, flexor pollicis brevis and opponens pollicis. Its palmar cutaneous branch supplies the radial side of the palm and, by digital branches, the palmar surface of the lateral 3½ digits, their fingertips and their nail beds. These digital branches lie anterior to the digital arteries, and the two lateral branches also supply the lateral two lumbrical muscles.

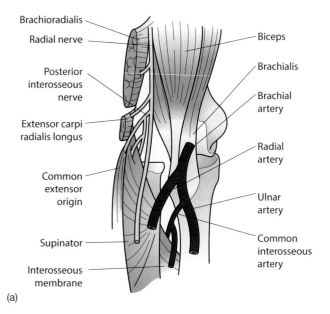

(a)

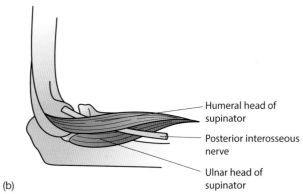

(b)

Figure 13.23 (a) Right cubital fossa, anterior aspect. (b) Passage of posterior interosseous nerve through the fibres of supinator muscle

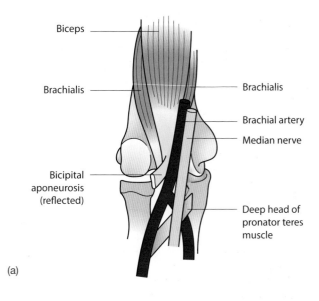

(a)

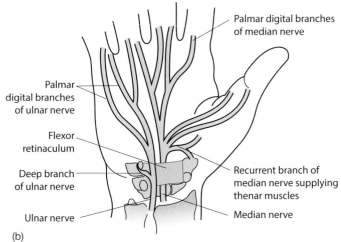

(b)

Figure 13.24 (a) Deep structures in the right cubital fossa. (b) Median and ulnar nerves in the hand

The ulnar nerve

From behind the medial epicondyle (Figs. 13.21a, 13.24 and 13.25) the **ulnar nerve** descends deep to FCU on the medial side of the forearm (Fig. 13.26). At the wrist it lies superficially, lateral to the tendon, and passes into the hand superficial to the flexor retinaculum, lateral to the pisiform, to end by dividing into superficial and deep branches (Fig. 13.24). In the forearm it supplies FCU and the ulnar half of FDP. Its dorsal cutaneous branch arises above the wrist and supplies the ulnar half of the dorsum of the hand and the medial 2½ fingers as far as the distal interphalangeal joints. In the hand digital branches supply the palmar surface of the medial 1½ fingers, their fingertips and their nail beds, and a deep branch supplies all the hypothenar muscles (p. 212), all the interossei, the third and fourth lumbricals and adductor pollicis.

Nerve injuries

Nerve injuries and clinical testing for the functional integrity of these nerves are described on pp. 235 and 236.

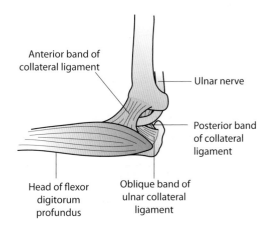

Figure 13.25 Medial view of the elbow joint – ulnar nerve passing behind the medial epicondyle of the right humerus and into the cubital tunnel

Lateral   Medial

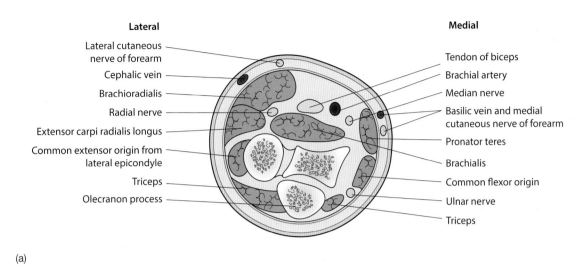

Lateral cutaneous nerve of forearm

Cephalic vein

Brachioradialis

Radial nerve

Extensor carpi radialis longus

Common extensor origin from lateral epicondyle

Triceps

Olecranon process

Tendon of biceps

Brachial artery

Median nerve

Basilic vein and medial cutaneous nerve of forearm

Pronator teres

Brachialis

Common flexor origin

Ulnar nerve

Triceps

(a)

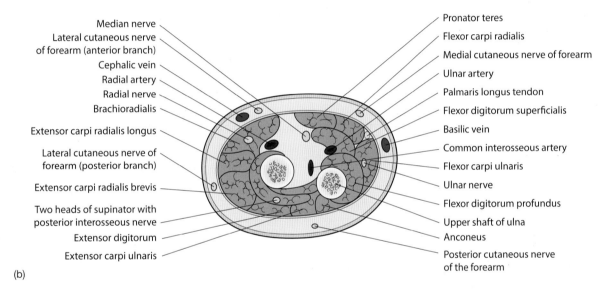

Median nerve

Lateral cutaneous nerve of forearm (anterior branch)

Cephalic vein

Radial artery

Radial nerve

Brachioradialis

Extensor carpi radialis longus

Lateral cutaneous nerve of forearm (posterior branch)

Extensor carpi radialis brevis

Two heads of supinator with posterior interosseous nerve

Extensor digitorum

Extensor carpi ulnaris

Pronator teres

Flexor carpi radialis

Medial cutaneous nerve of forearm

Ulnar artery

Palmaris longus tendon

Flexor digitorum superficialis

Basilic vein

Common interosseous artery

Flexor carpi ulnaris

Ulnar nerve

Flexor digitorum profundus

Upper shaft of ulna

Anconeus

Posterior cutaneous nerve of the forearm

(b)

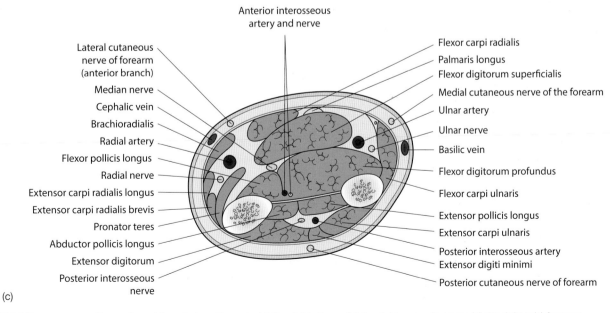

Anterior interosseous artery and nerve

Lateral cutaneous nerve of forearm (anterior branch)

Median nerve

Cephalic vein

Brachioradialis

Radial artery

Flexor pollicis longus

Radial nerve

Extensor carpi radialis longus

Extensor carpi radialis brevis

Pronator teres

Abductor pollicis longus

Extensor digitorum

Posterior interosseous nerve

Flexor carpi radialis

Palmaris longus

Flexor digitorum superficialis

Medial cutaneous nerve of the forearm

Ulnar artery

Ulnar nerve

Basilic vein

Flexor digitorum profundus

Flexor carpi ulnaris

Extensor pollicis longus

Extensor carpi ulnaris

Posterior interosseous artery

Extensor digiti minimi

Posterior cutaneous nerve of forearm

(c)

Figure 13.26 Transverse sections, viewed from below, through: (a) the right elbow; (b) the right upper forearm; (c) the right mid-forearm

MCQs

1. The anatomical snuffbox: **T/F**

a is bounded anteriorly by the tendons of extensor pollicis longus and brevis (____)

b is bounded posteriorly by the tendon of abductor pollicis brevis (____)

c overlies the scaphoid and the trapezium (____)

d contains the tendons of extensors carpi radialis longus and brevis in its floor (____)

e contains the basilic vein in its roof (____)

Answers

1.

a **F** – Its boundaries are, anteriorly, the tendons of abductor pollicis longus and extensor pollicis brevis, and posteriorly, the tendon of extensor pollicis longus.

b **F**

c **T** – Together with the radial styloid process, the wrist joint and the base of the first metacarpal bone.

d **T** – Together with the radial artery.

e **F** – The cephalic vein overlies the snuffbox.

2. The radial nerve: **T/F**

a is the main branch of the posterior cord of the brachial plexus (____)

b is derived from the posterior primary rami of C5, C6, C7, C8 and T1 nerve roots (____)

c is the main nerve supply to the extensor muscles of arm and forearm (____)

d gives rise to the anterior interosseous nerve (____)

e supplies the skin of the extensor aspect of the radial 3½ digits (____)

Answers

2.

a **T** – The other branches of the posterior cord are the axillary, thoracodorsal and upper and lower subscapular nerves.

b **F** – It arises from the anterior primary rami of these nerves.

c **T**

d **F** – In the supinator muscle the radial nerve gives rise to the posterior interosseous nerve. The median nerve gives rise to the anterior interosseous nerve.

e **T**

SBA

1. Three days after a dog bit her thumb the patient's wound was clearly infected and she also had a tender swelling on the radial side of her palm. What tendons are likely to be affected?

a Flexor digitorum profundus

b Flexor pollicis longus

c Flexor digitorum superficialis

d Flexor pollicis brevis

e Flexor carpi radialis

Answer

b An infective tenosynovitis has developed involving firstly the synovial sheath enveloping the tendon of flexor pollicis longus, also known as the radial bursa, which lies in the radial side of the palm. The flexor digitorum superficialis and profundus tendons lie within the common flexor sheath or ulna bursa, which lies lateral to this. Flexor pollicis brevis and flexor carpi radialis do not possess synovial sheaths.

2. An elderly lady presents after a fall that resulted in a painful deformity of her wrist. There is posterior displacement of the distal wrist and hand. What is the likely diagnosis?

a Colles' fracture

b Bennett's fracture

c Boxer's fracture

d Fracture of the distal ulna

e Scaphoid fracture

Answer

a This patient presents with a 'dinner fork deformity' typical of a Colles' fracture involving the distal end of the radius – the distal end of the radius is displaced posteriorly to present a deformity of the wrist comparable to the backward curve of a dinner fork.

EMQs

Each question has an anatomical theme linked to the chapter, and a list of 10 related items (A–J) placed in alphabetical order: these are followed by five statements (1–5). Match **one or more** of the items A–J to each of the five statements.

Muscles of the elbow and forearm
A. Brachioradialis
B. Extensor carpi radialis brevis
C. Extensor carpi ulnaris
D. Extensor digitorum
E. Flexor carpi radialis
F. Flexor carpi ulnaris
G. Flexor digitorum profundus
H. Flexor digitorum superficialis
I. Flexor pollicis longus
J. Pronator teres

Match the following attachments to the appropriate muscle(s) in the above list.
1. Flexor origin of the humerus
2. Extensor origin of the humerus
3. Distal phalanx
4. Mid-lateral border of the radius
5. Styloid process of the radius

Answers
1 EFHJ; 2 BCD; 3 DGI; 4 J; 5 A

Nerves of the elbow and forearm
A. Brachioradialis
B. Extensor carpi radialis brevis
C. Extensor carpi ulnaris
D. Extensor digitorum
E. Flexor carpi radialis
F. Flexor carpi ulnaris
G. Flexor digitorum profundus
H. Flexor digitorum superficialis
I. Flexor pollicis longus
J. Pronator teres

Match the following nerves to the appropriate muscle(s) in the above list.
1. Median
2. Ulnar
3. Radial
4. Ulnar nerve passes between its two heads
5. Crosses anterior to the median nerve at the level of the cubital fossa

Answers
1 EGHIJ; 2 FG; 3 ABCD; 4 F; 5 J

APPLIED QUESTIONS

1. What surface anatomical clues aid clinical diagnosis of a fractured distal radius?

1. A fall onto the outstretched hand may fracture the distal radius. In the common Colles' fracture the distal radial fragment is displaced posteriorly and impacted, shortening the bone. The radial styloid can usually be palpated approximately 1 cm distal to the ulnar styloid, but their palpation at the same horizontal level indicates bony displacement.

2. You notice in 'cops and robbers' films that, to make a person drop a knife, the defender often forces the attacker's hand into acute flexion. Why is this a very sensible move?

2. Try this yourself and you will find that the power grip is very weak in acute wrist flexion. Normally, the wrist extensors work synergistically with the flexors of the fingers. Flexion of the wrist deprives the long flexor tendons of the ability to contract further and make a strong grip. Flexing the wrist will therefore make someone relax their grip and drop whatever is in their hand.

Essential Clinical Anatomy · Bailey & Love · Essential Clinical Anatomy
essential Clinical Anatomy · Bailey & Love · Essential Clinical Anatomy · Bailey & Love
Bailey & Love · Essential Clinical Anatomy · Bailey & Love · Essential Clinical Anatomy

Chapter 14

The wrist and hand

THE BONES OF THE HAND

The carpus (Figs. 14.1 and 14.2) has eight carpal bones arranged as a proximal row of three, from lateral to medial the scaphoid, lunate and triquetral; a distal row of four, from lateral to medial the trapezium, trapezoid, capitate and hamate; and an anteromedially placed sesamoid bone – the pisiform.

The square flexor retinaculum is attached to the scaphoid, trapezium, pisiform and hamate. All its points of attachment are palpable, as is the scaphoid in the anatomical snuffbox.

The **metacarpals** have expanded bases that articulate with the distal row of carpal bones (Figs. 14.1 and 14.2) and the medial four also articulate with each other. Their slender bodies give attachment to the interossei, opponens pollicis and adductor pollicis muscles, and their heads articulate with the

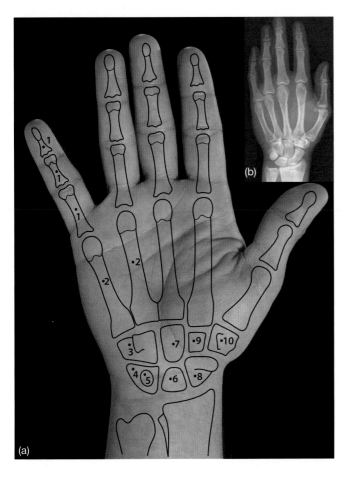

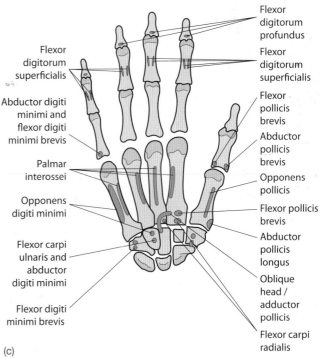

Figure 14.1 The hand. (a) Surface anatomy of the palmar surface: 1, proximal, middle and distal phalanges; 2, metacarpals; 3, hamate; 4, triquetral; 5, pisiform; 6, lunate; 7, capitate; 8, scaphoid; 9, trapezoid; 10, trapezium. (b) X-ray, dorsopalmar view. (c) Bones and muscle attachments, palmar aspect

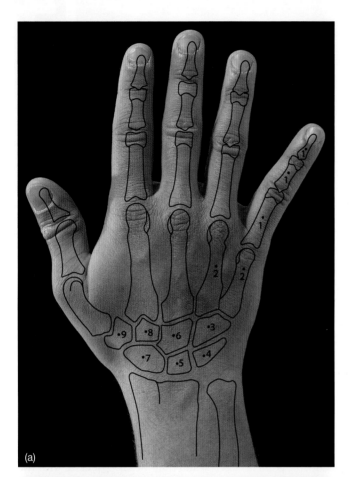

(a)

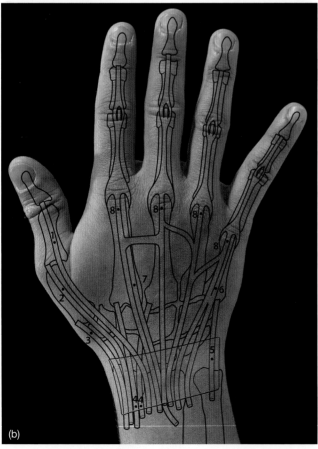

(b)

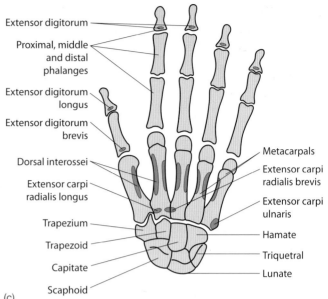

(c)

Figure 14.2 Dorsum of the hand. (a) Surface anatomy – bones, posterior view: 1, proximal, middle and distal phalanges; 2, metacarpals; 3, hamate; 4, triquetral; 5, lunate; 6, capitate; 7, scaphoid; 8, trapezoid; 9, trapezium. (b) Surface anatomy – extensor tendons: 1, extensor pollicis longus; 2, extensor pollicis brevis; 3, abductor pollicis longus; 4, extensor carpi radialis longus and brevis; 5, extensor carpi ulnaris; 6, extensor digiti minimi; 7, extensor indicis; 8, tendons of extensor digitorum. (c) Bones and muscle attachments

proximal phalanges. The 1 metacarpal is the shortest, strongest and most mobile; its axis is rotated to lie almost at a right angle to that of the other metacarpals. It articulates proximally with the trapezium.

The **phalanges** are long bones, three in each finger and two in the thumb. The proximal phalanges have cupped surfaces for proximal articulation with the metacarpals; the heads of the proximal and middle phalanges have paired articular condyles and the distal phalanges taper distally. The phalanges give attachment to the long flexors and extensors of the fingers and thumb and to all the small muscles of the hand, apart from the opponens muscles.

The wrist joint

The **wrist (radiocarpal) joint** is a biaxial synovial joint – the lower end of the radius and the fibrocartilaginous disc over the head of the ulna articulate with the proximal row of carpal bones (scaphoid, lunate and triquetral). The **capsule**, attached to the articular margins, is thickened by medial and lateral collateral ligaments. The triangular articular disc is intracapsular, its apex being attached to the base of the ulnar styloid and its base to the lower end of the radius. Only if the disc is perforated does the wrist joint communicate with the distal radioulnar joint.

The **intercarpal joints** are synovial joints; the extensive composite joint between the proximal and distal row of carpal bones is known as the **midcarpal joint**, and it is here that most of the flexion and abduction of the wrist occurs. The stability of the joints is dependent on ligaments: palmar, dorsal and interosseous.

Functional aspects

Flexion, extension, abduction, adduction and circumduction are possible and both the wrist and midcarpal joints contribute to each movement. **Flexion** (flexor carpi radialis and ulnaris aided by the long digital flexors) is greater than **extension** (extensor carpi ulnaris and radialis longus and bre-vis assisted by the long digital extensors). **Adduction** (extensor and flexor carpi ulnaris) is greater than **abduction** (flexor carpi radialis and extensor carpi radialis longus and brevis).

The stability of the wrist depends on capsular ligaments assisted by the many long tendons crossing it (Fig. 14.3). Very few dislocations occur.

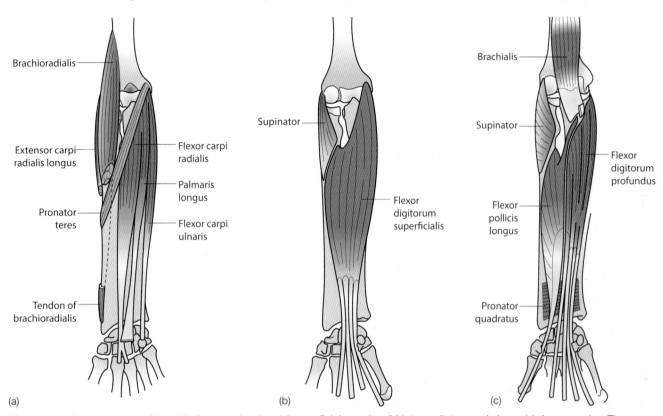

(a)   (b)   (c)

Figure 14.3 Anterior aspect of the right forearm showing: (a) superficial muscles; (b) intermediate muscle layer; (c) deep muscles. The tendons of these muscles cross the wrist joint to flex both wrist and fingers (Fig. 13.10, p. 215 and Tables 13.1 and 13.2)

A fall on the outstretched hand results in force being transmitted through the thenar eminence to the lateral bones of the carpus, the trapezoid, trapezium and scaphoid. In young adults the scaphoid may fracture across its waist (Fig. 14.4), and non-union of the fracture is not uncommon because of associated damage to the scaphoid's blood supply. In older people a similar fall may result in fracture of the lower end of the radius (Colles' fracture), producing a typical 'dinner fork' deformity in which the distal fragment is displaced dorsally. In a child, this injury may result in separation of the distal radial epiphysis.

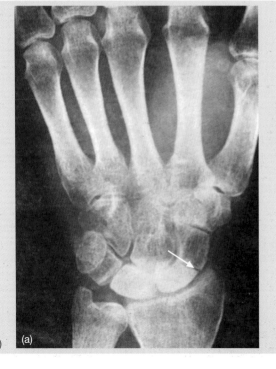

Figure 14.4 (a) Scaphoid fracture (arrow) (*continued*)   (a)

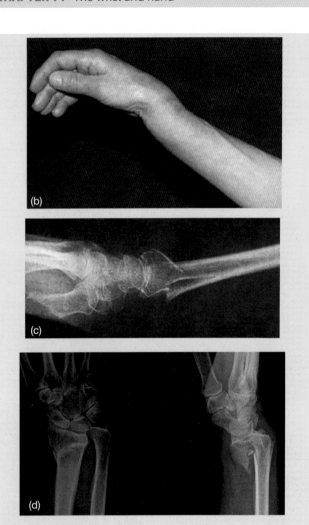

Figure 14.4 (*continued*) (b) Colles' fracture showing the 'dinner fork' deformity. (c) Colles' fracture, X-ray. (d) Fracture of distal radius with anterior displacement of the distal fragment, produced by a fall on the flexed wrist – this Smith's fracture is much less common that a Colles

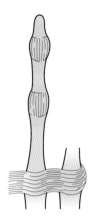

Figure 14.5 Deep transverse metacarpal ligament passing anterior to the metacarpophalangeal joints and anterior capsules of the interphalangeal joints

The fascia over the ventral surface of the wrist thickens to form the flexor retinaculum (Fig. 14.6b). Proximal to this the radial artery can be readily palpated as it lies on the radius. Medial to this are the tendons of flexor carpi radialis and palmaris longus, and under the latter the median nerve crosses the joint deep to the retinaculum. Medially the tendon of flexor carpi ulnaris lies over the ulnar artery and nerve. Lying centrally on a deeper plane are the tendons of flexor digitorum superficialis and profundus and flexor pollicis longus.

The carpometacarpal joint of the thumb

The carpometacarpal joint of the thumb is a synovial joint of considerable mobility owing to its lax capsule and saddle-shaped articulation. Because this joint's axis is at right angles to those of the fingers, flexion and extension occur in a plane at right angles to the thumbnail (and to the palm); abduction and adduction occur in the plane of the thumbnail. When these four movements combine, circumduction of the thumb can occur. The shape of the articular surfaces ensures that flexion is always accompanied by medial rotation, and extension by lateral rotation. One of the most specific thumb movements is that of **opposition**, in which the tip of the thumb is brought into contact with the tips of the fingers. It requires a combination of flexion, medial rotation and adduction of the thumb, and is very much a human attribute:

- **Flexion/medial rotation** – flexor pollicis longus and brevis and opponens pollicis
- **Extension/lateral rotation** – abductor pollicis longus and extensor pollicis longus and brevis
- **Abduction** – abductor pollicis longus and brevis
- **Adduction** – adductor pollicis
- **Opposition** – opponens pollicis.

The **carpometacarpal joints of the fingers** are synovial plane joints. The second and third are less mobile than the fourth and fifth, and all are less mobile than that of the thumb; the metacarpal heads articulate with the cupped bases of the proximal phalanges. The joint capsules have strong palmar thickenings, which are joined to each other by the deep transverse ligaments of the palm (Fig. 14.5). Flexion, extension, abduction, adduction and circumduction are all possible.

Relations of the wrist joint

These are complex but important (Fig. 14.6). Superficial veins and cutaneous nerves lie in the superficial fascia, the terminal branches of the radial nerve crossing the tendon of abductor pollicis longus. Dorsally the deep fascia thickens above the wrist joint to form the extensor retinaculum (Fig. 13.20, p. 220), which is attached to the lower ulna and radius. Beneath it pass the long extensor tendons and their synovial sheaths, each being retained by fibrous septae within fibro-osseous tunnels. The tendons bounding the anatomical snuffbox are visible when the thumb is extended (Figs. 13.18 and 13.19, p 220).

The metacarpophalangeal joints

The metacarpophalangeal joints are synovial joints, the metacarpal heads articulating with the cupped bases of proximal phalanges. The joint capsules have palmar thicken-

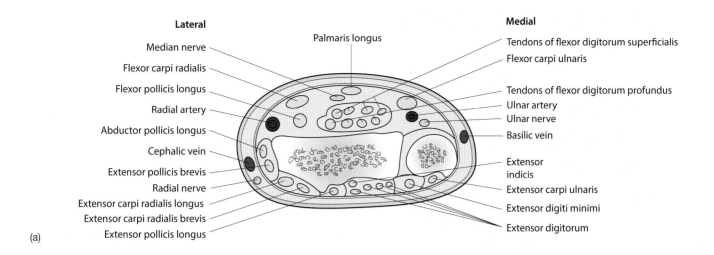

Lateral

Median nerve
Flexor carpi radialis
Flexor pollicis longus
Radial artery
Abductor pollicis longus
Cephalic vein
Extensor pollicis brevis
Radial nerve
Extensor carpi radialis longus
Extensor carpi radialis brevis
Extensor pollicis longus

Palmaris longus

Medial

Tendons of flexor digitorum superficialis
Flexor carpi ulnaris
Tendons of flexor digitorum profundus
Ulnar artery
Ulnar nerve
Basilic vein
Extensor indicis
Extensor carpi ulnaris
Extensor digiti minimi
Extensor digitorum

(a)

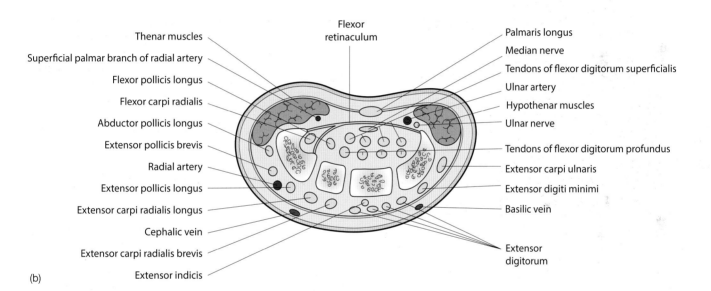

Thenar muscles
Superficial palmar branch of radial artery
Flexor pollicis longus
Flexor carpi radialis
Abductor pollicis longus
Extensor pollicis brevis
Radial artery
Extensor pollicis longus
Extensor carpi radialis longus
Cephalic vein
Extensor carpi radialis brevis
Extensor indicis

Flexor retinaculum

Palmaris longus
Median nerve
Tendons of flexor digitorum superficialis
Ulnar artery
Hypothenar muscles
Ulnar nerve
Tendons of flexor digitorum profundus
Extensor carpi ulnaris
Extensor digiti minimi
Basilic vein
Extensor digitorum

(b)

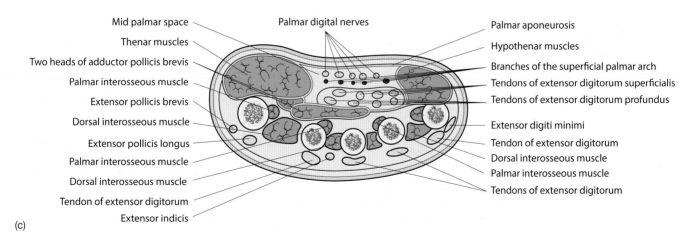

Mid palmar space
Thenar muscles
Two heads of adductor pollicis brevis
Palmar interosseous muscle
Extensor pollicis brevis
Dorsal interosseous muscle
Extensor pollicis longus
Palmar interosseous muscle
Dorsal interosseous muscle
Tendon of extensor digitorum
Extensor indicis

Palmar digital nerves

Palmar aponeurosis
Hypothenar muscles
Branches of the superficial palmar arch
Tendons of extensor digitorum superficialis
Tendons of extensor digitorum profundus
Extensor digiti minimi
Tendon of extensor digitorum
Dorsal interosseous muscle
Palmar interosseous muscle
Tendons of extensor digitorum

(c)

Figure 14.6 Transverse sections, viewed from below, through: (a) the right wrist; (b) the proximal carpus at the level of the flexor retinaculum (see Fig. 14.10); (c) the right palm at the mid-metacarpal level

ings, which join with each other to form the deep transverse ligaments of the palm.

Flexion, extension, abduction and adduction and circumduction are possible, except for the thumb, whose metacarpophalangeal joint is limited to flexion and extension:

- **Flexion** – long digital flexors and flexor pollicis longus, assisted by the interossei, lumbricals, flexor pollicis brevis and flexor digiti minimi
- **Extension** – in the fingers, extensor digitorum, extensor indicis and extensor digiti minimi; in the thumb, extensor pollicis longus and brevis
- **Abduction** – in the fingers, the dorsal interossei and abductor digiti minimi; in the thumb, abductor pollicis longus and brevis
- **Adduction** – palmar interossei and adductor pollicis.

The interphalangeal joints

The interphalangeal joints are synovial joints whose capsules are thickened by palmar and collateral ligaments and strengthened posteriorly by the extensor tendons and their expansions (Fig. 13.16, p. 219). Flexion is by the long digital flexors and extension mainly by the lumbrical and interosseous muscles with the long extensor tendons (Fig. 14.7).

THE PALM

To facilitate grasping, the skin of the palm is thick, ridged, without hairs or sebaceous glands and bound to the under-

lying palmar aponeurosis by strong fibrous attachments that give the palm its creases and the grip to unscrew a jar.

The **pahmar aponeurosis** comprises the strong central triangular part of the palm's deep fascia. Over the thenar and hypothenar muscles it is rather thinner and weaker. The aponeurosis, firmly attached to the palmar skin, overlies the superficial palmar arch and long flexor tendons (Fig. 14.3). Its proximal apex is continuous with the flexor retinaculum and receives the attachment of the tendon of palmaris longus; distally its base divides into four digital slips, which bifurcate around the long flexor tendons to be attached to the deep transverse ligaments of the palm.

Dupuytren's contracture (Fig. 14.8), an abnormal thickening of the palmar aponeurosis, is not uncommon in middle-aged and elderly individuals. Its cause is unknown, but it results in shortening and thickening of the digital bands, which then pull the fingers into flexion, especially the ring and little fingers. Eventually the metacarpophalangeal and proximal interphalangeal joints become permanently flexed. Surgical excision of the contracture is often effective.

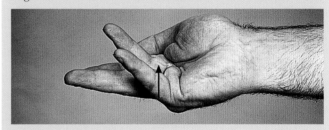

Figure 14.8 Dupuytren's contracture (arrow)

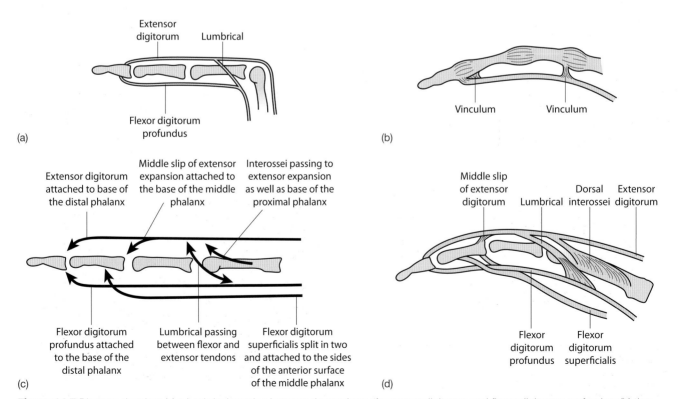

Figure 14.7 Diagram showing: (a) a lumbrical passing between the tendons of extensor digitorum and flexor digitorum profundus; (b) the vincula carrying fine vessels to the adjacent tendons; (c) the digital tendon attachments; (d) the long tendons and small digital muscles

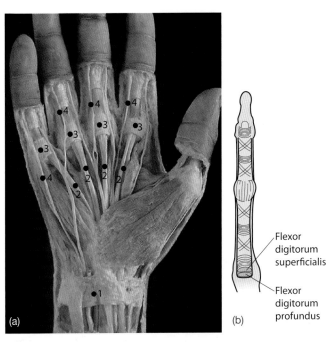

Figure 14.9 (a) Flexor surface of the hand, dissection: 1, flexor retinaculum; 2, long flexor tendons passing into, 3, fibrous sheaths; note the digital nerves, 4, lying superficially. (b) Fibrous digital sheaths of the long flexor tendons

The **flexor retinaculum** (Figs. 14.9 and 14.10) is a thickening of deep fascia, 2–3 cm square, which crosses the concavity of the carpus to form an osseofascial **carpal tunnel** to convey the long flexor tendons. Medially it is attached to the pisiform and hamate, and laterally to the scaphoid and trapezium. Thenar and hypothenar muscles arise from its superficial surface, and the ulnar artery and nerve and its palmar branches cross it. Beneath it the carpal tunnel conveys the long flexor tendons, the radial and ulnar bursae and the median nerve and its digital branches.

Whenever the size of the tunnel is reduced, as it may be following the tissue swelling of rheumatoid arthritis or pregnancy, symptoms are produced by compression of the median nerve deep to the retinaculum (carpal tunnel syndrome). Compression of its cutaneous digital branches produces pain, tingling (paraesthesia) and anaesthesia over the lateral 3½ digits. If the motor branches are affected then weakness, eventual paralysis and wasting of those small muscles of the hand supplied by the median nerve results. There will be progressive loss of coordination and strength in the thumb, and a loss of muscle bulk in the thenar eminence may be noted. Relief of symptoms is obtained by dividing the flexor retinaculum surgically.

The deep fasciae of the fingers and thumb form **fibrous flexor sheaths** (Fig. 14.9b) in continuity with the digital slips of the palmar aponeurosis. The tendons are confined within osseofascial tunnels that arch over the tendons and are attached to the sides of the phalanges. Each extends to the base of the distal phalanx. These sheaths, together with the palmar aponeurosis and the flexor retinaculum, prevent the long flexor tendons 'bowstringing' across the palm during contraction.

Septa pass from the lateral and medial margins of the palmar aponeurosis to the shafts of the 1 and 5 metacarpals to create three **palmar spaces** (Fig. 14.6c): the thenar, containing the thenar muscles; the hypothenar, containing the hypothenar muscles; and the central, containing the superficial palmar arch, median nerve, long flexor tendons and lumbricals, and deep palmar arch.

These potential fascial spaces may become infected, either by direct trauma from a puncture wound or by spread from a tendon sheath infection, and in these circumstances the infection can spread proximally deep to the flexor retinaculum to reach the lower forearm. The thick palmar fascia usually prevents the signs of infection appearing in the palm. The painful swelling is generally most evident on the dorsum where the fascia is thinner.

The fingertips are particularly liable to minor trauma and, should that cause infection (Fig. 14.11), then onset of pain soon follows because the soft tissue of the fingertip is tightly packed between firm fascial septa. Pus may spread from the fingertip proximally alongside the neurovascular bundle. Surgical drainage by an incision along the side of the finger may be required.

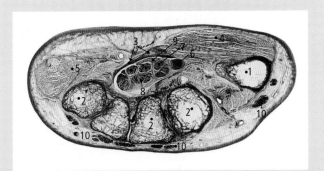

Figure 14.10 Axial plastination through the wrist to show the contents of the carpal tunnel: 1, base of 1 metacarpal; 2, row of carpal bones; 3, flexor retinaculum; 4, thenar eminence – ball of thumb; 5, hypothenar eminence; 6, flexor pollicis longus; 7, flexor digitorum superficialis; 8, flexor digitorum profundus; 9, median nerve; 10, extensor tendons

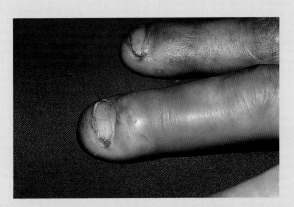

Figure 14.11 Acute paronychia (infection often starts under the edge of a nail)

Muscles of the palm

The **thenar muscles** (Fig. 14.12) are all supplied by the recurrent branch of the median nerve.

Abductor pollicis brevis lies superficially, immediately deep to the fascia. It is attached to the scaphoid and adjacent flexor retinaculum, and its tendon passes to the radial side of the base of the proximal phalanx of the thumb. It abducts the thumb.

Opponens pollicis is attached proximally to the trapezium and adjacent flexor retinaculum and distally to the radial side of the 1st metacarpal. It flexes, adducts and medially rotates the thumb (otherwise known as opposing the thumb) to bring the pulp of the thumb tip into contact with the tips of the flexed fingers.

Flexor pollicis brevis, attached proximally to the trapezium and adjacent flexor retinaculum, is attached distally to the base of the thumb's proximal phalanx. It flexes the carpometacarpal and metacarpophalangeal joints of the thumb.

The **hypothenar muscles** are small mirror images of the thenar muscles and are supplied by the deep branch of the ulnar nerve. They each arise from the medial side of the flexor retinaculum and pisiform or hamate bones. **Abductor digiti minimi** and **flexor digiti minimi** gain distal attachment to the base of the proximal phalanx of the little finger; **opponens digiti minimi** is attached distally to the ulnar margin of the 5 metacarpal shaft. Their action is indicated by their names.

The deep muscles of the hand

Adductor pollicis is attached laterally to the base of the thumb's proximal phalanx and, by a tendon, into the radial side of the same bone; medially it is attached by two heads into (a) the palmar surface of the base of the second and third metacarpals, and (b) the palmar surface of the body of the 3

metacarpal. It adducts and assists in opposition of the thumb. Its nerve supply is the deep branch of the ulnar nerve.

The **interossei** (Fig. 14.13) lie deep between the metacarpals: four dorsal and four palmar muscles. Proximally these are attached to the shafts of the metacarpals: the palmar to the palmar surfaces of the 1, 2, 4 and 5 bones; the larger, more powerful dorsal muscles are attached by two heads to adjacent metacarpals. Distally both palmar and dorsal muscles are attached to the base of the corresponding proximal phalanx

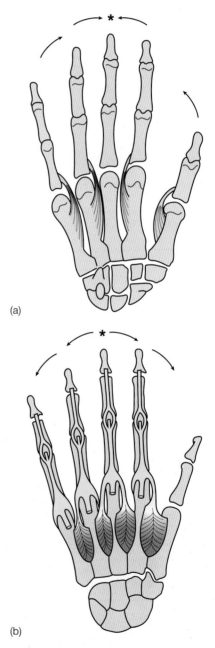

(a)

(b)

Figure 14.13 (a) Palmar interossei muscles pass from the sides of the metacarpals to the adjacent base of the proximal phalanx, the arrangement producing adduction of the thumb and fingers towards the central axis that passes through the middle finger*. (b) The dorsal interossei pass from adjacent sides of the metacarpals to be attached distally to the bases of the proximal phalanges and the dorsal digital expansions; their action serves to abduct the digits away from the central axis that passes through the middle finger*

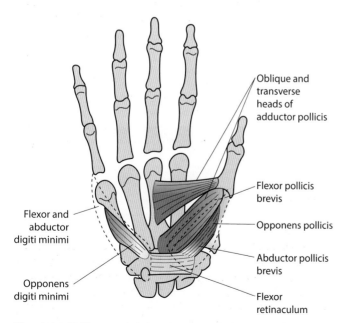

Oblique and transverse heads of adductor pollicis

Flexor pollicis brevis

Opponens pollicis

Abductor pollicis brevis

Flexor retinaculum

Flexor and abductor digiti minimi

Opponens digiti minimi

Figure 14.12 Thenar and hypothenar muscles; superficial muscles outlined (dashed)

and the extensor expansion. The **p**almar **ad**duct 'Pad' and the **d**orsal **ab**duct 'Dab' the fingers about the axis of the middle finger (Fig. 14.13). Both groups, acting with the lumbricals, flex the proximal phalanx and, by their attachment to the extensor expansion, help to extend the middle and distal phalanges. The nerve supply is the deep branch of the ulnar nerve.

The **lumbricals** (Fig. 14.14) are slender, worm-like muscles arising in the palm from the radial side of the four tendons of flexor digitorum profundus. Each is attached distally to the radial side of the extensor expansion of its tendon. Their action is similar to that of the interossei, but it is in the finer control of the upstroke in writing that they are most important. The two lateral lumbricals are supplied by the median nerve, the two medial by the ulnar nerve. The power grip involves the long finger flexors and intrinsic flexors of the four fingers, locked down and reinforced by thumb flexion

and adduction. A precision grip is much more a combination of mainly the interossei and lumbricals with assistance from the thenar and hypothenar opponens. In all hand movements it is a combination of ulnar, median and radial nerves as there is normally synergism between the wrist extensors and finger flexor groups.

BLOOD SUPPLY

The **superficial palmar arch** (Fig. 13.22, p. 221) provides an anastomosis between the radial and ulnar arteries in the hand. The superficial palmar branch of the ulnar artery passes laterally deep to the palmar aponeurosis to join the terminal branch of the radial artery superficial to the long flexor tendons. It provides four palmar digital branches which, by bifurcating, supply adjacent sides of the fingers and also join with the **deep palmar arch**, another anastomosis, formed largely by the radial artery and a smaller branch from the ulnar artery. It lies deep to the long flexor tendons and provides palmar metacarpal arteries and perforating arteries to the dorsum of the hand.

NERVES

The course of the nerves in the hand is described on pp. 197 and 198.

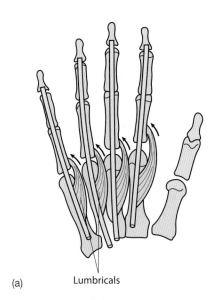

(a)   Lumbricals

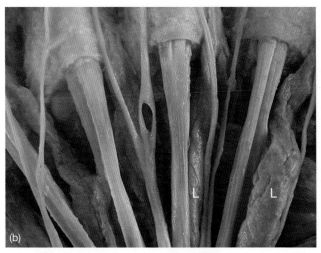

(b)

Figure 14.14 (a) Lumbrical muscles seen from the anterior aspect of the right hand, passing from the flexor digitorum profundus tendons around the lateral aspect of the four fingers to be attached to the dorsal digital expansion. They extend the interphalangeal joints by traction on the extensor tendons and flex the metacarpophalangeal joints by releasing tension in the digital aspect of the long flexor tendons. (b) Dissected right hand showing the lumbricals (L)

Upper limb sensory testing (with eyes closed) of dermatomes and individual nerves

Touch (cotton wool); pain (sterile needle); temperature (side of finger versus cold side of tuning fork); vibration (base of tuning fork on head of ulna); graphaesthesia (writing numbers on the forearm with a blunt instrument); stereognosis (recognizing a coin by touch); position sense (recognizing direction of movement – hold the sides of the index finger).

Motor testing

Power (grip); tone (passive flexion and extension of a relaxed elbow joint); coordination (finger to tip of nose – eyes open and then closed); reflexes (biceps C5/6; supinator, triceps C6/7); note wasting and abnormal movements; individual muscles – active and passive movements, and against resistance.

Peripheral nerve injuries

Radial nerve

In the arm, radial nerve injuries proximal to the attachment of triceps (most commonly in association with a fractured humerus) result in paralysis of triceps, brachioradialis, supinator, wrist and digital extensors. The characteristic deformity of wrist drop occurs and there is loss of sensation over the radial side of the dorsum of the hand and lateral 3½ fingers and a variable part of the posterior surface of the forearm.

In the axilla, the nerve may be injured by the pressure of a crutch or by pressure on the nerve when the patient falls asleep with their arm thrown over the back of a chair (such as commonly happens to drunken people). Wrist-drop and sensory loss over the radial side of the palm and lateral fingers result.

In the forearm, superficial injuries cause no more than a small area of diminished sensation over the radial side of the dorsum of the hand because the radial nerve contains no muscular branches. Deeper forearm injuries or fractures of the radial neck may damage the posterior interosseous nerve and result in inability to extend the thumb and the metacarpophalangeal joints of the fingers, because of the paralysis of the long extensors. Extension of the wrist is maintained because extensor carpi radialis is supplied by a branch of the radial nerve that arises above the elbow. In this case there is no sensory loss because the posterior interosseous nerve is entirely motor.

Median nerve

At the wrist (Figs. 14.15a,b), injuries are usually caused by lacerations over the wrist and result in paralysis of the thenar muscles and the first and second lumbricals and a loss of sensation over the radial two-thirds of the palm, the palmar surface of the thumb and the lateral 2½ fingers. No opposition of the thumb is possible and the index and middle fingers are flexed and partly 'clawed'.

At the elbow, a median nerve injury produces a serious disability; pronation of the forearm is lost and wrist flexion is weakened (being retained only by flexor carpi ulnaris and the ulnar half of flexor digitorum profundus; Fig. 12.19d, p. 200).

Ulnar nerve

At the wrist, lacerations may cause division of the nerve and produce the paralysis of many of the intrinsic hand muscles: the interossei, adductor pollicis, the hypothenar muscles and the third and fourth lumbricals, resulting in a clawed hand (similar to Fig. 12.19b, p. 200), with diminished sensation over the ulnar side of the palm. 'Clawed hand' is the result of the long digital flexors, now unopposed by the paralysed lumbricals and interossei, flexing the middle and distal phalanges. The consequent pull of the long digital extensors produces hyperextension of the metacarpophalangeal joints. Adduction of the thumb is lost. A damaged ulnar nerve may result in paralysis of adductor pollicis with a resultant positive Froment's sign – the long flexors compensating for adductor loss (Fig. 14.15c).

At the elbow, the ulnar nerve is vulnerable to trauma as it lies close to the subcutaneous medial epicondyle of the humerus, and injury results in paralysis of the ulnar half of flexor digitorum profundus and of flexor carpi ulnaris being added to the effects described above (Fig. 14.15d). This results in clawing of the hand and some radial deviation at the wrist (see Fig. 12.19b, p. 200, and Fig. 14.15d).

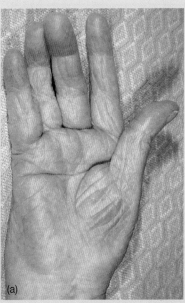
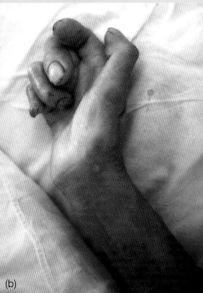
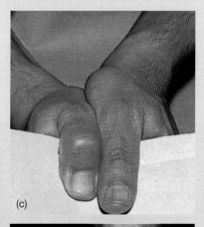
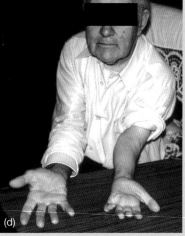

(a)   (b)   (c)   (d)

Figure 14.15 (a) Median nerve injury. (b) Median and ulnar nerve damage due to leprosy. (c) Ulnar nerve injury and inability to adduct the right thumb, which is replaced by flexing (Froment's sign). (d) Chronic ulnar nerve injury resulting in a left clawed hand and growth retardation

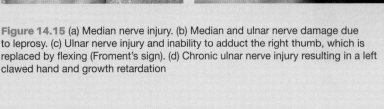

MCQs

1. The following muscles contribute to the extensor expansions of the fingers: T/F
- **a** extensor digitorum longus   (___)
- **b** extensor indicis   (___)
- **c** palmar interossei   (___)
- **d** extensor pollicis longus   (___)
- **e** the two medial lumbricals   (___)

Answers
1.
a T – The dorsal extensor expansion of the fingers has contributions from the ...
b T – ... extensor digitorum longus, extensor indicis, both the dorsal and palmar ...
c T – ... interossei and the four lumbrical muscles, which pass from the flexor digitorum longus into the dorsal hood and expansion.
d F – There is no extensor expansion in the thumb.
e T

2. The following structures pass superficial to the flexor retinaculum: T/F
- **a** palmar branch of the ulnar nerve   (___)
- **b** palmar branch of the median nerve   (___)
- **c** anterior interosseous nerve   (___)
- **d** the tendon of palmaris longus   (___)
- **e** the tendon of flexor pollicis longus   (___)

Answers
2.
a T – The ulnar nerve and its palmar branch lie superficial to the flexor retinaculum.
b T – Although the median nerve passes deep to the retinaculum, its palmar branch lies superficial to it.
c F – The anterior interosseous nerve ends proximal to the retinaculum in pronator quadratus.
d T – The tendon of palmaris longus passes superficial to the retinaculum to end in the palmar aponeurosis.
e F – The tendon of flexor pollicis longus lies in its own compartment deep to the retinaculum.

3. Palpation of the wrist reveals that: T/F
- **a** the palmaris longus tendon is present only in a minority of people   (___)
- **b** the median nerve can usually be rolled under the fingers over the tendons of flexor digitorum superficialis   (___)
- **c** the superficial branches of the radial nerve can be rolled over the flexor pollicis longus   (___)
- **d** the radial pulse is usually medial to the tendon of flexor carpi radialis   (___)
- **e** the scaphoid bone lies in the floor of the anatomical snuffbox   (___)

Answers
3.
a F – Palmaris longus is present in the great majority of people.
b F – The median nerve lies deep to palmaris longus tendon (in the minority, in whom the muscle is absent, the nerve can be rolled over the tendons of flexor digitorum).
c F – Branches of the radial nerve can be palpated over the tendon of extensor pollicis longus as it crosses the roof of the anatomical snuffbox.
d F – It is lateral to the tendon.
e T – Tenderness in the floor of the snuffbox may indicate a fracture of the scaphoid.

4. The median nerve: T/F
- **a** arises from medial and lateral divisions of the brachial plexus   (___)
- **b** passes between the two heads of pronator teres   (___)
- **c** is situated at the wrist between palmaris longus and flexor carpi radialis longus   (___)
- **d** lies on the centre of the flexor retinaculum   (___)
- **e** may, when subject to pressure in the carpal tunnel, produce anaesthesia over the thenar eminence   (___)

Answers
4.
a F – The median nerve arises from the medial and lateral cords of the plexus.
b T – To lie deep to the muscle.
c T – In this position it passes deep to the flexor retinaculum centrally.
d F – It lies deep to the retinaculum.
e F – Compression within the carpal tunnel does not affect the palmar branch of the median nerve, which passes into the hand superficial to the retinaculum. Its innervation of the skin of the thenar eminence is not affected.

SBA

1. A mid-term pregnant patient presents with a complaint of numbness in the middle three fingers of her right hand and some difficulty in grasping objects with that hand. Which of the following is most likely to be the cause?
a Carpal tunnel compression of the median nerve
b Wrist osteophytes compressing the ulnar nerve at the medial epicondyle of the humerus
c Osteoarthritis of the cervical spine
d Compression of the brachial plexus
e Rheumatoid arthritis, which is most marked in her fingers

Answer
a   *There is some fluid retention and oedema during pregnancy, which may narrow the carpal tunnel and compress the structures passing through it. The median nerve supplies motor fibres to the muscles of the thenar eminence and sensation to the thumb, index and middle finger and to the lateral half of the ring finger. Compression of the median nerve has produced symptoms and signs typical of the 'carpal tunnel' syndrome.*

2. A patient is admitted after a fall on his outstretched hand. He has no obvious deformity but exhibits tenderness in the anatomical snuffbox of the affected hand. Which carpal bone may have been fractured?
a Triquetral
b Scaphoid
c Capitate
d Pisiform
e Hamate

Answer
b   *The anatomical snuffbox on the posterolateral aspect of the hand is a triangular space walled by the tendons of extensor pollicis brevis, abductor pollicis longus and extensor pollicis longus. The scaphoid bone forms its floor and tenderness suggests that it is the bone fractured.*

EMQs

Each question has an anatomical theme linked to the chapter, and a list of 10 related items (A–J) placed in alphabetical order: these are followed by five statements (1–5). Match **one or more** of the items A–J to each of the five statements.

Relationships at the wrist
A. Flexor retinaculum
B. Median nerve
C. Pisiform bone
D. Radial artery
E. Radial nerve
F. Scaphoid bone
G. Styloid process of the radius
H. Styloid process of the ulna
I. Ulnar artery
J. Ulnar nerve

Match the following statements with the item(s) in the above list.
1. Lies in the floor of the anatomical snuffbox
2. Lies superficial to the median nerve
3. Passes medial to the pisiform bone
4. Overlain by the palmaris longus tendon
5. Gives attachment to the flexor retinaculum

Answers
1 DFG; 2 A; 3 IJ; 4 AB; 5 CF

Bones of the upper limb
A. Clavicle
B. Distal phalanx of the little finger
C. First metacarpal
D. Humerus
E. Pisiform
F. Proximal phalanx of the middle finger
G. Radius
H. Scaphoid
I. Scapula
J. Ulna

Match the following statements with the bone(s) of the above list
1. Has a styloid process
2. Gives attachment to the abductor pollicis longus
3. Gives attachment to flexor carpi ulnaris
4. Gives attachment to the short head of biceps
5. Gives attachment to the flexor digitorum profundus

Answers
1 GJ; 2 CGJ; 3 EJ; 4 I; 5 JB

APPLIED QUESTIONS

1. An old woman falls downstairs and sustains a mid-shaft fracture of the humerus, damaging the radial nerve in the spiral groove. What are the effects, both motor and sensory, on the hand and wrist?

1. Wrist drop is the most noticeable injury, owing to loss of action of all finger and wrist extensors. This also considerably weakens the power grip. The sensory loss, however, is often limited, owing to overlap of the nerves' sensory distribution, but may include a strip down the posterior aspect of arm and forearm as well as a small area of anaesthesia over the first dorsal interosseous muscle, in the posterior web between the thumb and index finger.

2. In the hand, which nerve lesion is the most serious, and why?

2. The median nerve lesion is the most disabling because thumb opposition is lost, as well as the sensation over the thumb, index and middle fingers. Consequently, all fine pincer movements, such as writing, are almost impossible.

3. How might a swelling proximal to the wrist joint be connected with infection in the tip of the thumb (tenosynovitis)?

3. The long flexor tendons of the thumb are surrounded by synovial sheaths. An infection in the pulp might readily spread proximally where, in some people, it joins the ulnar bursa, both of them passing deep to the retinaculum and extending for 2–3 cm to the level of the wrist.

4. A man who has attempted suicide has cut his wrists fairly deeply. After repair of the arteries, which other important structures would you also wish to test and how would you do this?

4. The two major nerves of the hand are both vulnerable. The median nerve lies just deep to palmaris longus, and the ulnar nerve lies between the ulnar artery and the pisiform bone. To test the median nerve, the patient is asked to abduct his thumb against resistance (note that thumb opposition can be mimicked by the long flexor tendons). True thumb opposition is impossible in long-standing median nerve lesions, as the thumb is laterally rotated and adducted and consequently looks like a monkey's or ape's hand. To test the ulnar nerve, the hand is placed palm downwards and the fingers straightened, and then abducted and adducted against resistance. Or try the paper-holding test between adducted fingers. When pulling on a sheet of paper held between thumb and side of index finger of both hands, adductor pollicis maintains the downward pressure; if the ulnar nerve is damaged additional pressure is applied by flexor pollicis with flexion of the interphalangeal joint (Froment's sign).

PART **5**

The lower limb

The hip and thigh

The lower limb, similar in structure to the upper, is modified by its functions of support and propulsion of the body. During its development there is rotation medially on its long axis, so that the flexor surface lies posteriorly and the sole of the foot faces backwards and then downwards. The pelvic girdle (Fig. 9.1a, p. 137), unlike the pectoral girdle, is firmly attached to the vertebral column, which allows transmission of the body's weight through it to the lower limb. In the standing position the centre of gravity passes behind the hip and in front of the knee and ankle joints. The weight is distributed between the heel and the balls of the toes, most of it being carried by bones and ligaments, with only a minimal amount of muscle activity being required to maintain balance.

THE FASCIA

The membranous layer of the superficial fascia of the abdomen extends into the thigh, fusing with the deep fascia at the level of the skin crease in front of the hip joint. The deep fascia of the gluteal region and thigh forms a firm investing layer, the **fascia lata**. Proximally it is attached in a continuous line to the inguinal ligament, iliac crest, posterior sacrum, sacrotuberous ligament, ischiopubic ramus and body of the pubis. Medial and lateral intermuscular septa spread from it to divide the thigh muscles into distinct compartments (Fig. 15.1).

Three centimetres below and 1 cm lateral to the pubic tubercle an oval deficiency in the fascia, the **saphenous opening** (Fig. 15.2a), transmits the great saphenous vein. The fascia lata

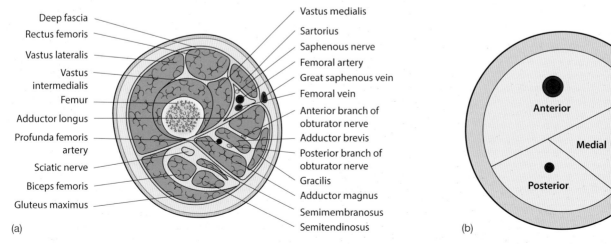

Figure 15.1 (a) Transverse section of the right thigh through the upper thigh, viewed from below (see dotted line in Fig. 15.2a for level): the deep fascia (fascia lata) divides the thigh into anterior, medial and posterior compartments, as shown in schematic (b)

is thickened on the lateral side of the thigh, forming the iliotibial tract, which is attached distally to the lateral tibial condyle. Gluteus maximus and tensor fasciae latae gain attachment to the tract and, because of this attachment, assist in extension and stabilization of the knee. Over the popliteal fossa the fascia is pierced by the small saphenous vein (**Fig. 15.3**).

The deep fascia of the lower leg is continuous with the fascia lata. It is attached to bone around the margins of the patella, to the medial surface of the tibia and, inferiorly, to both malleoli. It ensheaths the muscles and contributes to intermuscular septa that separate the anterior, lateral and posterior muscle compartments. The posterior muscles are further divided by a fascial envelope into superficial and deep compartments, the former enclosing gastrocnemius and soleus. Around the ankle the fascia thickens to form the retinacula, restraining the tendons as they enter the foot. On the dorsum of the foot the fascia is thin, but on the sole it is thickened to form the **plantar aponeurosis**. Throughout the leg and thigh, the fascia is pierced by perforating (communicating) veins joining the superficial to the deep veins, and by cutaneous nerves, arteries and lymph vessels.

The fascial compartments of the leg are rather rigid envelopes for the soft tissues contained within them; trauma and bleeding, such as may follow a leg fracture, can cause compartmental swelling and rise in pressure of sufficient severity to compromise the arterial supply to the contents of the compartment. It is essential in these circumstances that close observation is maintained on the pulses in the leg, and if the circulation is found to be threatened, a fasciotomy (incision along the length of the fascial sheath) must be urgently undertaken to relieve the pressure in that compartment.

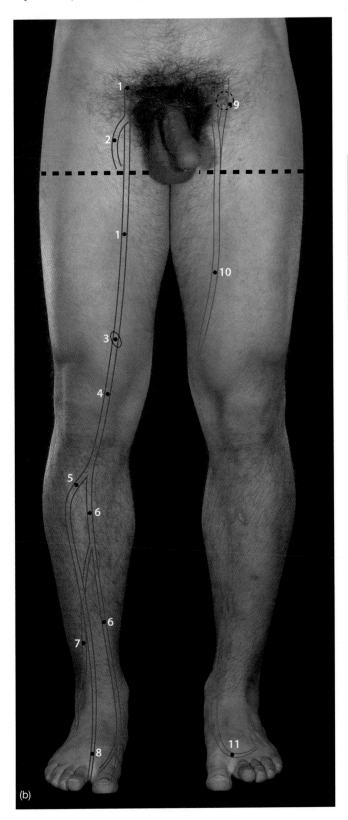

(b)

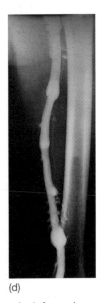
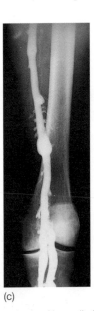
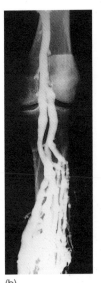

(b)   (c)   (d)

Figure 15.2 (a) Surface anatomy of lower limb vessels: 1, femoral artery; 2, profunda femoris; 3, adductor hiatus; 4, popliteal artery; 5, anterior tibial artery; 6, posterior tibial artery; 7, peroneal (fibular) artery; 8, dorsalis pedis artery; 9, saphenous opening; 10, great saphenous vein; 11, dorsal venous arch. NB: the dotted line indicates the level of the transverse section in Fig. 15.1a. (b–d) Lower limb venograms. (b) Numerous deep veins within soleus and gastrocnemius draining into the popliteal vein. (c) The popliteal vein becoming the femoral vein at the adductor hiatus. (d) The femoral vein on the medial side of the thigh – note the bulges above the valves

Venous drainage

There are three types of vein in the lower limb: superficial, deep and communicating (perforating) (Figs. 15.2 and 15.3). Valves are present in the larger veins and all the communicating veins; they direct blood flow towards the heart or from the superficial to the deep veins. The **superficial veins** drain skin and superficial fascia into two main channels, the great and small saphenous veins. These originate in the **dorsal** and **plantar venous arches** of the forefoot.

The **great saphenous vein** (Fig. 15.2a), from the medial end of the dorsal arch, ascends anterior to the medial malleolus, lying subcutaneously along the medial calf and thigh, accompanied in the calf by the saphenous nerve. It enters the deep venous system by passing through the saphenous opening into the femoral vein (Fig. 15.6a). It receives tributaries from the small saphenous vein and connects by communicating branches to the deep veins of the thigh and calf just behind the medial border of the tibia.

Just anterior and superior to the medial malleolus the great saphenous vein can readily be located and is frequently used for an emergency venous 'cutdown'. The great saphenous vein is also commonly used to bypass blocked coronary arteries in a coronary artery bypass graft (CABG) operation – known as a 'cabbage' procedure. It is reversed so that its valves do not obstruct the arterial blood flow.

The **small saphenous vein** (Fig. 15.3) originates at the lateral end of the dorsal venous arch, ascends behind the lateral malleolus up the posterior calf, and ends by passing through the fascia over the popliteal fossa into the popliteal vein. It receives cutaneous tributaries and communicates with the deep veins of the calf by perforating veins.

The **deep veins** comprise those of the foot and the soleal plexuses of veins, the popliteal and the femoral vein (p. 260). The superficial veins drain to them by communicating veins that perforate the deep fascia.

All the veins of the lower limb possess valves that permit blood flow only up the limb or from superficial veins to deep veins. Flow in the deep veins towards the heart is aided by the contraction of the calf muscles, the 'muscle pump'.

If the valves of the communicating veins become incompetent, the blood flow within them becomes reversed and the 'muscle pump' is less effective at helping the venous return to the deep veins. The result is that the superficial veins become distended (**varicose veins**) (Fig. 15.4) with the increased amount of venous return that they are carrying, and their valves become incompetent. The deep plexuses of veins are emptied by foot and calf muscle contraction, and in prolonged recumbency, when leg activity is minimal, stagnation of blood occurs within them, often followed by thrombosis (Fig. 15.5). This is one of the factors that accounts for the high frequency of **deep vein thrombosis** postoperatively. When deep

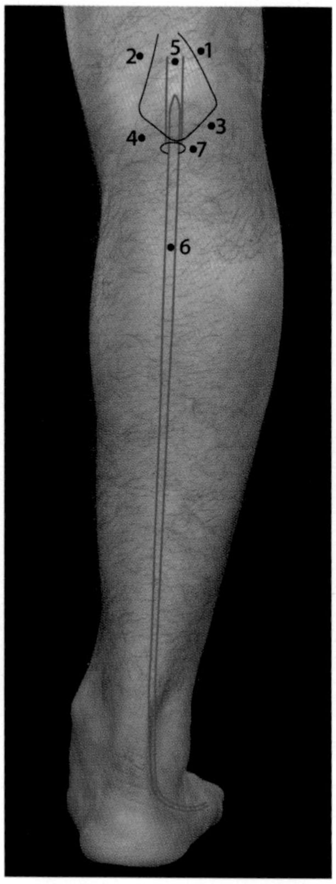

Figure 15.3 Surface anatomy of the small saphenous vein: 1, biceps femoris; 2, semitendinosus and semimembranosus; 3, lateral head of gastrocnemius; 4, medial head of gastrocnemius; 5, popliteal vein; 6, small saphenous vein; 7, opening for small saphenous vein in deep fascia

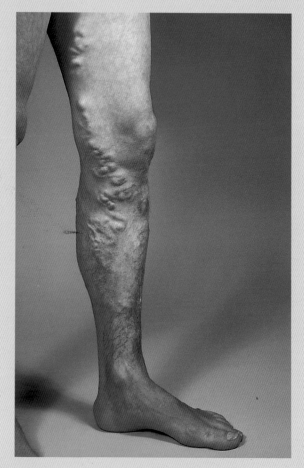

Figure 15.4 A varicose great saphenous vein distended with blood because the valves of the communicating veins are incompetent

venous thrombosis occurs there is always a risk that part of the thrombus can break off and cause a pulmonary embolus. More usually the thrombus resolves but damages the vein's valves, with the result that defective venous return from the lower limb may result in varicose veins, chronic leg swelling, skin changes and ulceration of the skin over the ankle – the postphlebitic limb.

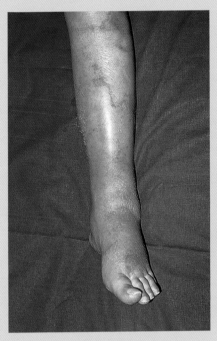

Figure 15.5 Deep venous thrombosis of left leg. Note the swelling and skin changes

Lymphatic drainage

There are two groups of lymph nodes in the lower limb, superficial and deep.

The **superficial groups** lie in the inguinal region (Fig. 15.6). The **upper superficial (horizontal) inguinal group** is in the femoral triangle, just below the inguinal ligament. It receives lymph from the lower abdominal wall, perineum, external genitalia, anal canal and gluteal region, and drains to the lower superficial inguinal group and the deep nodes. The **lower superficial inguinal (vertical) group** lies around the saphenous opening and receives lymph from the upper group and the skin of the thigh and the medial leg and foot. Its efferent vessels drain through the saphenous opening to the deep inguinal or external iliac group.

The **deep groups** lie under the deep fascia in the popliteal and inguinal regions. The **popliteal group**, a small group, lies in the popliteal fossa around the small saphenous vein and drains the skin of the lateral foot and calf and the deep tissues of the leg. Its efferents drain to the deep inguinal group. The **deep inguinal group** lies around the femoral canal and receives the lymph of all the superficial nodes and deep lymphatic vessels of the lower limb. Its efferents drain to the external iliac nodes.

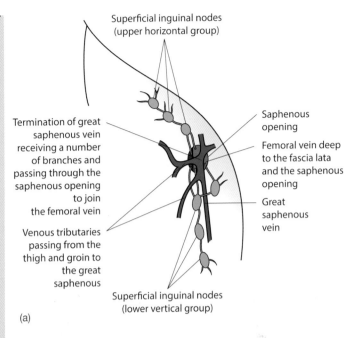

(a)

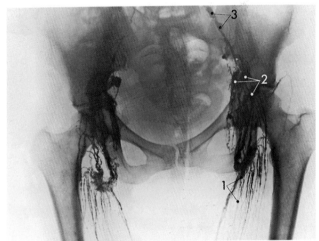

(b)

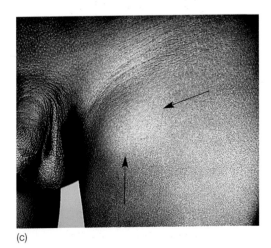

(c)

Figure 15.6 (a) Inguinal lymph nodes, the saphenous opening and the great saphenous vein. (b) Lower limb lymphangiogram: 1, lymphatic vessels of upper thigh; 2, inguinal lymph vessels; 3, external iliac lymph vessels. (c) Enlarged inguinal lymph nodes (arrows) from a foot infection

Enlargement of the inguinal nodes (Fig. 15.6c) follows soft tissue infection anywhere in the lower limb and perineum. Cancers arising in the external genitalia or anal canal may spread to and enlarge these inguinal nodes. Maldevelopment of the lymph vessels, or blockage of the vessels or nodes by disease, produces soft tissue swelling because of the interference with lymph flow. This is termed lymphoedema (Fig. 15.7).

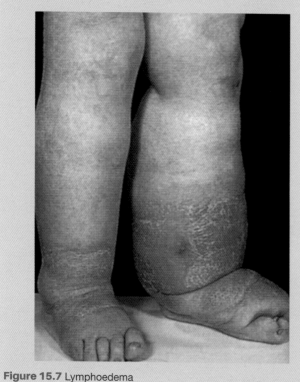

Figure 15.7 Lymphoedema

THE SKELETON

For the **hip bone (os innominatum)** (Figs. 15.8, 15.9 and 15.10), see also p. 136.

The lateral surface of the hip bone

The gluteal surface of the **ala of the ilium** is smooth and faces laterally; it is bounded by the iliac crest above and by the greater sciatic notch and the acetabulum below. It gives attachment to gluteus medius and minimus centrally and to gluteus maximus posteriorly. Rectus femoris gains attachment to its anterolateral border. The **ischial spine** separates the greater and lesser sciatic notches; below the lesser notch is the **ischial tuberosity**. The anterior border of the ilium has prominent **superior** and **inferior iliac spines**. The **obturator foramen** is bounded by the inferior and superior pubic rami (Fig. 15.10).

Fractures of the pelvis are the result of violent blows such as may result from road traffic accidents. Fractures of the acetabulum result from severe lateral forces; compression in an anteroposterior direction may cause fractures of the pubic rami, and if the fragments are displaced injuries to the adjacent bladder may occur.

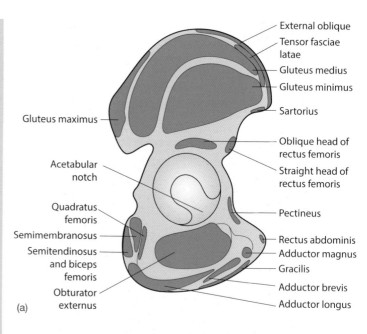

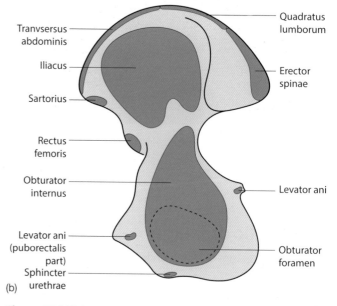

Figure 15.8 Right innominate bone showing muscle attachments: (a) lateral aspect (b) medial aspect

The femur

The femur (Fig. 15.11) possesses a proximal end, a shaft and a distal end. The **proximal end** consists of a head, a neck and greater and lesser trochanters. The **head** articulates with the **acetabulum** of the hip bone; in the centre of the head is a small pit (fovea) for the ligament of the head of the femur.

The narrow **neck** forms an angle of about 125 degrees with the shaft. Much of it lies within the hip joint capsule. The **greater trochanter**, a projection from the lateral part of the bone, gives attachment to the short rotators of the hip joint, gluteus medius and minimus, the obturator muscles and piriformis. The **lesser trochanter**, at the junction of the body and the neck, gives attachment to psoas major and iliacus;

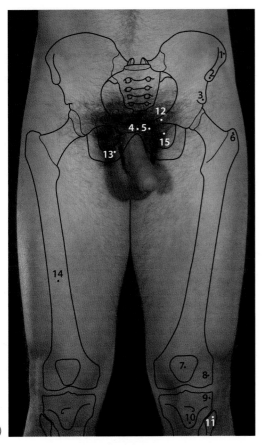

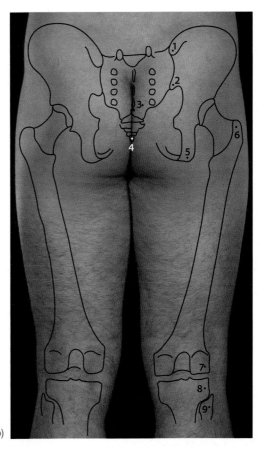

(a)   (b)

Figure 15.9 Surface anatomy of the pelvis and thigh. (a) Anterior view: 1, iliac crest; 2, anterior superior iliac spine; 3, anterior inferior iliac spine; 4, symphysis pubis; 5, pubic tubercle; 6, greater trochanter; 7, patella; 8, lateral condyle of femur; 9, lateral condyle of tibia; 10, tibial tuberosity; 11, head of fibula; 12, superior pubic ramus; 13, inferior pubic ramus; 14, shaft of femur; 15, obturator foramen. (b) Posterior view: 1, posterior superior iliac spine; 2, posterior inferior iliac spine; 3, posterior aspect of sacrum; 4, tip of coccyx; 5, ischial tuberosity; 6, greater trochanter; 7, lateral femoral condyle; 8, lateral condyle of the tibia; 9, head of fibula

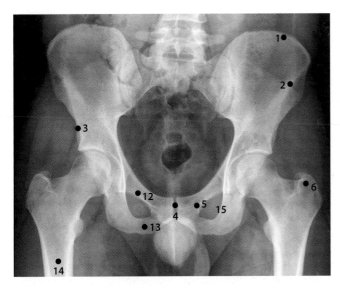

Figure 15.10 X-ray of hip joint and pelvis (labels as in Fig. 15.9a)

the **intertrochanteric line** joins it and the greater trochanter anteriorly, and the **intertrochanteric crest** joins them posteriorly (**Fig. 15.11**).

The **shaft** of the femur inclines medially at an angle of about 10 degrees. It is more oblique in the female because of the greater width of the female pelvis. It bears posteriorly, in its middle third, a longitudinal ridge, the **linea aspera**, which gives attachment to the adductors, short head of biceps and part of the quadriceps. In the lower third the linea aspera splays out into the **medial** and **lateral supracondylar lines**; the medial line ends at the **adductor tubercle** above the medial condyle.

The **distal end** is expanded into two masses, the **medial** and **lateral condyles**, for articulation with the tibial condyles and patella. The articular surfaces of the condyles are separated posteriorly by the intercondylar notch and united anteriorly by the concave articulation for the patella. The tibial articular surface of each condyle is markedly convex anteroposteriorly and slightly convex from side to side; the medial tibial surface is longer than the lateral. The side of each condyle bears a small elevation, the **epicondyle**, which gives attachment to the medial and lateral ligaments of the knee. Much of the lower end of the femur is subcutaneous and palpable (**Fig. 16.2a**, p. 267).

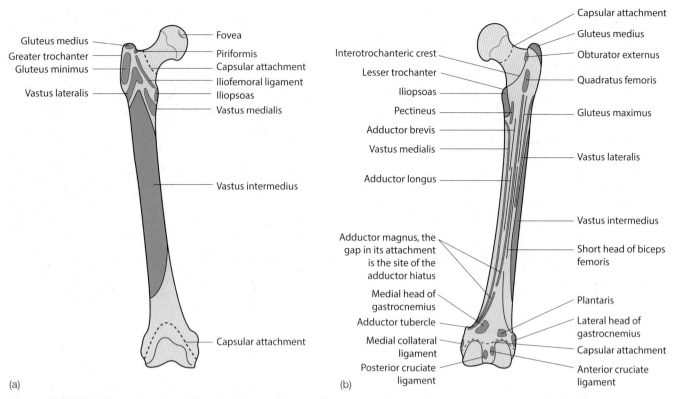

Figure 15.11 Right femur: (a) anterior view; (b) posterior view showing muscle and some ligament attachments

Fractures of the femoral neck are common in elderly individuals because of thinning of the bone structure (osteoporosis). It may fracture near to the trochanters, near the midpoint of the neck or below the head (subcapital; Figs. 15.12a–c). Subcapital fractures may be complicated by necrosis of the femoral head because of damage to the small arteries within the capsule supplying the femoral head. Pertrochanteric or midcervical fractures generally leave the retinacular vessels within the capsule undisturbed, and thus avascular necrosis does not occur and non-union is less frequent (Fig. 15.13).

Fractures of the shaft of the femur (Fig. 15.14) are accompanied by considerable blood loss because of associated injuries to the neighbouring muscles and blood vessels. A characteristic deformity is produced by fractures of the mid-shaft of the femur: namely a considerable shortening because of the now unresisted contraction of the strong thigh muscles, and the proximal fragment being flexed by the unopposed action of iliopsoas and abducted by the glutei, whereas the distal fragment is pulled medially by the adductors. Satisfactory reduction of the fracture must take account of these factors – strong traction to overcome the shortening, with the limb abducted to bring the distal fragment into line with the proximal fragment.

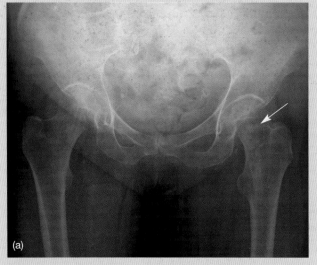

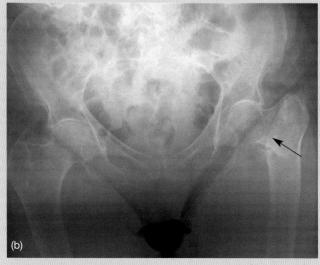

Figure 15.12 (a and b) Intra- and extracapsular fractures of neck of femur (arrows indicate site of fracture)

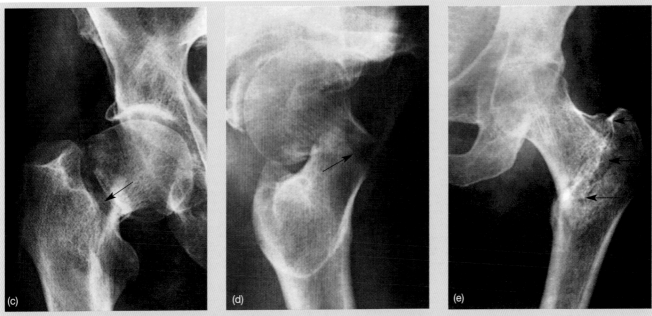

Figure 15.12 (*continued*) (c–e) Intra- and extracapsular fractures of neck of femur (arrows indicate site of fracture)

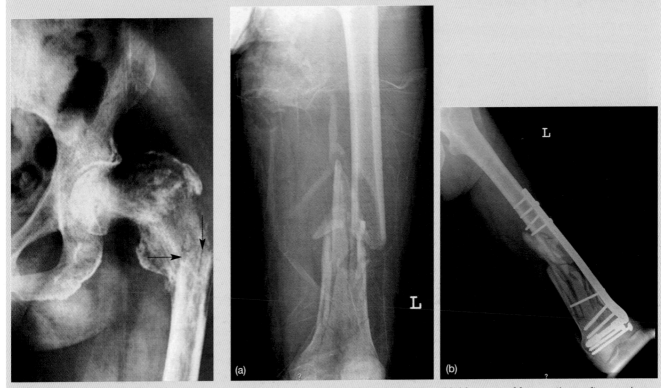

Figure 15.13 Subtrochanteric fracture of femur (arrows)

Figure 15.14 (a) and (b) Mid-shaft and lower-third fractures of femur – these often need internal nail fixation or external plates, as in (b)

THE HIP JOINT

The **hip joint** is a synovial joint of the ball and socket variety between the head of the femur and the acetabulum. The acetabular articular surface is horseshoe-shaped, being deficient below at the acetabular notch. It is deepened by the fibrocartilaginous **acetabular labrum** (Fig. 15.15), and bridging the acetabular notch is the transverse acetabular ligament. Figure 15.16 shows the surface anatomy of the lateral side of the hip joint.

Ligaments

The **capsule** is strong and dense, attached proximally to the acetabular labrum and rim, distally to the femur along the intertrochanteric line anteriorly and, posteriorly, above the

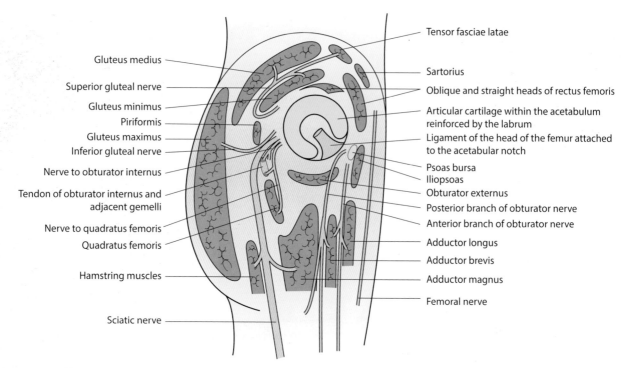

Figure 15.15 Diagram of lateral aspect of the right hip following removal of the femur

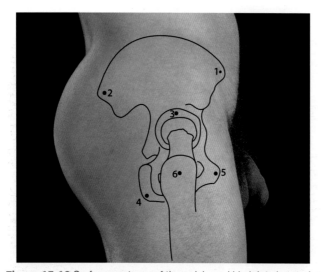

Figure 15.16 Surface anatomy of the pelvis and hip joint: 1, anterior superior iliac spine; 2, posterior superior iliac spine; 3, acetabulum; 4, ischial tuberosity; 5, symphysis pubis; 6, greater trochanter

intertrochanteric crest. In the reflection of the capsule on to the femoral neck are small blood vessels on which depends the nutrition of the femoral head.

The capsule is thickened by strong bands, namely the **iliofemoral ligament**, the **pubofemoral ligament** and the weaker **ischiofemoral ligament** (Fig. 15.17). These three ligaments spiral around the capsule in such a way as to limit extension of the joint. Note also:

- The ligament of the head of the femur – this passes from the fovea on the head of the femur to the acetabular notch.
- The acetabular labrum and transverse acetabular ligament , that completes the rim across the acetabular notch.

- The hip joint's synovial cavity may communicate with the psoas bursa.

Functional aspects

Movement

Flexion, extension, abduction, adduction, circumduction and medial and lateral rotation are possible. In the anatomical position the centre of gravity passes behind the axis of the joint, and thus gravity encourages extension of the joint, which is resisted by the capsular thickenings:

- **Flexion** – iliopsoas, helped by tensor fasciae latae, rectus femoris and sartorius. Flexion is limited to about 110 degrees by contact with the abdominal wall when the knee is flexed. Flexion is less when the knee is extended because of the tension in the hamstrings.
- **Extension** – limited to about 15–20 degrees, and is by gluteus maximus and the hamstrings, assisted by gravity.
- **Abduction** – gluteus medius and minimus, assisted by tensor fasciae latae. Abduction occurs during every step in walking, thus tilting the pelvis on the femur of the grounded leg to allow the opposite foot to clear the ground as it swings forward (pelvic tilt).

Damage to the abductors or their nerve supply results in a positive Trendelenburg sign: a patient standing on the affected leg, in the absence of satisfactory abductors, tilts the contralateral hip downwards. Such a disability makes the swing-through phase of walking very difficult and the patient walks with what is referred to as a waddling gait.

- **Adduction** – the thigh adductors and gracilis.
- **Medial rotation** – adductor magnus, longus and brevis, assisted by iliopsoas.

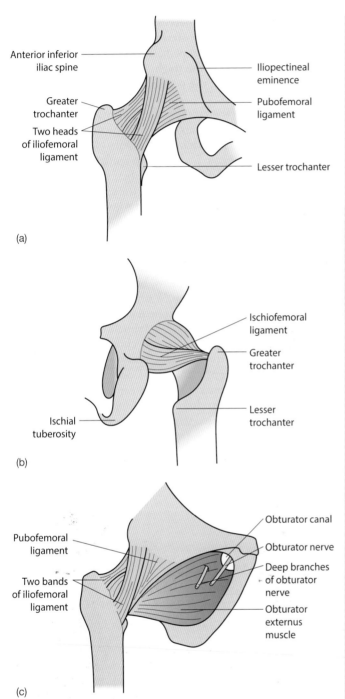

(a)

Anterior inferior iliac spine

Greater trochanter

Two heads of iliofemoral ligament

Iliopectineal eminence

Pubofemoral ligament

Lesser trochanter

(b)

Ischiofemoral ligament

Greater trochanter

Lesser trochanter

Ischial tuberosity

(c)

Pubofemoral ligament

Two bands of iliofemoral ligament

Obturator canal

Obturator nerve

Deep branches of obturator nerve

Obturator externus muscle

Figure 15.17 Ligaments of right hip joint. (a) Anterior aspect. (b) Posterior aspect of hip joint. (c) Anterior aspect of right hip joint showing the obturator externus muscle

Congenital dislocation of the hip (Fig. 15.18) is associated with a shallow acetabulum. Its incidence is less in babies who are carried astride the back with the hips strongly abducted. **A slipped upper femoral epiphysis** (Fig. 15.19) tends to occur in overweight boys of 10–15 years of age. It presents as a 'coxa vara' deformity, in which the angle of the femoral neck on the shaft is reduced. **Traumatic dislocation** is rare and almost always the result of a posterior force acting on the flexed hip (the joint is least stable when flexed and adducted), such as when the flexed knee hits the dashboard in a car accident. It is usually associated with a fracture of the posterior acetabular rim and, sometimes, with injury to the related sciatic nerve.

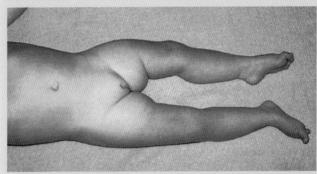

Figure 15.18 Congenital dislocation of the left hip – note the extra skin creases in the upper thigh

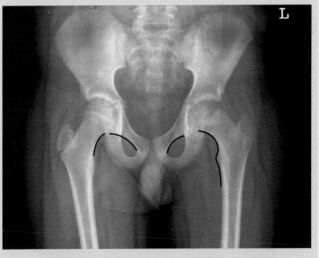

Figure 15.19 Slipped upper femoral epiphysis (left), showing that a line drawn along the upper border of the femoral neck remains superior to the femoral head (left) instead of passing normally through it (right)

- **Lateral rotation** – the short posterior muscles: piriformis, the obturator muscles, gemelli, quadratus femoris and gluteus maximus.

Stability

In spite of its great mobility the hip is a stable joint, its stability helped by the deep acetabulum, which clasps the femoral head, the strong capsule and its spiral thickenings, and the closely applied short lateral rotator muscles.

Blood supply

This is via anastomoses between the gluteal arteries and branches of the femoral artery. The vessels are conveyed to the joint in reflections of the capsule of the joint (retinacula).

Nerve supply

This is by branches of the femoral, obturator and sciatic nerves.

Relations

Anteriorly, iliopsoas and pectineus muscles separate the joint from the femoral vessels and nerve; posteriorly, the short lateral rotators, piriformis, obturator internus, gemelli and quadratus femoris separate the joint from the sciatic nerve. Rectus femoris is superior and obturator externus inferior (Fig. 15.15).

The psoas bursa lies between the iliopsoas tendon and the superior pubic ramus. It may communicate with the hip joint.

THE GLUTEAL REGION

The bulk of the buttock is composed of the three gluteal muscles (Table 15.1 and Fig. 15.20), which overlie smaller rotator muscles of the hip and the nerves and vessels leaving the pelvis for the lower limb. The gluteal muscles are supplied by branches of the internal iliac artery; the superior and inferior gluteal arteries traverse gluteus minimus to supply the muscles and contribute to the anastomosis around the hip joint; the internal pudendal artery briefly enters the region by the greater sciatic foramen before leaving it by the lesser sciatic foramen (Fig. 15.21a) to supply the perineum. The nerves, apart from the superior gluteal, all leave the pelvis below piriformis (Fig. 15.15); the **sciatic nerve** (Figs. 15.21b and 15.22) emerges below piriformis midway between the ischial tuberosity and the greater trochanter (a most important surface marking; Figs. 15.23 and 15.24). Lying alongside it, below piriformis, are the **inferior gluteal nerve** supplying gluteus maximus, the **pudendal nerve** supplying the muscles of the perineum, and the **nerves to quadratus femoris and obturator internus**. The **posterior femoral cutaneous nerve** emerges below piriformis superficial to the sciatic nerve and descends the midline of the thigh. It supplies the skin of the buttock, the perineum, the posterior thigh and the popliteal region.

The muscles of the buttock are frequently used for intramuscular injections. It is important that the needle is inserted into the upper outer quadrant of the buttock as far away as possible from the sciatic nerve. Up to 2 mL may be injected here. If the sciatic nerve is injured, there is paralysis of the hamstrings and all the muscles below the knee, together with a loss of sensation to the skin below the knee, except for that area supplied by the saphenous nerve (medial aspect of the leg and foot). Smaller injections may be made safely into the **deltoid site** on the lateral upper aspect of the arm.

Technique of intramuscular injection: Skin cleansing is not thought necessary by many, but if the region is soiled cleanse it with an alcohol swab. Wash your hands. The needle should be long enough to penetrate the muscle yet leave one-third of its length to permit removal should it snap at the hub – 21 or 23 gauge needles are usually chosen. Insert the needle at 90 degrees to the skin and gently aspirate to establish that the needle has not entered a blood vessel. When using the gluteal site a 'Z-track' technique can be used to prevent leakage – pull the skin downwards before injection so that the needle track is closed when the skin is released. Rotate the site of injection when frequent intramuscular injections are to be given.

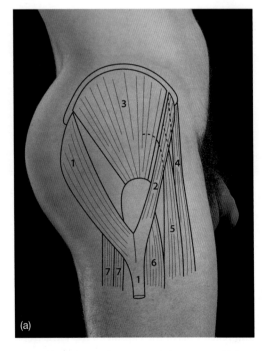

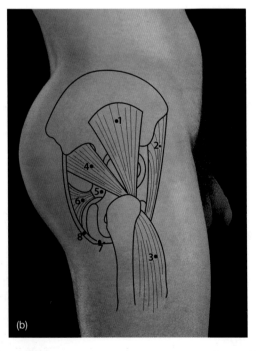

Figure 15.20 Surface anatomy of the gluteal region. (a) Most superficial muscles: 1, gluteus maximus has an extensive origin from pelvis and sacrum, the tendon to femur and iliotibial tract of fasciae latae; 2, tensor fasciae latae; 3, gluteus medius; 4, sartorius; 5, rectus femoris with straight and oblique heads; 6, vastus lateralis; 7, attachments of hamstring muscles to the ischium. (b) Gluteus maximus and medius removed: 1, gluteus minimus; 2, iliacus arising from superior aspect of the ilium; 3, vastus lateralis; 4, piriformis; 5, spine of the ischium; 6, sacrospinous ligament; 7, ischial tuberosity; 8, sacrotuberous ligament

TABLE 15.1 Muscles of the gluteal region (buttock)

Muscle	Proximal attachments	Distal attachments	Nerve supply	Actions
Gluteus maximus	Postero-external surface of ilium and sacrum	Majority of fibres attach to iliotibial tract and some into posterior upper femur	Inferior gluteal nerve (L5, S1, S2)	Extends and assists in lateral rotation of hip
Tensor fasciae latae	Anterior part of iliac crest	Iliotibial tract, a broad thickening of fasciae latae passing between iliac crest and upper end of tibia	Superior gluteal nerve (L4, L5, S1)	Flexes, abducts hip joint; extends and stabilizes knee joint (by iliotibial tract)
Gluteus medius	Gluteal surface of ilium, deep to gluteus maximus	Greater trochanter of femur	Superior gluteal nerve	Strong abductor and weak medial rotator of hip joint
Gluteus minimus	Gluteal surface of ilium deep to gluteus medius	Greater trochanter of femur	Superior gluteal nerve	Strong abductor and weak medial rotator of hip joint
Piriformis	Anterior surface of sacrum	Greater trochanter of femur	Branches of sacral plexus (S1, S2)	Lateral rotator of the hip joint
Quadratus femoris	Medially attached to ischial tuberosity	Laterally attached to intertrochanteric crest and posterior femur	Branch of sacral plexus (L5, S1)	Stabilization of hip joint; weak lateral rotator
Obturator externus	Outer surface of obturator membrane and adjacent bone	Greater trochanter of femur	Obturator nerve (L2, L3, L4)	Stabilization of hip joint; weak lateral rotator

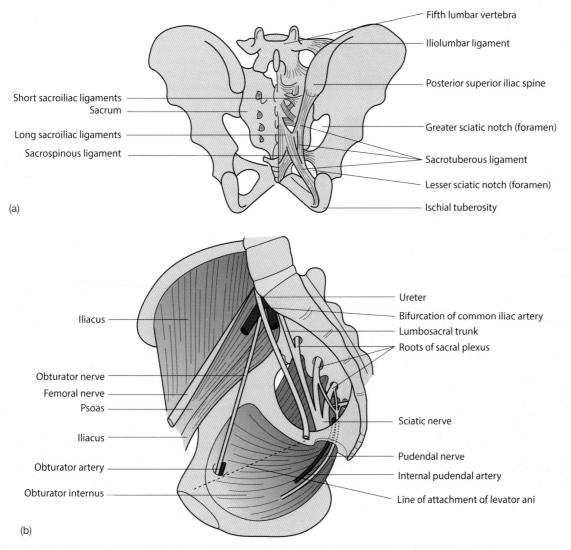

Figure 15.21 (a) Articulated pelvis – posterior aspect showing ligaments. (b) Muscles and nerves of lateral pelvic wall

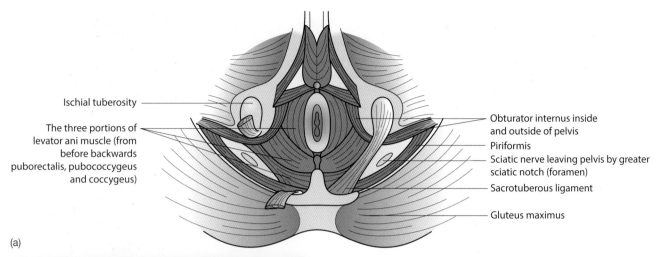

Ischial tuberosity

The three portions of levator ani muscle (from before backwards puborectalis, pubococcygeus and coccygeus)

Obturator internus inside and outside of pelvis

Piriformis

Sciatic nerve leaving pelvis by greater sciatic notch (foramen)

Sacrotuberous ligament

Gluteus maximus

(a)

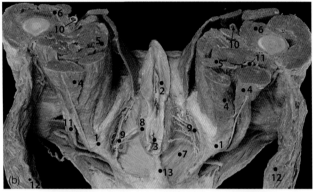

(b)

Figure 15.22 (a) Sciatic nerve passing through the male gluteal region from a perineal perspective. (b) Dissection of female perineum, seen in the lithotomy position: 1, ischial tuberosity; 2, labia and vestibule; 3, anus; 4, hamstring muscle group; 5, adductor muscle group; 6, quadriceps muscle group; 7, levator ani muscle; 8, puborectalis; 9, pudendal vessels and nerves in ischioanal fossae; 10, femoral artery; 11, sciatic nerve; 12, gluteus maximus (retracted laterally); 13, anococcygeal ligament

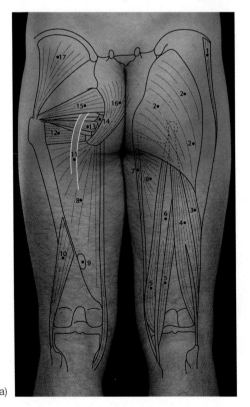

(a)

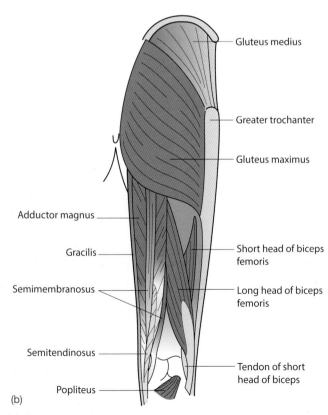

Gluteus medius

Greater trochanter

Gluteus maximus

Adductor magnus

Gracilis

Semimembranosus

Semitendinosus

Popliteus

Short head of biceps femoris

Long head of biceps femoris

Tendon of short head of biceps

(b)

Figure 15.23 (a and b) Surface anatomy of the muscles of the right gluteal region and posterior thigh: 1, tensor fasciae latae; 2, gluteus maximus; 3, vastus lateralis; 4, long head of biceps femoris; 5, semimembranosus; 6, semitendinosus; 7, gracilis; 8, adductor magnus; 9, adductor hiatus; 10, short head of biceps femoris; 11, sciatic nerve; 12, quadratus femoris; 13, obturator internus with the gemelli above and below; 14, sacrospinous ligament; 15, piriformis; 16, sacrotuberous ligament; 17, gluteus medius

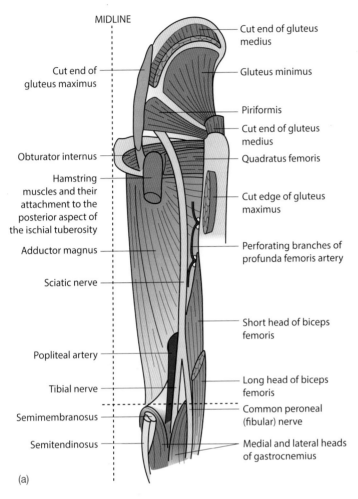

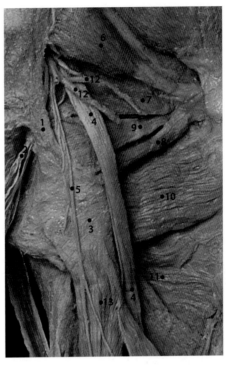

(b)

Figure 15.24 (a) Deep muscles of the posterior aspect of the right thigh (horizontal dashed line shows level of the cross-section in Fig. 15.25 below). (b) Dissection of posterior thigh and gluteal region with gluteus maximus muscle removed: 1, sacrotuberous ligament; 2, pudendal nerve in ischioanal fossa; 3, ischial tuberosity; 4, sciatic nerve; 5, posterior cutaneous nerve of the thigh; 6, piriformis; 7, superior gemellus; 8, inferior gemellus, 9, obturator internus muscle and tendon; 10, quadratus femoris; 11, adductor magnus; 12, inferior gluteal artery; 13, hamstrings

THE BACK OF THE THIGH

This contains the three hamstring muscles, semimembranosus, semitendinosus and biceps femoris (Table 15.2 and Fig. 15.23), and the sciatic nerve that supplies them. There are no large vessels in the back of the thigh – its contents are supplied by a deeply placed anastomotic chain fed by the gluteal and circumflex femoral arteries above, by the perforating branches of the profunda femoris artery (p. 259), and below by the popliteal artery.

The sciatic nerve

The sciatic nerve, the largest nerve in the body, originates from the lumbosacral plexus on the anterior surface of piriformis (Fig. 15.24). It descends through the greater sciatic foramen into the gluteal region, and thence through the posterior compartment of the thigh to end just above the popliteal fossa, by dividing into the tibial and common peroneal (fibular) nerves.

TABLE 15.2 Muscles of the back of the thigh

Muscle	Proximal attachment	Distal attachment	Nerve supply	Actions
Semitendinosus	Ischial tuberosity	Medial surface of upper tibia	Sciatic nerve (L5, S1)	Extends hip; strong flexor of knee. Also imparts slight medial rotation to knee
Semimembranosus	Ischial tuberosity	Posteromedial part of tibial condyle	Sciatic nerve (L5, S1)	Extends hip; strong flexor of knee. Also imparts slight medial rotation to knee
Biceps femoris	Long head: ischial tuberosity. Short head: linea aspera and lateral supracondylar line of femur	The two heads join to form a tendon attached to the head of the fibula	Sciatic nerve (S1)	Extends hip; strong flexor of knee. Also imparts lateral rotation to knee

Relations

It enters the gluteal region below piriformis, lying on the ischium and obturator internus and covered by gluteus maximus. In the thigh it is covered by the hamstring muscles and descends on the posterior surface of adductor magnus.

Branches

Muscular – to the hamstrings and the ischial part of adductor magnus; *articular* – to the hip and knee joints, and its terminal branches the **tibial and common peroneal (fibular) nerves** (Figs. 15.24 and 15.25).

THE FRONT AND MEDIAL SIDE OF THE THIGH

Sartorius separates the medially placed adductor muscles (Table 15.3) from the anterior muscles, the quadriceps (Fig. 15.28). Pectineus (Fig. 15.28b) and adductor longus lie anterior to adductor brevis, which is, in turn, anterior to the deeply placed adductor magnus. Gracilis lies medial to the other adductors (Fig. 15.28b). (Psoas and iliacus are described on pp. 127 and 140.) The femoral vessels (Fig. 15.29) pass deeply towards the femur in the adductor hiatus, leaving the anterior compartment by passing through the adductor hiatus into the popliteal fossa. The femoral nerve has a short course in the thigh before dividing into its several branches, just inferior to the inguinal ligament.

The **femoral triangle** is situated on the front of the upper thigh bounded by the inguinal ligament superiorly, the adductor longus medially and sartorius laterally (Fig. 15.28b). It is floored by adductor longus, pectineus and iliopsoas, and its roof is the fascia lata of the thigh. The roof contains an oval **saphenous opening** about 4 cm below and 1 cm lateral to the pubic tubercle, which conveys the great saphenous vein. In the triangle are the femoral vessels within the femoral sheath, with the femoral nerve and its branches laterally and outside

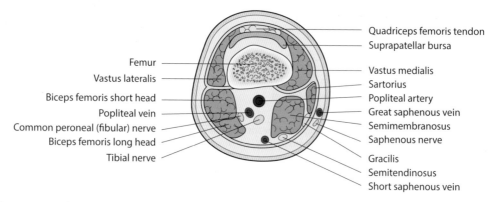

Figure 15.25 Transverse section through the right thigh at the level of the suprapatellar bursa, viewed from below (see the dotted line in Fig. 15.24)

Sciatica – pain in the leg extending down from the buttock towards the heel – is caused by pressure on the sciatic nerve or its nerve roots, commonly by intervertebral disc protrusion at the L4/L5 or L5/S1 level. The diagnosis is confirmed by noting that straight leg raising is diminished by the pain of the sciatica (Fig. 15.26), that the ankle reflex is absent and that there is sensory loss over the lateral side of the leg.

'Pulled hamstrings' are very common in athletes who sprint or run explosively, e.g. footballers and squash players. The severe muscular contraction required in this sudden exertion results in tears of the attachment to the ischial tuberosity, causing intramuscular bleeding and pain.

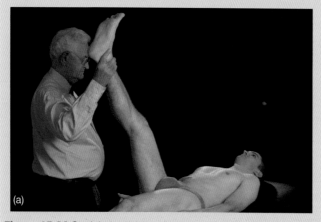
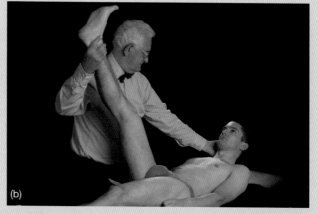

Figure 15.26 Straight leg raising. (a) The straightened leg is flexed at the hip. (b) The sciatic nerve is further stretched by extension of the ankle and neck flexion

the sheath. The **femoral sheath** (Fig. 15.27a) is a tube-like prolongation of transversalis fascia into the thigh, invaginated by the femoral vessels as they leave the abdomen. The sheath fuses with the vessels about 3 cm below the inguinal ligament; septa divide it into three compartments containing the femoral artery laterally and the femoral vein centrally and medially, the space known as the **femoral canal**, which contains fatty tissue and lymph nodes. The femoral canal communicates superiorly with the extraperitoneal tissue via a firm non-distensible **femoral ring**, which is bounded anteriorly by the inguinal ligament, medially by the pectineal part of the inguinal ligament, posteriorly by the thin pectineus muscle and pectineal ligament overlying the pubis, and laterally by the femoral vein.

The boundaries of the femoral ring are of considerable clinical importance, because when herniation of abdominal contents into the femoral canal occurs, the ring often provides a site of constriction for the contents of the hernial sac. Femoral hernias are rather more common in women because of their wider pelvis and larger femoral ring. They can be distinguished from inguinal hernias by their situation: they present below the inguinal ligament as a palpable, sometimes visible lump in the region of the saphenous opening, below and lateral to the pubic tubercle. They become subcutaneous by passing through the saphenous opening.

ANTERIOR GROUP OF THIGH MUSCLES

Sartorius is a long strap-like muscle that passes obliquely and medially down the thigh. Quadriceps is a large muscle mass forming the bulk of the anterior region of the thigh. The mass is divided into four separate muscles, each of which gains attachment to the patella (Table 15.4). The four parts of quadriceps are attached to the upper border and side margins in a single musculotendinous expansion. From the apex of the patella the strong **patellar ligament** (ligamentum patellae) descends to become attached to the tibial tubercle. On each side of the patellar tendon the capsule of the joint is strengthened by fibrous expansions (retinacula) of the quadriceps.

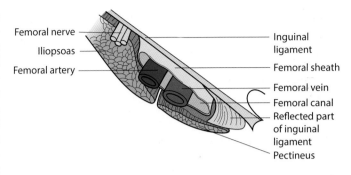

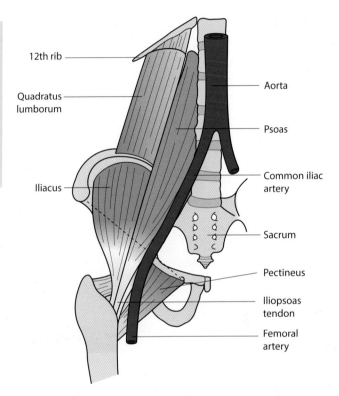

Figure 15.27 (a) Femoral sheath. (b) Deep thigh muscles showing the path of the femoral artery into the thigh. The dashed line marks the course of the inguinal ligament

TABLE 15.3 The adductor muscles

Muscle	Proximal attachment	Distal attachment	Nerve supply	Actions
Pectineus	Superior aspect of pubis	Posterior femur below lesser trochanter	Femoral nerve as well as obturator (L2, L3, L4)	Weak adductor and flexor of the hip
Adductor longus	Anterior body of pubis	Linea aspera of femur	Obturator nerve (L2, L3, L4)	Adductor of hip, medial rotation of femur
Adductor brevis	Body and inferior ramus of pubis	Upper half of linea aspera	Obturator nerve	Adductor of hip, medial rotation of femur
Adductor magnus	Wide attachment to outer surface of ischiopubic ramus and ischial tuberosity	Gluteal tuberosity, whole length of linea aspera, medial supracondylar line and, by a tendon, into adductor tubercle of femur	Obturator nerve	Strong adductor, medial rotation of femur; plus extension of hip
Gracilis	Lower border of ischiopubic ramus	Upper part of medial surface of tibia	Obturator nerve	Weak adductor of hip

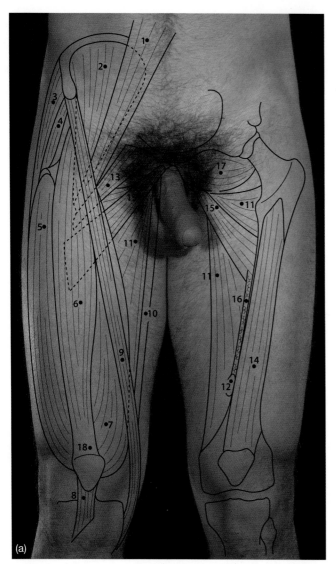

(a)

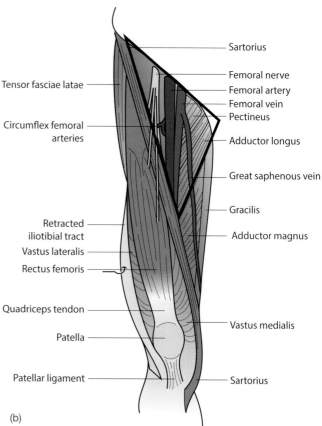

(b)

Figure 15.28 (a) Anterior aspect of the thigh, showing the superficial and deep muscles and femoral triangle: 1, psoas; 2, iliacus; 3, tensor fasciae latae; 4, gluteus medius; 5, vastus lateralis; 6, rectus femoris; 7, vastus medialis; 8, patellar ligament; 9, sartorius; 10, gracilis; 11, adductor magnus; 12, adductor hiatus; 13, pectineus; 14, vastus intermedialis; 15, adductor brevis; 16, adductor longus (central part of muscle excised on the left side); 17, obturator externus; 18, quadriceps tendon. (b) Anterior aspect of the thigh and femoral triangle (outlined)

In figure (b), the labels are:
Sartorius; Femoral nerve; Femoral artery; Femoral vein; Pectineus; Adductor longus; Great saphenous vein; Gracilis; Adductor magnus; Vastus medialis; Sartorius; Tensor fasciae latae; Circumflex femoral arteries; Retracted iliotibial tract; Vastus lateralis; Rectus femoris; Quadriceps tendon; Patella; Patellar ligament

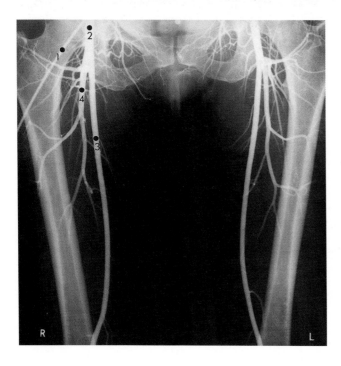

Figure 15.29 Femoral angiogram: 1, catheter; 2, femoral artery in groin; 3, femoral artery in adductor canal; 4, profunda femoris artery

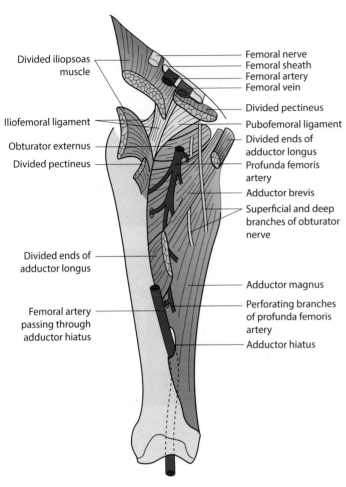

Divided iliopsoas muscle

Femoral nerve
Femoral sheath
Femoral artery
Femoral vein

Divided pectineus

Iliofemoral ligament

Pubofemoral ligament

Obturator externus

Divided ends of adductor longus

Divided pectineus

Profunda femoris artery

Adductor brevis

Superficial and deep branches of obturator nerve

Divided ends of adductor longus

Adductor magnus

Perforating branches of profunda femoris artery

Femoral artery passing through adductor hiatus

Adductor hiatus

Figure 15.30 Deep aspect of the medial thigh and relations of the profunda femoris artery

BLOOD SUPPLY

The femoral artery

The femoral artery (Figs. 15.27b, 15.30 and 15.31) is the continuation of the external iliac artery below the inguinal ligament. It descends vertically through the femoral triangle (Fig. 15.28b) and adductor canal to leave the latter by an opening in the adductor magnus (adductor hiatus) on the medial side of the lower femur.

Relations

At its origin it is deep to the inguinal ligament, halfway between the anterior superior iliac spine and the symphysis pubis (mid-inguinal point). It is palpable in the femoral triangle, being covered only by deep fascia and skin; the femoral vein lies medial to it. It leaves the triangle at its apex on adductor longus and enters the **adductor canal** with its vein and the saphenous nerve (p. 261); within the canal it is deep to sartorius. Three to four centimetres above the adductor tubercle of the femur the artery passes through the opening in the tendon of adductor magnus (adductor hiatus) to enter the popliteal fossa as the popliteal artery.

Branches

Just as the artery enters the femoral triangle it gives off three small branches to the skin of the lower abdominal wall and the inguinal region. The **profunda femoris artery** (Fig. 15.30) is the largest of its branches; it arises in the femoral triangle and descends close to the femur between the adduc-

TABLE 15.4 Anterior thigh muscles				
Muscle	**Proximal attachment**	**Distal attachment**	**Nerve supply**	**Actions**
Sartorius	Anterior superior iliac spine	Upper part of medial surface of tibia	Femoral nerve (L2, L3, L4)	Weak flexor abductor and lateral rotator of hip and knee flexor
Quadriceps a) Rectus femoris	By two heads: a) anterior inferior iliac spine; b) ilium, just above acetabulum	By a single tendon into upper border of patella	Femoral nerve	Powerful extensor of knee; flexor of hip
b) Vastus medialis	By a wide aponeurosis to lesser trochanter, linea aspera and medial supracondylar line of femur	To medial side of patella; some of its lower fibres are horizontal	Femoral nerve	Powerful extensor of knee. Prevention of lateral dislocation of patella by its horizontal fibres
c) Vastus lateralis	Greater trochanter and linea aspera	Lateral side of patella	Femoral nerve	Powerful extensor of knee
d) Vastus intermedius	Anterior and lateral surfaces of shaft of femur	Upper border of patella	Femoral nerve	Powerful extensor of the knee

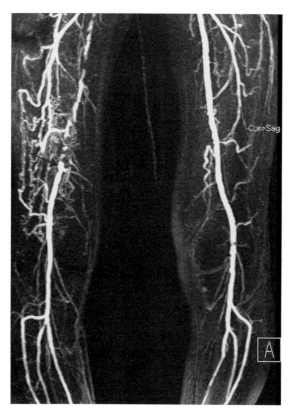

Figure 15.31 MR angiogram showing right femoral artery atherosclerosis, occlusion and narrowing, especially marked at the adductor hiatus (arrow)

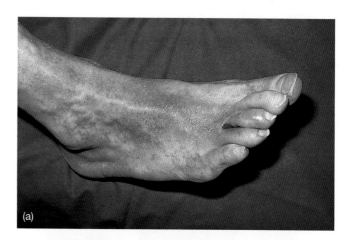

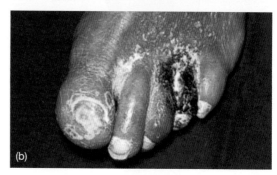

Figure 15.32 Ischaemic changes of the feet due to peripheral vascular disease blocking distal arteries: (a) ischaemic ulcer between third and fourth toes; (b) gangrenous fourth toe

tor muscles, giving off three or four perforating branches that pierce adductor magnus and supply the posterior part of the thigh, and contribute to anastomoses with branches of the popliteal artery. The **medial and lateral circumflex femoral arteries** encircle the upper femur and supply muscles and the hip joint, and contribute to the anastomoses around the femur and hip joint.

The femoral artery is very accessible in the femoral triangle; its pulsation is readily found below the mid-inguinal point, and first-aiders are taught to use it as a pressure point for the control of haemorrhage from the leg. Radiologists frequently use it for arterial catheterization, and clinicians for sampling arterial blood.

The femoral artery is one of the most common sites of peripheral arterial disease, the artery becoming blocked beyond the origin of profunda femoris down to the adductor hiatus (Fig. 15.31). The decrease in blood supply affects particularly the muscles of the calf, and exercise pain (intermittent claudication) may result. In more severe cases it results in ischaemic ulceration of the skin (Fig. 15.32).

The numerous branches of the femoral artery, but especially the medial circumflex femoral, with a contribution from the gluteal arteries, make a rich anastomosis around the hip joint, most branches of which pass to the head of femur via the retinacular fibres of the neck. A small branch of the obturator artery passes into the head of femur, and is considered more important in children.

The femoral vein

The femoral vein begins at the opening in the lower end of adductor magnus as the continuation of the popliteal vein. It ascends with the femoral artery to end under the inguinal ligament, as the external iliac vein. At first it lies behind the artery, but ends on its medial side.

The femoral vein is easily accessible on the medial side of the femoral artery. It is frequently used for venous access in shocked patients with a low blood pressure and collapsed veins.

Tributaries

The **profunda femoris vein** and **medial and lateral femoral circumflex veins** have a similar course to their arteries. The **great saphenous vein**, which drains the skin and subcutaneous tissues of much of the leg and thigh (p. 131), pierces the deep fascia over the saphenous opening in the roof of the femoral triangle to enter the femoral vein.

NERVES

The **femoral nerve** (Fig. 15.28b) is a branch of the upper part (L2, L3, L4) of the lumbosacral plexus (p. 129). It descends in the pelvis between iliacus and psoas, entering the thigh under the inguinal ligament lateral to the femoral artery and outside the femoral sheath. In the femoral triangle it immediately divides into terminal branches:

- **Cutaneous nerves** – supply skin on the medial and anterior aspect of the thigh.
- **Saphenous nerve** – the longest branch of the femoral nerve (L4) accompanies the femoral artery until the adductor hiatus, at which point it emerges from the adductor canal medial to sartorius to descend on the medial side of the knee. In the leg it entwines around the great saphenous vein to pass anterior to the medial malleolus. It supplies the skin over the medial side of the leg and foot.

It is often damaged when varicose veins are stripped, causing diminished and altered sensation over the medial ankle region.

- **Muscular branches** – to pectineus, sartorius and quadriceps.

The **obturator nerve** is a branch of the lumbosacral plexus (L2, L3, L4), whose pelvic course is described on p. 129. It enters the thigh through the obturator foramen, where it divides into anterior and posterior branches to supply all the adductors and pectineus, except the lateral half of adductor magnus (supplied by the sciatic nerve). Its cutaneous branches supply the skin over the medial thigh above the knee.

MCQs

1. The femoral nerve supplies: **T/F**
  a gluteus minimus muscle   (___)
  b rectus femoris   (___)
  c the skin over the lateral malleolus   (___)
  d iliacus muscle   (___)
  e pectineus muscle   (___)

Answers
1.
a **F** – *Gluteus minimus is supplied by the superior gluteal nerve.*
b **T**
c **F** – *The femoral nerve supplies the skin over the lower medial part of the leg and medial malleolus via its saphenous branch (L4).*
d **T**
e **T**

2. The hip joint: **T/F**
  a is supplied by the nerve to rectus femoris   (___)
  b is supplied by the obturator nerve   (___)
  c is supplied by the nerve to quadratus femoris   (___)
  d has a posterior capsule attached to the greater trochanter   (___)
  e is supported most strongly by the ischio-femoral ligament   (___)

Answers
2.
a **T** – *Hilton's law states that a joint receives its nerve supply from the same nerves that innervate ...*
b **T** – *... muscles acting across that joint. Hence the hip joint is innervated by the femoral, obturator, ...*
c **T** – *... the sciatic, and the nerve to quadratus femoris.*
d **F** – *The capsule of the hip joint is attached anteriorly to the trochanters and the intertrochanteric line between, but posteriorly it is attached halfway along the femoral neck.*
e **F** – *The ischiofemoral ligament is not as strong as the inverted Y-shaped iliofemoral ligament, which passes from the anterior inferior iliac spine to each end of the intertrochanteric line.*

3. In the mid-thigh region the: **T/F**
  a floor of the adductor canal is adductor magnus   (___)
  b roof of the adductor canal laterally is the vastus medialis   (___)
  c femoral artery lies medial to its vein   (___)
  d iliotibial tract lies along the medial aspect   (___)
  e gracilis muscle is often supplied by the femoral nerve   (___)

Answers
3.
a **F** – *The adductor canal (or subsartorial canal) is found medially in the middle third of the thigh. It commences at the apex of the femoral triangle and lies on adductor longus; it finishes below at the hiatus in the adductor magnus.*
b **T** – *Sartorius forms the medial roof.*
c **T** – *The contents of this canal are the femoral artery and vein, with the terminal cutaneous branch of the femoral nerve, the saphenous nerve and, occasionally, the nerve to vastus medialis and a sensory branch of the obturator nerve. The nerves lie anterior, the artery medial and the vein laterally.*
d **F** – *This notable thickening of the fascia lata lies along the lateral thigh from its proximal attachment to the tensor fasciae latae muscle to its distal attachment to the lateral condyle of the tibia.*
e **F** – *Gracilis is a member of the adductor group of muscles and innervated by the obturator nerve. It is also a weak flexor of the knee joint.*

SBA

1. A 30-year-old man is admitted with closed mid-shaft fractures of the tibia and fibula. The fracture is reduced and placed in a plaster cast. Three days later he complains of severe pain throughout the leg in the cast and, after removal of the cast, it is found that his foot is cold and swollen. No pulses can be felt. What is the likely cause of this?

a venous thrombosis
b arterial occlusion
c compartment syndrome
d injury to the posterior tibial nerve
e Raynaud's disease

Answer

c *The fascial compartments of the leg are rigid inelastic envelopes for the soft tissues contained within them. The muscle trauma and bleeding caused by a fracture may cause tissue swelling within a fascial compartment severe enough to compromise the arterial supply. Urgent surgical relief is required and lengthy incisions along the length of the lower leg (fasciotomy) are required to reduce the tissue pressure in that compartment.*

2. A confused, violent patient requires an urgent intra-muscular injection of a sedative. The nurse gives the injection into the upper lateral quadrant of the buttock. She chose this site in order to prevent damage to which nerve?

a sciatic nerve
b lateral femoral cutaneous nerve
c superior gluteal nerve
d obturator nerve
e inferior gluteal nerve

Answer

a *The sciatic nerve runs deeply through the lower medial quadrant and is sometimes injured by injections placed outside of the upper lateral quadrant.*

EMQs

Each question has an anatomical theme linked to the chapter, and a list of 10 related items (A–J) placed in alphabetical order: these are followed by five statements (1–5). Match **one or more** of the items A–J to each of the five statements.

Muscles of the hip and thigh
A. Adductor longus
B. Adductor magnus
C. Biceps femoris
D. Gluteus maximus
E. Obturator externus
F. Pectineus
G. Piriformis
H. Semitendinosus
I. Tensor fasciae latae
J. Vastus lateralis

Match the following statement to the muscle(s) in the above list.
1. Transmits the femoral artery
2. Forms the floor of the femoral triangle
3. Attached to the head of the fibula
4. Attached to the anteromedial upper tibia
5. Attached to the iliotibial tract

Answers
1 B; 2 AF; 3 C; 4 H; 5 DI

Nerves of the hip and thigh
A. Adductor longus
B. Adductor magnus
C. Biceps femoris
D. Gluteus maximus
E. Obturator externus
F. Pectineus
G. Piriformis
H. Semitendinosus
I. Tensor fasciae latae
J. Vastus lateralis

Match the following nerves to the muscle(s) in the above list.
1. Sciatic
2. Femoral
3. Lumbar plexus
4. Obturator
5. Superior gluteal

Answers
1 CH; 2 FJ; 3 ABEFJ; 4 ABEF; 5 I

APPLIED QUESTIONS

1. A butcher's knife slips and plunges into his thigh at the apex of the femoral triangle. Why is this likely to be particularly bloody?

1. Not only are the femoral artery and vein endangered as they pass down the front of the thigh towards the subsartorial canal, but so too are their branches and tributaries. Midway down the thigh a knife piercing sartorius and the femoral vessels also lacerates adductor longus, a fairly thin muscle, and may damage the profunda femoris vessels on its deep surface. The injury is therefore very bloody owing to damage to two large arteries and their accompanying veins.

2. An infected cut on the heel causes tenderness in which lymph nodes?

2. Lymph from the superficial tissues of the heel runs in the lymphatics that follow one or other of the saphenous veins. Those following the great saphenous vein eventually drain to the vertically disposed groups of superficial inguinal nodes around the termination of the vein, in the groin. The lymph vessels following the small saphenous vein pierce the deep fascia in the popliteal fossa and enter the popliteal nodes. From here lymph passes to the deep inguinal nodes around the femoral vein in the femoral triangle.

Chapter **16**

The knee, leg and dorsum of the foot

OSTEOLOGY

The **patella** (Fig. 16.1) is a sesamoid bone, triangular in shape with its apex inferior. Its anterior surface is subcutaneous; the posterior is smooth, with a smaller medial and a larger lateral facet for articulation with the femoral condyles. The quadriceps tendon is attached to the upper border and the patellar tendon or ligament to the apex; muscle fibres from vastus medialis are attached to its medial border and tendinous expansions from the vastus medialis and lateralis (retinacula) are attached to the medial and lateral borders and also to the neighbouring tibial condyles. In the standing position the lower border of the patella lies slightly proximal to the level of the knee joint.

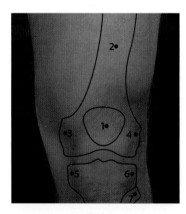

Figure 16.1 Surface anatomy of the bones of the knee: 1, patella; 2, femur; 3, medial femoral condyle; 4, lateral femoral condyle; 5, medial tibial condyle; 6, lateral tibial condyle; 7, head of fibula

The **tibia** (Fig. 16.2) is a long bone possessing an upper end, a shaft and a lower end. The **upper end** is expanded by the medial and lateral condyles and flattened superiorly, forming the **tibial plateau** with oval medial and lateral facets articulating with the femoral condyles. Between the articular facets is a rough intercondylar area that gives attachment to the two menisci and the anterior and posterior cruciate ligaments. The prominent anterior **tibial tuberosity** below the superior surface provides attachment for the patellar tendon; semimembranosus is attached along the side of the medial condyle. Beneath the lateral condyle is the articular facet for the head of the fibula.

The **shaft** is triangular in section, with medial, lateral and posterior surfaces. The upper part of the medial surface gives attachment to the tibial collateral ligament of the knee joint and to sartorius, gracilis and semitendinosus (see **Figs. 16.23b,c**); more distally the medial surface and sharp anterior border lie subcutaneously. To the lateral surface is attached tibialis anterior. The posterior surface is crossed by an oblique ridge, the **soleal line**, which gives attachment to soleus; attached to the surface above the line is popliteus, and to the area below the line tibialis posterior and flexor digitorum longus. The interosseous membrane is attached to a sharp ridge on the lateral border. The expanded lower end has a medial projection, the **medial malleolus**; its distal surface, together with the lateral surface of the malleolus, articulates with the talus. The posterior border of the lower end is grooved medially by the tendon of tibialis posterior. To the roughened lateral surface is attached the interosseous ligament of the inferior tibiofibular joint. The tibial condyles, its anterior border, the medial surface and the medial malleolus are palpable (Fig. 16.2a).

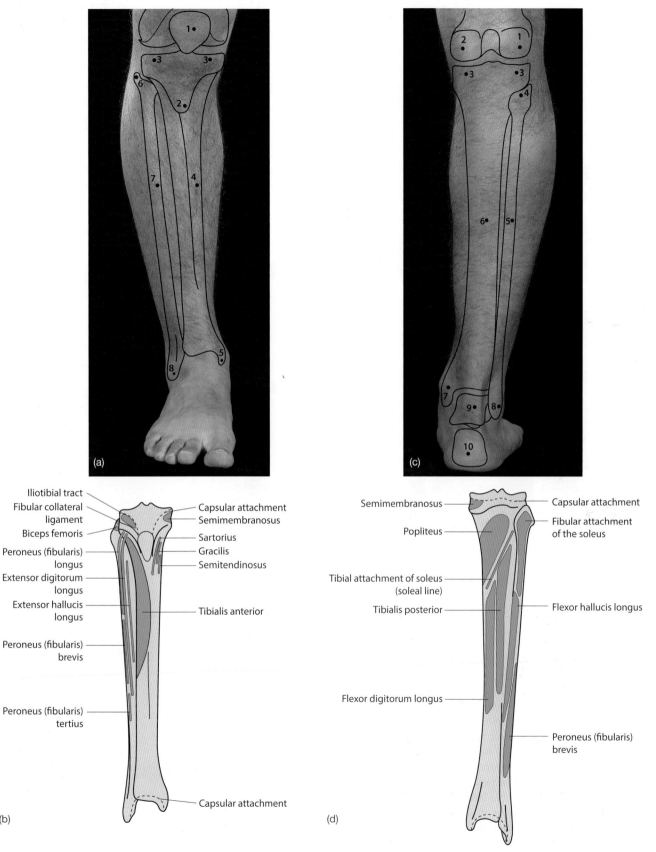

Figure 16.2 (a) Surface anatomy of bones of the leg, anterior aspect: 1, patella; 2, tibial tuberosity; 3, tibial plateau; 4, anterior subcutaneous surface of tibia; 5, medial malleolus; 6, head of fibula; 7, shaft of fibula; 8, lateral malleolus. (b) Anterior aspect of the tibia and fibula: muscle and capsular attachments. (c) Surface anatomy of the bones of the leg, posterior aspect: 1, lateral femoral condyle; 2, medial femoral condyle; 3, tibial plateau; 4, head of fibula; 5, shaft of fibula; 6, shaft of tibia; 7, medial malleolus; 8, lateral malleolus; 9, talus; 10, calcaneus. (d) Posterior aspect of the tibia and fibula: muscle and capsular attachments

Because of the bone's subcutaneous position, tibial shaft fractures due to direct trauma are frequently associated with skin wounds (compound fractures) (Figs. 16.3a,d) and are therefore prone to infection and poor union.

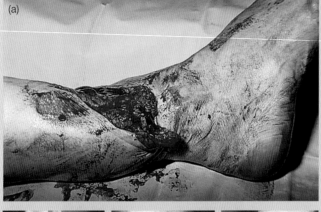

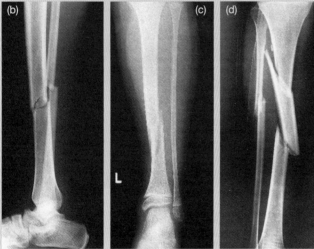

Figure 16.3 (a) Fractured shaft of the tibia with a compound wound. (b) Transverse fracture. (c) Spiral fracture. (d) Comminuted fracture of the tibia

The **fibula** (Figs. 16.2a,b) is a long bone with a head, a shaft and a lower end. It carries no weight but gives attachment to many muscles. The expanded **head** has an oval articular facet for the tibia; to its apex is attached the fibular collateral ligament of the knee joint and biceps tendon. The common peroneal nerve lying within peroneus longus is in close proximity to the neck of the fibula just below the head of the bone and can be palpated here. It is liable to damage by tight bandaging or a tight plaster cast. The **shaft** is long and slender; attached to its narrow anterior surface are the extensor muscles, to the posterior surface the flexor muscles and to the lateral surface the peroneal muscles. The expanded **lower end** forms the palpable **lateral malleolus** (Fig. 16.2a), which lies about 1 cm lower than the medial malleolus. Its medial side has an articular surface for the talus. Above the articular facet is the roughened area for the interosseous ligament of the inferior tibiofibular joint, and below it the bone gives attachment to the posterior talofibular ligament. The interosseous membrane is attached to its medial border. Both the head and the lateral malleolus are palpable.

A severe inversion of the ankle may result in ligamentous injury and talar pressure on the lateral malleolus severe enough to fracture the lower end of the fibula.

THE KNEE JOINT

The **knee joint** (Figs. 16.4a,b) is a synovial joint of a modified hinge variety between the lower end of the femur, the patella and the tibial plateau. The articular surface on the femur is formed of three continuous surfaces: a middle concave surface for the patella, and markedly convex medial and lateral condylar surfaces for articulation with the tibia. The posterior surface of the patella has a medial and a larger lateral facet for articulation with the femoral concavity. The upper surface of each tibial condyle is oval and slightly concave.

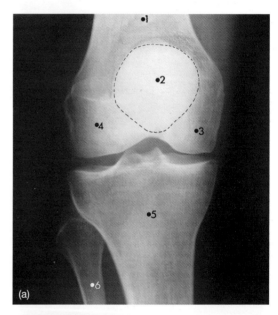

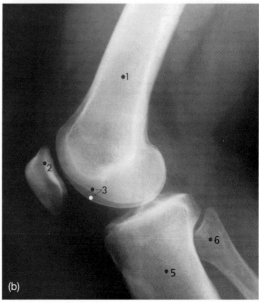

Figure 16.4 X-rays of the knee. (a) Anteroposterior view. (b) Lateral view. 1, femur; 2, patella; 3, femoral condyles; 4, lateral femoral condyle; 5, tibia; 6, fibula

Ligaments

Capsule

This is attached on the femur close to the articular margins medially and laterally, and above the intercondylar notch (Figs. 16.5 and 15.11b, p. 248). It is attached to the margins of the patella and to the periphery of the tibial plateau, except for anteriorly, where it descends below the tibial tuberosity, and posterolaterally where it is pierced by the tendon of popliteus.

Capsular thickenings

Coronary ligaments tether the margins of the medial and lateral menisci to the nearby margin of the tibial plateau.

Accessory ligaments

- **Patellar tendon**– from the apex of the patella to the tibial tuberosity.

> The knee jerk reflex is demonstrated by hitting the midpoint of this tendon with a tendon hammer, often with the knee hanging flexed over the bed or with the knees crossed. This should elicit contraction of the quadriceps muscle, which extends the knee and tests the integrity of the L3 and L4 nerve roots.

- **Patellar retinacula** – tendinous expansions of the vasti muscles passing to the patellar margins and to the tibial condyles.
- **Tibial collateral ligament** – a broad flat ligament passing from the medial epicondyle of the femur to the medial surface of the upper tibia. It is part of the capsule.
- **Fibular collateral ligament** – a round cord passing from the lateral epicondyle of the femur to the head of the fibula. It is separate from the capsule.
- **Anterior and posterior cruciate ligaments** – strong, intracapsular ligaments; the anterior passes upwards and backwards from the front of the tibial intercondylar area to the medial surface of the lateral femoral condyle (Fig. 16.5e); the posterior passes forwards and upwards from the back of the intercondylar area to the lateral surface of the medial condyle of the femur (Fig. 16.5a–e and 16.6). Forward displacement of the tibia on the femur is prevented by the anterior cruciate, posterior displacement by the posterior cruciate.

Intracapsular structures

The **synovial membrane** shows signs of the knee joint's development from three separate joint cavities; the patellofemoral joint communicates with each 'tibiofemoral

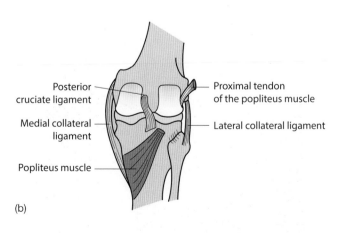

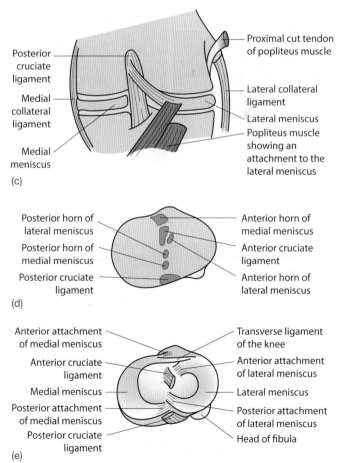

Figure 16.5 (a) Anterior aspect of the knee joint with the quadriceps muscle divided and the patellar ligament turned inferiorly. (b) and (c) Posterior aspect of the right knee joint. (d) and (e) Upper end of the right tibia showing ligamentous and meniscal attachments to the intercondylar region of the tibial plateau; superior view of the tibial plateau showing attachments of the cruciate ligaments and menisci

joint', but a remnant of the patellofemoral joint's membrane persists as the **infrapatellar fold**, connecting the lower border of the patella to the intercondylar notch. Both cruciate ligaments lie outside the synovial cavity in the fibrous septum between the tibiofemoral joints, but a communication between the joints exists in front of the ligaments. The synovial membrane is attached proximally to the articular margins of the femur, and distally to the margins of the tibial articular facets and the front of the intercondylar area. The synovium above the patella extends between quadriceps and the femur as the suprapatellar bursa (**Fig. 16.7**). The joint cavity communicates with this bursa and the popliteal and gastrocnemius bursae.

Rupture of the synovia of the knee joint as a consequence of osteoarthritis, or synovial herniation, results in a cystic swelling in the popliteal fossa (Baker's cyst). The lump is fluctuant but not tender, but if the cyst leaks, fluid may track down the calf, which becomes swollen and tender, mimicking a calf vein thrombosis.

The **menisci** are two crescentic pieces of fibrocartilage with thickened outer margins. Each lies on a tibial condyle attached by its ends, the anterior and posterior horns, to the intercondylar area (**Fig. 16.5e**) and by its outer margin to the capsule. The medial cartilage is larger and semicircular and

its central attachments embrace those of the lateral cartilage, which is smaller and forms three-fifths of a circle. The tendon of popliteus is attached to the posterior margin of the lateral meniscus.

The stability of the joint depends entirely on its ligaments and neighbouring muscles but, because it is a mobile weight-bearing joint, injuries are common, especially in sports involving running and physical contact such as soccer or rugby. Most injuries occur when a side force to the knee is applied while the leg is weight-bearing, i.e. when the foot is fixed to the ground. A blow to the lateral side may result in tearing of the medial tibial collateral ligament and, through the ligament's attachment to the medial meniscus, tearing of the medial meniscus (**Figs. 16.5c** and **16.8**). The knee is particularly prone to this injury when flexed, as it is then that the collateral ligaments are slack and making little contribution to the stability of the knee. Rupture of the cruciate ligaments is the result of severe anterior or posterior force being applied to the knee.

Tears of the anterior cruciate ligament are seen most frequently in young sportsmen; they are usually the consequence of violent abduction and twisting of the knee, such as may occur in a sliding football tackle. The diagnosis can be supported by a positive 'drawer' sign, i.e. the demonstration of excessive anterior movement of the tibia on the femur. The drawer test indicates the integrity or otherwise of the cruciate ligaments (**Fig. 16.9**).

The medial meniscus is the more liable to injury because it is fixed to the tibial collateral ligament. Presenting symptoms are pain and swelling of the knee, or locking of the knee owing to the partially detached cartilage becoming wedged between the tibial and femoral condyles. Tearing of the menisci is usually caused by forceful rotation of a flexed knee. In these circumstances external rotation causes the medial meniscus to be torn by being ground between the medial

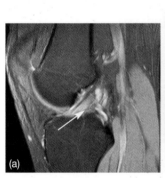
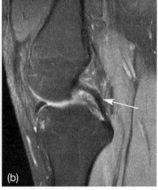

Figure 16.6 MR images of the knee. Sagittal views showing: (a) the anterior cruciate ligament (arrow); and (b) the posterior cruciate ligament (arrow)

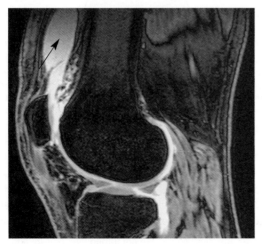

Figure 16.7 MR arthrogram of the knee (the suprapatellar bursa is arrowed)

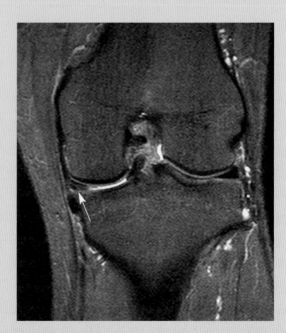

Figure 16.8 Coronal MR image of the knee showing a torn medial meniscus (arrow)

condyles of the femur and tibia. Internal rotation may tear the lateral meniscus. Displaced fragments of the meniscus lodged between the condyles prevent full extension of the knee.

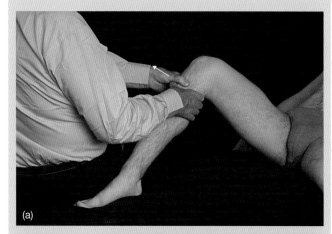

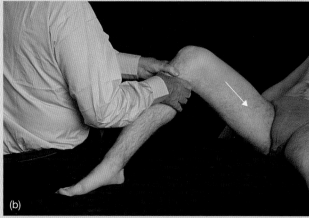

Figure 16.9 Drawer sign – testing laxity of the anterior and posterior cruciate ligaments. The lower leg is gripped around the upper tibia, with the knee flexed, and the tibia pushed backwards and pulled forwards (arrows). There should be no movement in these planes

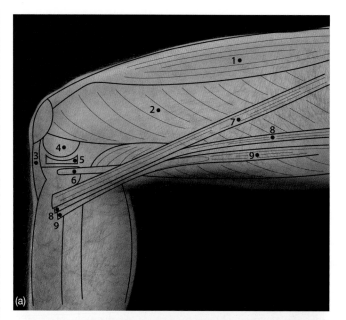

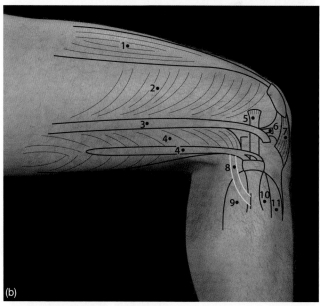

Figure 16.10 Muscles in the flexed knee. (a) Medial view: 1, rectus femoris; 2, vastus medialis; 3, patellar ligament; 4, medial condyle of femur; 5, medial meniscus; 6, tendon and muscle belly of semimembranosus; 7, sartorius; 8, gracilis muscle and tendon attachment; 9, semitendinosus muscle and tendon attachment. (b) Lateral view: 1, rectus femoris; 2, vastus lateralis; 3, iliotibial tract; 4, biceps femoris; 5, lateral collateral ligament of the knee; 6, lateral meniscus; 7, patellar ligament; 8, common peroneal (fibular) nerve; 9, peroneus (fibularis) longus; 10, extensor digitorum; 11, tibialis anterior

Functional aspects

Movements

The joint is capable of flexion, extension and a little rotation:

- **Flexion** – by hamstrings assisted by gastrocnemius.
- **Extension** – by quadriceps and the iliotibial tract (Figs. 16.10a,b). During movement the femoral condyles roll on the tibial condyles and also glide backwards. When the leg is almost straight the capsular and cruciate ligaments become taut and stop further backward gliding of the lateral femoral condyle. Further extension is only possible by backward movement of the medial condyle around the axis of the taut anterior cruciate ligament (medial rotation of the femur on the tibia). Rotation and extension are limited by the collateral ligaments of the knee. When fully extended the knee is in a 'locked' (i.e. stable) position, with almost no muscular contraction involved. At the start of flexion the femur rotates laterally on the tibia,

and the popliteus muscle pulls the lateral meniscus backwards, thereby preventing it being crushed between the lateral femoral and tibial condyles. This is the 'unlocking' movement of popliteus.

- **Rotation** – a small amount of rotation may be produced by the hamstrings when the knee is flexed.

Stability

The bony surfaces contribute little to the joint's stability, which is largely dependent on strong ligaments and powerful muscles. Its collateral ligaments are inextensible; the cruciate ligaments limit gliding and distraction of the bones; quadriceps anteriorly and gastrocnemius and hamstrings posteriorly stabilize the joint.

Quadriceps tends to pull the patella laterally because of the obliquity of the femur, but the displacement is limited by the projection of the lateral condyle of the femur and by the resistance provided by the horizontally attached fibres of vastus medialis into the medial border of the patella. When standing on the extended knee the centre of gravity passes in front of the axis around which the femoral condyles roll; the posterior cruciate ligaments thus take the strain.

Blood supply

There is an extensive anastomosis around the knee, contributed to by the popliteal, femoral and anterior tibial arteries (see Figs. 16.25a,b).

Nerve supply

This is by branches of the tibial, common peroneal (fibular), obturator and femoral nerves.

Relations

The joint is mainly subcutaneous, being separated from the skin by quadriceps, the patella and patellar ligament anteriorly, the biceps tendon laterally and semimembranosus and semitendinosus medially. To its posterior lie the popliteal vessels and, more superficially, the tibial and common peroneal (fibular) nerves in the popliteal fossa.

Dislocation of the patella usually occurs to the lateral side of the knee (Fig. 16.11a). It is often due to a flat lateral femoral condyle or weakness in the lower fibres of vastus medialis. Direct injury to the patella may cause it to fracture into several fragments, a stellate fracture (Fig. 16.11b). A transverse fracture into two fragments is more commonly the consequence of sudden acute contraction of quadriceps while attempting to correct a slip (Fig. 16.11c). In young adolescents the tibial tuberosity may become painful and reveal irregular ossification of the tendinous insertion at the tibial tuberosity (Osgood–Schlatter's disease; Fig. 16.12).

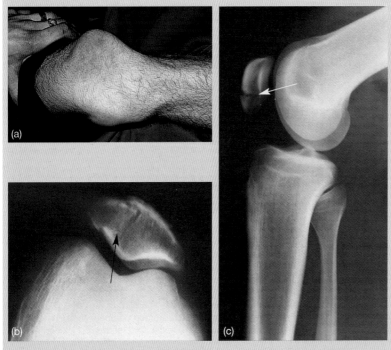

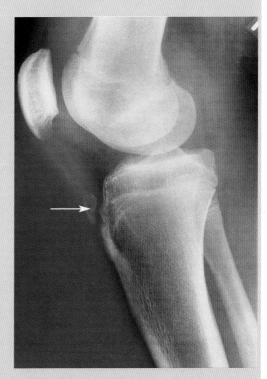

Figure 16.11 (a) Dislocated patella showing lateral displacement. (b) Stellate fracture of the patella (arrow). (c) Transverse fracture of the patella (arrow)

Figure 16.12 Osgood–Schlatter's disease showing irregular ossification of the bony attachment of the patellar ligament (arrow)

Bursae

These are numerous and variable. Anteriorly are the **supra-patellar**, which extends into the thigh deep to quadriceps and communicates with the knee joint, and the **prepatellar**, **superficial** and **deep infrapatellar**, which are related to the patellar ligament.

Posteriorly lie the **popliteal bursa**, deep to its muscle, and one associated with the **gastrocnemius** deep to its medial head. Both communicate with the knee joint and the **semimembranosus** bursa, which lies between the muscle and the medial head of gastrocnemius.

Suprapatellar 'bursitis': Because of the communication between it and the knee joint an effusion into the knee joint also involves the suprapatellar bursa. This can be detected by the patellar tap: pushing the patella towards the femoral condyle results in a palpable contact between the two bones, which is caused by fluid separating the patella and the femoral condyles, and indicates excessive fluid in the knee joint.

Prepatellar bursitis, more commonly known as 'plumber's' or 'housemaid's knee', results from chronic irritation of these bursae caused by constant kneeling on a hard surface. A tender fluctuant swelling is found over the patella (Fig. 16.13).

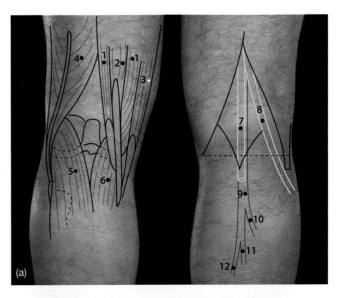

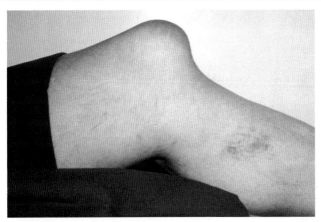

Figure 16.13 Prepatellar bursitis from constant kneeling down and scrubbing floors

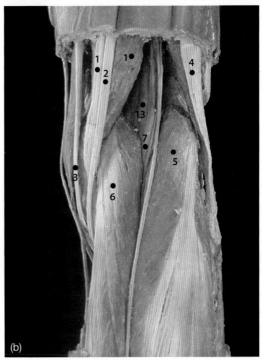

THE TIBIOFIBULAR JOINTS

Little movement occurs between the tibia and fibula.

The **superior tibiofibular joint** is a plane synovial joint between the undersurface of the lateral tibial condyle and the articular facet of the head of the fibula. Its synovia may be continuous with that of the knee joint.

The **inferior tibiofibular joint** is a fibrous joint between the adjacent inferior surfaces of the two bones. A strong, short, interosseous tibiofibular ligament unites them.

The **interosseous membrane** unites the interosseous borders of the two bones and gives attachment to the deep flexor and the extensor muscles of the leg.

The **popliteal fossa** is a diamond-shaped fossa behind the knee joint bounded superomedially by semitendinosus and semimembranosus, superolaterally by biceps femoris and

Figure 16.14 (a) Surface anatomy of the popliteal fossa: 1, semimembranosus; 2, semitendinosus; 3, gracilis; 4, biceps femoris; 5, lateral and, 6, medial head of gastrocnemius; 7, tibial nerve; 8, common peroneal (fibular) nerve; 9, popliteal artery; 10, anterior tibial artery; 11, peroneal (fibular) artery; 12, posterior tibial artery (the popliteal vein, 13, between the artery and main nerves has been omitted in the diagram) – the dashed line shows the level of the transverse section in Fig. 16.15. (b) Dissection of the right popliteal fossa with numbers corresponding to (a)

inferiorly by the medial and lateral heads of gastrocnemius (**Figs. 16.14a** and **16.15**). Its floor is the posterior surface of the femur, the knee joint capsule and the popliteus muscle, and it is roofed by thickened fascia lata that is pierced here by the small saphenous vein. It contains the popliteal vessels and branches, the tibial nerve, the common peroneal (fibular) nerve and branches and a few lymph nodes.

THE LEG AND DORSUM OF THE FOOT

The leg muscles are divided into anterior, lateral and posterior groups lying in fascial compartments separated by the tibia and fibula (**Figs. 16.16a,b**), interosseous membrane and anterior and posterior intermuscular septa, which pass inwards from

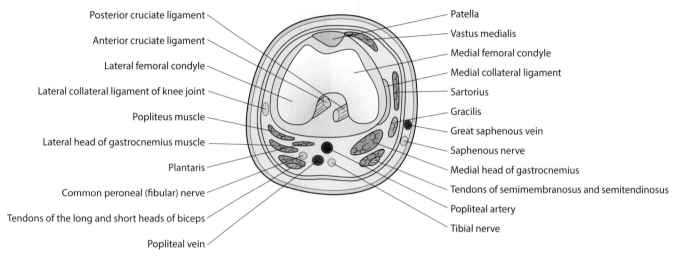

Figure 16.15 Transverse section through the right knee, viewed from below (at the level of the dashed line in Fig. 16.14a)

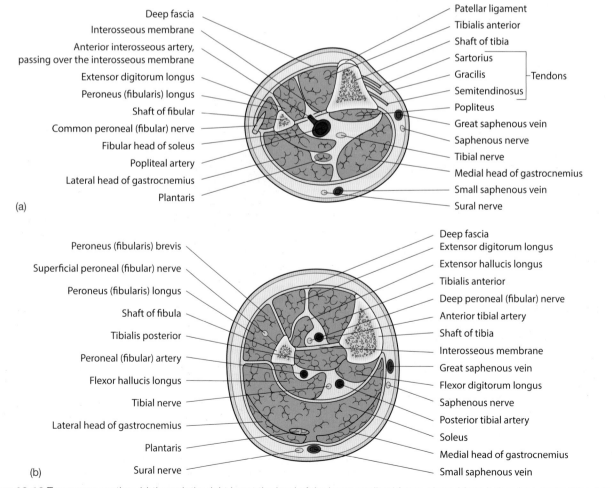

Figure 16.16 Transverse section: (a) through the right leg at the level of the lower popliteal fossa, viewed from below (see dashed line A in Fig. 16.17); (b) through mid-calf, viewed from below (see dashed line B in Fig. 16.17)

the investing deep fascia of the leg. Below, the deep fascia is thickened to form the superior extensor retinaculum (see Fig. 16.19b).

These fascial compartments are inextensible. Any swelling within the fascial compartment as a result of bleeding, infection or venous obstruction produces a rise in the intra-compartmental pressure that will hinder its blood supply and produce tender, swollen muscles (**compartment syndrome**). Surgical treatment is urgently required. A fasciotomy incision the length of the compartment is necessary to reduce the pressure within the fascial compartment.

The anterior (dorsiflexor) group of muscles

Only tibialis anterior is attached to the tibia; the others are each attached to the fibula (Table 16.1 and Fig. 16.17).

Only one, extensor digitorum brevis, is confined to the foot (Fig. 16.18). All are supplied by branches of the common peroneal (fibular) nerve. During walking these muscles pull the leg forwards over the grounded foot; when the foot is not bearing weight they dorsiflex the foot and toes.

In the foot is the **extensor digitorum brevis**, attached proximally to the anterior part of the upper surface of the calcaneus and distally by four small tendons to the medial four toes. It extends the medial four toes.

The two **extensor retinacula** lie across the extensor tendons in the lower leg and in front of the ankle joint. They prevent the tendons 'bowstringing' (**Figs. 16.18b** and **16.19b**). The **superior extensor retinaculum** is a thickening of deep fascia, about 3 cm wide, stretching between the anterior border of the tibia and fibula over the extensor tendons, the anterior tibial vessels and the deep peroneal (fibular) nerve. The **inferior extensor retinaculum** is thicker and bifurcates, extending medially from the upper surface of the calcaneus and then splitting into two parts in front of the ankle joint; the upper part is attached to the medial malleolus and the lower blends with the plantar aponeurosis. The **synovial sheaths** of the long extensors lie deep to the inferior retinaculum; only that of tibialis anterior extends proximally to the superior retinaculum (Fig. 16.19b).

Figure 16.17 Surface anatomy of the anterior lower leg showing the muscles: 1, patellar ligament; 2, sartorius; 3, gracilis; 4, semitendinosus; 5, soleus; 6, gastrocnemius; 7, tibialis anterior; 8, extensor digitorum; 9, peroneus (fibularis) longus; 10, extensor hallucis longus; 11, peroneus (fibularis) tertius; 12, subcutaneous tibial surface. Dashed lines A and B relate to the transverse sections in Fig. 16.16

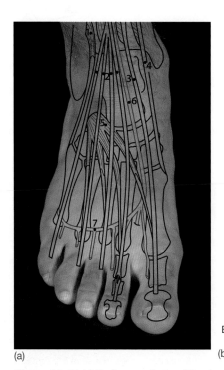
(a)

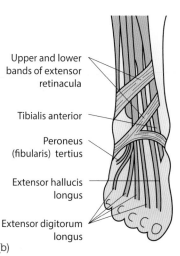
(b)

Upper and lower bands of extensor retinacula

Tibialis anterior

Peroneus (fibularis) tertius

Extensor hallucis longus

Extensor digitorum longus

Figure 16.18 (a) Surface anatomy of the dorsum of the foot showing the tendon attachments: 1, peroneus (fibularis) tertius; 2, the four tendons of extensor digitorum longus; 3, extensor hallucis longus; 4, tendon of tibialis anterior; 5, extensor digitorum brevis; 6, dorsalis pedis artery; 7, arcuate artery. (b) Anterior view of the ankle showing the extensor retinacula

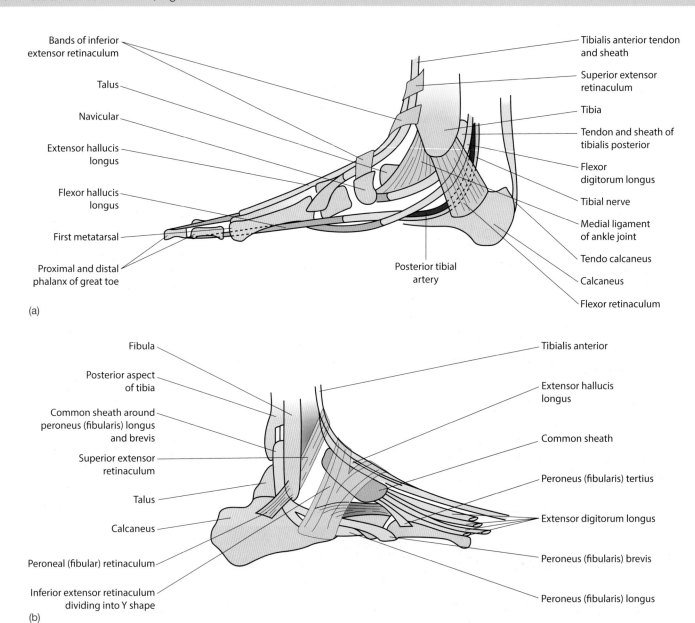

Figure 16.19 Right ankle region. (a) Medial aspect of the ankle. (b) Lateral aspect of the ankle showing the tendons and retinacula

TABLE 16.1 Muscles of anterior (extensor) compartment of leg

Muscle	Proximal attachment	Distal attachment	Nerve supply	Functions
Tibialis anterior (Figs. 16.17 and 16.18)	Lateral condyle and upper lateral surface of tibia	Medial cuneiform and base of 1st metacarpal	Peroneal (fibular) nerve (L4)	Dorsiflexion and inversion of foot
Extensor hallucis longus	Middle of anterior surface of the fibula and interosseous membrane	Base of distal phalanx of hallux	Peroneal (fibular) nerve (L5, S1)	Extension of hallux and dorsiflexion of ankle
Extensor digitorum longus	Lateral condyle of tibia and upper 3/4 of anterior interosseous membrane and fibula	Middle and distal phalanges of lateral four digits	Peroneal (fibular) nerve (L5, S1)	Extension of toes and dorsiflexion of ankle
Peroneus (fibularis) tertius	Lower anterior fibula and interosseous membrane	Base of 5th metacarpal	Peroneal (fibular) nerve (L5, S1)	Dorsiflexion of ankle, weak evertor of foot

The lateral (evertor) group of muscles

These are important in maintaining balance during standing (Table 16.2 and Figs. 16.20a–c). Both peroneal (fibular) muscles are supplied by the superficial peroneal nerve.

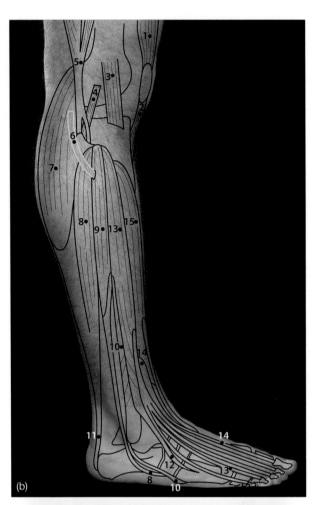

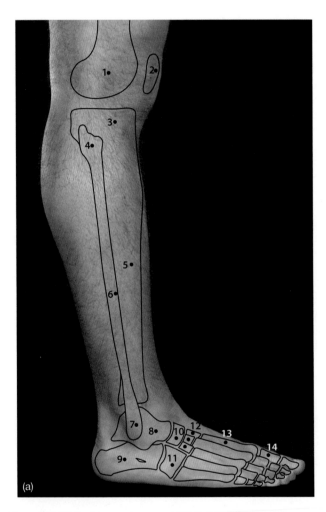

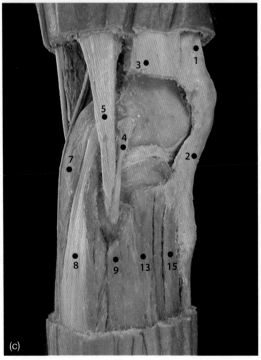

Figure 16.20 Surface anatomy and dissection of the lateral lower right leg. (a) Bones: 1, lateral condyle of femur; 2, patella; 3, tibial plateau; 4, head of fibula; 5, shaft of tibia; 6, shaft of fibula; 7, lateral malleolus; 8, talus; 9, calcaneus; 10, navicular; 11, cuboid; 12, medial, intermediate and lateral cuneiform; 13, metatarsals; 14, phalanges. (b) Muscles: 1, quadriceps; 2, patellar ligament; 3, iliotibial tract; 4, lateral collateral ligament of knee joint; 5, biceps femoris; 6, common peroneal (fibular) nerve; 7, gastrocnemius; 8, soleus; 9, peroneus (fibularis) longus; 10, peroneus (fibularis) brevis; 11, tendo calcaneus; 12, peroneus (fibularis) tertius; 13, muscle and four tendons of the extensor digitorum longus; 14, tendon of extensor hallucis longus; 15, tibialis anterior. (c) Dissection of the lateral side of the upper leg region (muscles labelled as in (b))

TABLE 16.2 Lateral muscles of the leg (peroneal (fibular) compartment)

Muscle	Proximal attachment	Distal attachment	Nerve supply	Functions
Peroneus (fibularis) longus	Head and upper 2/3 of fibula	Base of 1st metatarsal and medial cuneiform	Peroneal (fibular) nerve (L5, S1, S2)	Eversion of foot and weak plantar flexor of ankle
Peroneus (fibularis) brevis (Fig. 16.19b)	Lower 2/3 of lateral surface of fibula	Base of 5th metatarsal	Peroneal (fibular) nerve (L5, S1, S2)	Eversion of foot and weak plantar flexor of ankle

Forced inversion injuries – 'twisted ankles' – often result in avulsion of the base of the 5th metatarsal, the attachment of peroneus (fibularis) brevis (Fig. 16.21).

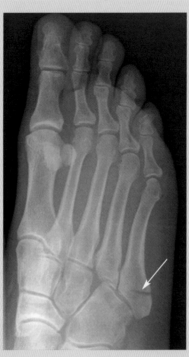

Figure 16.21 Fracture of the base of the 5th metatarsal (arrow)

The posterior (plantar flexor) group of muscles

These help in propelling the body forwards during walking by plantar-flexing the grounded foot (Table 16.3). Gastrocnemius is the most superficial, lying over popliteus and soleus, which in turn is superficial to flexor digitorum longus and flexor hallucis longus (Figs. 16.22 and 16.23a,b). Both gastrocnemius and soleus are powerful plantar flexors of the foot and are thus important in posture and locomotion. Between and within the muscles are extensive deep plexuses of veins; contraction of these calf muscles pumps the blood within them towards the heart against gravity. This muscle pump is sometimes known as the 'third heart'.

Branches of the tibial nerve supply all these muscles.

Rupture of the tendo calcaneus (Achilles tendon) usually occurs as the result of acute contraction of an unexercised muscle, such as may occur during a middle-aged person's first tennis game of the season or the parents' race at a school sports day. Rupture may be partial or complete; conservative treatment is adequate for partial tears but complete tears may require surgical treatment. The ankle reflex is demonstrated by tapping the tendon with a tendon hammer, easiest shown with the patient in the kneeling position. It tests the integrity of the S1 and S2 nerve roots.

TABLE 16.3 Posterior muscles of the leg

Muscle	Proximal attachment	Distal attachment	Nerve supply	Functions
Gastrocnemius (Fig. 16.22a)	By two heads Lateral head: lateral condyle of femur. Medial head: proximal to medial condyle of femur	Posterior surface of calcaneus by the Achilles tendon	Tibial nerve (S1, S2)	Flexion of knee, plantar flexion of ankle
Soleus	Head of fibula (soleal), line of femur	Posterior surface of calcaneus by the Achilles tendon	Tibial nerve (S1, S2)	Plantar flexion of ankle
Plantaris	Lateral supracondylar line of femur	Posterior surface of calcaneus by the Achilles tendon	Tibial nerve (S1, S2)	Weak assist to gastrocnemius
Popliteus	Lateral condyle of femur and lateral meniscus	Upper posterior surface of tibia	Tibial nerve (L4, L5)	Weak flexion of knee and unlocking of medial meniscus
Flexor hallucis longus	Lower 2/3 of posterior surface of fibula	Distal phalanx of hallux	Tibial nerve (S2, S3)	Flexion of hallux, plantar flexion of ankle, support to medial longitudinal arch
Flexor digitorum longus	Lower posterior surface of tibia and fibula	Distal phalanges of lateral four toes	Tibial nerve (S2, S3)	Flexion lateral four toes, plantar flexion of ankle and support of longitudinal arches of foot
Tibialis posterior	Posterior tibia below soleal line, posterior surface of fibula	Tuberosity of navicular, cuneiform and cuboid; bases of 2nd, 3rd and 4th metatarsals	Tibial nerve (L4, L5)	Plantar flexion of ankle, inversion of foot

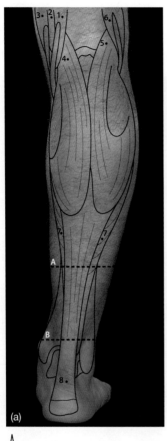

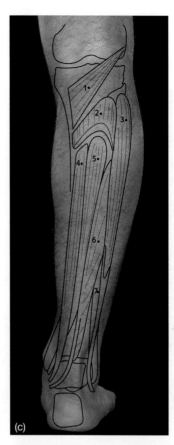

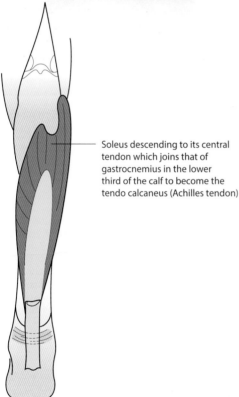

Soleus descending to its central tendon which joins that of gastrocnemius in the lower third of the calf to become the tendo calcaneus (Achilles tendon)

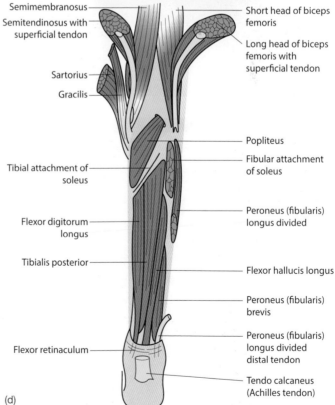

Semimembranosus

Semitendinosus with superficial tendon

Sartorius

Gracilis

Tibial attachment of soleus

Flexor digitorum longus

Tibialis posterior

Flexor retinaculum

Short head of biceps femoris

Long head of biceps femoris with superficial tendon

Popliteus

Fibular attachment of soleus

Peroneus (fibularis) longus divided

Flexor hallucis longus

Peroneus (fibularis) brevis

Peroneus (fibularis) longus divided distal tendon

Tendo calcaneus (Achilles tendon)

Figure 16.22 (a) Surface anatomy of the posterior aspect of the right calf: 1, semitendinosus; 2, semimembranosus; 3, gracilis; 4, 5, medial and lateral heads of gastrocnemius; 6, biceps femoris; 7, soleus; 8, tendo calcaneus (the dashed lines A and B relate to the transverse sections in Figs. 16.28a,b). (b) Posterior aspect of the right calf showing soleus (gastrocnemius has been removed). (c) Surface anatomy of the posterior aspect of the calf showing: 1, popliteus; 2, soleus; 3, peroneus (fibularis) longus; 4, flexor digitorum longus; 5, tibialis posterior; 6, flexor hallucis longus; 7, peroneus (fibularis) brevis. (d) Deep aspect of the posterior leg after removal of soleus and gastrocnemius

The **flexor retinaculum** (Figs. 16.19a and 16.24) is a thickened band of deep fascia passing from the medial malleolus to the medial side of the calcaneus, crossing from medial to lateral the tendons of tibialis posterior and flexor digitorum longus, the posterior tibial vessels, the tibial nerve and the tendon of flexor hallucis longus. Each tendon is enclosed in a separate synovial sheath, those of flexor hallucis longus and flexor digitorum longus passing into the sole of the foot.

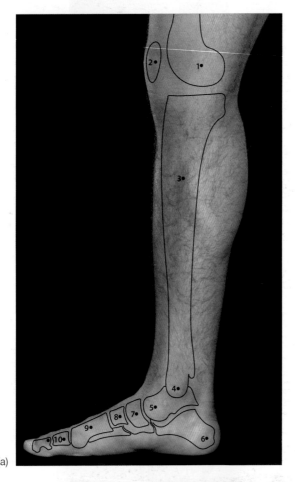

(a)

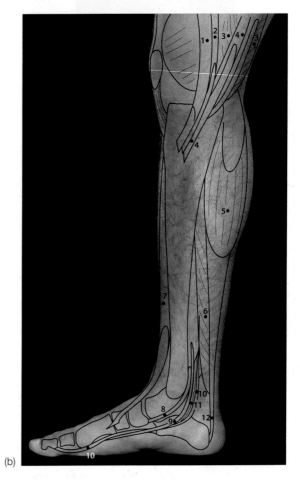

(b)

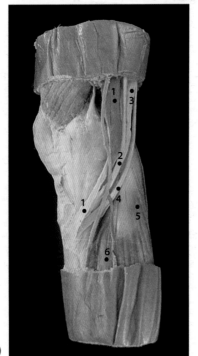

(c)

Figure 16.23 Surface anatomy and dissection of the medial aspect of right leg. (a) Bones: 1, medial femoral condyle; 2, patella; 3, shaft of tibia; 4, medial malleolus; 5, talus; 6, calcaneus; 7, navicular; 8, medial cuneiform; 9, metatarsal; 10, phalanges. (b) Muscles and tendons: 1, sartorius; 2, gracilis; 3, semimembranosus; 4, semitendinosus; 5, gastrocnemius; 6, soleus; 7, tibialis anterior; 8, tibialis posterior; 9, flexor digitorum longus; 10, flexor hallucis longus; 11, posterior tibial artery; 12, tendo calcaneus. (c) Dissection of medial aspect of upper leg (labels as in (b))

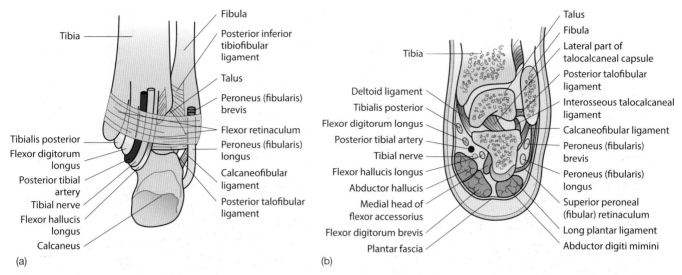

Figure 16.24 (a) Posterior aspect of the ankle showing relations of structures passing behind the right ankle. (b) Oblique coronal section through the ankle and talocalcaneal joints

VESSELS AND NERVES OF THE LEG

The popliteal artery

The popliteal artery (Figs. 16.25 and 16.26) is a continuation of the femoral artery. It descends from the adductor hiatus to the lower border of popliteus, where it divides into the anterior and posterior tibial arteries. Throughout its course its vein and the tibial nerve lie superficial to it.

The popliteal pulse is not easy to feel because the artery lies deep in the popliteal fossa. It is best felt in the middle of the popliteal fossa with the knee flexed.

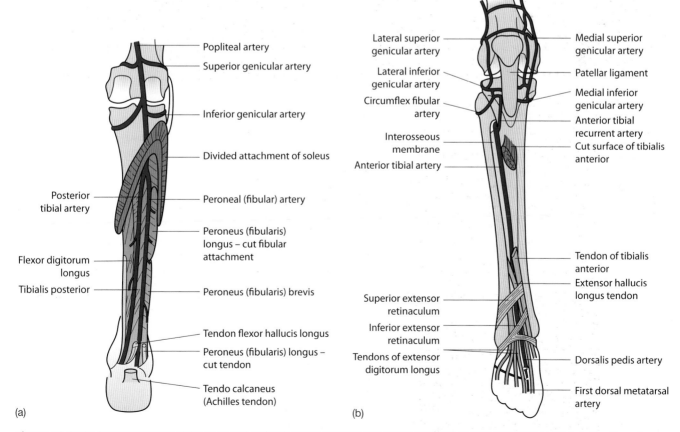

Figure 16.25 (a) Posterior aspect of the knee and calf with gastrocnemius and soleus removed to show the arteries. (b) Anterior dissection showing details of the anastomosis around the knee joint

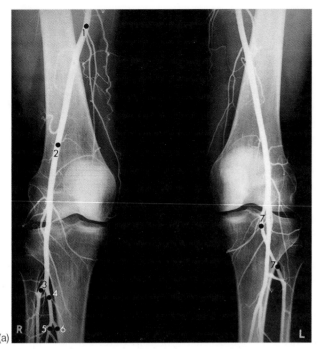
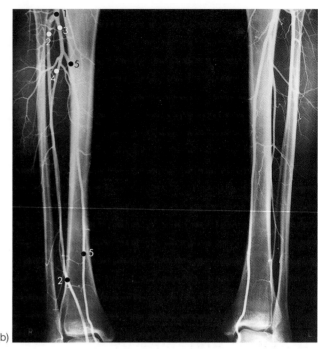

Figure 16.26 (a) Popliteal arteries filled with contrast material that has been injected into the abdominal aorta: 1, femoral artery; 2, popliteal artery; 3, anterior tibial artery; 4, tibioperoneal trunk; 5, peroneal (fibular) artery; 6, posterior tibial artery; 7, abnormally high origin of the left anterior tibial artery. (b) Arteriogram of the lower leg arteries: 1, distal popliteal artery; 2, anterior tibial artery; 3, tibioperoneal trunk; 4, peroneal (fibular) artery; 5, posterior tibial artery

Branches

The **anterior tibial artery** passes forwards above the interosseous membrane and descends the extensor compartment in company with the deep peroneal (fibular) nerve. Beyond the ankle it continues as the **dorsalis pedis artery**, which, in the foot, anastomoses with the lateral plantar artery. The dorsalis pedis artery can be palpated over the tarsal bones, just lateral to the extensor hallucis longus tendon. The **posterior tibial artery** descends through the flexor compartment of the leg alongside the tibial nerve. Its largest branch, the **peroneal (fibular) artery**, descends in the lateral (peroneal [fibular]) compartment. Behind the medial malleolus the posterior tibial artery divides into medial and lateral plantar arteries, which enter the sole of the foot (see **Fig. 16.29**). The posterior tibial artery is palpated on the medial aspect of the talus, just posterior to the medial malleolus (**Fig. 16.23b**).

The popliteal vein

The popliteal vein is formed by the union of the anterior and posterior tibial veins, crosses the popliteal fossa and passes through the adductor hiatus. Throughout its course it is superficial to its artery. Its tributaries correspond largely to the branches of the artery, but in addition the **small saphenous vein** (**Fig. 15.3**, p. 244) enters it by piercing the fascial roof of the popliteal fossa.

The tibial nerve

The tibial nerve is a terminal branch of the sciatic nerve (**Fig. 16.27**). Formed just above the popliteal fossa it descends

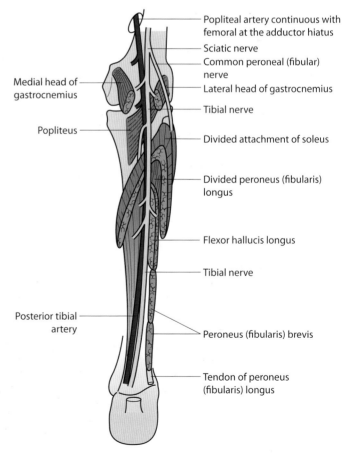

Figure 16.27 Posterior aspect of the knee and calf with gastrocnemius and soleus partly excised to demonstrate the distribution of the common peroneal (fibular) and tibial nerves

through the fossa, leaving it by passing deep to soleus, where it descends through the deep flexor compartment of the leg to the back of the medial malleolus. It divides into medial and lateral plantar nerves.

Relations

In the popliteal fossa it lies superficial to the popliteal vessels. In the calf it descends deep to soleus, on tibialis posterior at first and the ankle joint later. It divides distal to the flexor retinaculum (Figs. 16.24a and 16.28a).

Branches

It supplies all the muscles of the posterior compartment and sensation to the knee joint and lower leg. The **medial and lateral plantar nerves** are illustrated in Fig. 16.29. The **sural nerve**, a cutaneous branch, descends on gastrocnemius and unites with a branch of the common peroneal (fibular) nerve halfway down the calf to run alongside the small saphenous vein behind the lateral malleolus to the lateral side of the foot. It supplies the skin over the posterior calf, the ankle joint and the lateral surface of the foot.

The common peroneal (fibular) nerve

The common peroneal (fibular) nerve (Fig. 16.16) is also a terminal branch of the sciatic nerve that originates just above the popliteal fossa. It descends along the lateral margin of the fossa and enters peroneus (fibularis) longus, where it divides into superficial and deep peroneal (fibular) nerves.

Relations

It is overlapped by the biceps tendon in its upper course but is subcutaneous and easily palpated where it lies on the neck of the fibula (Fig. 16.20b).

Branches

- **Sural communicating branch** – pierces the roof of the popliteal fossa and joins the sural nerve halfway down the calf.
- **Lateral cutaneous nerve of leg** – supplies the lateral aspect of the leg.
- **Articular branches** – to the knee.

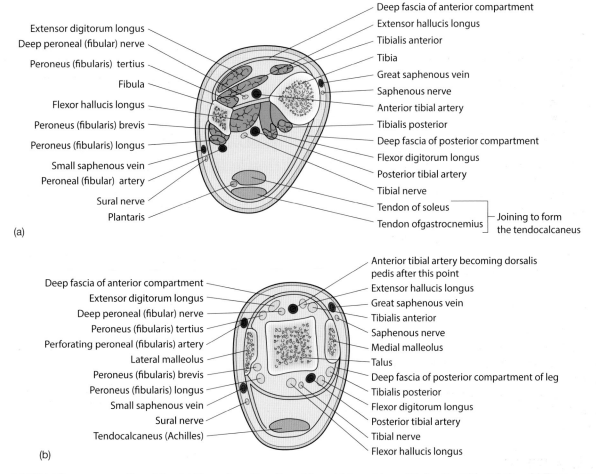

Figure 16.28 (a) Transverse section of the right lower leg at junction of the middle and lower thirds, viewed from below. (b) Transverse section through the right ankle showing the distribution of tendons, vessels and nerves, viewed from below. (These sections are at the levels shown by dashed lines A and B, respectively, in Fig. 16.22a)

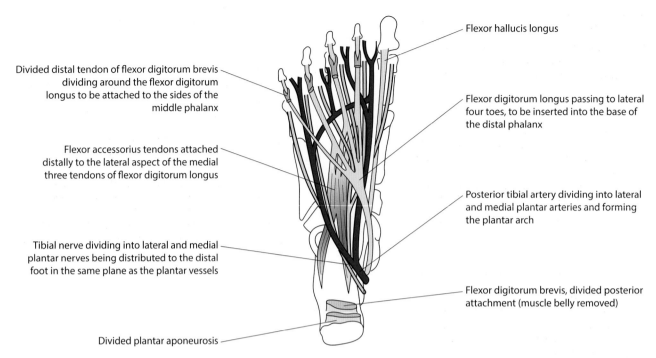

Flexor hallucis longus

Divided distal tendon of flexor digitorum brevis dividing around the flexor digitorum longus to be attached to the sides of the middle phalanx

Flexor digitorum longus passing to lateral four toes, to be inserted into the base of the distal phalanx

Flexor accessorius tendons attached distally to the lateral aspect of the medial three tendons of flexor digitorum longus

Posterior tibial artery dividing into lateral and medial plantar arteries and forming the plantar arch

Tibial nerve dividing into lateral and medial plantar nerves being distributed to the distal foot in the same plane as the plantar vessels

Flexor digitorum brevis, divided posterior attachment (muscle belly removed)

Divided plantar aponeurosis

Figure 16.29 Sole of the right foot; the bulk of flexor digitorum brevis has been removed to show the posterior tibial artery and tibial nerve and tendons in the sole of the foot

- **Superficial peroneal (fibular) nerve** – descends deep to peroneus (fibularis) longus and, in the lower leg, emerges through the deep fascia to divide into cutaneous branches. It supplies peroneus (fibularis) longus and brevis, and provides cutaneous branches to the lower lateral leg and, by its dorsal cutaneous branches, which descend over the extensor retinacula, the dorsum of the foot.
- **Deep peroneal (fibular) nerve** – passes around the neck of the fibula into the anterior compartment and descends in it together with the anterior tibial artery. It passes under the extensor retinacula to divide into medial and lateral terminal branches. It supplies the long dorsiflexors – extensor digitorum longus, extensor hallucis longus and tibialis anterior; its lateral terminal branch supplies extensor digitorum brevis and the ankle joint, and its medial terminal branch supplies skin in the web of the first toe on the dorsum of the foot.

Peripheral nerve injuries in the lower limb are described on pp. 294–297.

MCQs

1. You are invited to demonstrate the surface   **T/F**
markings of the lower limb. Not all the
landmarks you suggest are correct. Which
are correct?

a   the saphenous opening lies six finger   (___)
   breadths below the pubic symphysis

b   the tendon of adductor magnus can be   (___)
   palpated in the groin with the leg adducted

c   the site of the posterior inferior iliac spine   (___)
   is seen as a dimple

d   the common peroneal (fibular) nerve can   (___)
   be rolled against the head of the fibula

e   the lower fibres of vastus medialis lie   (___)
   horizontally

Answers

1.

a   **F** – *The saphenous opening lies some 3–4 finger breadths (3–4 cm) below and 1 cm lateral to the pubic tubercle.*

b   **F** – *The tendon that is so easily felt is that of adductor longus. Adductor magnus is much more fleshy and has no obvious tendon.*

c   **F** – *The 'dimples of Venus' seen or felt in the upper medial quadrant of the buttock are due to fascial adherence to the posterior superior iliac spines. This is also a useful landmark for the level of the 2nd sacral vertebra and the termination of the thecal sac.*

d   **F** – *The common peroneal (fibular) nerve winds around the neck of the fibula, where it may be easily felt.*

e   **T** – *It is these fibres that resist lateral dislocation of the patella.*

2. The knee joint: **T/F**

a   can only rotate when fully extended   (___)

b   is reinforced by numerous ligaments, the   (___)
   strongest of which is the tibial collateral
   ligament

c   contains cruciate ligaments that lie within   (___)
   the synovial cavity

d   has a nerve supply from the femoral and   (___)
   sciatic nerves only

e   has a meniscus to which popliteus is   (___)
   attached posteriorly

Answers

2.

a   **F** – *The knee joint has the ability to rotate, but only when flexed.*

b   **F**

c   **F** – *The intracapsular cruciate ligaments, which resist anteroposterior movements of the femur on the tibia, lie extrasynovially.*

d   **F** – *Its nerve supply follows Hilton's law and is therefore not only via the femoral and sciatic nerves, but also via a branch from the obturator nerve.*

e   **T** – *Popliteus pulls the lateral meniscus clear of the condyles at the initiation of knee flexion.*

SBA

1. A 50-year-old carpet fitter is complaining of a painful swelling close to his knee. On examination a tender fluctuant swelling is found in front of his left knee. What is the likely diagnosis?

a   infrapatellar bursitis

b   suprapatellar bursitis

c   prepatellar bursitis

d   lateral meniscus tear

e   anterior cruciate ligament tear

Answer

c   *Chronic irritation of this bursa caused by constant kneeling on hard surfaces results in inflammation and effusion of fluid into the bursa. This presents as a swelling in front of the patella and is commonly known as 'housemaid's knee'.*

2. The tendon of which muscle is stretched during the execution of the patellar reflex?

a   vastus medialis

b   quadriceps femoris

c   sartorius

d   biceps femoris

e   rectus femoris

Answer

b   *The patellar ligament provides the insertion of quadriceps femoris into the patella. The stretch reflex caused by the patella hammer is elicited by the femoral nerve carrying fibres from the L3 nerve roots.*

EMQs

Each question has an anatomical theme linked to the chapter, and a list of 10 related items (A–J) placed in alphabetical order: these are followed by five statements (1–5). Match **one or more** of the items A–J to each of the five statements.

Muscles of the lower leg
A. Extensor digitorum longus
B. Extensor hallucis longus
C. Flexor digitorum longus
D. Flexor hallucis longus
E. Gastrocnemius
F. Peroneus (fibularis) brevis
G. Peroneus (fibularis) longus
H. Soleus
I. Tibialis anterior
J. Tibialis posterior

Answers
1 E; 2 ABDFGHJ; 3 F; 4 EH; 5 B

Match the following statements with the muscle(s) in the above list.
1. Attached to the femoral condyles
2. Attached to the fibula
3. Attached to the styloid process of the fifth metatarsal
4. Forms the tendo calcaneus (Achilles tendon)
5. Lies medial to the dorsalis pedis artery

Nerves of the lower leg
A. Extensor digitorum longus
B. Extensor hallucis
C. Flexor digitorum longus
D. Flexor hallucis longus
E. Gastrocnemius
F. Peroneus (fibularis) brevis
G. Peroneus (fibularis) longus
H. Soleus
I. Tibialis anterior
J. Tibialis posterior

Answers
1 CDEHJ; 2 ABFGI; 3 CJ; 4 D; 5 G

Match the following nerves and statements with the muscle(s) in the above list.
1. Supplied by the tibial nerve
2. Supplied by the common peroneal (fibular) nerve
3. Medial to the tibial nerve at the ankle
4. Lateral to the tibial nerve at the ankle
5. Site of division of the common peroneal nerve

APPLIED QUESTIONS

1. Why is a knowledge of the suprapatellar bursa clinically important?

1. The superior extension of the knee joint, known as the suprapatellar bursa, may sustain an anterior penetrating wound which, because of its connection with the knee joint, may cause a septic arthritis. Any effusion in the knee, whether caused by trauma, inflammation or infection, is clinically evident by detectable swelling of the suprapatellar bursa.

2. Why is a popliteal pulse difficult to feel even in the normal individual?

2. The popliteal pulse is difficult to palpate in most people because it is the deepest lying structure in the popliteal fossa. Having pierced the adductor magnus at the adductor hiatus, it lies deep to its vein, which is in turn deep to the tibial nerve in the popliteal fossa. All these structures are embedded in fat, and both the artery and the vein are additionally surrounded by a tough fibrous sheath. Flexion of the knee, which allows relaxation of nerve and sheath, often facilitates palpation.

3. A young man is crossing the road and is knocked down by a bus. On his arrival at hospital it is noticed that he has a very swollen lateral side of the knee and lower leg, and that he cannot dorsiflex his foot. Can you explain his 'foot drop'?

3. This is a typical 'bumper-bar' injury or 'bumper fracture', which usually results in a fractured neck of the fibula and associated soft tissue damage. At this site the common peroneal (fibular) nerve winds into the lateral, and later the anterior, compartment of the lower leg and is easily damaged. The branches of the common peroneal (fibular) nerve are the superficial and deep peroneal (fibular) nerves. The deep nerve runs with the anterior tibial artery to supply the extensor group of muscles, including tibialis anterior, whereas the superficial peroneal (fibular) nerve supplies the peroneal muscles, which are the major evertors of the foot. Damage to the deep peroneal (fibular) nerve therefore results in an inability to dorsiflex the foot, whereas an injured superficial peroneal (fibular) nerve results in an inverted foot. A combination of these is 'foot drop', i.e. an inverted plantar flexed foot, which, if permanent, results in patients catching their big toe on the swing-through and scuffing the anterolateral part of their shoes when walking.

The foot

The foot is an arched platform formed of separate bones bound by ligaments and muscles; it supports the body's weight, acts as a rigid lever that can propel the body forwards and yet is resilient enough to absorb the shocks resulting from impact with the ground. The foot is also important as a source of proprioceptive information essential to the maintenance of balance during both standing and walking.

THE BONES OF THE FOOT

The skeleton of the foot comprises the tarsus, metatarsus and phalanges. The **tarsus** (Fig. 17.1) comprises the talus, calcaneus, navicular, cuboid and three cuneiform bones.

The **talus** carries the whole of the body weight. It has a body, neck and head, and no muscular attachments. The **body's** upper surface is markedly convex anteroposteriorly, slightly concave from side to side, and articulates with the inferior surface of the tibia. This broad articular facet is continuous with a facet on each side of the bone for articulation with the medial and lateral malleoli; the three articular surfaces are known as the **trochlear surface** of the talus. The concave inferior surface of the body articulates with the posterior facet on the calcaneus. The posterior margin bears a posterior tubercle that gives attachment to the posterior talofibular ligament. The **neck** bears a deep groove inferiorly. The hemispherical **head** articulates with the navicular bone, the calcaneus and the plantar calcaneonavicular (spring) ligament inferomedially (see Fig. 17.7).

The **calcaneus** (Figs. 17.1 and 17.2) is an irregularly rectangular bone forming the prominence of the heel and articulating with the talus above and the cuboid anteriorly. Its upper surface has posterior, middle and anterior articular facets for the talus. The middle facet lies medially on the prominent **sustentaculum tali**, which gives attachment to the calcaneonavicular ligament (spring ligament). Behind the facet is a deep groove, the **sulcus calcanei**, which, with the sulcus tali, forms a tunnel, the **sinus tarsi**, which houses the strong talocalcaneal ligament. These articulations with the talus constitute the 'subtalar' joint, which permits the movements of inversion and eversion of the ankle.

The inferior surface has an **anterior tubercle** to which is attached the short plantar ligament and, posteriorly, the **medial and lateral processes** on the weight-bearing **tuberosity**, to which are attached the long plantar ligament, the short muscles of the sole and the plantar aponeurosis. On the lateral surface is the **peroneal (fibular) tubercle**, separating the tendons of peroneus (fibularis) longus and brevis. The posterior surface gives attachment to the tendo calcaneus and the anterior surface articulates with the cuboid bone.

The **navicular bone** lies on the medial side of the foot and articulates with the talus posteriorly and the three wedged-shaped cuneiform bones anteriorly. Its medial surface extends down to form the prominent and palpable **navicular tuberosity**, to which are attached tibialis posterior and the calcaneonavicular ligament.

The wedge-shaped **cuboid** lies laterally. It articulates with the calcaneus posteriorly, the bases of the 4th and 5th metatarsals anteriorly and the lateral cuneiform medially. Its inferior surface gives attachment to the long plantar ligament, and it has a marked groove for the tendon of peroneus (fibularis) longus.

The three wedge-shaped **cuneiforms** articulate posteriorly with the navicular and anteriorly with the bases of the three medial metatarsals. To the medial cuneiform are attached the tendons of tibialis anterior and posterior and peroneus (fibularis) longus.

The **metatarsals and phalanges** of the foot resemble those of the hand, but the metatarsals are longer and more slender. The 1st metatarsal is thick and transmits the body weight in walking. The first toe usually has only two phalanges.

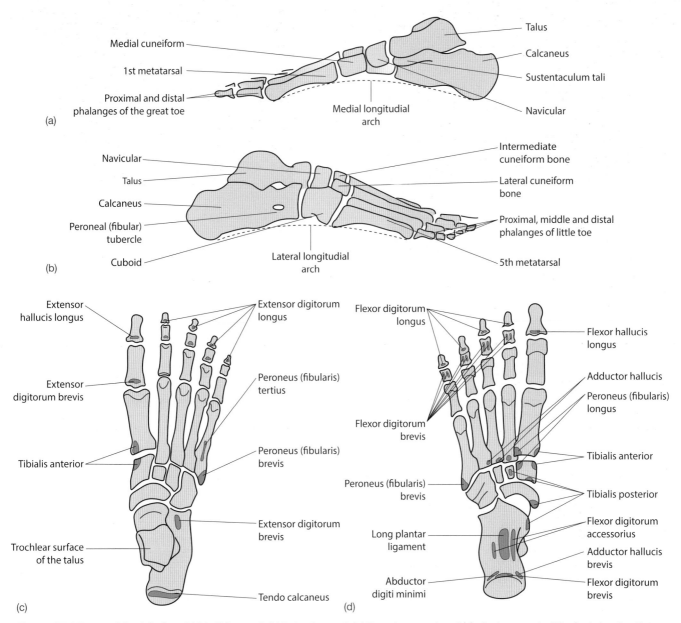

Figure 17.1 Bones of the right foot. (a) Medial aspect. (b) Lateral aspect. (c) Superior aspect and (d) plantar aspect of the foot showing the muscle attachments

THE ANKLE JOINT

The ankle joint is a hinged synovial joint between the mortise formed by the inferior surface of the tibia, the medial surface of the lower fibula and the trochlear surface of the talus (Fig. 17.2). Its stability rests on the medial and lateral malleoli lying alongside the talus. Its capsule, attached to the articular margins, possesses capsular thickenings that contribute considerably to the strength of the joint:

- **Medial (deltoid) ligament** – this is triangular in shape, with its apex attached to the medial malleolus and its base to the navicular, the neck of the talus, the plantar calcaneonavicular ligament and the medial side of the talus (Fig. 17.3), as well as the sustentaculum tali.

- **Lateral ligament** – this has three parts: an anterior talofibular ligament from the lateral malleolus passing horizontally to the neck of the talus; the calcaneofibular ligament passing back from the malleolar tip to the lateral side of the calcaneus; and the posterior talofibular ligament passing horizontally between the malleolar fossa of the lateral malleolus and the posterior tubercle of the talus (Figs. 17.4 and 17.5).

An accessory ligament, the **inferior transverse tibiofibular ligament**, a thick band between the two malleoli across the back of the talus, is covered with hyaline cartilage and deepens the articular surface between it and the talus.

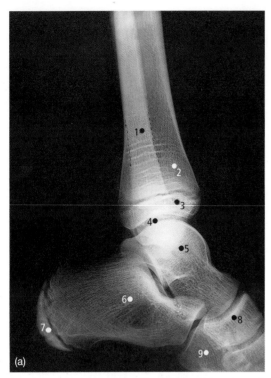

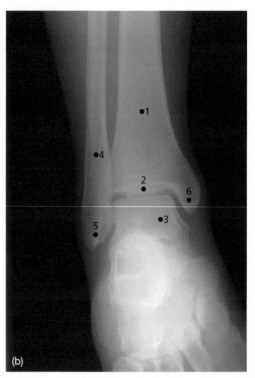

Figure 17.2 X-ray of the right ankle. (a) Lateral view: 1, outline of fibula overlapping tibia; 2, tibia; 3, tibial epiphysis; 4, line of the ankle joint; 5, talus; 6, calcaneus; 7, calcaneal epiphysis; 8, navicular; 9, cuboid. (b) Anteroposterior view: 1, tibia; 2, line of the ankle joint; 3, talus; 4, fibula; 5, lateral malleolus; 6, medial malleolus

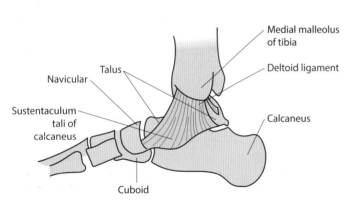

Figure 17.3 Medial aspect of the right ankle joint showing the deltoid ligament

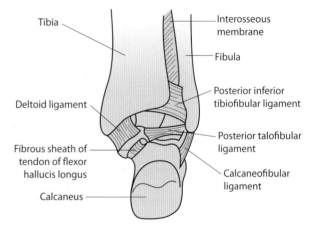

Figure 17.5 Posterior aspect of the right ankle joint showing the ligaments

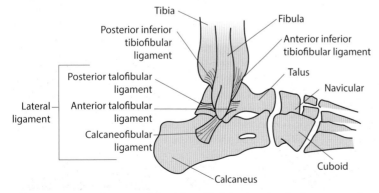

Figure 17.4 Lateral aspect of the right ankle joint showing the ligaments – the anterior talofibular, posterior talofibular and calcaneofibular ligaments combine to form the lateral ligament of the ankle

Functional aspects

Movement

Plantar flexion (downwards movement of the foot) and dorsiflexion (upwards movement) are possible, plantar flexion by the action of gastrocnemius and soleus, assisted by other flexor muscles and possibly the peronei. Dorsiflexion is produced by tibialis and other extensor muscles (plantar flexion is 'true flexion').

Stability

This is a stable joint maintained by the mortise arrangement of its bones and strong ligaments. The centre of gravity passes anterior to the joint, and as the foot is dorsiflexed on the grounded foot the tibiofibular mortise firmly grips the wider anterior talar surface, i.e. when walking up a slope. It is least stable in the plantar-flexed position, e.g. in a ballet dancer *en pointe*.

Relations

Medially and laterally the joint is subcutaneous (**Figs. 16.23a,b**, p. 280). Anteriorly it is crossed, medial to lateral, by the tendons of tibialis anterior and extensor hallucis longus, the anterior tibial vessels and deep peroneal (fibular) nerve, and the tendons of extensor digitorum longus. Posteromedially, from medial to lateral, it is crossed by tendons of tibialis posterior and flexor digitorum longus, the posterior tibial vessels and tibial nerve, and the tendon of flexor hallucis longus. The tendons of peroneus (fibularis) longus and brevis cross the joint posterolaterally. All the tendons are surrounded by synovial sheaths (**Figs. 16.19a,b**, p. 276).

The tarsal joints

The most important tarsal joints are:

- **Subtalar (talocalcaneal) joint** – a synovial joint between the inferior facet on the body of the talus and the posterior facet of the calcaneus. The capsule is partly thickened by talocalcaneal bands, but the strongest union is provided by the **interosseous talocalcaneal ligament** in the sinus tarsi, which is taut in eversion.
- **Talocalcaneonavicular joint** – a synovial joint of the ball and socket variety between the hemispherical head of the talus and the concavity formed by facets on the upper calcaneus, the concavity of the navicular and the plantar calcaneonavicular ligament. The capsule is reinforced by the spring ligament, the deltoid ligament and the bifurcate ligament (see below).
- **Plantar calcaneonavicular (spring) ligament** (**Fig. 17.7**) – a strong thick band between the sustentaculum tali and the navicular tuberosity; it is covered by articular cartilage and contributes to the articular surface for the head of the talus. It is important in maintaining the medial longitudinal arch of the foot.
- **Calcaneocuboid joint** – a synovial joint between the reciprocal concavo-convex facets of the two bones; the capsule is reinforced by the bifurcate and long and short plantar ligaments. The **bifurcate ligament** is attached proximally to the upper surface of the calcaneus and distally to the upper cuboid and navicular. The **long plantar ligament** passes between the posterior calcaneal processes to the ridges on the inferior surface of the cuboid and the bases of the lateral metatarsals. The **short plantar ligament** is more deeply placed and passes between the anterior process of the calcaneus and the adjacent cuboid (**Fig. 17.7**).

The collateral ligaments of the ankle, the deltoid and the lateral ligament can be partially or completely torn by forcible eversion or inversion injuries. The most severe injuries result in instability of the ankle joint. Inversion injuries are the most common and result in sprains or tears to the lateral ligament, especially its calcaneofibular and anterior talofibular components. More severe injuries result in associated bony injuries to the joint. A common fracture–dislocation of the ankle (Pott's fracture) (**Fig. 17.6**) occurs when the foot is forcibly everted. The lateral malleolus fractures first, followed by tearing of the medial collateral ligament; finally, the posterior margin of the lower tibia shears off against the talus. The three stages are referred to as first-, second- and third-degree Pott's fractures.

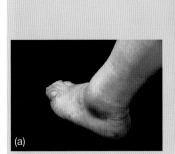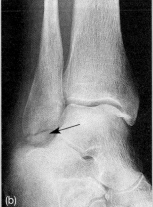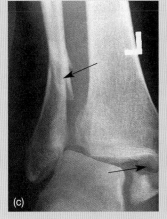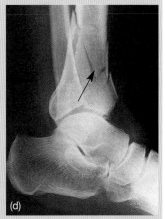

Figure 17.6 Fractures of the ankle joint (arrows): (a) shows swelling over the lateral malleolus; (b) fractured lateral malleolus; (c) fractured fibula and medial malleolus; (d) fractured lower tibia

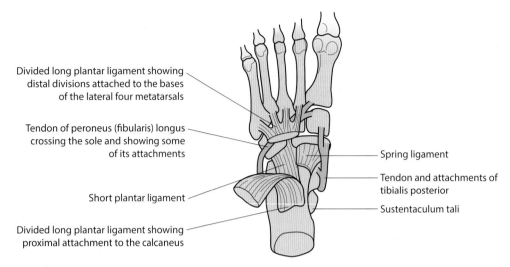

Divided long plantar ligament showing distal divisions attached to the bases of the lateral four metatarsals

Tendon of peroneus (fibularis) longus crossing the sole and showing some of its attachments

Short plantar ligament

Divided long plantar ligament showing proximal attachment to the calcaneus

Spring ligament

Tendon and attachments of tibialis posterior

Sustentaculum tali

Figure 17.7 Dissection of the sole of the right foot showing the plantar ligaments

Functional aspects

Inversion (the sole of the foot is turned inwards and its medial border raised) and **eversion** (the sole is turned outwards and its lateral border raised) are possible. Both movements occur not at the ankle joints but at the subtalar and talocalcaneonavicular joints. The calcaneus and the navicular, carrying the forefoot with them, move medially on the talus by a combination of rotary and gliding movements. The range of inversion and eversion is increased by movement at the **midtarsal (talonavicular and calcaneocuboid) joint**. Inversion is increased during plantar flexion because the narrow posterior end of the talus is not then so tightly fitted into the tibial mortise. Eversion is increased in dorsiflexion.

Inversion is produced by tibialis anterior and posterior, eversion by the peroneal (fibular) muscles. The interosseous talocalcaneal ligament limits inversion and the deltoid ligament limits eversion. These movements have been described with the foot off the ground; the same movements occurring when the foot is on the ground adjust the foot to uneven and sloping surfaces, as when walking across a steep incline or skiing down a mountain.

The **tarsometatarsal joints** and the remaining **intertarsal joints** are small plane synovial joints, capable only of slight gliding movements. They are tightly bound together by interosseous ligaments, and these are particularly strong on the **plantar aspect** of the foot.

Some children are born with the congenital deformity 'club foot' (Fig. 17.8), in which the toes most commonly point inwards and downwards (talipes equinovarus).

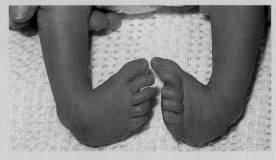

Figure 17.8 Talipes equinovarus

THE INTERPHALANGEAL JOINTS

The **metatarsophalangeal and interphalangeal joints** resemble those of the fingers but are less mobile, the metatarsal heads being bound together by deep transverse ligaments that unite all the plantar surfaces of the joint capsules. Plantar flexion and dorsiflexion occur at all these joints, as do a very limited amount of abduction and adduction. Plantar flexion is produced by flexor hallucis longus and brevis and flexor digitorum longus and brevis; dorsiflexion by extensor hallucis longus and the extensor digitorum longus and brevis muscles. The first metatarsophalangeal joint is much larger than the others. A sesamoid bone often lies within each tendon of flexor hallucis brevis, the tendons and sesamoids being incorporated into the joint capsule. The tendon of flexor hallucis longus lies in the groove between the sesamoid bones and is thus protected from pressure.

The natural angle between the long axis of the 1st metatarsal and its proximal phalanx may be accentuated by tight shoes (**hallux valgus**) (Fig. 17.9). Hallux valgus is one of the most common foot deformities and is often seen in elderly individuals, possibly owing to loss of muscle tone. There is

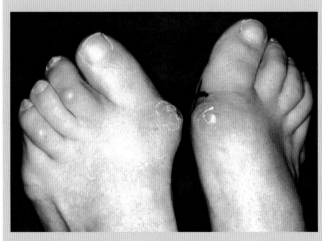

Figure 17.9 Bilateral hallux valgus

lateral deviation of the big toe, increased angulation of the first metatarsophalangeal joint and prominence of the metatarsal head. A protective bursa may develop on the medial side of the joint, and persistent trauma from shoes produces inflammation within it, with attendant swelling, redness and pain (bunion). Surgical correction may be required to relieve pain or deformity.

THE ARCHES OF THE FOOT

The arched foot is a human characteristic and is present from birth. Although a baby's foot appears flat because of the prominent fat pad on the sole of its foot, the skeletal basis for an arch can be seen radiologically. The arch becomes visible once the child begins to walk. The arches distribute the body weight over a larger area and prevent crushing of the vessels and nerves that cross the sole. The jointed pattern of the arch gives the foot resilience to absorb the impact of the body's weight when the foot comes into contact with the ground, yet still allows its use as a semirigid lever to propel the body forwards in walking. There are medial, lateral and transverse arches, which are collectively involved in these functions.

The maintenance of each arch depends on bony, ligamentous and muscular factors: the short ligaments and muscles tie adjacent bones together, and the long ligaments, the plantar aponeurosis and the long muscle tendons tighten the ends of the arch together. Some long tendons act as slings, supporting the centre of the arch. The ligaments and muscles on the plantar surface are stronger and more numerous than on the dorsum.

The **medial longitudinal arch** (Fig. 17.1a) is visible and obvious; it extends from the medial process of the calcaneus via the talus, navicular and three cuneiforms to the heads of the three medial metatarsals. Some support to the arch is given by the sustentaculum tali to the talus and by the wedge shape of some of the bones, but their contribution is not as significant as that made by the ligaments and muscles:

- The **plantar calcaneonavicular (spring) ligament** (Fig. 17.7), which supports the head of the talus
- **Interosseous ligaments**
- The **plantar aponeurosis**, which binds the ends of the arch together
- The **short muscles** of the foot, especially abductor hallucis, flexor hallucis brevis and flexor digitorum brevis
- **Tibialis anterior**, which is attached to the centre of the arch
- **Flexor hallucis longus** and the medial part of **flexor digitorum longus**, which span across the arch
- **Tibialis posterior**, which ties the posterior bones of the arch together.

The **lateral longitudinal arch** (Fig. 17.1b) is lower than the medial; it extends from the lateral process of the calcaneus via the cuboid to the heads of the 4th and 5th metatarsals. Its shape is maintained largely by ligaments and to a lesser extent by muscles, namely:

- The **plantar aponeurosis**
- The **long and short plantar ligaments**, which unite the calcaneus, the cuboid and the bases of the 4th and 5th metatarsals
- **Interosseous ligaments**
- The **short muscles of the foot**, especially flexor digitorum brevis
- **Peroneus (fibularis) longus**, which passes below the centre of the arch deep to the cuboid, which it supports.

The **transverse arch** lies across the distal row of the tarsus, the cuneiform and cuboid bones and the adjacent metatarsals. Its shape is maintained by the wedge-like shape of the cuneiform, the interosseous ligaments and the peroneus (fibularis) longus, tibialis posterior and adductor hallucis muscles.

Flat feet (pes planus) (Fig. 17.10) are caused by a flattening of the medial longitudinal arch – the result of excessive ligamentous laxity, particularly in the plantar calcaneonavicular 'spring' ligament, loss of muscle power or abnormal load distribution. Flat feet are common in older people, especially if excessive weight gain has occurred. Diagnosis is readily made by examination of wet footprints on the bathroom floor, where it is revealed that the normally raised medial arch has disappeared. The underlying cause is often inherited and the condition is usually asymptomatic, but it may cause chronic foot strain.

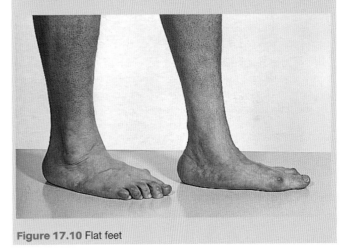

Figure 17.10 Flat feet

THE SOLE OF THE FOOT

The skin over the weight-bearing areas of the heel and 'ball' of the foot is thickened in its superficial layers and firmly attached to the deep fascia. The superficial fascia is fat-filled and serves to cushion the deeper structures. The deep fascia has a thickened central portion, the **plantar aponeurosis**, and thin medial and lateral portions. The aponeurosis is attached posteriorly to the back of the undersurface of the calcaneus and divides anteriorly into five digital expansions. These are attached to the fibrous flexor sheaths and to the deep transverse ligaments between the metatarsal heads. When the toes are dorsiflexed the aponeurosis tightens and the longitudinal arch is accentuated.

Inflammation in the attachments of the plantar aponeurosis (**plantar fasciitis**) occasionally occurs and is accompanied by acute pain on pressure over the calcaneus, especially during weight-bearing and standing. It is a condition often suffered by those doing a lot of walking because of their job, e.g. postmen and postwomen.

Muscles of the sole

These include counterparts to those of the hand, in the short flexors, abductors and adductor of the great toe, and lumbrical and interosseous muscles, but there is no opponens muscle (Fig. 17.11). These small muscles help to maintain the arches and flex and extend the toes, but have little abductor or adductor function. A sesamoid bone is present on each side of the head of the 1st metatarsal, embedded in the tendons of the short muscles passing to the phalanges of the great toe. They form a protective groove for the tendon of flexor hallucis longus.

Flexor accessorius has no counterpart in the hand. Attached to calcaneus posteriorly and to the tendons of flexors digitorum and hallucis longus anteriorly, it maintains tension in the long tendons and can flex the toes even when the long flexors must relax, e.g. when the leg, during the supporting phase of walking, is pulled forward over the ankle joint by tibialis anterior and the extensor muscles.

The long flexor tendons pass in the sole into the long flexor sheaths, to be attached to the terminal phalanges. Three calf muscles are inserted on the medial side of the foot: **tibialis posterior** (Fig. 17.7; see also Fig. 16.29, p. 284) to the tuberosity of the navicular and then to most of the other tarsal bones and to the metatarsal bases; **peroneus (fibularis) longus** crosses the foot inferiorly from the lateral side to attach to the medial cuneiform and the base of the 1st metatarsal; and **tibialis anterior** is attached to the same two bones. They each give good support to the arches of the foot.

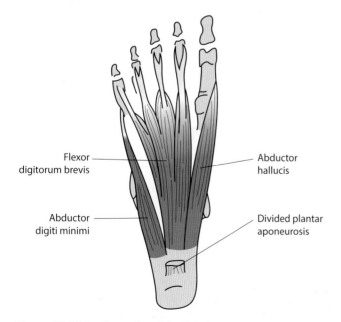

Figure 17.11 Small muscles of the right foot

Flexor digitorum brevis

Abductor hallucis

Abductor digiti minimi

Divided plantar aponeurosis

Rollerblading and inline skating often cause **tendinitis** in these long flexors as they battle to keep the feet balanced when turning corners.

Nerves of the sole

- **Medial plantar nerve** (Fig. 16.29, p. 284) – this begins under the flexor retinaculum and passes forwards, accompanied by its vessels. It supplies flexor hallucis brevis, abductor hallucis, flexor digitorum brevis and the 1st lumbrical, and supplies cutaneous branches to the medial part of the sole and the medial three and a half toes.
- **Lateral plantar nerve** – this is a terminal branch of the tibial nerve. Accompanied by its artery, it passes obliquely forwards across the sole to the base of the 5th metatarsal, to divide into deep and superficial branches, which supply the remaining short muscles of the sole, and cutaneous branches to the skin over the lateral side of the foot and the lateral one and a half toes.

Cutaneous nerve supply

This is outlined in Figs. 17.12–17.14. To summarize: we kneel on skin supplied by L3/4, and the dorsum of the foot is supplied by L5. We stand on skin supplied by S1 and sit on S3. Autonomic nerves, mainly sympathetic, are contained in the branches of the lumbosacral plexus and supply blood vessels, sweat glands and erector pili muscles.

Lower limb sensory testing (with the patient's eyes closed) of dermatomes and individual nerves: touch (cotton wool); pain (sterile needle); temperature (side of warm finger versus side of cold tuning fork); vibration (base of a tuning fork on the medial malleolus); graphaesthesia (writing numbers on the shin with a blunt instrument); position sense (recognizing direction of movement – hold the sides of the big toe).

Motor testing: power (dorsiflexion of foot against resistance); tone (passive flexion and extension of a relaxed knee joint); coordination (running the heel up and down the opposite shin – eyes open and then closed); reflexes (knee L3, L4; ankle S1, S2); note wasting and abnormal movements; individual muscles – active and passive movements, and movement against resistance.

PERIPHERAL NERVE INJURIES IN THE LOWER LIMB

Femoral nerve

Injuries to this nerve produce loss of knee extension (quadriceps), some loss of hip flexion (iliacus and pectineus) and loss of sensation over the front of the thigh and the medial side of the thigh, leg and foot (anterior and medial femoral cutaneous nerves and saphenous nerves) (Fig. 17.15).

Damage to the lateral femoral cutaneous nerve of the thigh, which may follow its entrapment just below the inguinal ligament close to the anterior superior iliac spine by, for example, a psoas abscess, often results in pain and sensory loss over the lateral thigh (meralgia paraesthetica).

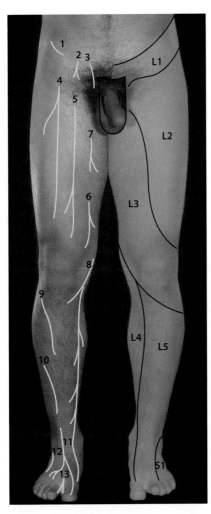

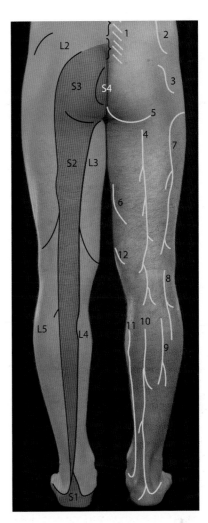

Figure 17.12 Surface anatomy showing lower leg dermatomes (left leg) and cutaneous nerves (right leg), anterior aspect: 1, subcostal; 2, femoral branch of genitofemoral; 3, ilioinguinal; 4, lateral cutaneous of thigh; 5, intermediate cutaneous of thigh; 6, medial cutaneous of thigh; 7, obturator; 8, saphenous; 9, lateral cutaneous of calf; 10 and 11, superficial peroneal (fibular); 12, sural; 13, deep peroneal (fibular)

Figure 17.13 Surface anatomy of lower limb dermatomes (left leg) and cutaneous nerves (right leg), posterior aspect: 1, dorsal rami; 2, subcostal; 3, posterior lumbar rami; 4, posterior cutaneous nerve of thigh; 5, gluteal and perineal branch; 6, obturator; 7, lateral cutaneous nerve of thigh; 8, lateral cutaneous nerve of calf; 9, sural communicating; 10, sural; 11, saphenous; 12, medial cutaneous nerve of thigh

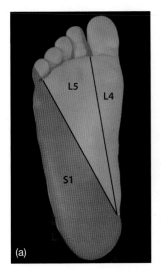

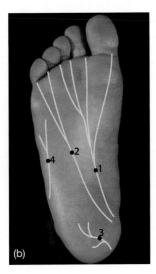

Figure 17.14 Surface anatomy of the sole. (a) Dermatomes. (b) Cutaneous nerves: 1, medial plantar; 2, lateral plantar; 3, medial calcaneal branch of the tibial nerve; 4, sural. L = lumbar, S = sacral

Obturator nerve

Injury to this nerve will produce some loss in the power of adduction, but this is not complete because adductor magnus is partly supplied by the sciatic nerve. Occasionally there is an associated slight loss of sensation over the middle of the medial thigh. This is often related to lateral pelvic wall malignancy.

Sciatic nerve

A proximal injury, e.g. following a posterior dislocation of the hip, produces an almost flail limb (hip flexion is retained)

but there is often no or only minimal loss of sensation (Fig. 17.16).

Tibial nerve

Injury in the leg causes loss of plantar flexion and sensory loss over the sole of the foot. Injury proximal to the sural nerve produces sensory loss over the lateral side of the leg and foot similar to that produced by leprosy affecting the tibial nerve (Fig. 17.17). Injury at the ankle paralyses the small muscles of the foot, and the unopposed action of the long flexors and extensors produces a highly arched foot and claw toes.

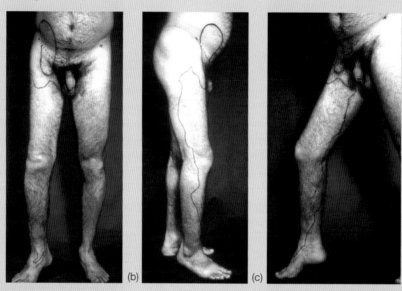

(a)   (b)   (c)

Figure 17.15 (a–c) Femoral nerve palsy caused by a haematoma within the psoas muscle sheath – note the outline of the swelling marked in black across the inguinal region causing right quadriceps wasting and sensory loss over the anteromedial thigh and following the course of the saphenous nerve towards the ankle. The area of sensory loss is marked by the red line

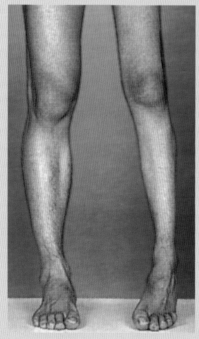

Figure 17.16 Left sciatic nerve palsy with severe muscle wasting below the knee

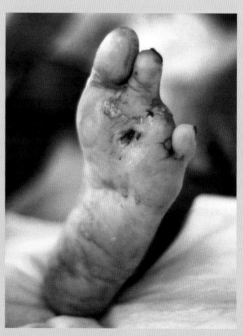

Figure 17.17 Peripheral neuropathy affecting the tibial nerve causing toe loss and ulceration of the sole due to loss of sensation. In developed countries, this palsy is most commonly seen with diabetes mellitus

Common peroneal (fibular) nerve

This is a relatively common injury because of its superficial and vulnerable position as it winds around the neck of the fibula. Dorsiflexion (extensor muscles) and eversion (the peronei) are lost; the foot drops and becomes inverted. There is sensory loss over the medial side of the dorsum of the foot.

Superficial peroneal (fibular) nerve

Eversion (the peronei) is lost and the foot becomes inverted. There is loss of sensation over the medial side of the dorsum of the foot.

Deep peroneal (fibular) nerve

Dorsiflexion of the foot and toes is lost and there may be sensory loss between the first and second toes.

POSTURE AND WALKING

Posture

The body weight is transmitted through the pelvic girdle to both femoral heads. In each limb the weight is transmitted through bones whose internal architecture is adapted to withstand compressive stresses to the foot, whose arches distribute the weight between the calcaneal tubercles and the metatarsal heads. The head of the 1st metatarsal takes more than a third of the metatarsal load.

In the normal stance the line of weight (centre of gravity) in the anatomical position lies in front of the 2nd sacral vertebra and passes slightly behind the hip joints and in front of the knee and ankle joints. The erect posture is maintained by muscles and ligaments. In the anatomical position the body's weight causes hyperextension at the hip and knee, which is resisted at the hip by the iliofemoral ligament and by contraction of iliopsoas. Hyperextension at the knee is resisted by the collateral and cruciate ligaments and contraction of the hamstrings and gastrocnemius. The ankle joint mortise contributes more than the ligaments to the stability of the joint. Slight changes in posture may bring the line of weight behind the knee, and flexion is resisted by contraction of quadriceps. The long digital flexors help by holding the toes firmly to the ground.

Walking

In each limb the cycle of movement has a stance (supporting) phase and a swing phase. The cycle begins as the heel touches the ground and ends as the same heel touches the ground again.

In the **stance (supporting) phase** the body weight is taken on the grounded leg and muscle contraction increases the forward momentum of the body. As the heel touches the ground, extension of the hip joint gives a forward thrust and medial rotation maintains the direction of progress. Meanwhile, hip abduction by gluteus minimus, gluteus medius and tensor fasciae latae tilts the pelvis on the grounded leg, giving the swinging leg some height to move forward. The knee of the grounded leg is extended and locked, so that weight is carried by bones and ligaments, and at the end of this swing the grounded knee is unlocked by lateral rotation of the femur on the tibia. At the ankle joint, plantar flexion, which is partly passive, gives way to active dorsiflexion, so that the body weight is pulled over the ankle and the foot becomes slightly everted, and the body weight is transferred from the heel along the lateral border of the foot to the metatarsal heads.

The swing phase

In this, the leg swings through from a trailing to a leading position. At the hip joint, there is flexion, lateral rotation and adduction. At the knee joint, flexion occurs until the swinging foot has passed the supporting foot and then extension occurs, at the end of which some lateral rotation of the tibia may lock the knee joint in preparation for weight-bearing. At the ankle joint, the foot is first dorsiflexed but then becomes plantar-flexed as the knee extends. The foot itself becomes inverted and the heel touches the ground (heel strike) in readiness for the next supporting phase.

Starting to **walk** involves a forward tilting of the body, thus advancing the centre of gravity and the line of weight. The supporting limb is extended, the pelvis is tilted on the supporting limb and the heel is raised by the calf muscles. The opposite limb flexes and then extends until the heel touches the ground. Thus it becomes the supporting limb after a very short swing phase. Turning to left or right involves most of the trunk muscles as well as the rotators at the hip joint. They largely determine the route followed by the swinging leg and the position of the touch-down of the swinging heel.

In **running**, the centre of gravity is usually further forward due to flexion of the vertebral column, thus altering the total posture. There is considerable time between the end of the stance phase and the heel strike of the foot of the swinging leg, so that the body is clear of the ground (unsupported) for this time. In running, active plantar flexion at the ankle joint at the end of the stance phase increases the forward momentum of the body.

Although described separately, these movements merge indistinguishably into one another. Limitation of the movement at any joint results in a marked alteration in gait. The individuality of the gait depends on the length of the stride, the extent of pelvic rotation (swinging the hips) and the impetus at the end of the stance phase.

MCQs

1. In the adult foot: **T/F**
  a inversion is increased in plantar flexion   (___)
  b eversion is increased in plantar flexion   (___)
  c eversion is produced by tibialis anterior   (___)
  d inversion is produced by the peroneal   (___)
     (fibular) muscles
  e eversion is limited by tension in the deltoid   (___)
     ligament

Answers

1.

a **T** – *The movement is greatest in plantar flexion because the narrower posterior part of the talus allows more movement in the plantar-flexed ankle joint.*
b **F** – *The range of eversion is greatest in dorsiflexion.*
c **F** – *It is produced by the peroneal (fibular) muscles.*
d **F** – *It is produced by the synergistic action of tibialis anterior and posterior muscles and limited by tension in the peroneal (fibular) muscles and the interosseous talocalcaneal ligament ...*
e **T** – *... and also by tension in the tibialis muscles.*

---

2. The arches of the foot: **T/F**
  a cause the weight of the body to be concen-   (___)
     trated in a small area of the sole
  b give the foot rigidity   (___)
  c are dependent on bony factors alone   (___)
  d are not present at birth   (___)
  e are supported by prominent plantar capsu-   (___)
     lar thickenings

Answers

2.

a **F** – *They allow weight to be spread over a wide area.*
b **F** – *They make it resilient and well suited to absorb impacts when jumping.*
c **F** – *The maintenance of the arches is dependent on muscular, ligamentous and bony factors.*
d **F** – *They are present but masked by fat.*
e **T** – *They are stronger and more numerous than the dorsal capsular thickenings.*

---

3. In the lower limb damage to: **T/F**
  a L4 results in an absent ankle jerk   (___)
  b L2 results in weakened hip flexion   (___)
  c the obturator nerve results in little or no   (___)
     sensory loss
  d the tibial nerve results in loss of sensation   (___)
     on the sole of the foot
  e S1 may result in weakness of eversion   (___)

Answers

3.

a **F** – *L4 is the spinal nerve involved in the knee jerk.*
b **T** – *Damage to L2 affects the contraction of iliopsoas, attached to the lesser trochanter, and is a powerful flexor of the hip.*
c **T** – *Remember that all cutaneous sensory supply involves much overlapping between nerves.*
d **T** – *And also loss of the ankle jerk reflex.*
e **T** – *Damage to S1 also involves a loss of sensation posterior to the lateral malleolus, as well as causing problems with plantar flexion and an absent ankle jerk.*

SBA

1. A young man was admitted having fallen while running downhill over rough ground. His right ankle was swollen and there was tenderness over his medial malleolus and the lateral side of his right lower leg. X-rays showed a fracture of the medial malleolus and a spiral fracture of the lower third of the fibula. What is the probable mechanism that caused this type of injury?

a forced inversion of the ankle
b an upward compressive force from the talus hitting the lower articular surface of the tibia
c forced eversion and external rotation of the ankle
d forced dorsiflexion of the foot
e extreme plantar flexion of the foot

Answer

c *This is the typical injury following forceful eversion of the ankle and is known as a Pott's fracture; the talus is forced laterally and, by its attachment to the strong deltoid ligament, causes a fracture of the medial malleolus, together with forceful lateral displacement of the external malleolus producing a spiral fracture of the shaft of the fibula.*

2. An elderly man with bladder cancer begins to have difficulty walking. Examination reveals some weakness in the adductor muscles of his right thigh and loss of sensation over the middle of the medial aspect of his right thigh. What nerve do you suspect has been affected?

a obturator
b femoral
c sciatic
d tibial
e peroneal

Answer

a *The obturator nerve lies on the lateral wall of the pelvis, where an advanced bladder cancer may compress and infiltrate it. Damage to the nerve will cause some loss of adduction of the hip but this is not complete because adductor magnus is supplied in part by the sciatic nerve. There may also be a slight loss of sensation over the middle part of the medial surface of the thigh.*

EMQs

Each question has an anatomical theme linked to the chapter, and a list of 10 related items (A–J) placed in alphabetical order: these are followed by five statements (1–5). Match **one or more** of the items A–J to each of the five statements.

Cutaneous innervation of the lower leg
A. 1st sacral dermatome
B. 2nd lumbar dermatome
C. 3rd lumbar dermatome
D. 3rd sacral dermatome
E. 4th lumbar dermatome
F. 5th lumbar dermatome
G. Lateral cutaneous nerve of thigh
H. Obturator nerve
I. Saphenous nerve
J. Sural nerve

Answers
1 C; 2 EI; 3 A; 4 D; 5 BCH

Match the following cutaneous innervation to the nerve(s) and dermatome(s) in the above list.
1. Front of the patella
2. Medial aspect of the ankle
3. Sole of the foot
4. Buttock
5. Medial aspect of the thigh

APPLIED QUESTIONS

1. Describe the anatomical basis for 'flat feet'.

1. In infants the flat appearance of the feet is normal, a result of the subcutaneous fat pads in the soles. Bony arches are present at birth, but only become visible after the baby has walked for a few months. Flat feet in adolescents and adults are caused by 'fallen arches', usually the medial longitudinal. During long periods of standing, older persons, or those who rapidly gain weight, stretch the plantar ligaments and aponeurosis, which are non-elastic structures, with the loss of their important bowstringing effect in the stationary foot. The strain on the spring ligament eventually makes it unable to support the head of the talus, and as a result flattening of the medial longitudinal arch occurs, with lateral deviation of the forefoot. Fallen arches are painful owing to stretching of the plantar muscles and strained plantar ligaments. Pes planus is a true flattening from osteomuscular causes.

2. Why is it not uncommon to find that the patient with a severe sprain of the ankle has an avulsion fracture of the 5th metatarsal?

2. In severe inversion injuries tension is exerted on the laterally placed muscles, in particular the peronei. Peroneus (fibularis) brevis, originating from the fibula, inserts into the tuberosity of the 5th metatarsal. Tension on this insertion often results in its fracture. It is not uncommon to find, in younger patients, that the normal radiological appearances of the epiphysis in this region are wrongly thought to represent a fracture of the tuberosity.

Bailey & Love · Essential Clinical Anatomy
Essential Clinical Anatomy · Bailey & Love
Bailey & Love · Essential Clinical Anatomy

PART **6**

The head and neck

Chapter **18**

The skull, scalp and face

THE SKULL

The skull, a term that includes the mandible, is described viewed from above, from in front, from the side and from below.

Superior aspect

The vault (roof of the cranium) is crossed by three sutures (Fig. 18.1). The **coronal suture** separates the frontal bone from the two parietal bones posteriorly. The midline **sagittal suture** separates the two parietal bones. Its junction with the coronal suture, the **bregma**, is incompletely ossified at birth and can be felt as a diamond-shaped deficiency known as the **anterior fontanelle**. This closes at about 18 months of age. The **lambdoid suture** separates the two parietal bones and the occipital bone posteriorly, and meets the sagittal suture at the **lambda**. This, too, is not ossified at birth and presents as a small bony deficiency, the **posterior fontanelle**, which closes by the 3rd to 6th month.

An early fusion of fontanelles may cause a restriction of brain growth; a late closure of the fontanelles may be an indication of an increased intracranial pressure that has resulted from an accumulation of cerebrospinal fluid (CSF) (hydrocephalus) (**Fig. 18.2**). Hydrocephalus is the result of (a) overproduction of CSF, (b) obstruction to its flow, or (c) a decrease in its absorption. Surgical treatment usually involves draining the CSF into the venous system by means of an indwelling shunt.

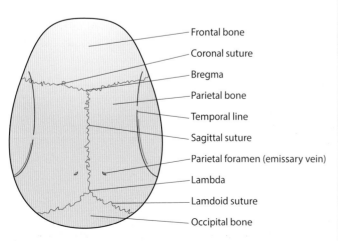

Figure 18.1 Bones and sutures of vault

- Frontal bone
- Coronal suture
- Bregma
- Parietal bone
- Temporal line
- Sagittal suture
- Parietal foramen (emissary vein)
- Lambda
- Lamdoid suture
- Occipital bone

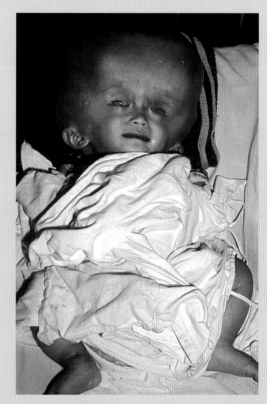

Figure 18.2 Severe untreated hydrocephalus

Anterior aspect

The smooth convexity of the frontal bone lies superiorly; below it are the openings of the orbital, nasal and oral cavities (Figs. 18.3a–c). The **supraorbital margin** possesses a supraorbital notch or foramen in its inner third, which transmits the supraorbital vessels and nerve. The lateral orbital margin is formed by the frontal and zygomatic bones (the frontozygomatic suture is subcutaneous and palpable), the medial margin by the frontal bone and the frontal process of the maxilla, the inferior margin by the maxillary bone medially, and the lateral margin by the zygomatic bone. Above the supraorbital margins are the palpable superciliary arches, between which lies the **glabella**.

The prominence of the cheek is produced by the zygomatic bone. One centimetre below the orbit on the maxilla, in line with the supraorbital notch, is the **infraorbital foramen**, from which emerge the infraorbital vessels and nerve. The **nasal aperture** is bounded above by the nasal bones, and below and laterally by the maxillae. The opening of the oral cavity is surrounded by the alveolar margins of the maxillae and mandible, which bear sockets for the teeth. The **mental foramen** on the mandible is in line with the supra- and infraorbital foramina, and from it emerge the mental vessels and nerve.

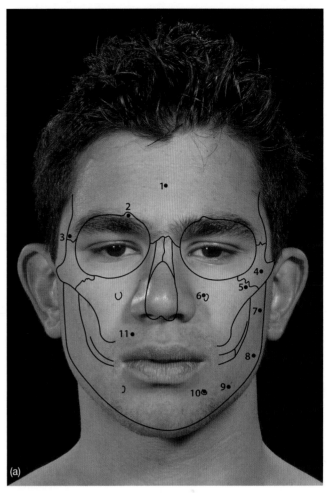

(a)

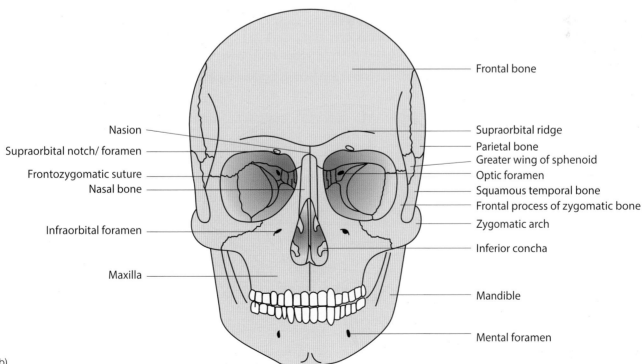

(b)

Figure 18.3 (a) Surface anatomy of the facial skeleton: 1, frontal bone; 2, supraorbital notch; 3, frontozygomatic suture; 4, zygomatic bone; 5, zygomaxillary suture; 6, infraorbital foramen; 7, ramus of mandible; 8, angle of mandible; 9, body of mandible; 10, mental foramen; 11, maxilla. (b) Skull – anterior view. (*continued*)

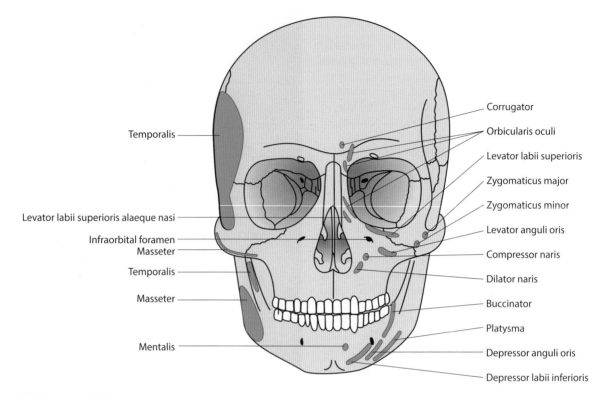

(c)

Figure 18.3 (*continued*) (c) Anterior view showing muscle attachments

Lateral aspect

The **zygomatic arch** is formed by the zygomatic process of the temporal bone and the temporal process of the zygomatic bone (Fig. 18.4). The temporal superior line curves upwards and backwards from the zygomatic process of the frontal bone across the parietal bone, and then down and forwards over the squamous temporal bone to end above the external acous-

tic meatus. The region below the temporal line, deep to the zygomatic arch, is the **temporal fossa**, which is roofed by the temporal fascia attached to the temporal line and the upper border of the zygomatic arch. The medial wall of the fossa is formed by the frontal, parietal, temporal and greater wing of the sphenoid bones. Their H-shaped union, the **pterion**, lies about 4 cm above the midpoint of the zygomatic arch.

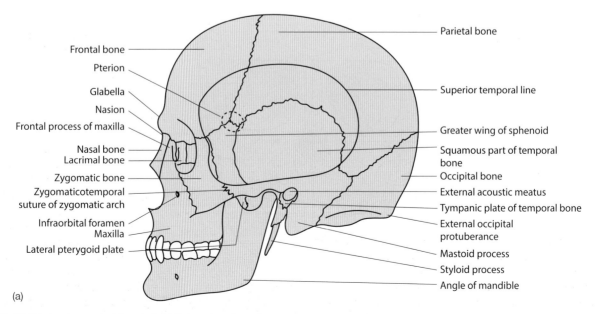

(a)

Figure 18.4 Lateral aspect of the skull: (a) Bones. (*continued*)

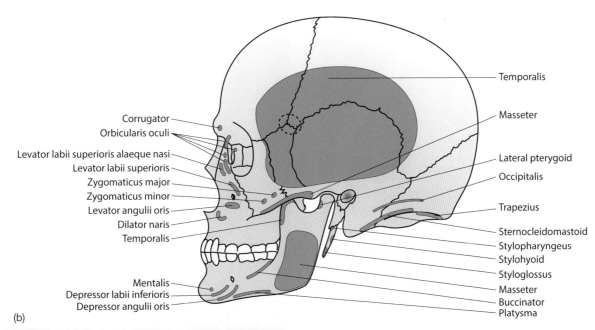

Corrugator
Orbicularis oculi
Levator labii superioris alaeque nasi
Levator labii superioris
Zygomaticus major
Zygomaticus minor
Levator angulii oris
Dilator naris
Temporalis

Mentalis
Depressor labii inferioris
Depressor angulii oris

Temporalis
Masseter
Lateral pterygoid
Occipitalis
Trapezius
Sternocleidomastoid
Stylopharyngeus
Stylohyoid
Styloglossus
Masseter
Buccinator
Platysma

(b)

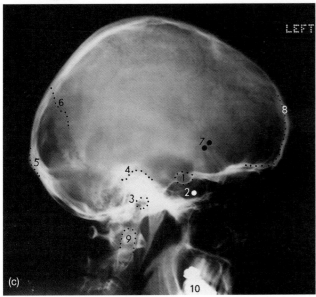

(c)

Figure 18.4 (*continued*) (b) Muscle attachments. (c) X-ray: 1, pituitary fossa; 2, sphenoidal air sinus; 3, external acoustic (auditory) meatus; 4, petrous temporal bone; 5, external occipital protuberance; 6, parieto-occipital suture; 7, meningeal vessel markings; 8, frontal bone; 9, dens of axis; 10, dental fillings

Below the temporal fossa is the **infratemporal fossa**, limited medially by the lateral pterygoid plate, which communicates with the pterygopalatine fossa through the pterygomaxillary fissure and with the orbit through the inferior orbital fissure. The **external acoustic meatus** opens below the posterior zygomatic arch and the palpable **mastoid process** is prominent behind the meatus.

The pterion overlies where the middle meningeal artery grooves the inner surface of the bone and is therefore an important clinical landmark. A blow to the side of the head may fracture the thin bones of the pterion and rupture the middle meningeal vessels. The resulting haematoma lies outside the dural covering of the brain but exerts pressure and compression on the underlying brain (Fig. 18.5). If the hae-matoma continues to grow, death may follow in hours without surgical treatment, which involves raising a flap of skin (whose base lies inferiorly, because it is from this direction that all vessels and nerves reach the scalp) over the pterion and drilling a burr hole. The haemorrhage from the middle meningeal artery may be stopped and the haematoma evacuated through this burr hole.

Hard blows to the head result in fractures that usually radiate out from the site of impact in rather straight lines. A severe blow, such as from a hammer or a bullet, may cause a depressed fracture in which several small pieces of skull detach and are driven into the brain. The depressed fragments require surgical elevation (Fig. 18.6). Fractures of the cranial base will be discussed later (p. 310).

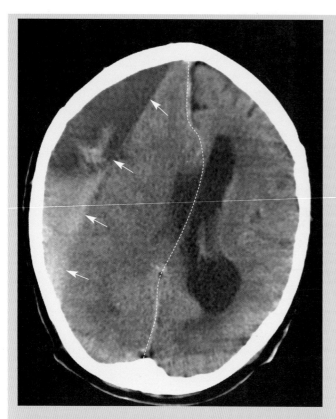

Figure 18.5 Extradural haematoma (arrows) showing a cerebral shift – the dotted line shows the midline shift

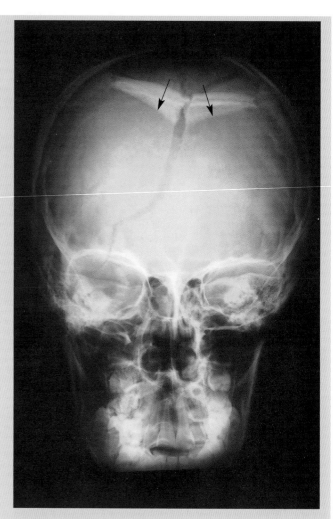

Figure 18.6 Depressed fracture of the skull (arrows)

Inferior aspect

Anteriorly is the hard palate, formed by the palatine processes of the maxillae in front of the horizontal plates of the palatine bones (Fig. 18.7). It is bounded anterolaterally by the alveolar processes of the maxillae, whose rounded posterior extremity is the maxillary tuberosity. Anteriorly a midline incisive foramen communicates with the nasal cavity and transmits the greater palatine arteries and nasopalatine nerves; on the posterolateral palate are the greater and lesser palatine foramina, which convey vessels and nerves of the same name. The **posterior nasal apertures (choanae)** open above the palate, bounded above by the body of the sphenoid bone, below by the horizontal plates of the palatine bones and laterally by the medial pterygoid plates. The apertures are separated by the thin, wedge-shaped midline **vomer**. From the medial pterygoid plate projects the **hamulus** (Fig. 18.8), which gives attachment to the pterygomandibular raphé. Behind the base of the lateral pterygoid process is the foramen ovale, which transmits the mandibular nerve, and posterolateral to the foramen are the spine of the sphenoid and the foramen spinosum, which transmits

the middle meningeal artery. To the spine of the sphenoid is attached the sphenomandibular ligament, and lateral to the spine is the **mandibular fossa**, with which the mandibular condyle articulates. The petrous temporal bone lies between the occipital and sphenoid bones and contains the carotid canal, whose inferior opening lies behind the spine of the sphenoid. Posterolateral to the carotid opening is the **jugular foramen**, which transmits the internal jugular vein and the glossopharyngeal, vagus and accessory nerves. Posterolateral to the styloid process is the stylomastoid foramen, which transmits the facial nerve. The occipital bone contains the **foramen magnum**, bounded on each side by the occipital condyles, and a foramen transmitting the hypoglossal nerve.

Posterior aspect

Behind the foramen magnum are the superior and inferior nuchal lines, between which are attached the postvertebral muscles. In the middle of the superior line is the prominent and palpable **external occipital protuberance**.

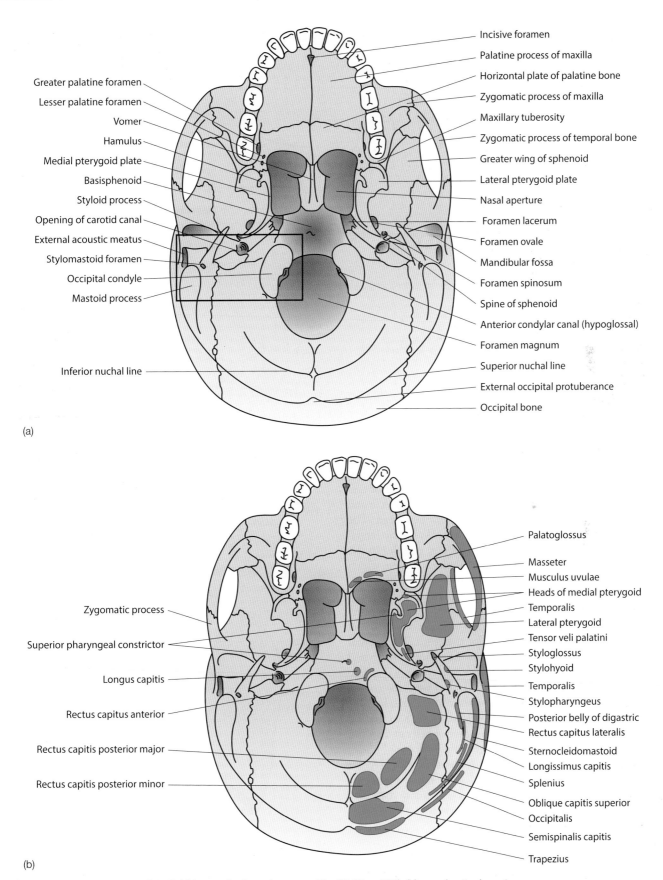

Greater palatine foramen
Lesser palatine foramen
Vomer
Hamulus
Medial pterygoid plate
Basisphenoid
Styloid process
Opening of carotid canal
External acoustic meatus
Stylomastoid foramen
Occipital condyle
Mastoid process

Inferior nuchal line

Incisive foramen
Palatine process of maxilla
Horizontal plate of palatine bone
Zygomatic process of maxilla
Maxillary tuberosity
Zygomatic process of temporal bone
Greater wing of sphenoid
Lateral pterygoid plate
Nasal aperture
Foramen lacerum
Foramen ovale
Mandibular fossa
Foramen spinosum
Spine of sphenoid
Anterior condylar canal (hypoglossal)
Foramen magnum
Superior nuchal line
External occipital protuberance
Occipital bone

(a)

Zygomatic process

Superior pharyngeal constrictor

Longus capitis

Rectus capitus anterior

Rectus capitis posterior major

Rectus capitis posterior minor

Palatoglossus
Masseter
Musculus uvulae
Heads of medial pterygoid
Temporalis
Lateral pterygoid
Tensor veli palatini
Styloglossus
Stylohyoid
Temporalis
Stylopharyngeus
Posterior belly of digastric
Rectus capitus lateralis
Sternocleidomastoid
Longissimus capitis
Splenius
Oblique capitis superior
Occipitalis
Semispinalis capitis
Trapezius

(b)

Figure 18.7 Inferior aspect of skull: (a) bones (for boxed area see Fig. 21.17, p. 366); (b) muscle attachments

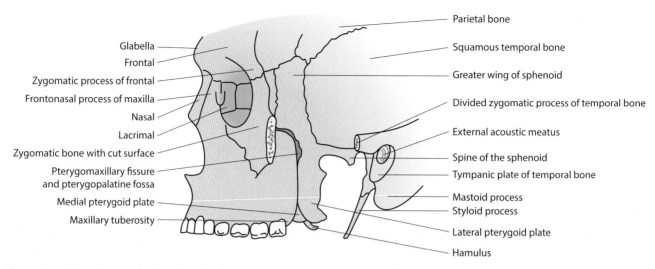

Figure 18.8 Lateral view of the skull showing the styloid process and pterygoid plate

THE INDIVIDUAL BONES OF THE SKULL

The mandible

The mandible (**Fig. 18.9**) is formed by the midline union of two halves, each with a horizontal body and a vertical ramus whose posterior junction forms the palpable **angle** of the mandible. The **ramus** is flat and rectangular. Superiorly it has two processes separated by the **mandibular notch**; the anterior **coronoid process** gives attachment to the temporalis muscle and the posterior **condylar process** bears an articular head. The lateral pterygoid muscle is attached to its neck. To the lateral surface of the ramus is attached the masseter muscle. In the centre of the medial surface is the **mandibular foramen**, which transmits the inferior alveolar vessels and nerve; its lower lip, the **lingula**, gives attachment to the sphenomandibular ligament. The medial pterygoid muscle is attached below the foramen. The **body** has a smooth inferior border and an upper alveolar border containing sockets for the teeth. The **mental foramen** is on the lateral surface below the premolar teeth and transmits the mental vessels and nerve. On the inner surface the **mylohyoid line** passes downwards and forwards to the midline and gives attachment to the mylohyoid muscle. This separates the fossa for the sublingual gland above from that for the submandibular gland below. The anterior belly of digastric muscle is attached in the midline below the mylohyoid line.

Loss of teeth in old age results in absorption of alveolar bone, so that the mental foramen, which lies midway between the upper and lower borders in adult life, is nearer to the lower border at birth and nearer to the alveolar border in old age.

Maxilla

Each maxilla (**Figs. 18.3, 18.4** and **18.8**) consists of a body and four processes. The **body** contains the **maxillary air sinus**. Its thin superior (orbital) surface forms the larger part of the orbital floor. The **zygomatic process** (**Fig. 18.7b**) extends lat-

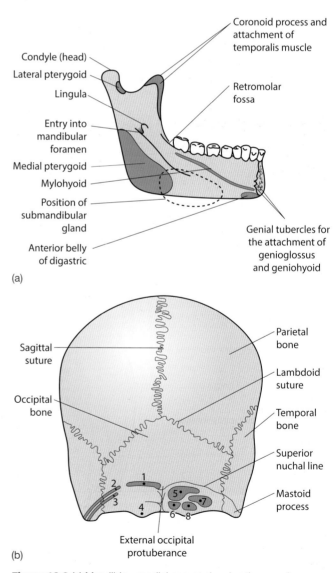

Figure 18.9 (a) Mandible – medial aspect showing the muscle attachments. (b) Posterior aspect of the skull, showing the bones and muscle attachments: 1, trapezius; 2, sternocleidomastoid; 3, splenius capitus; 4, occipital condyle; 5, semispinalis capitis; 6, rectus capitis posterior minor; 7, superior oblique; 8, rectus capitis posterior major

erally to the zygomatic bone. The **alveolar process** projects downwards and bears the upper teeth, and its posterior extension forms the **maxillary tuberosity**. The horizontal **palatine process** contributes to the hard palate. The **frontal process** articulates with the frontal bone and forms part of the medial wall of the orbit.

The infraorbital nerve may be damaged in fractures of the maxilla and produce sensory loss over the cheek. An associated fracture of the zygomatic bone is common and may be marked by painful limitation of movement in the temporomandibular joint. Fractures involving the orbital floor (Fig. 18.10) may give rise to 'double vision'.

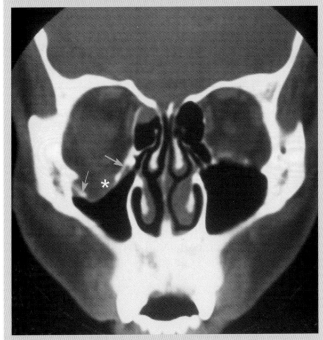

Figure 18.10 Coronal CT scan of face showing a 'blow-out' orbital floor fracture (arrows) with protrusion of orbital contents into the maxillary sinus (*). This type of fracture is usually a sports injury, squash being one of the most common causes – see also Fig. 19.2, p. 316

The sphenoid

The sphenoid (see p. 358 and Fig. 20.10, p. 346) consists of a central body from which two pairs of processes (the greater and lesser wings) extend laterally and two processes, the pterygoid processes, pass inferiorly. The cube-shaped **body** encloses the paired sphenoidal air sinuses. The inferior surface roofs in the nasopharynx. The superior surface is indented to form the **pituitary fossa** (sella turcica), anterior to which is the **optic groove** and posterior to which is the **dorsum sellae**, bearing the **posterior clinoid processes** projecting upwards over the fossa.

Each greater wing has four surfaces: the concave upper surface supports the temporal lobe of the brain; the lower surface, which overlies the infratemporal fossa, bears the **spine of the sphenoid** (Figs. 18.7a and 18.8); the anterior region is the posterolateral wall of the orbit; and the lateral surface contributes to the medial wall of the temporal fossa.

A swelling within the fossa from a pituitary tumour may produce pressure on the optic nerve or chiasma, causing visual defects (Fig. 18.11).

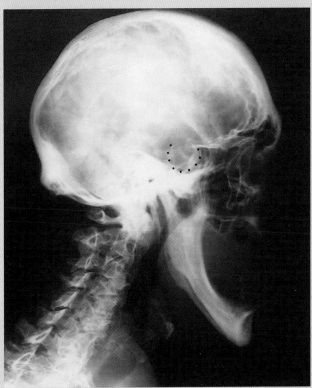

Figure 18.11 Lateral view of skull showing pituitary enlargement in a patient with acromegaly (pituitary fossa outlined with dots)

The lesser wing of the sphenoid extends laterally and forms the posterior limit of the floor of the anterior cranial fossa. The **anterior clinoid process** projects medially from the posterior border. Between the lesser wing and the body is the **optic canal**, and between the lesser and greater wings is the **superior orbital fissure**. From the **pterygoid process** hang downward projecting medial and lateral **pterygoid plates**, which unite anteriorly to bound the pterygoid fossa.

The temporal bones

Each **temporal bone** consists of four parts: squamous, petromastoid, tympanic and styloid. The **squamous part** (Fig. 18.4a) is a thin plate of bone on the lateral skull, articulating with the greater wing of the sphenoid and the parietal bone. Its zygomatic process extends forwards from the lateral surface and contributes to the zygomatic arch. Below the process is the **mandibular fossa** (Fig. 18.7a) for the condyle of the mandible. The thin squamous part contributes to the external acoustic meatus. The dense **petromastoid part** contains the middle and inner ears and extends medially between the sphenoid and occipital bones. Its upper surface forms part of the floor of the middle and posterior cranial fossae. The part forming the front of the posterior fossa is pierced by the **internal acoustic meatus**, which transmits the facial and vestibulocochlear nerves. The inferior surface contains the **carotid** canal for the internal carotid artery, and the **jugular fossa** lies between it and the occipital bone. The bony **auditory tube** opens anteriorly on to the inferior surface of the petrous temporal bone. The **mastoid process** (see Figs. 18.4 and 18.7a) is prominent posteriorly and contains the tympanic antrum and mastoid air cells.

Before the advent of antibiotics, and even nowadays in the developing world, infection in the mastoid air cells (mastoiditis) was difficult to eradicate owing to the spongy nature of this bony cavity, which usually provides a barrier to easy drainage of the infection (Fig. 18.12).

Fractures of the skull base usually tear the dura and arachnoid mater and thereby cause leakage of CSF externally by the ear or nose. More rarely they may tear the internal carotid artery as it lies within the cavernous sinus, producing an acute arteriovenous fistula. This becomes clinically evident as the pressure within the draining ophthalmic veins increases to produce a protruding pulsating eye. There may also be injuries to the cranial nerves lying close to the sinus – III, IV, V and VI.

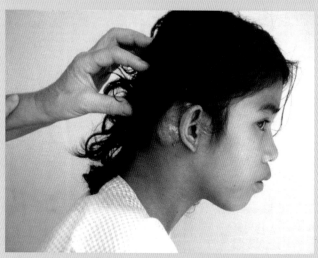

Figure 18.12 Mastoiditis in a child – note pus exuding from the swollen, inflamed mastoid process, which is pushing the pinna forwards

The **tympanic part** of the temporal bone is a curved plate forming the anterior wall and floor of the bony external acoustic meatus. The **styloid process** develops from the second arch cartilage (Fig. 18.8) and is a slender downward projection of the petrous part. About 2 cm long, it gives attachment to stylopharyngeus, stylohyoid, and styloglossus, and the stylohyoid and stylomandibular ligaments. The **stylomastoid foramen** (Fig. 18.7a), between it and the mastoid process, transmits the facial nerve.

The occipital bone

The **occipital bone** (Figs. 18.4, 18.7a and 18.9b) has a basilar, a squamous and two lateral portions around the **foramen magnum**. The **squamous part**, a flat plate, extends backwards and upwards to articulate with the parietal and mastoid part of the temporal bone. The outer part is marked by the **superior** and **inferior nuchal lines** and the

external occipital protuberance; it gives attachment to the postvertebral muscles. The intracranial surface is grooved by the superior sagittal and transverse venous sinuses. The **lateral parts** bear, inferiorly, the **occipital condyles** for articulation with the atlas. Anteriorly the **hypoglossal canal** conveys the hypoglossal nerve.

The parietal bones

The **parietal bones** (Figs. 18.1 and 18.4) are two convex quadrilateral plates the form the posterior skull vault. They meet at the sagittal suture and articulate anteriorly with the frontal bone at the coronal suture, and posteriorly with the occipital bone at the lambdoid suture.

The measurement across the fetal skull – the 'biparietal distance' – is used in ultrasonography to monitor intrauterine growth.

The frontal bone

The **frontal bone** (Figs. 18.1 and 18.4) has a domed superior portion forming the anterior skull vault, and its inferior horizontal **orbital plates** contribute to the roof of each orbit. It articulates superiorly with the parietal bones at the coronal suture and inferiorly with the sphenoid, zygomatic, nasal and ethmoid bones and frontal process of the maxilla. The orbital plates meet the lesser wings of the sphenoid posteriorly. The paired **frontal air sinuses** are within the bone above the nose and the medial part of the orbit. In a small proportion of individuals a persistent frontal (metopic) suture remains throughout adult life and should not be mistaken for a fracture.

The zygomatic bones

The **zygomatic bones** (Figs. 18.3, 18.4a and 18.7) form the prominence of each cheek. Their orbital surface contributes to the lateral wall of the orbit, their lateral surface forms the prominence of the cheek and their temporal surface forms the anterior limit of the temporal fossa. The temporal process forms the anterior part of the zygomatic arch, the frontal process articulates with the frontal bone and the zygoma articulates with the maxilla and with the greater wing of the sphenoid in the lateral wall of the orbit.

A fracture of this bone or the orbital plate of the maxillary bone may result in 'double vision' (diplopia) as a result of the eyeball being displaced downwards (Fig. 18.10).

The nasal bones

The **nasal bones** (Figs. 18.3 and 18.4a) meet anteriorly in the midline and form the skeleton of the upper part of the external nose. They articulate with the frontal bone, and with the frontal processes of the maxillae.

The **ethmoid bone** (Fig. 21.8, p. 359) consists of a midline **perpendicular plate** and a perforated horizontal **cribriform plate** uniting its two **ethmoidal labyrinths**. Between the two cribriform plates a median ridge – the crista galli – projects superiorly. The cribriform plate conveys the olfactory nerves from the forebrain to the nose.

A fracture involving the cribriform plate may result not only in loss of the sense of smell (**anosmia**), but also in tearing of the dura mater that covers the nerve, resulting in a leak of CSF from the nose (**CSF rhinorrhoea**).

Each ethmoidal labyrinth contains the ethmoidal air cells, which lie in the lateral wall of the nose (Figs. 19.18 and 19.19, p. 322) and are the immediate medial relation of the orbit.

The **lacrimal bones** (Fig. 19.1, p. 315) are small thin bones lying on the medial wall of the orbit and each, with the frontal process of the maxilla, surrounds the lacrimal sac and duct.

THE SCALP

The scalp covers the vault of the skull, extending from the supraorbital margins anteriorly to the superior nuchal line posteriorly. It consists of five layers (**SCALP**):

- Thick **S**kin containing many hair follicles and sweat glands.
- Fibrous **C**onnective tissue that is adherent to the skin and to the underlying aponeurosis. It is richly supplied with vessels and nerves embedded within it.
- Musculofibrous epicranial **A**poneurosis containing the **occipitalis muscle** posteriorly and the **frontalis muscle** in front. Laterally the aponeurosis is attached to the temporal fascia. Anteriorly the frontalis has no bony attachment but blends with the fibres of the orbicularis oculi muscles. Occipitalis is attached to the superior nuchal line. Occipitofrontalis draws the scalp backwards in frowning and raises the eyebrows. It is innervated by the facial nerve.
- **L**oose areolar tissue, which allows free movement of the aponeurosis and overlying skin over the periosteum.

Scalping injuries, such as those caused by long hair catching in moving machinery, pull the outer layers of the scalp away from the skull along this layer.

- The **P**eriosteum (pericranium) of the bones of the vault, which is continuous through the sutures of the vault with the endocranium.

The scalp is richly supplied by anastomosing branches of the external carotid (occipital, posterior auricular and superficial temporal arteries) and ophthalmic arteries (supraorbital and supratrochlear arteries). Veins accompany the arteries and drain to the external and internal jugular veins. They may communicate with the diploic veins of the skull via numerous emissary veins, and hence with the intracranial dural venous sinuses.

Scalp wounds bleed profusely but usually heal without hindrance or infection because of the rich blood supply. As the vessels are supported by the surrounding connective tissue, they do not retract as readily as do other vessels. Bleeding will continue from a scalp wound until local pressure or sutures closes the vessels. Surgeons have devised numerous skin flaps based on the vascular pedicles of the dozen or so branches that anastomose within the scalp, and employ these to fashion skin flaps that, attached to an underlying segment of the cranium, allow craniotomies to be performed. Blood or pus collecting under the scalp is limited posteriorly by the attachment of occipitalis and the temporal fascia and cannot spread into the occipital or subtemporal regions. A scalp

infection can spread via the diploic and emissary veins to involve the skull bones, the meninges or even occasionally the dural venous sinuses.

The sensory innervation of the scalp is by the trigeminal, lesser and greater occipital nerves and the dorsal rami of the second and third cervical nerves (Fig. 23.9, p. 394). Lymph vessels pass to lymph nodes in the circular chain around the base of the skull; posteriorly to the occipital and mastoid nodes and anteriorly to the preauricular nodes. All eventually drain to the deep cervical nodes.

THE FACE

The face contains the external openings of the mouth, nose and orbit. Facial skin is thin, sensitive and hairy. In males, facial hair is very dense over the temporal fossa, the zygomatic arch and the mandibular region. Voluntary facial muscles are attached to it. The subcutaneous tissue is very vascular and has a varying amount of fat; there is no fat in the eyelids. There is no deep fascia in most of the face, and sweat and sebaceous glands are abundant. The mucocutaneous junction around the mouth is on the facial aspect of the lips (the red margin). Mucous and small salivary glands are present on the inner aspect of the lips and cheeks.

The **facial muscles** (Figs. 18.4b and 18.13) are the muscles of facial expression and are arranged as sphincters and dilators around the mouth, nose and orbit. They are all innervated by the facial nerve.

Orbicularis oris is the sphincter around the mouth and forms the greater part of the substance of the lips. Contraction produces pouting lips, as in whistling and kissing. Other muscles blend with it, such as the buccinator and the levator and depressor muscles, which are attached to the angles of the mouth (anguli) and to the middle of the lips (labii).

Buccinator forms the greater part of the cheek. It has a continuous lateral attachment to the pterygomandibular raphé and the outer surfaces of the maxillae and mandible adjacent to the last molar tooth. Its fibres pass forwards and medially,

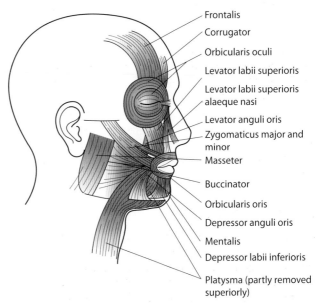

Frontalis
Corrugator
Orbicularis oculi
Levator labii superioris
Levator labii superioris alaeque nasi
Levator anguli oris
Zygomaticus major and minor
Masseter
Buccinator
Orbicularis oris
Depressor anguli oris
Mentalis
Depressor labii inferioris
Platysma (partly removed superiorly)

Figure 18.13 The facial muscles

decussate behind the angle of the mouth and enter the lips, blending with orbicularis oris. The muscle keeps food out of the vestibule and between the teeth in chewing, and is used to increase the pressure in forced blowing (e.g. in trombone players).

Orbicularis oculi surrounds the opening of the orbit and has palpebral and orbital parts. The central palpebral fibres lie within the eyelids; the peripheral orbital fibres surround the orbital margin and are attached by the medial palpebral ligament to the frontal process of the maxilla. The fibres blend with frontalis above the orbit. The palpebral part closes the eyelid in sleep, winking and blinking; the orbital part closes the eye more forcefully and is used in frowning.

Platysma is a broad flat sheet of muscle lying in the superficial fascia on each side of the neck. Superiorly it passes over the mandible to blend with muscles around the mouth; inferi-

orly it blends with the superficial fascia over the upper part of the chest. It is a weak depressor of the jaw.

Vessels and nerves

The face is supplied mainly by the facial and transverse facial arteries and is drained by the facial and retromandibular veins (p. 393 and Fig. 23.6, p. 393). Lymph drainage is to the submental nodes, that of the medial part of the cheek and face to the submandibular nodes and that of the forehead and lateral part of the cheek to the parotid nodes. Sensory nerves are conveyed by the three divisions of the trigeminal nerve (Table 18.1) and, over the jaw, by the great auricular nerve. Their distribution is illustrated in Fig. 23.9, p. 394. Motor innervation is by the facial nerve.

TABLE 18.1 Practical cranial nerve functions: a clinical anatomist's guide to testing

Nerve	Site of injury or disease	How to test	Abnormal signs
I. Olfactory **	Fracture across cribiform plate	Odour to each nostril	Anosmia (no sense of smell)
II. Optic ***	1 Optic foramen fracture 2 Extrasellar extension of pituitary tumour 3 Disease of optic tract and visual cortex	Shine light in affected eyes Assess visual fields Assess visual fields	Loss of direct + consensual pupil constriction Bitemporal hemianopia Homonymous hemianopia
III. Oculomotor **	Fracture across middle cranial fossa and raised intracranial pressure	Shine light in affected eye Shine light in normal eye	Direct pupil reflex absent Consensual reflex present Direct reflex present Consensual reflex absent Eye turned down and out Ptosis and dilated pupil
IV. Trochlear *	Brainstem tumour or orbital fracture	Needs specialist ocular testing	Eye fails to look down and out Patient has diplopia
V. Trigeminal **	Direct injury to maxillary and mandibular nerves in head and neck surgery and trauma	1 Sensation to cornea 2 Sensation to cheek 3 Sensation to chin 3a Sensation to lips and cheek 4 Motor – 'Clench your teeth'	Numbness or paraesthesia Masseter and temporalis fail to contract
VI. Abducens **	Fractures across both the orbit and the middle cranial fossa Raised intracranial pressure	Follow finger from side to side	No lateral movement Diplopia on lateral gaze
VII. Facial *****	Peripherally: 1 Malignant parotid tumours and surgery 2 Skull base fractures across temporal bone (often bilateral) 3 Upper motor lesions	'Smile' 'Whistle' 'Wrinkle the forehead – frown'	1 Facial muscle paralysis: no forehead wrinkle 2 As 1, + loss of taste in anterior two-thirds of tongue and hearing abnormal 3 Forehead can wrinkle but otherwise facial paralysis present
VIII. Acoustic ***	Fractures of temporal bone (VII often also affected)	Clap hands near ear Tick of watch Weber test – tuning fork Rinne test – tuning fork	No hearing Sound travels to good ear only Bone/air conduction
IX. Glossopharyngeal *	Deep laceration of neck Skull base tumour Brainstem lesion	Touch anterior pillar of fauces with spatula	No gag reflex
X. Vagus **	Deep laceration of neck Skull base tumour Brainstem lesion	'Open your mouth' – look at soft palate	Uvula deviated to normal side Vocal cord paralysed – hoarse voice Cannot sing high notes
XI. Spinal accessory **	Laceration or operation in posterior triangle of neck	'Shrug your shoulders' 'Push your chin against my hand' 'Take a deep breath in'	Trapezius fails to contract Sternomastoid muscle not seen or felt to contract
XII. Hypoglossal *	Laceration, surgery and tumours in region of carotid bifurcation	'Stick your tongue out'	Tongue protrudes to side of lesion Difficulty in speaking (dysarthria)

Range: * = very rare; ***** = very common

MCQs

1. In the skull: **T/F**

a the sutures are all fibrous joints   (____)

b the sagittal suture separates the frontal from   (____)
the parietal bones

c the lambda (posterior fontanelle) lies   (____)
between the sagittal and lambdoid sutures

d the anterior fontanelle is usually closed at   (____)
birth

e the posterior fontanelle usually closes 18   (____)
months after birth

Answers

1.

a **T** – *And after middle age they begin to ossify from the cranial surface.*

b **F** – *At birth the frontal bone is separated from the parietal bones by the coronal suture.*

c **T** – *The lambda (posterior fontanelle) is in this position. The bregma (anterior fontanelle) is between the sagittal, coronal and frontal sutures.*

d **F** – *The diamond-shaped anterior fontanelle is usually open until 18 months after birth.*

e **F** – *The posterior fontanelle usually closes between 3 and 6 months of age.*

---

2. The scalp: **T/F**

a is attached by the occipitalis muscle to the   (____)
skull

b is attached by the frontalis muscle to the   (____)
skull

c receives sensory innervation from the dorsal   (____)
rami of the second and third cervical nerves

d is supplied, in part, by the ophthalmic artery   (____)

e drains directly to the subcutaneous lymph   (____)
nodes at the base of the skull

Answers

2.

a **T** – *Occipitalis is attached to the superior nuchal line.*

b **F** – *Frontalis is attached to orbicularis oculi and not to bone.*

c **T** – *These nerve fibres, conveyed in the greater and lesser occipital nerves, supply the posterior scalp.*

d **T** – *Through its supraorbital and supratrochlear branches.*

e **T** – *A superficial circle of lymph nodes around the base of the skull receives all lymph from the scalp.*

SBA

1. A young man is brought to the emergency department after a fight in the street. He exhibits right periorbital bruising, and X-rays confirm the presence of an inferior 'blow-out' fracture of the orbit. Which of the following nerves is at risk of injury in this case?

a frontal

b inferior alveolar

c infraorbital

d supratrochlear

e optic

Answer

c *A fracture of the inferior orbital wall is likely to be associated with damage to the infraorbital nerve. This is more likely to be the case when the fracture results in an inferior 'blow-out' of the orbital contents because the nerve leaves the orbit immediately inferior to the orbital floor. The patient will exhibit loss of sensation over the cheek.*

---

2. An unconscious man is admitted after being struck on the head with a club. A CT scan reveals a depressed fracture in the region of the pterion and an underlying epidural haematoma. Which of the following arteries is most likely to have been injured?

a maxillary

b deep temporal

c middle meningeal

d external carotid

e superficial temporal

Answer

c *The middle meningeal artery, a branch of the maxillary artery, runs between the dura mater and the skull deep to the pterion and is likely to be injured in any fracture close to this region. The pterion lies 4 cm above the midpoint of the zygomatic arch.*

EMQ

Each question has an anatomical theme linked to the chapter, and a list of 10 related items (A–J) placed in alphabetical order: these are followed by five statements (1–5). Match **one or more** of the items A–J to each of the five statements.

Bones of the skull
A. Frontal
B. Mandible
C. Maxilla
D. Nasal
E. Occipital
F. Palatine
G. Parietal
H. Sphenoid
I. Temporal
J. Zygomatic

Match the following statements with the bone(s) in the above list.
1. Gives passage to the mandibular branch of the trigeminal nerve
2. Surrounds the foramen magnum
3. Gives passage to the middle meningeal artery
4. Crossed by the superficial temporal artery
5. Contains the middle ear

Answers
1 H; 2 E; 3 H; 4 I; 5 I

APPLIED QUESTIONS

1. A fracture in the region of the pterion may have serious consequences. What structure is at greatest risk in this injury?

    1. The pterion is the meeting point of the temporal, parietal and frontal bones with the greater wing of the sphenoid bone. In the fetal skull it is occasionally seen as a fontanelle. In the adult it lies some 4 cm above the midpoint of the zygomatic arch. The bone is relatively thin in this area and it overlies the anterior division of the middle meningeal artery, which may be lacerated in a fracture at this site. Thus an extradural haematoma and cerebral compression may follow a direct hit.

2. A full sailor's beard overlies which bones?

    2. The normal beard overlies the zygomatic portion of the temporal bone, zygomatic bone, ramus, angle and body of the mandible and maxilla. A very long beard may overlie the manubrium and body of the sternum.

Essential Clinical Anatomy · Bailey & Love · Essential Clinical Anatomy
ential Clinical Anatomy · Bailey & Love · Essential Clinical Anatomy · Bailey & Love
ley & Love · Essential Clinical Anatomy · Bailey & Love · Essential Clinical Anatomy

Chapter 19

The orbit, nose and mouth

THE ORBITAL CAVITY AND EYEBALL

The two pyramid-shaped **orbital cavities** (Fig. 19.1) lie within the facial skeleton. Each has a roof, a floor and medial and lateral walls, and contains the eyeball, extraocular muscles, vessels, nerves, lacrimal gland and fat. The periosteum of the orbit is continuous at the back of the orbit with the dura mater and sheath of the optic nerve.

The relations of the orbit are important for the clinician. The **roof**, formed by the orbital plate of the frontal bone and, posteriorly, the lesser wing of the sphenoid, separates the orbit from the anterior cranial fossa. The **floor**, formed largely by the maxilla and zygoma, separates the orbit from the maxillary air sinus and has an inferior orbital fissure posteriorly. The **lateral wall**, formed by the zygomatic bone and the greater wing of the sphenoid, separates the orbit from the temporal fossa. The **medial wall** consists of, from anterior to posterior, the maxilla, the lacrimal bone, the orbital plate of the ethmoid and the body of the sphenoid. It separates the orbit from the ethmoidal air sinuses and the nasal cavity.

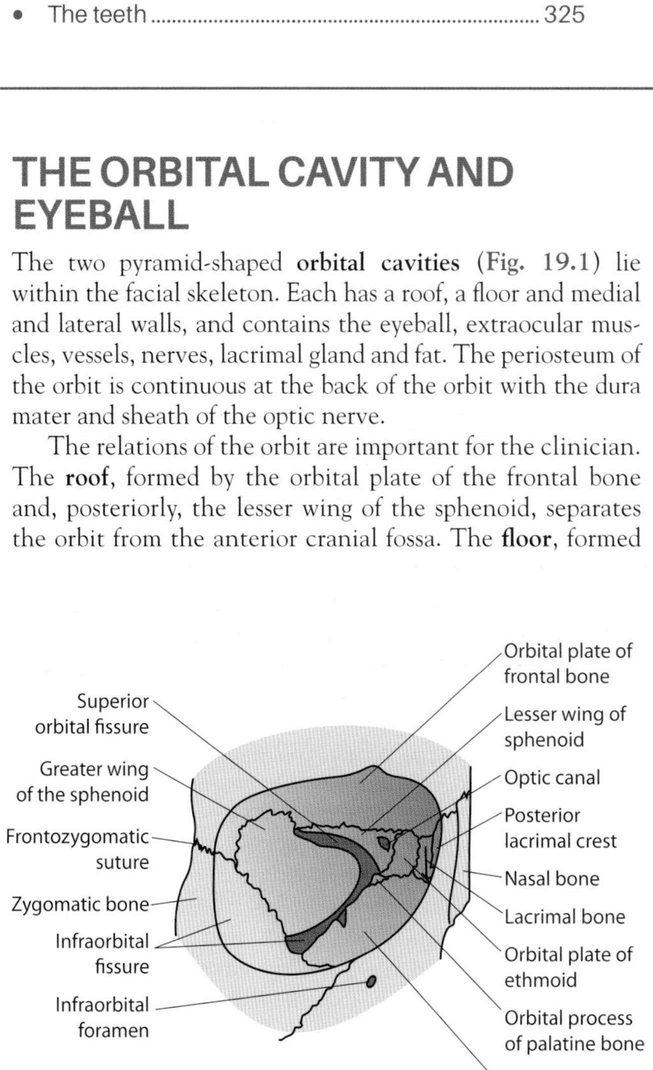

The **orbital cavity** has three posterior openings, the superior and inferior orbital fissures laterally and the optic canal medially.

The **superior orbital fissure** (Fig. 19.1, see also 19.8 and 19.9), between the greater and lesser wings of the sphenoid, opens into the middle cranial fossa and is divided by the tendinous attachment of the extraocular muscles into a narrow lateral and a wider medial part. The lateral part transmits the lacrimal, trochlear and frontal nerves, the medial, superior and inferior divisions of the oculomotor nerve, the nasociliary nerve and the abducent nerve. Ophthalmic veins pass posteriorly to enter the cavernous sinus.

The **inferior orbital fissure**, between the floor and lateral wall, opens into the pterygopalatine fossa medially and the infratemporal fossa laterally. It transmits the maxillary nerve, which in the canal becomes the infraorbital nerve, and its zygomatic branch, together with communicating veins.

The **optic canal** opens into the apex of the cavity and conveys the optic nerve and ophthalmic artery from the middle cranial fossa. Anteriorly a wide canal passes downwards from the cavity's inferomedial angle to the nose; it contains the nasolacrimal duct. Superolaterally is the fossa for the lacrimal gland.

Superior orbital fissure
Greater wing of the sphenoid
Frontozygomatic suture
Zygomatic bone
Infraorbital fissure
Infraorbital foramen

Orbital plate of frontal bone
Lesser wing of sphenoid
Optic canal
Posterior lacrimal crest
Nasal bone
Lacrimal bone
Orbital plate of ethmoid
Orbital process of palatine bone
Maxilla

Figure 19.1 Bones of the orbital cavity

A blow to the eye may, because of the thinness of the medial and inferior orbital walls, fracture the orbit (**Fig. 19.2**). A fracture of the medial wall may involve the ethmoidal and sphenoidal sinuses; a fracture of the lower margin may involve the maxillary sinus and infraorbital nerve, resulting in loss of sensation over the cheek. Diplopia may also occur.

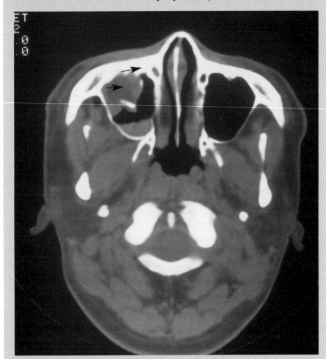

Figure 19.2 Axial CT scan of a 'blow-out' orbital fracture – arrows show bony fragments pushed by orbital contents that have sunk into the maxillary air sinus below – see also Fig. 18.10, p. 309

THE EYEBALL

The eyeball is situated in the anterior orbital cavity and is almost spherical, but is distorted anteriorly by the projecting cornea (**Fig. 19.3**). The optic nerve leaves it posteromedially. The wall of the eyeball has three coats. From without inwards these are:

- An outer fibrous coat forming the dense white **sclera**, which covers the posterior five-sixths of the eyeball and the transparent **cornea** anteriorly.
- The pigmented **choroid**, which, anteriorly, has a circular thickening, the **ciliary body**, containing the ciliary muscle. In front of the ciliary body the choroid thins to form the **iris**, with its central aperture, the **pupil**. The iris contains the circular sphincter pupillae and the radial dilator pupillae muscles.
- The **retina** contains the light receptors, which relay impulses along the optic nerve. There are several layers of nervous elements (**Fig. 19.4**). Medially on the posterior wall is a pale area, the **optic disc**, where the optic nerve leaves the eyeball (**Fig. 19.5**). About 3 mm lateral to the disc, at the visual axis, is a small depression, the **fovea centralis**. The area around it, the **macula**, is used mainly for daylight vision.

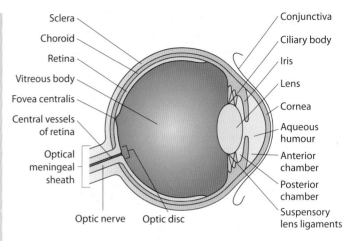

Figure 19.3 Cross-section through the eyeball

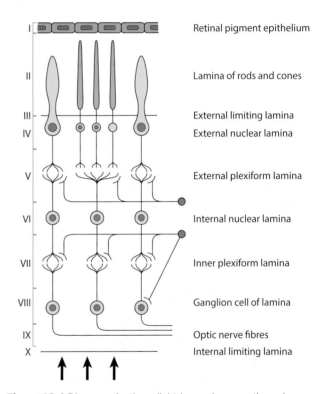

Figure 19.4 Diagram of retina – light (arrows) passes through numerous layers as shown, before impinging on the photoreceptors (rods and cones)

Detachment of the retina: trauma to the eye may cause fluid to track between the deeper pigmented layer and the overlying neural layer of the retina, resulting in detachment of the inner layer. The patient complains of 'starburst' flashes of light, and urgent laser treatment is required to prevent permanent loss of vision.

The biconvex **lens** divides the eyeball cavity into a posterior part filled with the jelly-like **vitreous body** and an anterior part filled with the more fluid **aqueous humour**. The iris further divides the anterior part into an anterior chamber between the iris and cornea and a posterior chamber between the iris and lens. These two chambers are in continuity through the pupil. The lens is held in position by its

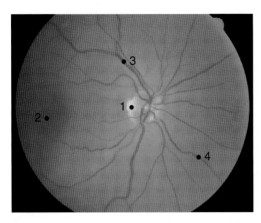

Figure 19.5 Ophthalmoscopy of a normal retina: 1, optic disc; 2, macula; 3, superior temporal branches of central vein and artery; 4, inferior nasal vessels

suspensory ligament passing from its periphery to the ciliary body. Accommodation, the process by which near objects are focused on the retina, is achieved by contraction of the ciliary muscle drawing the ciliary body forwards and relaxing the suspensory ligament. The lens, because of its inherent elasticity, then becomes more convex.

The lens becomes harder and less elastic with age and there is a gradual loss of focusing power in the elderly (**presbyopia**). Loss of transparency of the lens occurs in some people (**cataract**) (Fig. 19.6), a condition that can be cured by lens extraction or a lens implant. In a proportion of elderly people the reabsorption of aqueous humour diminishes and the accumulation of the contents of the eye increases intraocular pressure and with it causes some compression of the retina, with the effect that there is a slow but progressive loss of visual acuity (**glaucoma**).

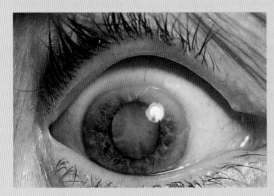

Figure 19.6 Cataract – note the milky opacity of the lens behind the pupil

Blood supply

This is by the central artery of the retina and ciliary branches, both branches of the ophthalmic artery. Veins pass to the ophthalmic veins.

Occlusion of the central artery of the retina may occur as the result of arterial disease or because of embolism (the trapping of free-floating clots) in the artery. It produces permanent blindness.

Ophthalmoscopy allows examination of the retina (Fig. 19.5) and its structures: the optic disc, the macula, radiating retinal vessels and fovea centralis. Abnormalities such as **papilloedema** (swelling of the optic disc; Fig. 19.7), which results from an increase in intracranial pressure, aneurysms, exudates along the path of the arterial branches and 'nipping' of the veins by the arteries in patients with hypertension can be identified ophthalmoscopically. In diabetes mellitus after some years it is not uncommon to find deterioration of eyesight that may be due to the accumulation of protein exudates covering the macular region, as seen in Fig. 19.7a.

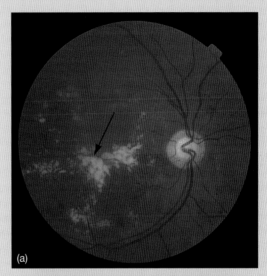

(a)

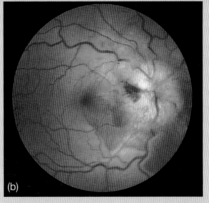

(b)

Figure 19.7 (a) Retinoscopy of diabetes mellitus with the macula destroyed by exudates (arrow). (b) Papilloedema – note and compare this with Fig. 19.5. In this case the patient has no clear optic disc due to vascular congestion and swelling

Nerve supply

The optic nerve carries sensory fibres from the retina. Ciliary nerves carry autonomic fibres to the muscles of the iris and the ciliary muscles and sensory fibres from the conjunctiva; the long ciliary nerves carry sympathetic fibres and arise from the nasociliary nerve. The short ciliary nerves arise from the ciliary ganglion and carry postganglionic parasympathetic fibres.

The **corneal reflex**, the 'blink reflex' when a speck of dirt touches the cornea, is mediated by trigeminal sensory fibres causing facial nerve activity to close the eyes. The **pupillary** reflex is a constriction of the pupil on exposure to bright light. The sensory component is the optic nerve, and the motor component comprises parasympathetic fibres carried within the oculomotor nerve. The sympathetic fibres cause pupillary dilatation related to fear and excitement.

THE ORBIT

Orbital (bulbar) fascia

The eyeball behind the cornea is closely surrounded by the orbital fascia, which separates it from the orbital fat. Thickenings of the fascia attached to the lacrimal and zygomatic bones form the medial and lateral **check ligaments** of the eye, and a thickening below the eyeball forms the **suspensory ligament** that provides a hammock-like support for the eye.

Extraocular muscles

The four **rectus muscles** (Fig. 19.8) – superior, inferior, medial and lateral – are attached posteriorly to the common tendinous ring surrounding the optic canal and the medial end of the superior orbital fissure. Anteriorly the muscles pass forwards, in positions implied by their names, to be attached to the sclera just in front of the equator of the eyeball.

The **superior oblique** is attached posteriorly above the common tendinous ring (Fig. 19.9), and passes forwards for its tendon to hook around a fibrocartilaginous pulley, the **trochlea**, on the superomedial border of the front of the orbit. It then passes backwards and laterally to gain attachment to the posterolateral surface of the eyeball, behind the equator.

The **inferior oblique** is attached anteriorly to the anteromedial floor of the orbit and passes backwards to be attached to the posterolateral surface of the eyeball, behind the equator.

Nerve supply

Lateral rectus is served by the abducent nerve, superior oblique by the trochlear nerve and the remaining muscles by the oculomotor nerve.

Functions

The muscles of each eye work together in a coordinated manner so as to fix both eyes on to an object. There is an angle

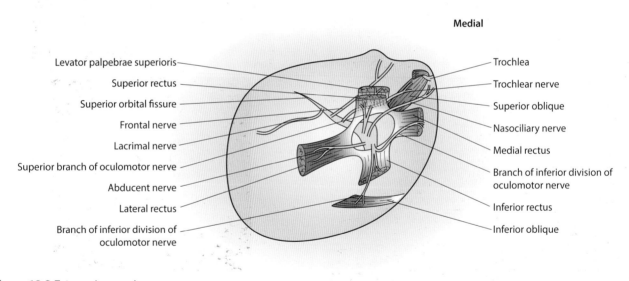

Medial

Levator palpebrae superioris
Superior rectus
Superior orbital fissure
Frontal nerve
Lacrimal nerve
Superior branch of oculomotor nerve
Abducent nerve
Lateral rectus
Branch of inferior division of oculomotor nerve

Trochlea
Trochlear nerve
Superior oblique
Nasociliary nerve
Medial rectus
Branch of inferior division of oculomotor nerve
Inferior rectus
Inferior oblique

Figure 19.8 Extraocular muscles

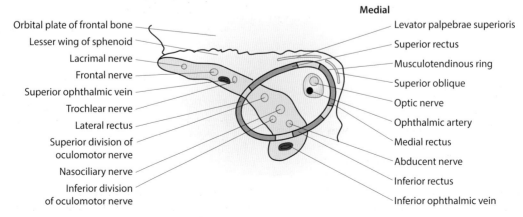

Medial

Orbital plate of frontal bone
Lesser wing of sphenoid
Lacrimal nerve
Frontal nerve
Superior ophthalmic vein
Trochlear nerve
Lateral rectus
Superior division of oculomotor nerve
Nasociliary nerve
Inferior division of oculomotor nerve

Levator palpebrae superioris
Superior rectus
Musculotendinous ring
Superior oblique
Optic nerve
Ophthalmic artery
Medial rectus
Abducent nerve
Inferior rectus
Inferior ophthalmic vein

Figure 19.9 Extraocular tendinous ring and relations in the right eye

between the visual or optic axis and the orbital axis, and all movements other than horizontal involve some rotation as well as angular deviation of the eyeball. Looking left involves contraction of the left lateral rectus and right medial rectus; looking down and to the right involves the left superior oblique and the right inferior rectus; looking up and to the left involves the left inferior oblique and the right superior rectus. An easy way to remember these complex vectors is that cranial nerve IV (the trochlear nerve, formerly known as the pathetic nerve) makes you look 'down and out'.

Incoordination of the muscles of the two eyes results in a squint and 'double vision' (diplopia). **Oculomotor palsy,** when complete, results in paralysis of most of the eye muscles, together with levator palpebrae superioris and the sphincter pupillae. Consequently the upper lid droops (ptosis), there is a fully dilated pupil and the eyeball tends to look downwards and outwards owing to the unopposed action of lateral rectus and superior oblique muscles, which are not paralysed (Fig. 21.13a, p. 362). **Abducent nerve palsy** (Fig. 19.10) results in paralysis of the lateral rectus muscle and the eye cannot be moved laterally in the horizontal plane. The palsy may result from viral infection, but occasionally it may be a non-localizing sign of increased intracranial pressure (because the long intracranial course of the nerve renders it particularly susceptible to stretching by the raised pressure). **Trochlear nerve palsy** is rare; patients attempt to minimize the diplopia it causes by tilting the head.

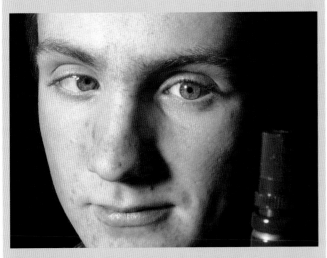

Figure 19.10 Left IVth nerve palsy – the patient is looking at the red marker: the left eye cannot abduct but right eye movement is normal

Levator palpebrae superioris

Levator palpebrae superioris raises the upper eyelid. It is attached posteriorly above the common tendinous origin and anteriorly to the conjunctiva and tarsal plate. It is supplied by the oculomotor nerve. Some smooth muscle fibres are also present, and are innervated by sympathetics from the superior cervical ganglion (Müller's muscle). This is the reason why there is a mild ptosis in Horner's syndrome when the sympathetic fibres to the Müller's muscle are compromised.

Sympathetic denervation, which usually follows trauma or neoplastic infiltration of the cervical sympathetic trunk, causes a partially drooped eyelid (ptosis), a small pupil due to paralysis of dilator pupillae and a hot, flushed and dry face on that side (Horner's syndrome) (Fig. 19.11).

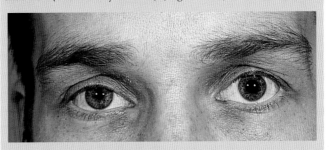

Figure 19.11 Right Horner's syndrome

Blood supply of the orbit

The **ophthalmic artery** arises as the first branch of the internal carotid artery in the middle cranial fossa above the cavernous sinus. It enters the orbit through the optic canal, and gives ciliary branches, the central artery of the retina and muscular branches before ending behind the medial side of the upper eyelid by dividing into supratrochlear, supraorbital and dorsal nasal branches.

Superior and inferior **ophthalmic veins** drain the orbit and pass through the superior orbital fissure to the cavernous sinus. They communicate through the inferior orbital fissure with the pterygoid venous plexus posteriorly and with the facial vein anteriorly near the medial angle of the eye.

Thus infection may pass from the central part of the facial skin to involve the cavernous sinus; for example, the spread of an infection from a squeezed pimple on the face may lead to a thrombosis in the cavernous sinus, with resultant oedema of the conjunctiva and possible damage to the cranial nerves traversing the sinus (Fig. 25.9, p. 437).

Nerves of the orbit

The **nerves of the orbit** are described more fully on p. 360.

THE EYELIDS

The eyeball is protected anteriorly by two movable skin folds, the larger upper and the smaller lower eyelids, which are united medially and laterally and limit the **palpebral fissure** at its medial and lateral angles. Within the medial angle of each eyelid is a pink elevation, the **lacrimal caruncle**. On the medial margin of each lid is a small elevation, the **lacrimal papilla**, on the apex of which is the **lacrimal punctum**, the opening of the lacrimal canaliculus (Fig. 19.12). Each eyelid has five layers:

- Skin
- Superficial fascia, devoid of fat
- Palpebral fibres of orbicularis oculi and levator palpebrae superioris (Fig. 18.13, p. 311)

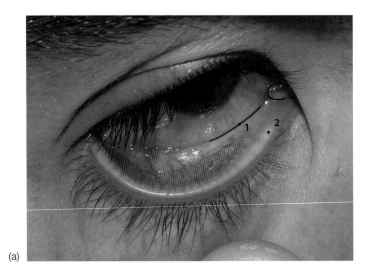

(a)

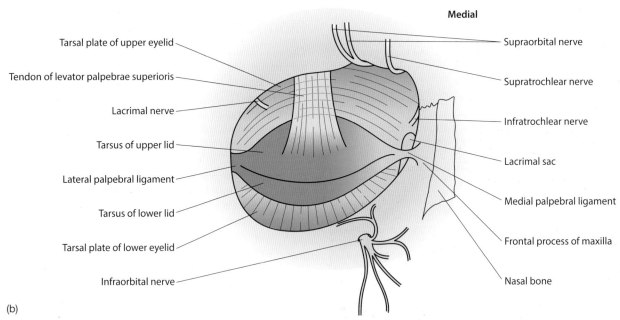

Medial

Tarsal plate of upper eyelid

Tendon of levator palpebrae superioris

Lacrimal nerve

Tarsus of upper lid

Lateral palpebral ligament

Tarsus of lower lid

Tarsal plate of lower eyelid

Infraorbital nerve

Supraorbital nerve

Supratrochlear nerve

Infratrochlear nerve

Lacrimal sac

Medial palpebral ligament

Frontal process of maxilla

Nasal bone

(b)

Figure 19.12 (a) Right lower eyelid everted to show the lacrimal punctum: 1, conjunctival fornix; 2, lacrimal punctum. (b) Diagram of tarsal plates in the closed right eye – skin, superficial fascia and palpebral muscles removed

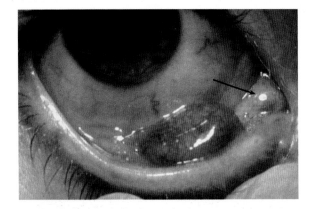

Figure 19.13 Chalazion (Meibomian cyst) caused by blockage of the tarsal glands – these open on the inside of the eyelid and are readily misdiagnosed as a stye (an infection of the root of an eyelash). The arrow points to the lacrimal caruncle.

- Tarsal plate, an elliptical plate of dense fibrous tissue attached to the orbital margin by medial and lateral palpebral ligaments (Fig. 19.12b). On the plate's deep surface lie tarsal (Meibomian) glands, which are modified sebaceous glands. Their ducts open onto the lid margin (Fig. 19.13)
- Conjunctiva, a thin layer of epithelium lining the inner surface of both lids and which is reflected over the front of the eyeball. When the lids are closed the conjunctiva encloses a narrow sac containing a small amount of lacrimal fluid. The upper and lower pouches between the lids and the eyeball are known as the conjunctival fornices.

The eyelashes emerge through the skin of the lid margin, and small sebaceous glands are associated with them.

Eye closing is effected by orbicularis oculi, and the upper lid is raised by levator palpebrae superioris.

When the sensory innervation of the cornea, the trigeminal nerve, is damaged and the cornea is thus anaesthetized, it is prone to injury by particles that may cause corneal ulcers. The rash of herpes zoster (shingles) infection of the Vth cranial nerve will produce corneal ulcers.

THE LACRIMAL APPARATUS

The structures producing and removing tears are collectively termed the lacrimal apparatus (Fig. 19.14). They comprise the lacrimal gland and its ducts, the conjunctival sac, the lacrimal sac and the nasolacrimal duct. The front of the eyeball and its conjunctival covering is constantly washed by tears that are essential to ensure the conjunctiva remains moist and viable. The tears are drained by blinking, when the increased intraconjunctival pressure produced by the closed lids forces the fluid into the lacrimal puncta and thence into the lacrimal sacs (Figs. 19.12a and 19.15).

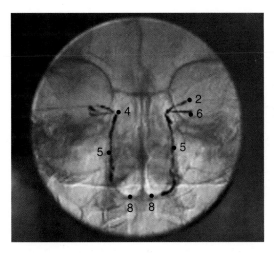

Figure 19.14 Lacrimal apparatus: 1, upper lid; 2, superior lacrimal canaliculus; 3, lacrimal caruncle; 4, lacrimal sac; 5, nasolacrimal duct; 6, inferior lacrimal canaliculus; 7, lower lid eyelashes

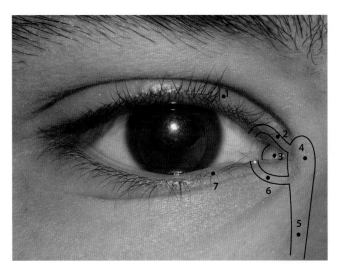

Figure 19.15 Macrodacryocystogram – this contrast medium study outlines both sets of lacrimal apparatus (labels correspond to those in Fig. 19.14 above, with 8, hard palate)

The **lacrimal gland** is a serous gland in the superolateral angle of the orbit behind the upper lid. It is almond-shaped, with a palpebral process between the conjunctiva and the tarsal plate, and it has 6–12 ducts opening into the superior conjunctival fornix. It is supplied by a branch of the ophthalmic artery and innervated by the facial nerve through the pterygopalatine ganglion; postganglionic parasympathetic secretomotor fibres pass in the lacrimal and zygomatic nerves. Its lymph drains to the parotid nodes. Each **lacrimal canaliculus** is about 10 mm long and passes from the lacrimal punctum in each eyelid to the **lacrimal sac**. This is a thin fibrous sac on the medial side of the orbit in the lacrimal fossa; it receives both lacrimal canaliculi and drains to the **nasolacrimal duct**. The duct descends in the medial wall of the orbit and opens into the inferior meatus of the nasal cavity. Its opening is guarded by a flap of mucous membrane that prevents air passing up the duct when the nose is blown.

The first action one takes when crying is to blow the nose as a response to increased secretions pouring into the inferior meatus.

THE NOSE

The nose warms and moistens inspired air and has olfactory receptors. It comprises the external nose and the two nasal cavities. The **external nose** bears the anterior nostrils (nares). Its skeleton is formed superiorly by nasal bones, which articulate with the frontal bone and the frontal process of the maxillae, and inferiorly by several cartilages that surround the anterior nares. The skin covering the external nose is firmly attached over these cartilages. Just within the external nose is the **vestibule** (Fig. 19.16), from which project coarse hairs (vibrissae), whose function is to keep dirt particles from entering the upper airways.

The **nasal cavities**, between the anterior nares and the nasopharynx, are lined by ciliated columnar epithelium and, superiorly, by olfactory epithelium. They are separated by a midline septum and each possesses a roof, floor, lateral and medial walls, and anterior and posterior apertures. The narrow arched **roof** lies below the anterior cranial fossa. It is formed, from anterior to posterior, by the nasal cartilages, nasal and frontal bones, the cribriform plate of the ethmoid and the body of the sphenoid (Fig. 19.17). The horizontal **floor** forms part of the roof of the oral cavity and is formed by

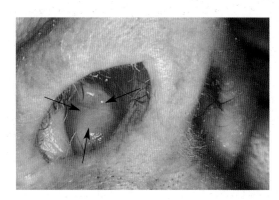

Figure 19.16 View through the anterior nostrils showing a polyp (arrows)

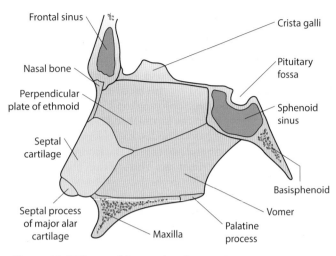

Figure 19.17 Bones of the nasal septum

the palatine process of the maxilla and the horizontal plate of the palatine bone. Anteriorly the midline incisive canal transmits the greater palatine artery and the nasopalatine nerve. The **medial wall** of the cavity is the nasal septum. It is largely formed, from anterior to posterior, by the septal cartilage, the perpendicular plate of the ethmoid and the vomer. The **lateral wall** (Fig. 19.18) lies medial to the orbit, the ethmoid and maxillary air sinuses and the pterygopalatine fossa. Its surface area is greatly increased by three horizontal bony projections, the superior, middle and inferior **nasal conchae** (turbinates), and by diverticula, the **paranasal air sinuses**. The inferior concha is the largest and lies about 1 cm above the floor of the nose. Beneath each concha is a **meatus**, and above the superior concha the **sphenoethmoidal recess**. The sphenoid air sinus opens into the recess, the posterior ethmoidal air cells into the superior meatus and the nasolacrimal duct into the inferior meatus. The middle meatus possesses the **bulla ethmoidalis**, which contains the middle ethmoidal air cells. A semicircular groove below the bulla, the **hiatus semilunaris**, has openings for the frontal, anterior ethmoidal and maxillary air sinuses (**Fig. 19.19**).

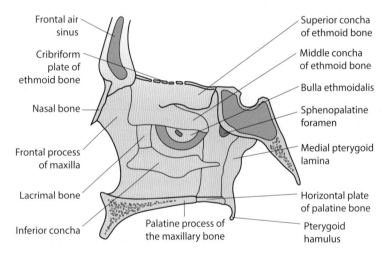

Figure 19.18 Bones of the lateral wall of the nasal cavity

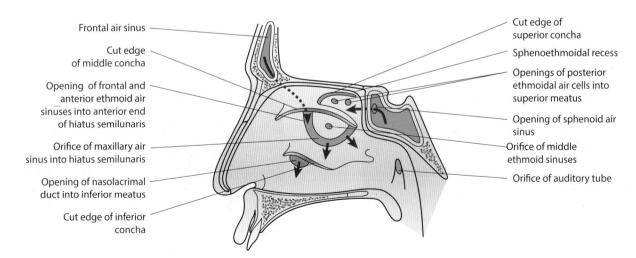

Figure 19.19 Lateral wall of the nasal cavity showing the openings of the paranasal air sinuses (arrows indicate the directions of mucus drainage)

Nerve supply

Branches of the maxillary nerve and the anterior ethmoidal branch of the ophthalmic nerve supply the nose (**Fig. 19.20**). The olfactory mucosa – the sensory organ of smell – is in the upper cavity, supplied by the olfactory nerves.

Blood supply

The ophthalmic, palatine and maxillary arteries are the main supply, but the anterior inferior part of the cavity receives additional branches from the facial artery. The veins drain to the pterygoid venous plexus and the facial vein.

Lymphatic drainage

The anterior cavity drains to the submandibular nodes, the posterior part to the retropharyngeal nodes.

THE PARANASAL AIR SINUSES

Paired frontal and maxillary sinuses and numerous ethmoidal and sphenoidal air sinuses lie within the corresponding bones. They develop as diverticula from each nasal cavity and are lined by its mucoperiosteum. They are small at birth and enlarge during eruption of the second dentition, to reach adult size after puberty. They lighten the front of the skull and may increase the resonance of the voice. Their lymphatics drain mainly to the deeply placed retropharyngeal nodes.

The **frontal sinus**, situated above the medial end of the superciliary arch, is separated by a bony septum from its fellow. It lies anterior to the anterior cranial fossa and above the orbit. Each sinus opens into the middle meatus of the nasal cavity through the long frontonasal duct (**Fig. 19.19**).

The **maxillary sinus** (**Fig. 19.21**) – the largest of the paired air sinuses – is pyramidal. Its base forms part of the lateral wall of the nose, and its apex projects laterally into the zygomatic process of the maxilla. The roof separates the sinus from the orbit and conveys the infraorbital vessels and nerve in the infraorbital canal. The floor is the alveolar margin, containing molar teeth, the roots of which project into the cavity. The posterior wall contains the posterior superior alveolar nerve and lies in front of the infratemporal and pterygopalatine fossae. The anterior wall forms the facial surface of the maxilla and is covered in part by the mucous membrane of the vestibule of the mouth.

The sinus opens into the hiatus semilunaris from high on its medial wall. Its lymph drains to the submandibular and retropharyngeal nodes.

The maxillary sinuses are the most commonly infected because their openings, well above the floor of the sinus, are not well positioned for natural drainage.

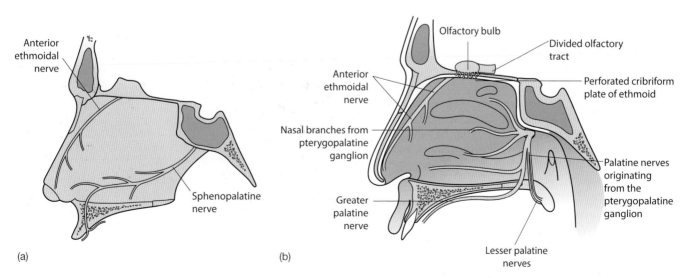

(a)   (b)

Figure 19.20 Nerve supply of: (a) the septum; (b) the lateral wall of the nose

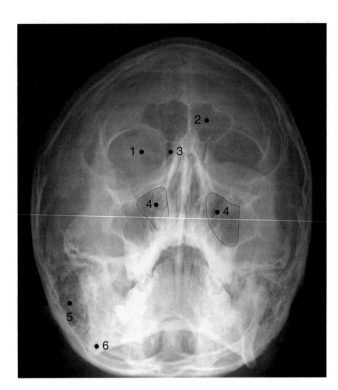

Figure 19.21 X-ray (an upwardly oblique view) showing the paranasal air sinuses: 1, orbital cavity; 2, frontal sinus; 3, ethmoidal sinus; 4, maxillary sinus; 5, mastoid air cells; 6, angle of mandible

Because of the close relationship between frontal and maxillary sinus openings, an infection in the frontal sinus will often drain by gravity into the maxillary sinus (sinusitis). The most effective way to drain the maxillary sinus is to kneel in the Muslim praying position, which brings the opening of the sinus into a dependent position for drainage. Infection of a carcinoma of the maxillary sinus may, because of the close relation of the sinus floor to the upper teeth, produce pain referred to those teeth.

Each ethmoidal labyrinth, lying between the orbit and the upper part of the nasal cavity, contains numerous air cells, the **ethmoidal sinuses**; these are divided into anterior, middle and posterior groups.

An infection or abscess in these cells may readily invade the thin medial wall of the orbit and optic canal, causing optic neuritis and the risk of blindness.

The **sphenoidal sinuses** are contained within the body of the sphenoid and usually communicate with each other through an incomplete bony septum. They lie below the sella turcica and pituitary gland, above the nasal cavity, and medial to the cavernous sinus and its contents. Each sinus opens into the sphenoethmoidal recess.

Blood supply

The main supply is by the sphenopalatine branch of the maxillary artery. It anastomoses on the anterior lower part of the septum (Little's area) with labial and palatine branches; this area is a common site for a nosebleed (epistaxis).

Lymphatic drainage

Drainage is to the submandibular, retropharyngeal and deep cervical nodes.

Nerve supply

The olfactory nerve supplies the roof and upper parts of the lateral walls. The lateral nasal wall is supplied by anterior ethmoidal branches superiorly and the superior alveolar nerve inferiorly.

Surgeons have devised an approach to the pituitary, which lies immediately above the sphenoidal sinus, via the nose and sphenoidal sinus (trans-sphenoidal hypophysectomy).

THE ORAL CAVITY

This, the first part of the alimentary tract, extends from the lips to the isthmus of the fauces (Fig. 19.22). It contains the tongue and the alveolar arches, with gums and teeth. Into it open the salivary glands. The alveolar arches, gums and teeth divide the cavity into an outer vestibule and an inner oral cavity. The **vestibule**, a slit-like cavity limited externally by the lips and cheeks, opens on to the face between the lips at the oral fissure; internally it is limited by the gums and teeth. It communicates with the mouth between the teeth or, when the teeth are occluded, by the retromolar space. The parotid duct opens into the vestibule just above and opposite to the upper second molar tooth. The vestibule is emptied by the actions of buccinator.

Paralysis of buccinator causes the most distressing symptom for sufferers of a facial nerve paralysis. They must keep a tissue in their hand to wipe the saliva that drools out from the corner of the mouth.

The **oral cavity** is limited anteriorly and laterally by the maxilla and mandible and teeth; it possesses a roof, a floor and a posterior opening. The roof is formed by the palate, which separates the mouth from the nasal cavities. Much of

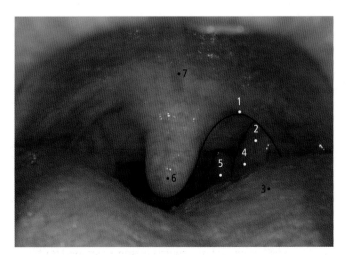

Figure 19.22 Oral cavity showing the pillars of the fauces: 1, palatoglossal fold (anterior arch of fauces); 2, palatine tonsil, upper pole; 3, tongue; 4, palatine tonsil; 5, palatopharyngeus (posterior arch of fauces); 6, uvula; 7, palate

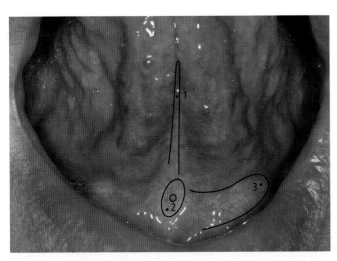

Figure 19.23 Undersurface of tongue showing: 1, frenulum; 2, opening of submandibular duct; 3, sublingual gland – just below the mucous membrane

the floor is occupied by the tongue, from which mucous membrane spreads to the body of the mandible. A midline fold of mucous membrane, the **frenulum** (Fig. 19.23), connects the undersurface of the tongue to the floor. On each side of the frenulum is a **sublingual papilla**, on to which opens the submandibular duct. Behind and lateral to the papillae are the sublingual glands (Fig. 19.23). The posterior opening, the **fauceal isthmus**, is bounded laterally by the palatoglossal fold (the anterior arch of the fauces), superiorly by the soft palate, and inferiorly by the back of the tongue (Fig. 19.22). The **gums (gingivae)** surround the necks of the teeth. They are composed of fibrous tissue covered by a vascular mucous membrane and are firmly attached to the alveolar margins.

Nerve supply

Much of the inside of the cheeks and lips is supplied by buccal branches of the mandibular nerve with contributions from the mental branch of the inferior alveolar nerve and the infraorbital branch of the maxillary nerve.

THE TEETH

Each tooth has a projecting crown, a neck surrounded by the gum and one or more roots embedded in the alveolar bone. Its central cavity opens on to the apex of the root and is filled with **pulp** (loose connective tissue, vessels and nerves). The cavity is surrounded by **dentine**, a hard, calcified material. The dentine of the crown is covered by **enamel**, a very hard inorganic layer. The periodontal membrane – modified periosteum of the alveolar socket – holds the root in position. The teeth are named, from the front and moving laterally: incisor (I), canine (C), premolar (P) and molar (M). They vary in size, shape and function, as follows:

- **Crowns** – incisors have sharp cutting edges used for biting food, whereas the cutting edges of the canines are large and conical. Premolars, which are bicuspid, and molars, with three to five tubercles, are used in chewing.

- **Roots** – incisors, canines and premolars possess a single root (with the exception of the first upper premolar, which has two); lower molars have two roots and upper molars three.

Humans have two sets of teeth, which erupt at different times. The deciduous (milk) teeth appear between the 6th and 24th months. They are replaced by permanent teeth, which appear between the 6th and 24th years. Each half of each jaw contains five deciduous teeth (I2, C1, M2) and eight permanent teeth (I2, C1, P2, M3). The average time of eruption of the teeth in each half of the upper and lower jaws is shown in Table 19.1.

The first deciduous tooth to appear is a lower central incisor, the first permanent tooth a first molar. The third molars (wisdom teeth) appear between the 17th and 25th years. Lower teeth tend to appear slightly earlier and in girls generally before boys.

TABLE 19.1 The dates of appearance of both deciduous (in months) and permanent (in years) teeth. There are five deciduous and eight permanent teeth in each quadrant of the mouth. The dates indicate the appearance of the individual teeth

Deciduous (months)	Incisor	Canine	Molar	
	7–8	18	12–24	
	6–9	18	12–24	
Permanent (years)	Incisor	Canine	Premolar	Molar
	7–8	12	9–10	6–12 18+
	7–8	12	9–10	6–12 18+

Nerve and blood supply

The **teeth** of the upper jaw are innervated by numerous anterior and posterior superior alveolar branches of the maxillary nerve, the lower by the single inferior alveolar branch of the mandibular nerve. The central incisors have bilateral innervation. Blood supply is by the corresponding arteries. The labial surface of the **upper gums** is supplied by the infraorbital and posterior superior alveolar nerves, the lingual surface by the nasopalatine and greater palatine nerves. The labial surface of the **lower gums** is supplied by the mental and buccal nerves, the lingual surface by the lingual nerve.

Imperfect oral hygiene leads to the development of cavities in the enamel and subsequent infection of the pulp cavity (**dental caries**). The cavity is inextensible and the pain (toothache) caused by the rise in pressure is severe. **Inferior alveolar nerve block** (usually known as an inferior dental block) is very commonly used in dentistry. The anaesthetic agent is injected around the site of the nerve's entry into the mandible, adjacent to the lingula. All the teeth of that half of the mandible are anaesthetized, together with the lower lip, which is supplied by the mental branch of the nerve. NB: the upper jaw teeth require a separate injection for each tooth because of their individual innervation. The pain of upper jaw toothache may easily be confused with that of **maxillary sinusitis** because of the identical innervation – many a filling has been carried out on a normal tooth in patients whose 'dental' pain originated in the maxillary sinus.

Lymphatic drainage

Drainage is from the maxillary teeth and gums to the upper deep cervical nodes, and from the mandibular teeth and gums to the submental, submandibular and deep cervical nodes.

THE PALATE

The palate (Figs. 18.7, p. 307 and 20.5, p. 342) forms the roof of the mouth and separates it from the nasal cavities. It comprises the hard palate anteriorly and the soft palate posteriorly.

The **hard palate** is formed by the palatine processes of the maxillae and the horizontal plates of the palatine bones. The anterior midline **incisive foramen** transmits the nasopalatine nerve and a branch of the greater palatine artery. The greater and lesser palatine foramina lie posterolaterally and convey nerves and vessels of the same name. The hard palate is covered by mucoperiosteum rich in mucous glands. It is supplied by the greater and lesser palatine nerves and vessels, apart from an area behind the incisors, which is supplied by the nasopalatine nerve. Its lymph drains to the deep cervical nodes.

The **soft palate** (Fig. 19.22) is a mobile partition between the nasopharynx and oropharynx, consisting of several paired muscles attached to the back of the hard palate that are covered by mucous membrane. It plays an important role in swallowing and in modulating speech. On its posterior free border is the midline conical projection, the **uvula**. On each side two vertical folds, the anterior and posterior arches of the fauces, descend from its inferior surface to the tongue and pharynx. They contain the palatoglossus and, posteri-orly, the palatopharyngeus muscles, with the palatine tonsil in between.

Muscles of the soft palate

Tensor veli palatini, known also as **tensor palati**, is attached superiorly to the base of the skull close to the spine of the sphenoid. Its fibres converge on to a narrow tendon that hooks around the hamulus. In the palate the tendon fans out and joins with that of the opposite side to form the **palatine aponeurosis**, 'the skeleton' of the soft palate, into which the other palatal muscles are attached. **Levator veli palatini** descends from the petrous temporal bone in the lateral wall of the nasopharynx to blend into the soft palate (Fig. 19.25a).

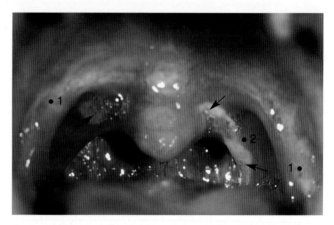

Figure 19.24 Ulcerated fauces (arrows) due to immunosuppression – note the ulcers on the: 1, palatoglossal and 2, palatopharyngeal folds

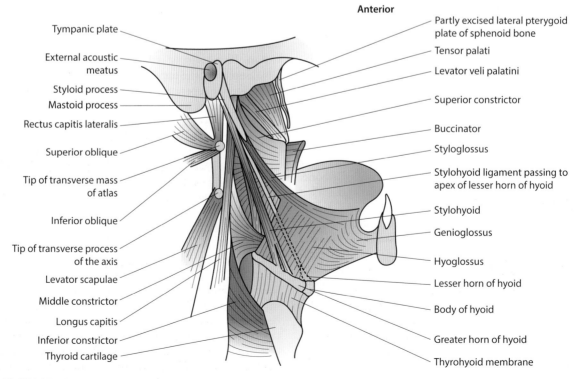

Figure 19.25 (a) Extrinsic muscles of the tongue. (*continued*)

Anterior

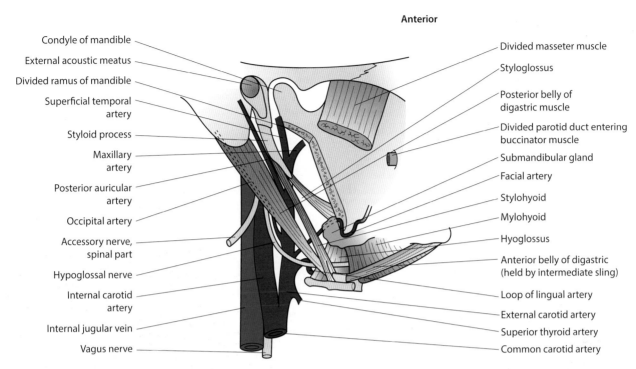

Condyle of mandible
External acoustic meatus
Divided ramus of mandible
Superficial temporal artery
Styloid process
Maxillary artery
Posterior auricular artery
Occipital artery
Accessory nerve, spinal part
Hypoglossal nerve
Internal carotid artery
Internal jugular vein
Vagus nerve

Divided masseter muscle
Styloglossus
Posterior belly of digastric muscle
Divided parotid duct entering buccinator muscle
Submandibular gland
Facial artery
Stylohyoid
Mylohyoid
Hyoglossus
Anterior belly of digastric (held by intermediate sling)
Loop of lingual artery
External carotid artery
Superior thyroid artery
Common carotid artery

Figure 19.25 (*continued*) (b) Extrinsic muscles of the tongue and blood vessels of the neck revealed by removal of the posterior mandible

Palatoglossus descends from the palate to the lateral tongue. **Palatopharyngeus** descends from the palate to blend with the constrictor muscles of the pharynx before gaining attachment to the thyroid cartilage. Its upper horizontal fibres form a functional palatopharyngeal sphincter.

Nerve supply

Tensor palatini is innervated by a branch of the mandibular nerve and all the other muscles via the pharyngeal plexus. The mucous membrane is innervated by the greater and lesser palatine nerves and branches of the glossopharyngeal nerve. Taste fibres may be carried in these sensory nerves.

Blood supply

This is by palatine branches of the maxillary, facial and lingual arteries; venous drainage is to the pharyngeal venous plexus.

Lymphatic drainage

This is to the deep cervical nodes.

THE TONGUE

The muscular tongue, covered with mucous membrane, lies in the floor of the mouth and oropharynx (Fig. 19.23). It is used in chewing, swallowing, articulation and, in the infant, suckling. It is also a sensory organ of taste and common sensation. It is the shape of an inverted shoe and is attached posteriorly mainly to the hyoid bone and the mandible, lying on the geniohyoid and mylohyoid muscles. The upper surface

(dorsum) is divided by a V-shaped groove, the **sulcus terminalis**, into an anterior two-thirds and a posterior third. In the centre of the sulcus is a pit, the **foramen caecum**, the origin of the thyroglossal duct.

Extremely rarely thyroid glandular tissue can be found at the foramen caecum, as this is the embryological site of origin of the thyroid gland, which develops from the distal end of the thyroglossal duct.

The mucous membrane of the oral anterior two-thirds of the dorsum of the tongue is covered with papillae. Taste buds are most numerous around the sides of the tongue and in front of the sulcus terminalis.

The mucous membrane is raised posteriorly in a midline glossoepiglottic fold that separates two shallow fossae, the **valleculae**, limited laterally by the pharyngeal wall. The lower surface also has a midline fold anteriorly, the **frenulum** (Fig. 19.23), which attaches it to the floor of the mouth.

Very occasionally the frenulum is short and restricts tongue movement (tongue tie). This is simply treated by surgical division of the frenulum.

Within the posterior tongue are nodules of lymphatic tissue, the **lingual tonsils**, which give this part of the tongue a cobblestone appearance.

Muscles of the tongue

Intrinsic and extrinsic muscles lie on each side of a midline fibrous septum. The **intrinsic muscles**, arranged in vertical, horizontal and transverse bundles, lie within the tongue and have no attachment to bone. The **extrinsic muscles** (Fig. 19.25) are attached to the mandible, hyoid bone, styloid process and palate. They alter the position of the tongue; the intrinsic muscles alter its shape.

Genioglossus is attached to the mental spine of the mandible and its fibres pass backwards to fan out towards the midline of the tongue along its length.

If the genioglossus is paralysed or totally relaxed, for example as occurs in general anaesthesia or when the patient is in coma, there is a tendency for the tongue to fall back and obstruct the airway. Insertion of a tube ensures that the airway is maintained. Pulling the mandible forwards helps to protect the airway by pulling the tongue anteriorly, because of its attachment to the mental spine.

Hyoglossus, a thin quadrilateral muscle, attaches to the hyoid bone and passes up into the side of the tongue (Fig. 19.24). On the upper medial surface of hyoglossus lie the tongue, lingual artery, middle constrictor muscle, stylohyoid ligament and glossopharyngeal nerve. Laterally and below lie styloglossus, the lingual nerve, the submandibular gland and duct, the sublingual gland and the hypoglossal nerve. **Styloglossus** passes between the superior and middle constrictors to the side of the tongue. **Palatoglossus** passes downwards and forwards from the palate to the side of the tongue forming the anterior pillar of the fauces (Fig. 19.25).

Blood supply

This is from the lingual artery. Venous drainage is by the lingual vein, which drains into the internal jugular vein.

Nerve supply

The lingual nerve supplies sensation to the anterior two-thirds of the tongue, the glossopharyngeal sensation to the posterior third. Taste fibres are conveyed by the facial nerve from the chorda tympani to the anterior two-thirds of the tongue and by the glossopharyngeal nerve to the posterior third. All muscles are supplied by the hypoglossal nerve, except palatoglossus, which is supplied by the pharyngeal plexus.

When one side of the tongue is paralysed, as may follow a hypoglossal nerve paralysis, the protruded tongue deviates to that side (Fig. 19.26).

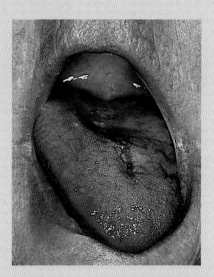

Figure 19.26 Left XIIth nerve palsy – when the tongue is protruded, it deviates to the side of the nerve lesion

Lymphatic drainage

It should be noted that the lymph from any part of the tongue may drain to nodes on both sides of the neck. The tip of the tongue drains to the submental nodes or directly to the deep cervical nodes; the side of the tongue drains to the submandibular nodes and the dorsum to the submandibular and jugulodigastric nodes. Efferent vessels then pass to the deep cervical nodes.

With **lingual cancer**, cancers arising in the posterior third of the tongue spread to the superior group of deep cervical glands on both sides of the neck. However, cancers arising from the anterior tongue spread first to the submandibular and submental nodes and only later to the inferior deep cervical nodes.

MUSCLES OF THE FLOOR OF THE MOUTH

- **Mylohyoid** (Figs. 19.25b and 19.27) – the two mylohyoid muscles form a diaphragm across the floor of the mouth between the mandible and the hyoid bone. Each is attached anterolaterally to the mylohyoid line on the mandible (Fig. 18.9a, p. 308) and its fibres pass downwards and medially, the posterior to the hyoid bone, the anterior to a midline raphé between the hyoid and the midline of the mandible. They are supplied by branches of the inferior alveolar nerve.
- **Geniohyoid** – this lies above mylohyoid, passing from the mental spine of the mandible to the hyoid bone. It is supplied by C1 fibres carried in the hypoglossal nerve.
- **Digastric** – this consists of two muscle bellies united by an intermediate tendon, which is slung by a fibrous sheath to the greater horn of the hyoid (Fig. 19.25b). The posterior belly is attached to the medial side of the mastoid process and the anterior belly to the digastric fossa on the mandible. The posterior belly is supplied by the facial nerve, the anterior by the inferior alveolar nerve.

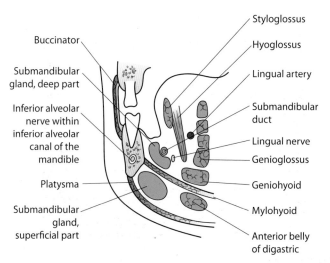

Figure 19.27 Coronal section through the tongue and floor of the mouth

Functions

The three muscles act together; they raise the hyoid bone during swallowing or, when the hyoid bone is fixed, depress the mandible, thereby opening the mouth.

SALIVARY GLANDS

There are three paired glands – parotid, submandibular and sublingual – and numerous small ones around the mouth cavity (Fig. 19.28). Their secretions clean and moisten the mouth, assisting in chewing, swallowing, phonation and digestion.

The parotid and submandibular ducts can be demonstrated radiographically after contrast medium has been injected into them (Fig. 19.29).

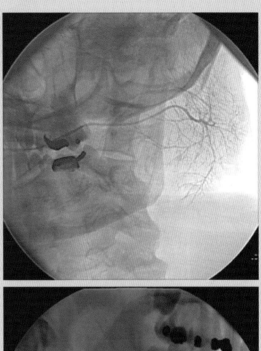

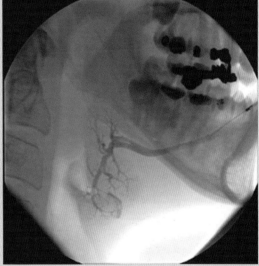

Figure 19.29 Parotid sialogram: 1, syringe inside the mouth; 2, cannula within the parotid duct just above the second upper molar tooth; 3, contrast within the glandular ducts

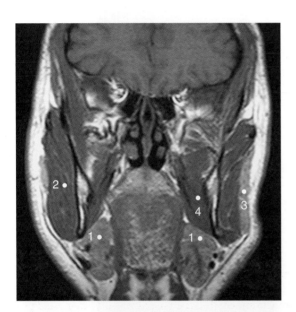

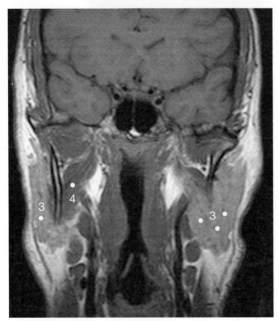

Figure 19.28 (a) and (b) Coronal MR images showing the salivary glands: 1, submandibular glands; 2, masseter muscle; 3, parotid gland; 4, medial pterygoid muscle

The parotid gland

The parotid gland (Fig. 19.30) is the largest salivary gland and lies wedged between the mandibular ramus, the mastoid process, and the styloid process medially covered by the deep investing layer of cervical fascia that invests the gland. It is irregular in shape and described as having anteromedial, posteromedial and superficial surfaces. The anterior border overlies masseter, and from it emerges the duct to pass forwards across masseter before turning medially around the anterior border of the muscle to pierce buccinator and open on to the mucous membrane of the cheek, opposite the second upper molar tooth. It is about 5 cm long.

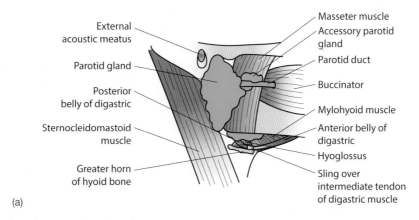

(a)

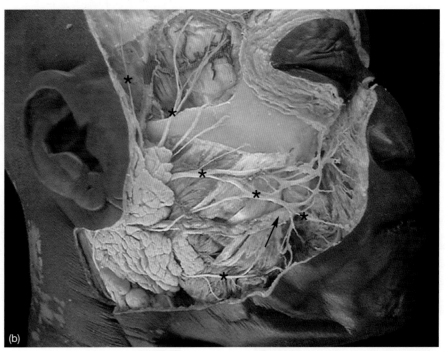

(b)

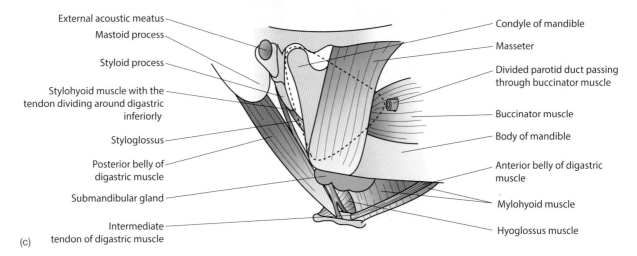

(c)

Figure 19.30 (a) Diagram of parotid gland – superficial view. (b) Detailed dissection of parotid gland showing its duct (arrow) and the numerous VIIth nerve branches (*) that emerge from its anterior border. (c) Diagram of the parotid 'bed' (parotid shown by the dashed line)

Relations

The superficial surface is covered by skin and fascia. The superficial parotid lymph nodes are buried in its surface. The anteromedial surface is wrapped around the mandibular ramus, extending on to masseter laterally and the medial pterygoid muscle medially (**Fig. 19.31**). The posteromedial surface lies on the mastoid process, the sternocleidomastoid muscle and the posterior belly of digastric muscle. Medially the deep part of the gland is separated by the styloid process and its muscles from the carotid sheath and the pharynx. The upper part of the gland lies between the external auditory meatus and the temporomandibular joint. The gland is traversed by the external carotid artery deeply, the retromandibular vein and the facial nerve superficially.

Blood supply

This is by branches of the external carotid artery. Venous blood drains to the retromandibular vein.

Nerve supply

Sympathetic fibres from the superior cervical ganglion pass with the external carotid artery; parasympathetic fibres are conveyed by the glossopharyngeal nerve via the otic ganglion and the auriculotemporal nerve. The parasympathetic nerves are secretomotor, producing saliva, and the sympathetic fibres vasoconstrictor, giving rise to a dry mouth.

Lymphatic drainage

The superficial part of the gland drains to the parotid nodes, the deep part to the retropharyngeal nodes.

Mumps, an acute viral infection, causes inflammation and swelling of the parotid and submandibular glands (**Fig. 19.32b**). It is particularly painful because the parotid gland is encased in an inextensible envelope of the deep investing cervical fascia. The pain is worsened by chewing and opening the mouth, because of the attachments of this fascia to the jaw.

A malignant **tumour** of the parotid may involve the structures lying within it, such as the retromandibular vein or – more significantly – the facial nerve, resulting in a facial palsy (**Fig. 19.32a**). Pain arising from a parotid tumour may be referred to the temporomandibular joint because of the common innervation of the gland and joint by the auriculotemporal nerve. The fine branches of the facial nerve that traverse the gland (**Fig. 19.30b**) are at risk of damage during surgical excision of the parotid and care must be taken to avoid this.

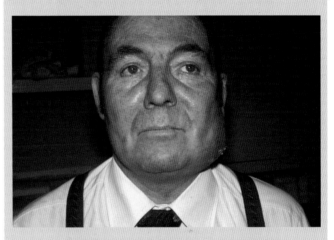

Figure 19.32 (a) Parotid tumour due to adenoma (*continued*)

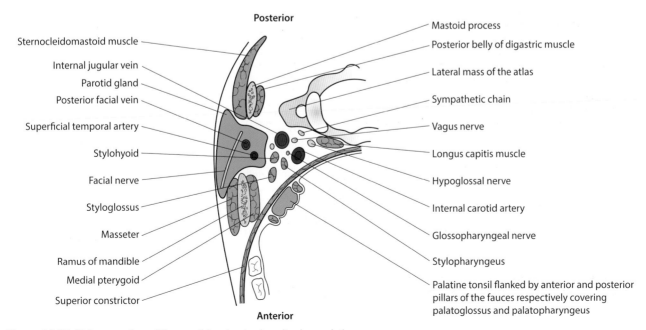

Figure 19.31 Oblique section of the parotid region to show its deep relations

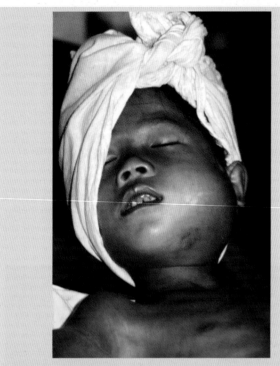

Figure 19.32 (*continued*) (b) Mumps showing extensive swelling of the submandibular and parotid glands

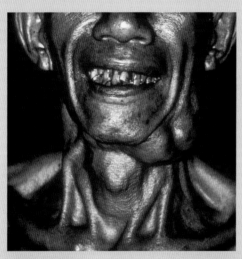

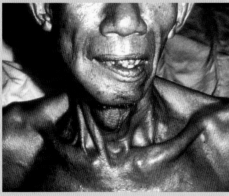

Figure 19.33 Tumour of submandibular gland: (a) preoperative; (b) postoperative, showing facial nerve palsy of mandibular branch, damaged during tumour removal and causing drooping of the lower lip and salivary drooling

The submandibular gland

The submandibular gland (Figs. 19.25b, 19.27, 19.30c and 19.33) lies in the floor of the mouth. It has a fibrous capsule and is divided into superficial and deep parts by the posterior border of mylohyoid. The submandibular duct arises from the deep part and passes forward between mylohyoid and hyoglossus, medial to the sublingual gland, to open on the sublingual papilla in the floor of the mouth at the base of the frenulum. The lingual nerve crosses the submandibular duct laterally from above and then turns upwards medial to it.

Relations

Superficial part – superomedially are mylohyoid and the anterior belly of digastric; superolaterally are the body of the mandible and medial pterygoid; inferiorly lies the deep investing layer of cervical fascia, the submandibular lymph nodes and superficial fascia containing platysma. The facial artery grooves its posterior surface and passes lateral to the gland to reach the inferior border of the mandible.

The *deep part* is wedged between mylohyoid and hyoglossus, separated from the latter by the lingual nerve and, below it, the hypoglossal nerve. Posteriorly it lies on the middle constrictor close to the lingual artery and hypoglossal nerve (Fig. 19.27).

Blood supply

This is from the facial and lingual arteries. Venous blood drains to the facial and lingual veins.

Nerve supply

Sympathetic fibres from the superior cervical ganglion are conveyed along arteries; parasympathetic fibres are carried in the facial nerve via the chorda tympani and hitch-hike on to the lingual nerve before synapsing in the submandibular ganglion.

Lymphatic drainage

Drainage is to the overlying submandibular nodes.

Salivary calculi may form in the salivary gland ducts. They are most common in the submandibular duct and cause painful swelling of the gland; this is exacerbated when salivary flow is increased, such as during eating. Submandibular duct stones may be removed surgically via the floor of the mouth, or, if this is impossible, the submandibular gland requires removal. The operation runs the risk of damage to the mandibular branch of the facial nerve (Fig. 19.33). If the incision for this operation is made about 3 cm below the angle of the mandible, such damage to the facial nerve should not occur.

The sublingual glands

The sublingual glands (Fig. 19.23) are paired, almond-shaped glands lying beneath the mucous membrane of the floor of the mouth. They drain either to the neighbouring submandibular duct or directly into the mouth cavity via 15–20 small ducts. Each gland lies on mylohyoid, medial to the mandible and lateral to the submandibular duct, the lingual nerve and hyoglossus. Its blood and nerve supply and its lymphatic drainage are similar to those of the submandibular gland.

DEVELOPMENT OF THE FACE AND PALATE

The face develops from five primordia that grow around the developing mouth (stomodeum) (Fig. 19.34). These include the singular large midline frontonasal process and the left and right maxillary and mandibular processes, which derive from first pharyngeal arch tissues. Defects in the formation of the first pharyngeal arch therefore result in facial deformity that may involve the maxilla, zygoma and mandible. Defects can occur in the degree of closure of the stomodeum, resulting in either macrostomia (too little closure) or microstomia (too much closure). The frontonasal process forms the forehead, premaxilla (the central anterior part of the maxilla associated with the incisor teeth) and nasal region, including the nostrils, nasal septum, nose, ethmoid, cribriform plate and philtrum (Fig. 19.34). The left and right maxillary processes grow and fuse with the frontonasal process and form the upper cheek, palate and upper jaw. The left and right mandibular processes fuse in the anterior midline to form the chin, lower jaw and lower cheek. Incomplete mandibular process fusion is often seen as a dimple in the skin of the chin.

The palate (hard and soft) develops from the primary and secondary palates. The medial nasal prominences of the frontonasal process form the median palatine process/primary palate, which eventually forms the premaxillary part of the maxilla (Figs. 19.34 and 19.35). The secondary palate is formed by the left and right lateral palatine processes, which arise from their respective maxillary prominences. The palatine processes grow to meet and join each other and the nasal septum in the midline and the primary palate anteriorly. The posterior parts of the lateral palatine plates grow posteriorly to form the soft palate and uvula.

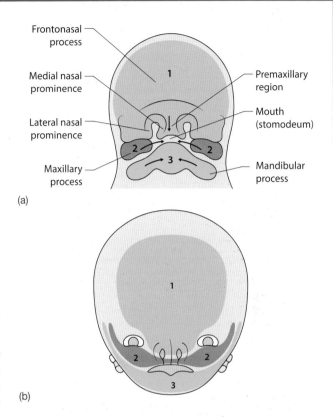

(a)

(b)

Figure 19.34 (a) Facial development the tissue primordia situated around the primitive mouth (stomodeum). The maxillary (2) and mandibular (3) primordia/processes grow and move toward the midline. The anterior midline premaxillary part of the frontonasal process (1) is met on either side by the maxillary processes. Arrows indicate the direction of tissue movement. (b) The completed face showing the approximate regions formed from the tissue primordia

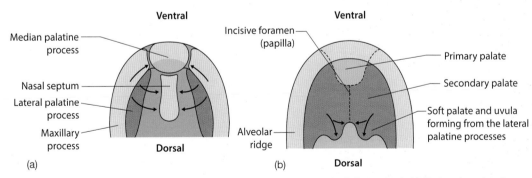

(a)   (b)

Figure 19.35 Formation of the palate from the median and lateral palatine processes (inferior view). (a) Early palate development showing the median and lateral palatine processes. Arrows indicate the direction of tissue growth towards their points of fusion. (b) Later stage of palate development showing the normal location of the lines of fusion. Palate clefting can occur if growth or fusion does not complete normally

Defects in the growth and/or fusion of the palatine processes and premaxilla can result in various forms of cleft palate, which can be unilateral or bilateral and may be associated with a cleft in the lip and/or uvula (Figs. 19.36 and 19.37). Cleft palate can be classified as anterior or posterior depending upon the position of the cleft relative to the incisive fossa/ papilla. A cleft lip most often occurs either side of the midline philtrum and represents a failure of fusion of the maxillary process with the medial nasal prominence (Fig. 19.34). Cleft lip may be associated with a cleft palate, and can extend towards the nose or eye (Fig. 19.37).

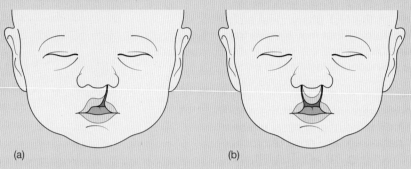

(a)

(b)

Figure 19.36 Clefting of the lip represents an anterior cleft defect due to failure of complete fusion between the median palatine process and the tissues from the maxillary prominences. (a) Left unilateral cleft lip. (b) Bilateral cleft lip

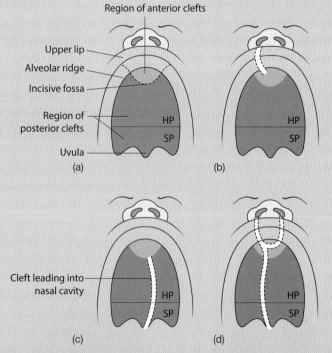

Region of anterior clefts

Upper lip
Alveolar ridge
Incisive fossa
Region of posterior clefts
Uvula

HP
SP

(a)

HP
SP

(b)

Cleft leading into nasal cavity

HP
SP

(c)

HP
SP

(d)

Figure 19.37 Developmental defects of the palate (inferior view) can be unilateral or bilateral. (a) Normal soft (SP) and hard (HP) palate showing the regions for anterior clefts and posterior clefts (separated by dashed line). (b) Anterior right unilateral cleft palate with left unilateral cleft lip. (c) Posterior left unilateral cleft palate. (d) Bilateral anterior cleft palate and cleft lip with posterior right unilateral cleft palate

MCQs

1. With regard to the paranasal sinuses: **T/F**

  a the maxillary sinus of the newborn is relatively large compared with that of the adult   ( )

  b the mucous membrane of the maxillary sinus and the upper premolar teeth have the same nerve supply   ( )

  c pain may be referred from the frontal sinus to the scalp   ( )

  d the sphenoidal sinuses are supplied by the posterior ethmoidal nerves   ( )

  e the frontal, sphenoidal, maxillary and anterior ethmoidal sinuses drain into the middle meatus   ( )

Answers

1.

a F – *Paranasal air sinuses are rudimentary in the newborn. The mastoid air cells, for example, because of their lack of development, offer no protection to the facial nerve as it leaves the stylomastoid foramen. Facial nerve palsy occasionally occurs after forceps delivery.*

b T – *The superior alveolar (dental) nerve supplies both structures, and it is quite common for a dentist to perform some dental procedure, such as a filling, when the real cause of the pain he thinks he is treating is within the sinus.*

c T – *The nerve supply is by the supraorbital nerve, which also supplies the scalp as far as the vertex. Referred pain to the scalp may therefore be a feature of frontal sinusitis.*

d T

e F – *The sphenoidal sinus drains into the sphenoethmoidal recess and not into the middle meatus.*

2. The parotid gland: **T/F**

  a is a serous gland   ( )

  b is in direct contact with the internal carotid artery   ( )

  c possesses a deep lobe in contact with the external acoustic meatus   ( )

  d envelops the branches of the facial nerve   ( )

  e lies within the deep cervical fascia   ( )

Answers

2.

a T

b F – *The gland is in contact with the external carotid artery and its branches but is separated from the internal carotid artery by the posterior belly of digastric, stylohyoid and the styloid process.*

c T

d T – *The facial nerve divides within the substance of the gland into its five terminal branches.*

e T – *The gland is enclosed within the parotid fascia, an extension of the investing layer of the deep cervical fascia.*

SBA

1 A 50-year-old woman was complaining of left-sided dental pain in her upper teeth. No dental abnormality could be found but she had pain in the left maxillary area when that region was tapped by the doctor. What is the likely diagnosis?
  a frontal sinusitis
  b posterior ethmoidal sinusitis
  c sphenoid sinusitis
  d maxillary sinusitis
  e anterior ethmoidal sinusitis

Answer

d *The maxillary sinus lies in the body of the maxillary bone. Infection produces pain in the sinus, which lies in close proximity to those teeth that arise from the maxillary bone. This is because the roots of these upper jaw teeth have exactly the same nerve supply as the maxillary sinus – the superior alveolar nerves, branches of the maxillary nerve.*

2 An unconscious patient is admitted after sustaining a head injury. The physician performs an ophthalmoscopic examination and finds that the pupil of the left eye constricts when the light is shone into that eye. Pupillary constriction on stimulation by light indicates which two cranial nerves are intact?
  a optic and oculomotor
  b optic and facial
  c ophthalmic and facial
  d maxillary and facial
  e ophthalmic and oculomotor

Answer

a *The physician has confirmed the presence of an intact pupillary light reflex, which is mediated by afferent impulses carried by the intact optic nerve sensing the light impulses. Efferent impulses carried by parasympathetic fibres lying in the intact oculomotor nerve then cause contraction of the sphincter pupillae muscle of the iris to result in constriction of the pupil.*

EMQs

Each question has an anatomical theme linked to the chapter, and a list of 10 related items (A–J) placed in alphabetical order: these are followed by five statements (1–5). Match **one or more** of the items A–J to each of the five statements.

Orbit and nose
A. Bulla ethmoidalis
B. Ethmoid bone
C. Greater wing of sphenoid
D. Inferior concha
E. Lacrimal bone
F. Lesser wing of sphenoid
G. Maxilla
H. Palatine bone
I. Septal cartilage
J. Vomer

Answers
1 CF; *2* F; *3* D; *4* BIJ; *5* ABG

Match the following statements with the bone(s) in the above list.
1. Borders the superior orbital fissure
2. Transmits the ophthalmic artery
3. Overlaps the opening of the nasolacrimal duct
4. Forms the nasal septum
5. Contains paranasal air sinuses

Muscles of the mouth
A. Anterior belly of the digastric muscle
B. Buccinator
C. Hyoglossus
D. Intrinsic muscles of the tongue
E. Longus capitis
F. Masseter
G. Medial pterygoid
H. Orbicularis oris
I. Palatopharyngeus
J. Styloglossus

Answers
1 BH; *2* I; *3* AFG; *4* CDJ; *5* A

Match the following nerves to the muscle(s) in the above list.
1. Facial
2. Vagus
3. Trigeminal
4. Hypoglossal
5. Inferior alveolar

APPLIED QUESTIONS

1. Why might a simple jaw fracture result in a numb lower lip?

1. *The mental nerve that provides the sensory supply to the lower lip is a branch of the inferior alveolar nerve, which lies inside the mandible, supplying the teeth. Any jaw fracture may damage the nerve and cause loss of sensation over the chin and lower lip.*

2. Following removal of a submandibular gland for a cancerous growth, why might the patient have a 'drooping' lower lip?

2. *The lower lip musculature is supplied by the cervical and marginal mandibular branches of the facial nerve. When operating on a submandibular growth it may be impossible to avoid cutting through either or both of these nerves, leaving the patient with a drooping lip (Fig. 19.33b).*

3. Where would a radiologist insert his cannula to perform a sialogram of the submandibular gland?

3. *When the tip of the tongue is put up to the roof of the mouth, a prominent midline fold of mucous membrane – the frenulum – can be seen. On either side of the frenulum are the sublingual papillae, on the surface of which can be found the opening of the submandibular (Wharton's) duct. Lying lateral to the papillae are the sublingual folds, beneath which lie the sublingual glands, whose numerous ducts open along the crest of the folds. A few drops of lemon juice on the tongue will increase salivation. Clinicians sometimes employ this to identify the small submandibular duct orifices.*

4. What have the mastoid, ethmoid, sphenoid and maxilla in common?

4. *They are hollow bones containing air-filled spaces. The mastoid air cells lead into the middle ear while the ethmoid, sphenoid and maxillary paranasal air sinuses all open into the lateral wall of the nasal cavity. These air spaces are said to lighten the weight of the skull and give the voice resonance.*

Bailey & Love · Essential Clinical Anatomy · Bailey & Love · Essential Clinical Anatomy
Essential Clinical Anatomy · Bailey & Love · Essential Clinical Anatomy · Bailey & Love
Bailey & Love · Essential Clinical Anatomy · Bailey & Love · Essential Clinical Anatomy

Chapter **20**

The temporomandibular joint, pharynx and larynx

THE TEMPOROMANDIBULAR JOINT

The **temporomandibular joint** (Fig. 20.1) is a synovial joint of a modified hinge (condyloid) variety between the condyle of the mandible and the mandibular fossa of the temporal bone. The hemicylindrical condyle is directed medially and the temporal articular surface is convexo-concave from front to back. The articular surfaces are covered with fibrocartilage.

Ligaments

- **Capsular** – attached to the neck of the mandible and to the articular margins of the temporal bone.
- **Lateral ligament** – a strong thickening of the capsule, passes down and back from the inferior zygomatic arch to the back of the mandible, thus limiting backwards movement.
- **Accessory ligaments** – the **sphenomandibular ligament** from the spine of the sphenoid to the mandibular lingula;

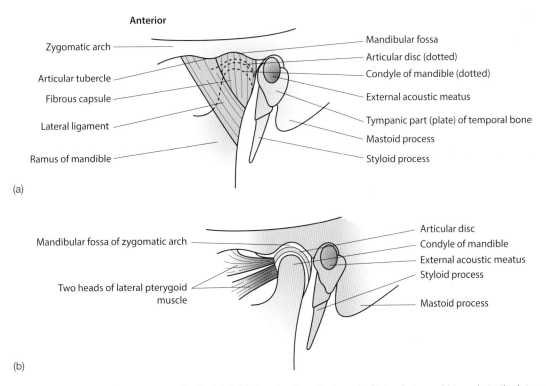

Anterior

(a) Zygomatic arch — Articular tubercle — Fibrous capsule — Lateral ligament — Ramus of mandible

Mandibular fossa — Articular disc (dotted) — Condyle of mandible (dotted) — External acoustic meatus — Tympanic part (plate) of temporal bone — Mastoid process — Styloid process

(b) Mandibular fossa of zygomatic arch — Two heads of lateral pterygoid muscle

Articular disc — Condyle of mandible — External acoustic meatus — Styloid process — Mastoid process

Figure 20.1 Lateral view of the (a) temporomandibular joint, (b) showing the attachment of lateral pterygoid muscle to the intracapsular disc

the **stylomandibular ligament**, a thickening of the deep layer of the cervical fascia, passes from the styloid process to the posterior border of the mandibular ramus.

- **Intracapsular structures** – a fibrocartilaginous disc, concave on its undersurface, is attached by its margins to the capsule, dividing the joint cavity into superior and inferior compartments. This increases the range of the joint's movements.

Functional aspects

Movement

Movement has two components, each occurring in different compartments of the joint (Fig. 20.2): **gliding** occurs in the upper compartment as the condyle of the mandible and the articular disc move together over the articular surface; a **hinge movement** occurs in the lower compartment, the mandibular condyle articulating with the undersurface of the articular disc. These components are never completely dissociated during mandibular movements, and movement in one compartment must be accompanied by movement in the other. Both movements are involved in depression and elevation, but in protrusion, retraction and grinding the gliding movement is predominant.

Depression occurs about an axis passing through the mandibular lingula; the condyles are pulled forwards by lateral pterygoid and the body is pulled downwards by geniohyoid, digastric and mylohyoid acting from a fixed hyoid bone. **Elevation**, around the same axis, is produced by masseter, temporalis and medial pterygoid; **protrusion** by the two lateral pterygoids acting together; **retraction** by the posterior fibres of temporalis; and **grinding movements** by alternating protrusion and retraction of the two sides. In chewing the mandible is moved from side to side while being elevated by masseter and temporalis. The tongue and the cheeks keep the food between the teeth.

Stability

This varies with the position of the mandible. The joint is most stable when the mandible is fully elevated and the mouth closed; the condyles then lie in the articular fossae, occlusion of the teeth prevents further upward movement and the taut lateral ligament prevents posterior dislocation. Contraction of the muscles is necessary to maintain this position; in sleep the jaw drops open, owing to gravity. In the resting position the teeth are slightly separated. When the mandible is depressed the condyle lies on the articular tubercle and the joint's stability depends on muscular tone and capsular strength.

Forward dislocation is the most common form of dislocation, often occurring when the jaw is totally relaxed in a wide yawn. Excessive contraction of the lateral pterygoids causes the heads of the mandible to be pulled anterior to the articular tubercles. Traumatic dislocations are caused by blows to the open mouth. Reduction of the dislocation is achieved by pressing down onto the molars, with or without the relaxation provided by general anaesthesia, and guiding the mandibular condyle backwards into the mandibular fossa.

Blood supply

This is via the superficial temporal and maxillary arteries.

Nerve supply

This is via the auriculotemporal nerve.

Relations

Laterally – skin and superficial fascia; medially – the sphenomandibular ligament, auriculotemporal nerve and middle meningeal artery; anteriorly – the lateral pterygoid; posteriorly – the parotid gland, auriculotemporal nerve and tympanic plate of the temporal bone.

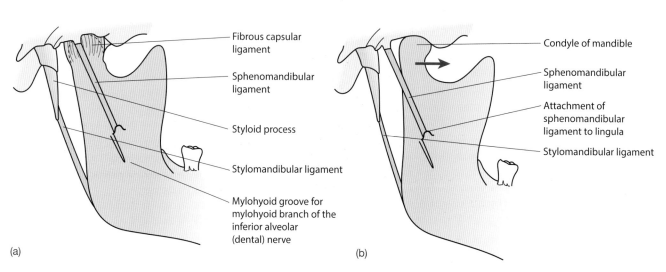

(a)   (b)

Figure 20.2 Movements of the temporomandibular joint around the sphenomandibular ligament attachments: (a) mouth closed and (b) mouth open, viewed from the medial aspect. The arrow shows the forward movement of the condyle onto the convexity of the temporal articular surface

THE MUSCLES OF MASTICATION

All are supplied by the mandibular division of the trigeminal nerve.

- **Masseter** (Fig. 18.13, p. 311) – attached superiorly to the lower border of the anterior zygomatic arch and inferiorly to the lateral surface of the angle and ramus of the mandible. It elevates the mandible.
- **Temporalis** (Fig. 20.3) – attached superiorly to the lateral surface of the skull below the temporal line; inferiorly the fibres converge on to a narrow tendon attached to the coronoid process and anterior border of the mandible. The anterior fibres are vertical, the posterior horizontal. The anterior fibres elevate and the posterior fibres retract the mandible.

- **Medial pterygoid** – attached above by two heads: the deep head to the medial surface of the lateral pterygoid plate, and the superficial head to the maxillary tuberosity; inferiorly it is attached to the medial surface of the ramus and the angle of the mandible. It elevates and protrudes the mandible.
- **Lateral pterygoid** (Fig. 20.1b) – anteriorly attached by two heads, the upper to the infratemporal surface of the greater wing of the sphenoid and the lower from the lateral surface of the lateral pterygoid plate; posteriorly it is attached to the neck of the mandible and the capsule and intra-articular disc of the temporomandibular joint. It protrudes and depresses the mandible and is the muscle that produces forced opening against resistance.

THE INFRATEMPORAL FOSSA

This lies below the base of the skull and behind the maxilla and the pterygoid plates of the sphenoid, in front of the carotid sheath (Fig. 20.4). It is limited medially by the pharynx and laterally by the temporalis muscle and ramus of the mandible. Inferiorly it is continuous with the fascial spaces of the neck. It contains the lateral and medial pterygoid muscles, the mandibular division of the trigeminal nerve and its branches, the maxillary artery and its branches (for a full description of this artery see p. 390), the pterygoid venous plexus and the sphenomandibular ligament. The **temporal fascia**, a dense sheet, covers the temporalis muscle and has a continuous attachment to the temporal line above and the zygomatic arch below. It is continuous with the epicranial aponeurosis.

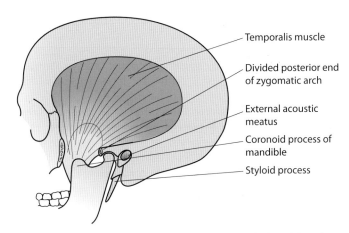

Temporalis muscle

Divided posterior end of zygomatic arch

External acoustic meatus

Coronoid process of mandible

Styloid process

Figure 20.3 Tendon of temporalis muscle revealed by excision of the zygomatic arch

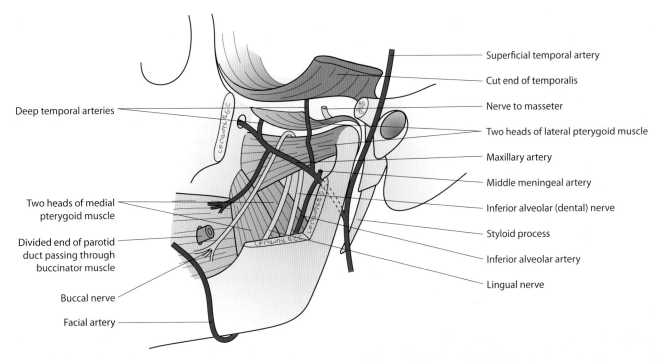

Deep temporal arteries

Two heads of medial pterygoid muscle

Divided end of parotid duct passing through buccinator muscle

Buccal nerve

Facial artery

Superficial temporal artery

Cut end of temporalis

Nerve to masseter

Two heads of lateral pterygoid muscle

Maxillary artery

Middle meningeal artery

Inferior alveolar (dental) nerve

Styloid process

Inferior alveolar artery

Lingual nerve

Figure 20.4 Infratemporal fossa – left zygomatic arch and coronoid process of the mandible removed (lateral view)

THE PHARYNX

The pharynx is a muscular tube about 14 cm long with a largely deficient anterior wall that communicates with the nose, mouth and larynx. It extends from the skull base to the level of the 6th cervical vertebra, where it becomes the oesophagus (Fig. 20.5). It is divided into three parts: the nasopharynx, oropharynx and laryngopharynx. Posteriorly it lies on the prevertebral fascia and muscles; laterally it is related, from above downwards, to the auditory tube, the styloid process and its muscles, the carotid sheath and its contents, and the thyroid gland.

Its thin walls have mucous, submucous and muscular coats. The **mucous coat** is continuous with those of the nose, auditory tube, oral cavity, larynx and oesophagus; it is lined in the nasopharynx with respiratory epithelium and elsewhere with stratified squamous epithelium. The **submucosa** is thickened superiorly, where the muscular coat is deficient, to form the **pharyngobasilar fascia** attached to the base of the skull. The **muscular coat** comprises the superior, middle and inferior constrictor muscles, blending with and reinforced by salpingo-, stylo- and palatopharyngeus muscles (Fig. 20.6).

The **superior constrictor** is attached anteriorly to the medial pterygoid plate, the retromolar fossa of the mandible and, between these two points, to the pterygomandibular raphé (Fig. 20.6).

The **middle constrictor** is attached anteriorly to the stylohyoid ligament and the lesser and greater horns of the hyoid. The **inferior constrictor** has two parts: one attached anteri-orly to the oblique line on the thyroid cartilage and the other, lower, part attached to the fascia over cricothyroid and the cricoid cartilage. The gap between these two parts, known as the dehiscence of Killian, is a weak point in the pharyngeal wall. This muscle acts as a sphincter at the lower end of the pharynx. It is always closed apart from a short relaxation during the onset of swallowing (see below).

Each constrictor fans out from its anterior attachment and passes posteriorly around the pharynx to join its opposite fellow in a fibrous midline raphé that extends from the occipital bone to the oesophagus (Fig. 20.6b). The pairs of muscles overlap; the inferior lies outside the middle, which is outside the superior constrictor, rather like three flowerpots or glasses stacked one inside the other.

Salpingopharyngeus, **stylopharyngeus** and **palatopharyngeus** are attached to the auditory tube, styloid process and soft palate, respectively. They descend to blend with the inner surfaces of the constrictors and gain attachment to the lamina of the thyroid cartilage. All pharyngeal muscles elevate the pharynx and are concerned in swallowing (p. 345). They are supplied by the vagus and cranial accessory nerves via the pharyngeal plexus, apart from stylopharyngeus, which is supplied directly by the glossopharyngeal nerve.

Between the superior constrictor and the skull base the pharyngobasilar fascia is pierced by the auditory tube. Stylopharyngeus and styloglossus, and the glossopharyngeal nerve, enter between the superior and the middle constrictors and the recurrent laryngeal nerve enters below the inferior constrictor.

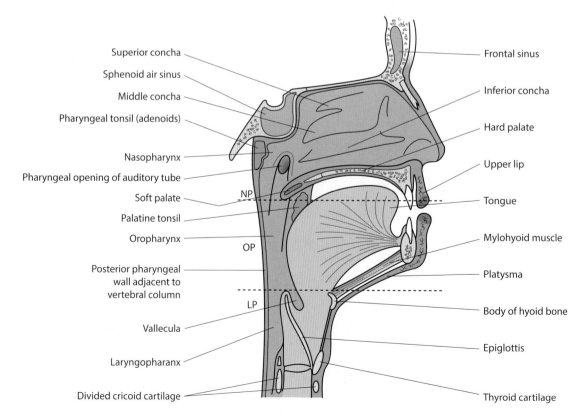

Figure 20.5 Sagittal section showing the subdivisions of the pharynx: NP, naso-; OP, oro-; LP, laryngopharynx

Rarely the pharyngeal mucosa may bulge through between the thyroid and cricoid components of the inferior constrictor (Killian's dehiscence) to produce an acquired pharyngeal pouch, in which food may become lodged.

The interior of the pharynx

The **nasopharynx** lies behind the two posterior nasal openings (**choanae**). On each lateral wall are the openings of the auditory tube (Fig. 20.5). Posteriorly a small aggregation of lymphoid tissue, the nasopharyngeal tonsils (**adenoids**), is present. The nasopharynx is limited superiorly by the base of the skull; below it communicates with the oropharynx through the pharyngeal isthmus, a constriction that can be closed by the mobile soft palate (Fig. 20.5).

The **oropharynx** extends down to the upper border of the epiglottis, where it is continuous with the laryngopharynx. Anteriorly it communicates through the **faucial isthmus or**

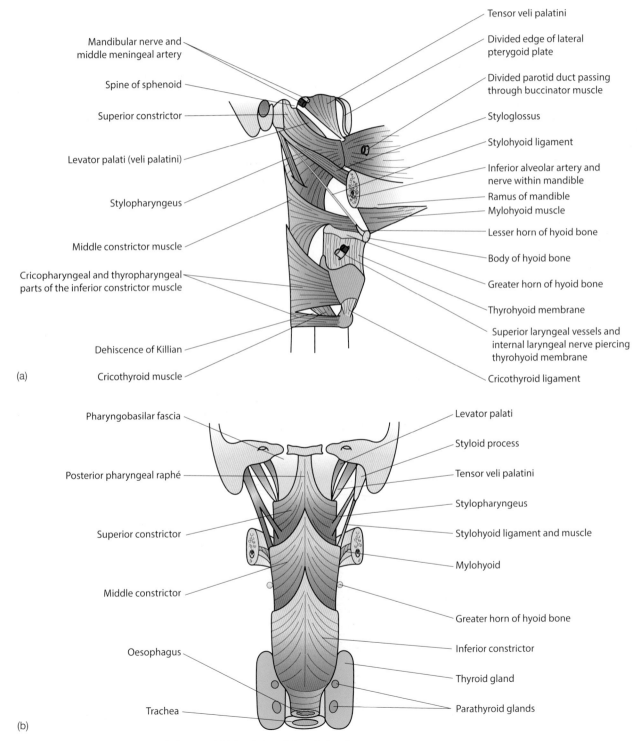

(a)

Labels (lateral view):
- Mandibular nerve and middle meningeal artery
- Spine of sphenoid
- Superior constrictor
- Levator palati (veli palatini)
- Stylopharyngeus
- Middle constrictor muscle
- Cricopharyngeal and thyropharyngeal parts of the inferior constrictor muscle
- Dehiscence of Killian
- Cricothyroid muscle
- Tensor veli palatini
- Divided edge of lateral pterygoid plate
- Divided parotid duct passing through buccinator muscle
- Styloglossus
- Stylohyoid ligament
- Inferior alveolar artery and nerve within mandible
- Ramus of mandible
- Mylohyoid muscle
- Lesser horn of hyoid bone
- Body of hyoid bone
- Greater horn of hyoid bone
- Thyrohyoid membrane
- Superior laryngeal vessels and internal laryngeal nerve piercing thyrohyoid membrane
- Cricothyroid ligament

(b)

Labels (posterior view):
- Pharyngobasilar fascia
- Posterior pharyngeal raphé
- Superior constrictor
- Middle constrictor
- Oesophagus
- Trachea
- Levator palati
- Styloid process
- Tensor veli palatini
- Stylopharyngeus
- Stylohyoid ligament and muscle
- Mylohyoid
- Greater horn of hyoid bone
- Inferior constrictor
- Thyroid gland
- Parathyroid glands

Figure 20.6 Constrictor muscles of pharynx: (a) lateral view; (b) posterior view

fauces with the oral cavity. Below the isthmus is the tongue, partly in the pharynx and partly in the oral cavity (Figs. 20.5 and 20.7). In the lateral wall of the isthmus are two vertical folds of mucous membrane, the **anterior and posterior arches of the fauces**, formed by palatoglossus and palatopharyngeus. The **palatine tonsil**, more commonly known as 'the **tonsil**', lies between them (Fig. 19.22, p. 324). Behind the tongue a median and two lateral glossoepiglottic folds define two shallow depressions, the valleculae.

The **laryngopharynx** extends from the oropharynx to the oesophagus. Anteriorly lie the laryngeal opening and the arytenoid and cricoid cartilages, and the cavity passes forwards on each side of the larynx to form the **piriform fossae**. Each fossa is bounded by mucous membrane-covered cartilages and is related to the thyroid and thyrohyoid membrane laterally and the aryepiglottic fold medially.

The piriform fossae are danger sites for perforation during rigid endoscopy and have acquired some notoriety as sites where malignancies may develop silently without symptoms before presentation with secondary deposits in the deep cervical lymph nodes. The pharyngeal lumen is narrowest at its junction with the oesophagus, the **cricopharyngeal sphincter**.

Blood supply

This is via branches of the external carotid, lingual, facial and maxillary arteries. Veins drain to the pharyngeal venous plexus and thence to the internal jugular vein.

Nerve supply

This is via the pharyngeal plexus on the side of middle constrictor. The **pharyngeal plexus** is formed by:

- Sensory fibres from branches of the glossopharyngeal nerve
- Motor fibres carried in the vagus, and cranial accessory nerves from the nucleus ambiguus (supplying all muscles apart from stylopharyngeus, which is supplied by the glossopharyngeal nerve)
- Branches from the cervical sympathetic chain via the superior cervical ganglion.

The simplest way to test the integrity of the pharyngeal plexus and its cranial nerves is by touching the posterior part of the tongue or the fauces, which should induce a 'gag'. This is due to the sensory glossopharyngeal portion stimulating the vagus and cranial accessory nerves, which are motor to the early phase of gagging or vomiting (gag reflex) – a simple way to test the three cranial nerves simultaneously (p. 366).

Lymphatic drainage

The nasopharynx drains to the retropharyngeal nodes, the remainder of the pharynx to the deep cervical nodes.

Aggregations of lymph tissue surround the upper part of the pharynx: a pair of palatine tonsils below the soft palate (see below), the lingual tonsil in the posterior tongue, the

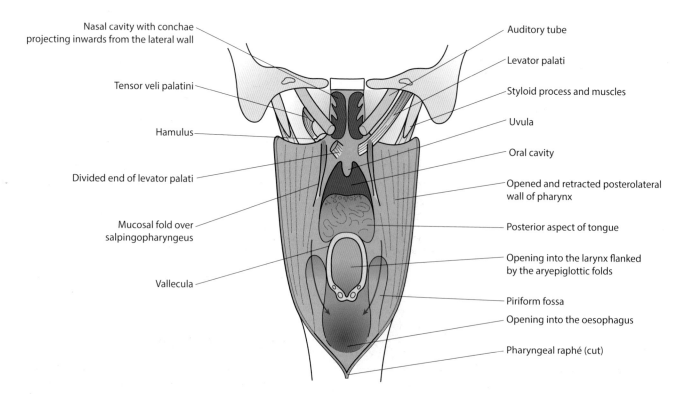

Figure 20.7 Interior of the pharynx, viewed from behind – the arrows lie in the piriform fossae on each side

tubal tonsil around the opening of the auditory tube, and the nasopharyngeal tonsil (adenoids) in the roof and posterior wall of the nasopharynx.

In young children the adenoids and tubal tonsils are prone to infection and enlargement, and the resultant swelling may cause blockage of the auditory (Eustachian) tube. This results in infection of the middle ear (otitis media) and is often the cause of mouth-breathing and nasal speech. Surgical removal of tonsils and adenoids must occasionally be performed to improve hearing and developmental problems caused by long-standing 'glue ear'. The effects of auditory tube blockage are appreciated by airline passengers, who learn to relieve it by sucking and swallowing sweets, thus using levator palati and salpingopharyngeus to 'pop open' the auditory tube.

Damage to the pharyngeal plexus may be the result of a stroke or a neurological disease process within the brainstem, known as the bulb. The resulting 'bulbar palsy' may cause difficulty in swallowing.

The tonsil

Each **tonsil** (palatine tonsil; **Figs. 19.22**, p. 324, **19.31**, p. 331, and **20.5**) is a body of lymph tissue in the fossa on the lateral wall of the fauces. It is oval in shape, with upper and lower poles. Its size varies but it is always larger in children. A well-marked **supratonsillar cleft** lies between the upper pole and the upper wall of the fossa. The deep surface is attached to a fibrous capsule, which separates it from the superior constrictor muscle and facial artery. The tonsil's blood vessels enter it inferiorly. Anteriorly lies the palatoglossal arch and posteriorly the palatopharyngeal arch. Above it is the soft palate and below it is the tongue.

Blood supply

There are tonsillar branches from the facial, lingual and ascending pharyngeal arteries. The veins drain to the pharyngeal venous plexus.

Lymphatic drainage

This is to the deep cervical chain, particularly the jugulodigastric node.

Infection of the palatine tonsils (tonsillitis; **Fig. 20.8**) is common in children. The gland is seen to be swollen and its surface marked by exudates of pus. Pain is often referred to the ear (referred otalgia) via the glossopharyngeal nerve, which lies in the tonsillar bed, and swallowing is difficult because of the pain. Rarely the infection may develop into a peritonsillar abscess (quinsy), which requires surgical drainage. Tonsillectomy is occasionally required for repeated bouts of infection.

The auditory tube

The auditory (Eustachian) tube (**Figs. 20.7** and **21.4a**, p. 357) connects the lateral pharyngeal wall of the nasopharynx and the middle ear. It is about 4 cm long and directed upwards, backwards and laterally. The lateral third lies within the temporal bone; the remainder is largely cartilaginous and

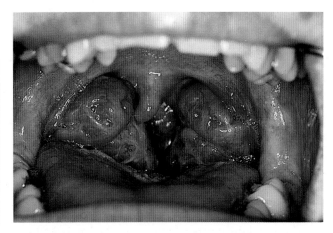

Figure 20.8 Tonsillitis – note the enlarged, swollen palatine tonsils

completed by fibrous tissue. It is supplied by the pharyngeal branch of the maxillary nerve and the tympanic branch of the glossopharyngeal. Its lymph vessels drain to the retropharyngeal nodes.

The tube passes between the middle ear and nasopharynx and serves to equalize the pressure on the two sides of the tympanic membrane. Salpingopharyngeus and tensor and levator veli palatini pull on the medial part of the tube during swallowing and thus open the tube.

In children the tube is wider and more horizontal, and infection is thus more likely to spread from the nasopharynx to the middle ear. The auditory tube allows intubation of the middle ear and the opportunity to clear it of inflammatory exudates. A catheter is passed along the nasal floor to the posterior nasopharynx and then manipulated into the tube. Infection of the mucous membrane is the most common cause of **blockage of the auditory tube** and this results in absorption of the air and a reduction of air pressure in the middle ear. Hearing is diminished.

The styloid muscles

The styloid process gives attachment to three muscles and a ligament (**Figs. 19.25a,b**, pp. 326 and 327). The muscles are active in swallowing.

Stylopharyngeus descends to enter the pharynx between superior and middle constrictors, and blends with the latter before attaching to the thyroid cartilage. It is supplied directly by the glossopharyngeal nerve. **Stylohyoid** descends to the hyoid bone and is supplied by the facial nerve. **Styloglossus** passes between the superior and middle constrictors to be attached to the side of the tongue. It is supplied by the hypoglossal nerve. The **stylohyoid ligament**, a second branchial arch derivative, passes to the lesser horn of the hyoid bone and gives attachment to the middle constrictor.

Deglutition (swallowing)

The **first (oral) phase** of swallowing is voluntary and involves the food passing from the mouth to the oropharynx. The mandible is fixed, with the teeth occluded by the muscles of mastication; the tongue is tensed by its intrinsic muscles and raised by the palatoglossus and the muscles attached to the hyoid bone (geniohyoid, mylohyoid, stylohyoid and digastric). The tongue is pressed against the hard palate, from before backwards, so forcing the food into the oropharynx.

The **second (pharyngeal) phase** is largely involuntary. Food is passed to the lower end of the pharynx. The phase is initiated by food touching the arches of the fauces, the soft palate, the posterior oropharynx or the epiglottis. The nasopharynx is closed off, as is the larynx, with coincident cessation of respiration. The pharyngeal isthmus is closed by levator and tensor veli palatini raising and tensing the soft palate; there is simultaneous approximation of the pharyngeal walls to the posterior free border of the soft palate by palatopharyngeus and the superior constrictor. The larynx is closed by approximation of the epiglottis and arytenoid cartilages; contraction of the arytenoid muscle and the passive bending backwards of the epiglottis both contribute to this. Liquids flow around the sides of the epiglottis and, with the food bolus, pass down into the piriform fossae of the laryngopharynx (this is known as 'the lateral food channel'). The larynx is raised and the pharynx shortened by the palatopharyngeus, salpingopharyngeus, stylopharyngeus and thyrohyoid muscles. The vocal folds are adducted and respiration inhibited.

In the **final (oesophageal) phase** food is passed into the oesophagus by the momentary relaxation of the inferior constrictor. This is involuntary and initiated by food stimulating the lower pharyngeal walls. Peristaltic waves convey food onwards to the stomach, the soft palate and larynx return to their positions, and respiration recommences.

Because of the multiple innervation and complex coordination of the several muscles used it is not a good idea to talk or laugh while swallowing, otherwise the food or drink may appear in the nose or go 'down the wrong way' into the airway.

THE LARYNX

The larynx (Fig. 20.9) provides phonation in the human and, equally importantly, a protective sphincter in the respiratory

passage between the pharynx and trachea. It lies opposite the 3rd to 6th cervical vertebrae, being covered anteriorly by the deep (investing) layer of cervical fascia and the infrahyoid or strap muscles. The thyroid gland and carotid sheath lie on either side. The skeleton of the larynx is formed of cartilages surrounding its lumen: the unpaired thyroid, cricoid and epiglottic and the paired arytenoid, cartilages (Fig. 20.10; see also Fig. 20.12). Articulations occur at the cricothyroid and cricoarytenoid joints.

The **thyroid cartilage** comprises two thin quadrilateral laminae united anteriorly at an angle of 120 degrees in the female and 90 degrees in the adult male, forming the midline subcutaneous **laryngeal prominence**, more commonly known as the 'Adam's apple', above which is the V-shaped **thyroid notch**. From the posterior border of each lamina extend the superior and inferior horns of the thyroid. The outer surface of each lamina bears an oblique line. The inferior horn articulates with the cricoid cartilage. To the upper border is attached the **thyrohyoid membrane**. The thyrohyoid, sternothyroid and inferior constrictor muscles are attached to

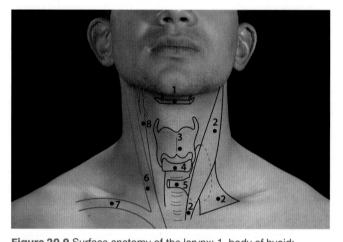

Figure 20.9 Surface anatomy of the larynx: 1, body of hyoid; 2, sternocleidomastoid; 3, thyroid cartilage; 4, cricoid cartilage; 5, divided isthmus of thyroid gland; 6, internal jugular vein; 7, subclavian vein; 8, common carotid artery

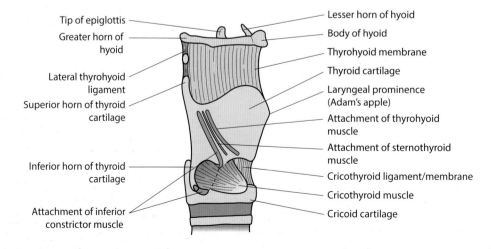

Figure 20.10 Cartilages of the larynx: (a) lateral view (*continued*)

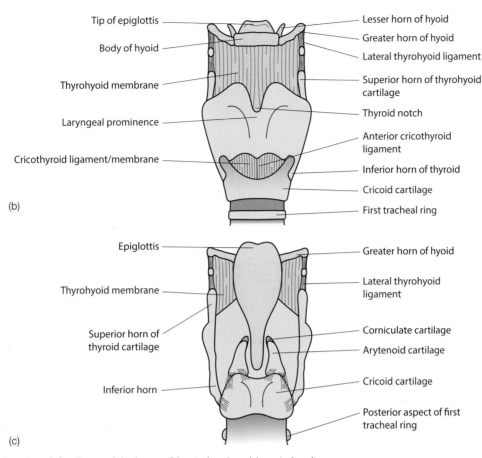

(b)

- Tip of epiglottis
- Body of hyoid
- Thyrohyoid membrane
- Laryngeal prominence
- Cricothyroid ligament/membrane
- Lesser horn of hyoid
- Greater horn of hyoid
- Lateral thyrohyoid ligament
- Superior horn of thyrohyoid cartilage
- Thyroid notch
- Anterior cricothyroid ligament
- Inferior horn of thyroid
- Cricoid cartilage
- First tracheal ring

(c)

- Epiglottis
- Thyrohyoid membrane
- Superior horn of thyroid cartilage
- Inferior horn
- Greater horn of hyoid
- Lateral thyrohyoid ligament
- Corniculate cartilage
- Arytenoid cartilage
- Cricoid cartilage
- Posterior aspect of first tracheal ring

Figure 20.10 (*continued*) Cartilages of the larynx: (b) anterior view; (c) posterior view

the oblique line, and the small muscles of the pharynx to the posterior border. The cricothyroid muscle is attached to the inferior horn. To the posterior of the laryngeal prominence is attached the epiglottis, and below it the vocal ligament and cricothyroid ligament (**Fig. 20.12**).

The **cricoid cartilage** completely encircles the lower larynx; signet ring-shaped, it is broader posteriorly. The lateral surface articulates with the inferior horn of the thyroid, its upper border with the arytenoid cartilages. The conus elasticus and cricothyroid ligament are attached to the upper border of the arch, to the cricothyroid and lateral cricoarytenoid muscles laterally and to the posterior cricoarytenoid muscle posteriorly.

The **epiglottic cartilage (epiglottis)** is a leaf-shaped cartilage whose narrow inferior end is attached to the back of the laryngeal prominence of the thyroid cartilage (**Fig. 20.10c**). Its broad upper end projects behind the tongue. The sides give attachment to the aryepiglottic membrane and small laryngeal muscles.

Viral infections of the laryngeal mucous membrane may be serious in that they cause epiglottitis, an inflammatory swelling of the epiglottis with a resultant narrowing of the laryngeal opening. Stridor and laryngeal spasm may result, which may require the production of an emergency airway (**Fig. 20.11**).

Cricothyroidotomy ('mini-trach') is the usual emergency procedure used to alleviate an upper airway obstruction. A needle or knife is inserted through the cricothyroid ligament,

its tip pointing downwards away from the vocal cords, and a small tracheostomy tube or catheter is inserted. Positive-pressure ventilation may then be administered.

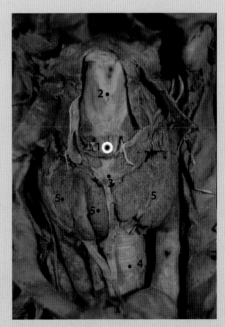

Figure 20.11 Cricothyroidotomy dissection: 1, site for emergency airway (cricothyroid membrane); 2, laryngeal prominence (Adam's apple); 3, cricoid cartilage; 4, trachea; 5, thyroid gland

The **arytenoid cartilages** are each pyramid-shaped (Fig. 20.12). The inferior base of each articulates with the cricoid and to it are attached the lateral and posterior cricoarytenoid muscles and the vocal ligament; to the anterior border is attached the aryepiglottic fold or membrane.

Joints, membranes and ligaments

The **cricothyroid joints** are synovial joints between the inferior horn of the thyroid and the cricoid. The **cricoarytenoid joints** are synovial joints between the arytenoids and the cricoid lamina.

The **conus elasticus** (Fig. 20.12) is a ligament of yellow elastic tissue joined anteriorly and contributing to the cricothyroid ligament. Each side has an upper free border behind the thyroid lamina and is attached inferiorly to the cricoid; the free borders reach posteriorly to the vocal process of the arytenoid cartilages and form the **vocal folds (true vocal cords)**.

The **arytenoid (quadrangular) membrane** extends from the side of the epiglottis to the arytenoids; its free upper border is the aryepiglottic fold and the lower border forms the **vestibular fold (false vocal cords)** (Fig. 20.13; see also Fig. 20.15a).

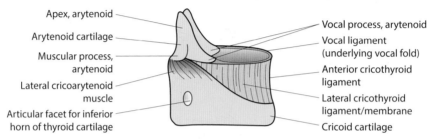

Figure 20.12 Conus elasticus, made up of the two lateral cricothyroid membranes

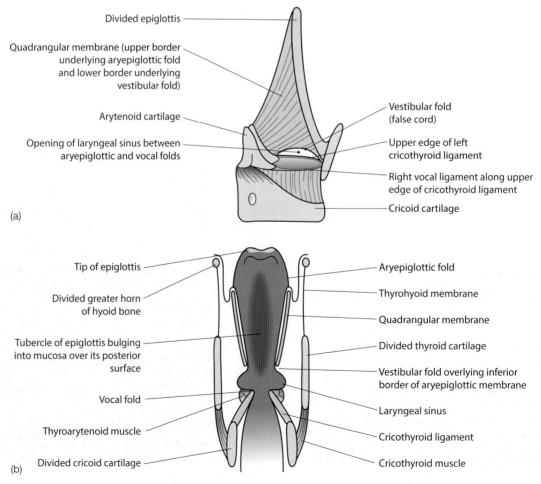

Figure 20.13 Quadrangular membrane: (a) external; (b) internal coronal cross-section

The **thyrohyoid membrane** unites the upper border of the thyroid cartilage with the hyoid bone. It is pierced by the internal laryngeal nerve.

Muscles

All, apart from the transverse arytenoid, are paired muscles (Fig. 20.14). **Cricothyroid** extends from the lower border of the thyroid to the lateral border of the cricoid; the **posterior cricoarytenoid** passes between the posterior surface of the cricoid and the arytenoid, and the **lateral cricoarytenoid** between the outer lateral cricoid and the arytenoid; the **transverse arytenoid** attaches to each arytenoid. The **aryepiglottic muscle** passes between the lateral borders of the epiglottis to the arytenoid. **Thyroarytenoid** passes from the back of the laryngeal prominence to the arytenoid outside the conus elasticus, and also gains attachment to the free border of the ligament, forming the **vocalis muscle**.

Interior of the larynx

The upper opening of the larynx is bounded anteriorly by the epiglottis, laterally by the aryepiglottic folds, and posteriorly by the arytenoid cartilages and transverse arytenoid muscle. Within the larynx two pairs of horizontal folds lie on its lateral walls: the upper **vestibular fold** (false vocal cord) and the lower **vocal fold** (true vocal cord) (Fig. 20.15). The gap between the vocal folds is known as the **rima glottidis**.

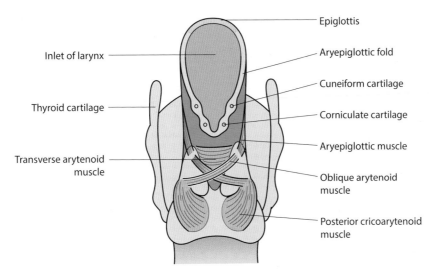

- Epiglottis
- Inlet of larynx
- Aryepiglottic fold
- Cuneiform cartilage
- Thyroid cartilage
- Corniculate cartilage
- Aryepiglottic muscle
- Transverse arytenoid muscle
- Oblique arytenoid muscle
- Posterior cricoarytenoid muscle

Figure 20.14 Muscles of the larynx from the posterior aspect

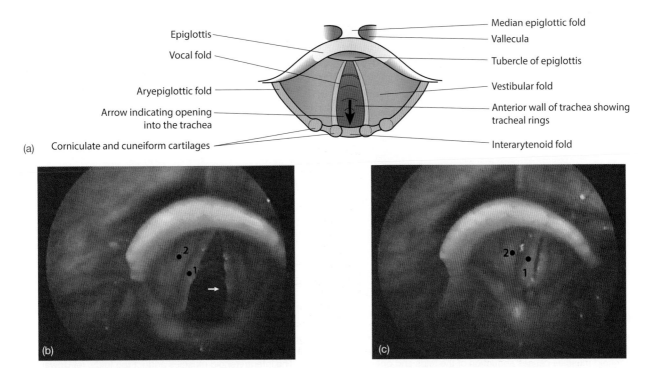

- Epiglottis
- Median epiglottic fold
- Vocal fold
- Vallecula
- Tubercle of epiglottis
- Aryepiglottic fold
- Vestibular fold
- Arrow indicating opening into the trachea
- Anterior wall of trachea showing tracheal rings
- (a) Corniculate and cuneiform cartilages
- Interarytenoid fold

Figure 20.15 Gap between the vocal folds. (a) Diagrammatic view from above (arrow indicating the upper trachea). Laryngoscopic views: (b) open (with the arrow in the same position as in 'a'), (c) closed. 1, vocal fold; 2, vestibular fold

Nerve supply

The sensory supply to the mucous membrane above the vocal folds is by the internal laryngeal nerve; the area below the vocal folds is supplied by the recurrent laryngeal nerve. All muscles are supplied by the recurrent laryngeal nerve, apart from cricothyroid (external branch of the superior laryngeal nerve).

Lymphatic drainage

This is to deep cervical and pretracheal nodes.

The larynx can be inspected either indirectly with a laryngeal mirror or directly with a laryngoscope. The base of the tongue, epiglottis, aryepiglottic folds and piriform fossae, together with the false and true cords, can be seen (**Figs. 20.15b,c**). **Laryngoscopy** is frequently performed prior to anaesthetic intubation of the airway. It demands that the axes of the mouth, oropharynx and larynx are in one plane. This is achieved by flexing the neck forwards and extending the head at the atlanto-occipital joint, i.e. having the patient adopt the position of 'sniffing the morning air'.

The vestibular folds have an important protective function. The vestibule is very sensitive to the presence of inhaled foreign objects, and a cough reflex is the immediate response. If this fails to dislodge the object, choking occurs if the rima glottidis is obstructed. First-aid treatment must attempt to force air from the lungs up through the larynx, and this is best achieved by the Heimlich manoeuvre – standing behind the patient and wrapping both arms around their lower chest prior to forcefully compress it. This expels the air in the lungs out through the larynx with such force that the foreign body is dislodged.

The **laryngeal nerves** are vulnerable to injury during thyroid surgery and may be infiltrated by cancerous nodes in the neck. This results, in both cases, in paralysis of the relevant vocal cord. The voice becomes weaker and more hoarse. Involvement of both laryngeal nerves produces a lack of adduction of both vocal cords, a very weak voice and exertional dyspnoea. Tracheostomy (p. 377) may be necessary.

Movements of the larynx

Vocalization is achieved by movements of the thyroid and arytenoid cartilages altering the length, tension and position of the vocal folds. Swallowing results from the raising and lowering of the larynx and the approximation of the epiglottis to the arytenoids, preventing food from entering the airway (**Fig. 20.16**).

Forward rotation of the **thyroid cartilages** at the cricothyroid joints lengthens and tenses the vocal folds. It is produced by the cricothyroid muscle and reversed by the posterior thyroarytenoid.

Movements of the **arytenoid cartilage** occur at the cricoarytenoid joints and are gliding and rotatory: the posterior cricoarytenoid is the single cord abductor and thus vital in airway patency, especially when this has been threatened by recurrent laryngeal nerve injury.

- **Gliding** – lateral gliding separates the cartilages, abducts the vocal folds and produces an inverted V-shaped rima glottidis. Lateral and posterior cricoarytenoid muscles are involved and are counteracted by the transverse arytenoid.
- **Rotation** – lateral rotation separates the vocal processes, abducting the vocal folds to produce a diamond-shaped rima glottidis. This is only produced by the posterior cricoarytenoid, i.e. it is the single cord abductor and vital in airway patency. It is counteracted by nearly all the other intrinsic muscles, especially the lateral cricoarytenoid. Vocalis increases tension in the vocal fold. Closure of the epiglottis against the arytenoids may be helped by the aryepiglottic muscles, but passive pressure from the food bolus is probably more important. Raising and lowering of the larynx is shown in **Fig. 20.16e**.

The prime function of the larynx is as a sphincter. Sphincter action prevents food entering the trachea and also closes the larynx when increased intrathoracic pressure is required before coughing or to help increase intra-abdominal pressure, e.g. during micturition, defecation or vomiting. Abdominal straining is made more effective by closure of the glottis during contraction of the anterior abdominal

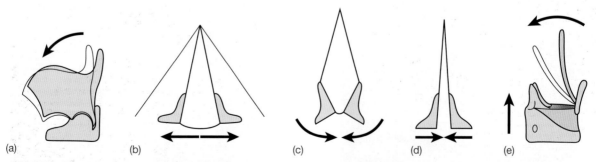

Figure 20.16 Movements of larynx. (a) Rocking the thyroid cartilage on the cricoid lengthens the vocal folds and changes the pitch. (b) Gliding of the arytenoids down the cricoid causes abduction of the folds. (c) Lateral rotation of the arytenoids by the posterior cricoarytenoid muscles causes abduction of the folds and opens the airway. (d) The interarytenoid muscles adduct the folds. (e) Upwards movement of the larynx assists in the closing of the inlet as in swallowing and certain speech patterns

wall muscles. Sound is produced by columns of air passing through the larynx, usually during expiration. Vocalization is achieved by frequency modulation of the movements, length and tension of the vocal folds, and its intensity by the volume and speed of the expired air. Resonance is increased by the large air-filled spaces in the lungs, pharynx, mouth and nose.

Hoarseness or loss of voice results from swelling of the vocal folds as a result of infection, overuse, changes in its contour by a benign or malignant tumour (Fig. 20.17), or laryngeal muscle paralysis.

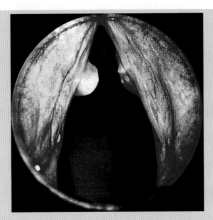

Figure 20.17 Singer's nodules on both vocal folds

MCQs

1. The palatine tonsil: **T/F**
  a lies on the middle constrictor muscle   (____)
  b lies anterior to the palatopharyngeal muscle   (____)
  c drains to the submandibular lymph nodes   (____)
  d is innervated by the glossopharyngeal nerve   (____)
  e is supplied by the facial artery   (____)

Answers

1.

a **F** – The superior constrictor separates it from the facial artery and the carotid sheath.

b **T** – This muscle lies posterior to the tonsil in the palatopharyngeal arch, the posterior pillar of the fauces.

c **F** – The lymphatic drainage is to the deep cervical nodes, particularly the jugulodigastric ...

d **T** – ... plus a small contribution from the lesser palatine nerve ...

e **T** – ... plus a contribution from the ascending palatine and lingual arteries. The gland's main arterial supply enters at its anteroinferior angle, an important fact for surgeons undertaking tonsillectomy.

2. The temporomandibular joint: **T/F**
  a has articular surfaces covered with hyaline   (____)
     cartilage
  b is most frequently dislocated anteriorly   (____)
  c contains an intra-articular fibrous disc   (____)
  d is more stable when the teeth are occluded   (____)
  e is protruded by the anterior belly of the   (____)
     digastric muscle

Answers

2.

a **F** – The articular surfaces are covered with fibrocartilage.

b **T** – This most commonly occurs in overwide opening of the mouth, as in yawning.

c **T** – During protrusion and depression of the mandible the lateral pterygoid also pulls forward the intra-articular disc.

d **T**

e **F** – Protrusion is by the lateral pterygoids. The anterior belly of the digastric muscle assists gravity to open the mouth.

SBA

1. A 7-year-old girl is brought to the doctor complaining of a cough with fever and right-sided earache. Otoscopy is performed and reveals a reddened tympanic membrane beyond which can be seen a yellowish-brown fluid. What is the most likely route by which an upper respiratory tract infection can spread to the middle ear?

a choanae
b facial canal
c tonsillar fossae
d pharyngotympanic tube
e posterior nares

Answer

d A respiratory infection may travel from the upper respiratory tract to the oropharynx or nasopharynx via the auditory (Eustachian or pharyngotympanic) tube, which provides a direct connection from the nasopharynx to the middle ear cavity.

2. A middle-aged woman was brought to the emergency room fighting for breath. Her companion said that she had experienced a worsening sore throat for several days and for the previous 12 hours had been having increasing difficulty in breathing. Attempts to perform endotracheal intubation have been unsuccessful due to widespread soft tissue swelling of her oropharynx and it has been decided to perform an urgent cricothyroidotomy. At which point should an incision be made?

a the cricothyroid membrane, which is situated between the cricoid and the first tracheal ring
b the cricothyroid membrane, which is situated between the thyroid cartilage and the cricoid cartilage lying immediately below it
c the sternal notch
d the trachea between the third and fourth tracheal rings
e the thyrohyoid membrane lying between the thyroid cartilage and the hyoid bone above

Answer

b If endotracheal intubation cannot be performed, acute laryngeal obstruction demands an urgent cricothyroidotomy. This is performed by making an incision in the cricothyroid membrane, which lies between the thyroid cartilage and the cricoid cartilage below. A large-bore needle or knife is inserted through the membrane, its tip pointing downwards away from the vocal cords, and a small endotracheal tube or catheter is inserted. Positive-pressure ventilation is then commenced. When there is laryngeal obstruction this is the easiest, quickest and most certain way of establishing an emergency airway.

EMQs

Each question has an anatomical theme linked to the chapter, and a list of 10 related items (A–J) placed in alphabetical order: these are followed by five statements (1–5). Match **one or more** of the items A–J to each of the five statements.

Muscles of the pharynx and larynx
A. Lateral cricoarytenoid
B. Cricothyroid
C. Inferior constrictor
D. Levator veli palate
E. Middle constrictor
F. Palatopharyngeus
G. Posterior cricoarytenoid
H. Stylohyoid
I. Stylopharyngeus
J. Superior constrictor

Answers
1 AG; 2 B; 3 I; 4 H; 5 ABCDEFJ

Match the following nerve(s) to the muscles in the above list.
1. Recurrent laryngeal nerve
2. Superior laryngeal
3. Glossopharyngeal
4. Facial
5. Vagus

APPLIED QUESTIONS

1. Why might a child with recurrent ear infections benefit from an adenoidectomy?

1. An enlarged nasopharyngeal tonsil or adenoid is a cause of auditory tube blockage, leading to recurrent middle ear infections. If it is particularly large, its removal may improve mucous drainage of the tympanic cavity and thus reduce the number of middle ear infections.

2. Where is the most likely site for a fish bone to impact in the pharynx?

2. The classic sites for a fish bone to stick are the piriform fossae or recesses. These are the shallow channels of the laryngopharynx on either side of the laryngeal inlet, and it is down these two channels that food passes, having been deflected from the larynx by the elevated epiglottis. A less common site in which a fish bone might impact is in the vallecula, the small depression between tongue and epiglottis.

3. During an indirect laryngoscopy, what structures may be visible?

3. The structures seen on indirect laryngoscopy are, first, the base of the tongue and the lingual surface of the epiglottis, and then, if the patient is instructed to produce a high pitched 'ee-ee', the aryepiglottic fold and vocal cords, which are brought into view by this. On cessation of phonation the cords abduct, revealing the upper tracheal rings through the opened rima glottidis. The vestibular folds above the true cords are pink, fleshy folds of mucous membrane compared with the normal pearly white of the vocal cords. Before withdrawing the mirror, the piriform fossae and vallecula should be checked for abnormalities.

Essential Clinical Anatomy · *Bailey & Love* · Essential Clinical Anatomy
sential Clinical Anatomy · *Bailey & Love* · Essential Clinical Anatomy · *B*
iley & Love · Essential Clinical Anatomy · *Bailey & Love* · Essential Clinical Anatomy

Chapter 21

The ear, intracranial region and cranial nerves

THE EAR

The organ of hearing and balance is divided into an external ear, conveying sound waves to the tympanic membrane, a middle ear, relaying the membrane's vibrations to the internal ear, and the cochlea of the internal ear, which translates these vibrations into nerve impulses. The semicircular canals, the organ of balance, are also in the inner ear.

The **external ear** consists of the auricle (pinna) (Fig. 21.1) and the external acoustic meatus. The **auricle** is formed of an irregularly shaped piece of fibrocartilage covered by firmly adherent skin. It has a dependent lobule – used for earrings – and an anterior tragus, which projects and overlaps the opening of the meatus. The **external acoustic meatus** passes almost horizontally with an S-shaped curve from the tragus to the tympanic membrane in a slightly anterior direction. It is about 3 cm long. Its cartilaginous lateral third is continuous with the cartilage of the auricle; the bony medial two-thirds are formed mainly by the temporal bone. The meatus is lined by skin containing many wax-secreting (ceruminous) glands. It is innervated by the auriculotemporal nerve anteriorly and the vagus nerve posteriorly. The translucent **tympanic membrane** (eardrum) (Fig. 21.2) separating the external and middle ears is oval in shape and lies obliquely, with its outer (lateral) surface facing downwards and forwards. The handle of the malleus is attached to its medial surface and produces a small elevation on the drum, which can be seen with an auriscope as the umbo.

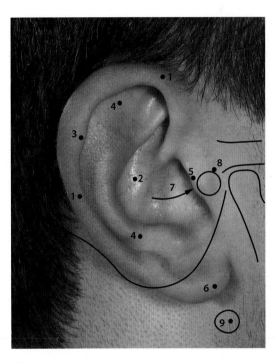

Figure 21.1 External ear: 1, helix; 2, concha; 3, auricular tubercle (of Darwin); 4, antihelix; 5, tragus; 6, lobule; 7, external acoustic meatus; 8, (circle) position of external acoustic meatus; 9, (circle) position of transverse process of atlas

The external meatus is straightened to facilitate otoscopic examination by pulling the auricle upwards and backwards. The earpieces of a stethoscope are angulated to accommodate the anteromedial direction of the external acoustic meatus.

Auriscopically the tympanic membrane appears as oval, glistening and semiopaque, and the handle of the malleus can be seen attached to its deep surface. A 'cone of light' is seen on the anteroinferior part of the membrane. A reddened, bulging membrane is indicative of otitis media (infection of

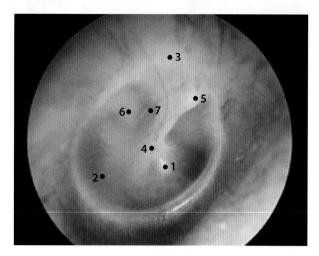

Figure 21.2 Auriscopic view of right tympanic membrane: 1, cone of light (reflex); 2, pars tensa; 3, pars flaccida; 4, umbo; 5, malleus; 6, incus; 7, chorda tympani

the middle ear) (Fig. 21.3). Perforation of the membrane is sometimes a consequence of otitis media. Bleeding or escape of cerebrospinal fluid (CSF) through a ruptured membrane may occur after a fracture of the skull base involving the middle cranial fossa.

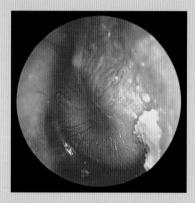

Figure 21.3 Otitis media – note the loss of the normal anatomical landmarks shown in Fig. 21.2 due to inflammation and swelling

The **middle ear (tympanic cavity**; Fig. 21.4a) lies within the temporal bone. It is about 15 mm high and 15 mm long, and its medial and lateral walls curve inwards, being about 2 mm apart in their middle and 6 mm apart at the roof. The cavity, lined in part by ciliated columnar epithelium, contains three small bones, the malleus, incus and stapes – the auditory ossicles (Fig. 21.4c). The **lateral wall** is formed mainly by the tympanic membrane. Above and behind the membrane is an upward extension of the cavity, the **epitympanic recess**, which contains part of the malleus and incus. The **medial wall** has a central bulge, the **promontory**, overlying the base of the cochlea (see below). Above and behind it is the **fenestra vestibuli** (oval window) and below it the **fenestra cochleae** (round window). Both these foramina lead to the inner ear.

The fenestra vestibuli is closed by the footplate of the stapes, and the fenestra cochleae by a fibrous membrane. The **anterior wall** has two openings, the upper for tensor tympani muscle, which attaches to the handle of the malleus, and the lower for the auditory (Eustachian) tube (Fig. 21.4a), which communicates with the nasopharynx. High on the **posterior wall** is the **aditus**, the opening into the mastoid antrum. Below it foramina transmit the stapedius muscle to the stapes and the chorda tympani. The facial nerve grooves the medial wall and then descends the medial and part of the posterior wall in a bony canal.

The three small ossicles, the malleus, incus and stapes, are connected to each other by fibrous tissue; they extend from the tympanic membrane to the fenestra vestibuli and transmit vibrations from the membrane to the inner ear. The two muscles, **tensor tympani** (supplied by the mandibular nerve) and **stapedius** (facial nerve), attached to the malleus and stapes, respectively, modify the transmission of vibrations. Decreased mobility of the ossicles in middle and old age produces degrees of conductive deafness. The middle ear is innervated by the glossopharyngeal nerve via the tympanic plexus. Lymphatic drainage is to the preauricular and retropharyngeal nodes.

The **mastoid (tympanic) antrum** is a cavity within the mastoid process. It communicates with the middle ear by the aditus (Fig. 21.4a). At birth the mastoid process is small and the facial nerve lies more superficially, but as air cells develop the process enlarges to surround the antrum. Posteromedially the antrum is separated from the posterior cranial fossa and cerebellum by a thin plate of bone; above it is the temporal lobe of the brain. The auditory tube, by providing a communication between the middle ear and nasopharynx, allows equalization of air pressure on both sides of the tympanic membrane; it also provides a pathway for infection to ascend from the throat to the antrum and mastoid air cells.

An abscess may develop in the mastoid (Fig. 18.12, p. 310), following a middle ear infection, with potentially serious consequences, as it may spread to the neighbouring cerebellum and temporal lobe of the brain and result in meningitis and/or brain abscess.

Earache (otalgia) is a symptom that has several causes; it is usually the result of otitis media, but may also be due to an infection of the external acoustic meatus (otitis externa). The middle and external ear are supplied by branches of the trigeminal, glossopharyngeal and vagus nerves, so pain in the ear may be referred from other structures supplied by these nerves: pharynx, larynx, sinuses, teeth or posterior tongue. Referred otalgia is therefore frequently a complex diagnostic challenge.

The **internal ear**, within the temporal bone, is a complicated membranous sac (the membranous labyrinth) filled with fluid (endolymph) contained within a bony cavity (the bony labyrinth). The **bony labyrinth** (Fig. 21.5) comprises, in continuity, the cochlea, the vestibule and the semicircular canals. The **cochlea** is a coiled bony tube of 2½ turns around a central pillar, the modiolus. The coil is partially divided by a narrow plate of bone, the **spiral lamina**, which projects into its cavity (Fig. 21.7). The base of the cochlea

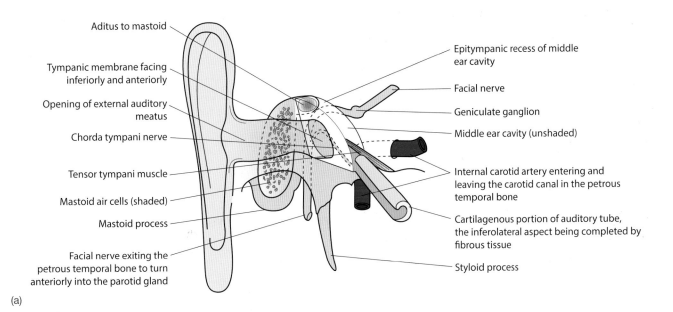

Aditus to mastoid

Tympanic membrane facing inferiorly and anteriorly

Opening of external auditory meatus

Chorda tympani nerve

Tensor tympani muscle

Mastoid air cells (shaded)

Mastoid process

Facial nerve exiting the petrous temporal bone to turn anteriorly into the parotid gland

Epitympanic recess of middle ear cavity

Facial nerve

Geniculate ganglion

Middle ear cavity (unshaded)

Internal carotid artery entering and leaving the carotid canal in the petrous temporal bone

Cartilagenous portion of auditory tube, the inferolateral aspect being completed by fibrous tissue

Styloid process

(a)

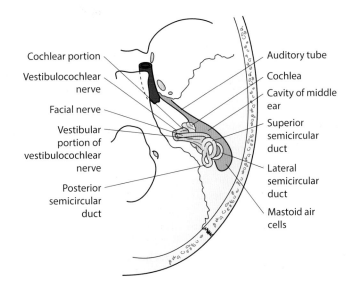

Cochlear portion

Vestibulocochlear nerve

Facial nerve

Vestibular portion of vestibulocochlear nerve

Posterior semicircular duct

Auditory tube

Cochlea

Cavity of middle ear

Superior semicircular duct

Lateral semicircular duct

Mastoid air cells

(b)

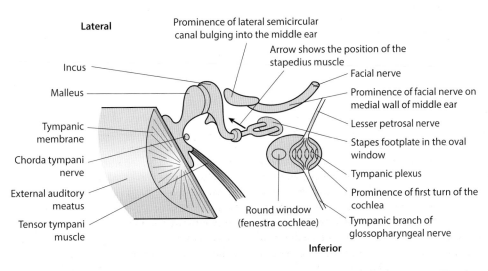

Lateral

Prominence of lateral semicircular canal bulging into the middle ear

Arrow shows the position of the stapedius muscle

Incus

Malleus

Tympanic membrane

Chorda tympani nerve

External auditory meatus

Tensor tympani muscle

Facial nerve

Prominence of facial nerve on medial wall of middle ear

Lesser petrosal nerve

Stapes footplate in the oval window

Tympanic plexus

Prominence of first turn of the cochlea

Tympanic branch of glossopharyngeal nerve

Round window (fenestra cochleae)

Inferior

(c)

Figure 21.4 (a) The external and middle ear sectioned in the coronal plane viewed from the anterolateral aspect. The mastoid process has also been sectioned. (b) The middle and internal ear within the temporal bone viewed from above. (c) The middle ear cavity: the tympanic membrane laterally and the prominences and windows medially. The ossicles are within the cavity of the inner ear

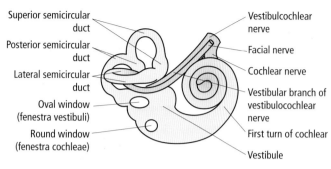

Figure 21.5 Bony labyrinth

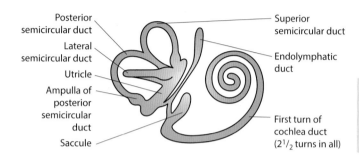

Figure 21.6 Membranous labyrinth

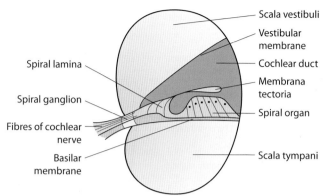

Figure 21.7 Section through the cochlea

The vestibular and cochlear nerves (Figs. 21.4b, 21.5 and 21.7), although separate, are frequently both involved in the same pathological process. Vertigo (loss of balance), deafness and abnormal noises in the ears (tinnitus) often occur concurrently.

THE INTRACRANIAL REGION

The skull vault covers the cerebral hemispheres, and inferiorly the base of the skull forms the anterior, middle and posterior cranial fossae containing the frontal lobes, temporal lobes and cerebellum and brainstem, respectively (Fig. 21.8).

The **vault** is formed by the frontal, parietal, squamous temporal and occipital bones. There are two foramina for emissary veins near the vertex (Fig. 18.1, p. 302). The inner surface is grooved in the sagittal plane by the superior sagittal sinus as far back as the internal occipital protuberance. On each side of the groove can be seen pits, the **lateral recesses**, containing **arachnoid granulations**. Laterally the vault is grooved by the anterior and posterior middle meningeal vessels.

The **anterior cranial fossa** covers the orbits, ethmoidal sinuses and nasal cavity. It is formed by the frontal bone, the cribriform plate of the ethmoid and the sphenoid. Anteriorly 15–20 filaments of the olfactory nerve perforate the dura over the cribriform plate to enter the olfactory bulb. The posterior border of the lesser wing of the sphenoid separates the anterior from the middle cranial fossa (Fig 21.8).

The **middle cranial fossa** has a median part and two larger lateral compartments (Fig. 21.8). The **median part**, formed by the body of the sphenoid, is hollowed above by the **pituitary fossa** (sella turcica). Anteriorly a transverse ridge, the tuberculum sellae, separates the fossa from the optic nerve in its groove. A posterior plate of bone, the dorsum sellae, bears two posterior clinoid processes, attachments for dura mater. On each side of the body of the sphenoid a shallow carotid groove leads posteriorly to the foramen lacerum. The body of the sphenoid contains sphenoidal air sinuses, which lie inferior to the pituitary gland and cavernous venous sinuses. Each **optic canal** conveys the optic nerve and its meningeal coverings and the ophthalmic artery. The **foramen lacerum**, between the occipital bone and the greater wing of the sphe-

opens into the **vestibule**, whose lateral wall communicates with the middle ear at the vestibular and cochlear fenestrae. The anterior, posterior and lateral **semicircular canals** each form two-thirds of a circle and open at each end into the vestibule. The canals lie in three planes at right angles to each other.

The **membranous labyrinth** (Fig. 21.6) lies within the bony labyrinth and comprises the duct of the cochlea, the saccule, the utricle and the three semicircular ducts. All are in continuity. The **duct of the cochlea** divides the cavity of the bony cochlea into three: an upper **scala vestibuli** containing perilymph; a **scala media**, the cavity of the duct containing endolymph; and a lower **scala tympani** containing perilymph. On the basilar membrane between the scala media and tympani are hair cells supporting the **membrana tectoria**. The hair cells move with the disturbances of the perilymph set up by movements of the stapes at the fenestra vestibuli. The **spiral organ** (end-organ of hearing) consists of the hair cells and the tectorial membrane and is supplied by the cochlear nerve (Fig. 21.7).

The **saccule and utricle** are two sacs within the vestibule, united by the narrow Y-shaped endolymphatic duct. Both contain a small area of projecting hairs, the **maculae**, the end-organ of static balance. The narrow **semicircular ducts** each possess a dilated ampulla containing a sensory area, the **crista**, the organ of kinetic balance. Both maculae and cristae contain nerve fibres from the vestibular division of the VIIIth cranial nerve, which are stimulated when the supporting hair cells are deformed by movement of the endolymph or by movement of the otoliths, small crystals of calcium carbonate in the fluid.

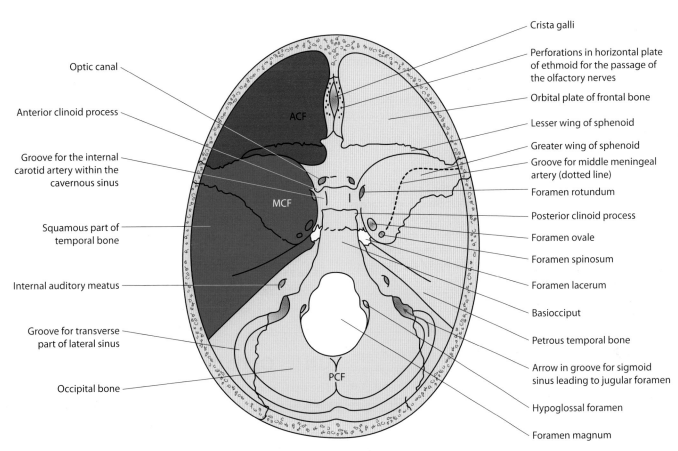

Optic canal

Anterior clinoid process

Groove for the internal
carotid artery within the
cavernous sinus

Squamous part of
temporal bone

Internal auditory meatus

Groove for transverse
part of lateral sinus

Occipital bone

ACF

MCF

PCF

Crista galli

Perforations in horizontal plate
of ethmoid for the passage of
the olfactory nerves

Orbital plate of frontal bone

Lesser wing of sphenoid

Greater wing of sphenoid

Groove for middle meningeal
artery (dotted line)

Foramen rotundum

Posterior clinoid process

Foramen ovale

Foramen spinosum

Foramen lacerum

Basiocciput

Petrous temporal bone

Arrow in groove for sigmoid
sinus leading to jugular foramen

Hypoglossal foramen

Foramen magnum

Figure 21.8 Intracranial fossae: ACF – anterior; MCF – middle; PCF – posterior

noid, is filled with fibrocartilage. The internal carotid artery crosses above it.

The **lateral parts**, formed by the greater and lesser wings of the sphenoid and the temporal bone, support the temporal lobe of the brain. One fissure and three foramina are found on the medial aspect of each side:

- The **superior orbital fissure** (see Figs. 19.8 and 19.9, p. 318).
- The **foramen rotundum** in the greater wing of the sphenoid behind the superior orbital fissure opens into the pterygopalatine fossa and transmits the maxillary nerve.
- The **foramen ovale**, also in the greater wing of the sphenoid, about 1.5 cm behind and below the foramen rotundum, opens into the infratemporal fossa and transmits the mandibular nerve and lesser petrosal nerve.
- The **foramen spinosum** is posterolateral to the foramen ovale. It transmits the middle meningeal vessels and meningeal branches of the mandibular nerve. The vessels groove the bones of the vault of the skull as they pass laterally (the anterior branch lies deep to the pterion; Fig. 18.7a, p. 307).

Posterolaterally, in the middle cranial fossa, a thin plate of bone, the **tegmen tympani**, overlies the mastoid antrum, the middle ear and the **auditory** tube.

The posterior cranial fossa

This, the largest of the fossae, is deeply concave and lies above the foramen magnum. It is formed by the sphenoid, temporal, occipital and parietal bones (Fig. 21.8) and limited anteriorly by the dorsum sellae and the petrous temporal bones. Posterolaterally grooves for the transverse sinus on the inner surfaces of the occipital and parietal bones form the fossa's upper limit. The fossa contains the cerebellum, pons and medulla, and is roofed by the dural **tentorium cerebelli** (p. 431), on which lie the occipital lobes of the cerebrum. It possesses the following foramina:

- The large midline **foramen magnum** in the floor of the fossa is bounded on each side by the occipital condyles. This transmits the spinal cord and its meninges, the vertebral and spinal arteries and the spinal root of the accessory nerves.
- The **jugular foramen**, between the occipital and temporal bones, is irregular in outline. It contains the bulb of the jugular vein and the inferior petrosal dural venous sinus, and transmits the glossopharyngeal, vagus and accessory nerves.
- The **internal acoustic meatus** is on the posterior aspect of the temporal bone. Each is directed laterally and transmits the facial and vestibulocochlear nerves surrounded by a meningeal sheath.

- The **hypoglossal canal**, above the occipital condyle, transmits the hypoglossal nerve.
- The **condylar canal** and the **mastoid foramen** transmit emissary veins.

The internal occipital protuberance lies at the point of union of the two transverse sinuses in the midline posteriorly.

THE CRANIAL NERVES

The 12 pairs of cranial nerves originate in the brain and leave the cranial cavity through its basal foramina. Each carries one or more of the following fibres: general sensory, visceral sensory (parasympathetic and sympathetic), special sensory (sight, hearing, balance), motor and visceral motor (parasympathetic and sympathetic). The attachments of the nerves to the brainstem are shown in Fig. 21.9.

CN I – Olfactory nerve

The olfactory nerve is an outgrowth of the forebrain and supplies the olfactory mucous membrane of the upper nasal cavity (Fig. 21.10). The fibres originate in the mucosa and join to form 15–20 bundles, which pass through the cribriform plate of each ethmoid and overlying dura and arachnoid to reach the olfactory bulb.

Fractures of the anterior cranial fossa involving the cribriform plates may be accompanied by a loss of CSF from the nose (CSF rhinorrhoea) and, if the nerves are also damaged, long-term anosmia (loss of sense of smell).

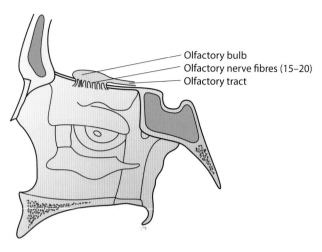

Olfactory bulb
Olfactory nerve fibres (15–20)
Olfactory tract

Figure 21.10 Sagittal section of the anterior cranial fossa and nasal cavity showing the olfactory nerve

CN II – Optic nerve

The optic nerve is the sensory nerve of vision. Its fibres originate in the ganglion layer of the retina and converge on the posterior part of the eyeball (Fig. 21.11). It passes back through the orbit and optic canal to the middle cranial fossa, where it unites with that of the opposite side to form the **optic chiasma** lying on the body of the sphenoid. Here the medial or nasal fibres (carrying the temporal visual field) cross to the opposite optic tract while the lateral or temporal fibres, con-

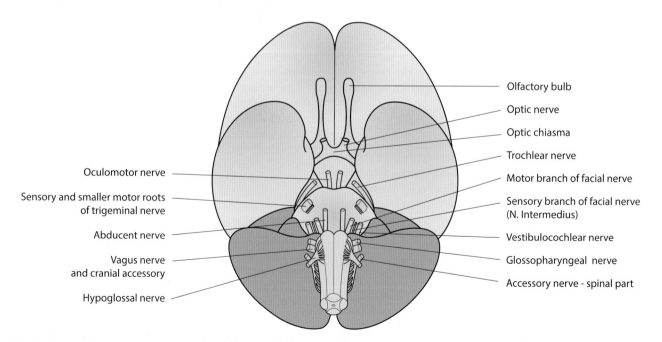

Oculomotor nerve

Sensory and smaller motor roots of trigeminal nerve

Abducent nerve

Vagus nerve and cranial accessory

Hypoglossal nerve

Olfactory bulb

Optic nerve

Optic chiasma

Trochlear nerve

Motor branch of facial nerve

Sensory branch of facial nerve (N. Intermedius)

Vestibulocochlear nerve

Glossopharyngeal nerve

Accessory nerve - spinal part

Figure 21.9 Base of the brain showing the attachment of the cranial nerves to the brainstem

cerned with the nasal visual field, pass backwards in the optic tract of the same side.

Relations

Within the orbit, enclosed in its meningeal sheath, the nerve lies surrounded by the cone of extraocular muscles. The ciliary ganglion is posterolateral and the ophthalmic artery and nasociliary nerve medial. The central artery of the retina (a branch of the ophthalmic artery) enters the nerve in this part of its course. **In the optic canal** the nerve is accompanied by the ophthalmic artery. **The intracranial course** is short and lies on the sphenoid bone medial to the internal carotid artery. The optic chiasma lies above and anterior to the pituitary gland.

Because of the meninges surrounding the nerve, an increase in CSF pressure causes some venous stasis and oedema (swelling) of the optic nerve and retina, and this can be recognized ophthalmoscopically as **papilloedema** (Fig. 19.7b, p. 317). Visual defects may result from pressure on the optic nerves or chiasma from pituitary tumours or aneurysms (swellings) of the internal carotid arteries. Figure 21.11 explains the particular visual field defects that follow damage to the optic nerves, optic chiasma and optic tracts.

CN III – Oculomotor nerve

The oculomotor nerve (Fig. 21.12) has somatic motor and parasympathetic motor fibres. The somatic fibres supply the extrinsic eye muscles, except for superior oblique and lateral rectus. The parasympathetic fibres synapse in the ciliary ganglion and supply the sphincter pupillae and ciliary muscle. The oculomotor nerve leaves the midbrain between the cerebral peduncles and passes through the posterior and middle cranial fossae to divide into superior and inferior divisions near the superior orbital fissure.

Relations

In the posterior cranial fossa, the nerve, medial to the trochlear nerve, lies close to the tentorium cerebelli. In the middle cranial fossa it passes forwards on the lateral wall of the cavernous sinus.

Branches

The **superior division** traverses the superior orbital fissure within the tendinous ring of the extraocular muscles (**Figs. 19.8** and **19.9**, p. 318) and supplies superior rectus and levator palpebrae superioris. The **inferior division** has the same course through the fissure, and supplies the medial and inferior recti and inferior oblique muscles. It also carries a parasympathetic branch to the ciliary ganglion (**Fig. 21.12**).

The **ciliary ganglion** lies in the posterior orbit lateral to the optic nerve and receives preganglionic parasympathetic fibres, sympathetic fibres from the internal carotid plexus and sensory fibres from the nasociliary nerve. Efferent fibres from the ganglion supply the ciliary muscle and muscles of the iris. Parasympathetic stimulation produces pupillary constriction; sympathetic stimulation produces pupillodilatation.

Because of its close relationship to the edge of the tentorium cerebelli the oculomotor nerve may be damaged if there is a lateral shift of the brain, as may occur with an intracranial haemorrhage. One of the earliest localizing signs of increasing intracranial pressure may be a selective palsy of the parasympathetic fibres; dilatation of the pupil is due to damage to the parasympathetic fibres passing to the ciliary ganglion. Signs of a complete palsy of the nerve are: ptosis (drooping eyelid); loss of pupillary light reflexes; dilatation of the pupil, because of loss of the parasympathetic supply to sphincter pupillae; abduction and downward deviation of the eye, because of the unopposed action of superior oblique and lateral rectus; and loss of accommodation in the eye, because of paralysis of ciliary muscles (**Figs. 21.13a,b**).

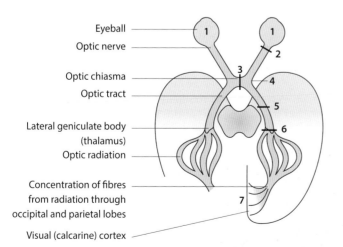
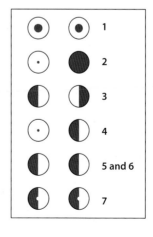

Figure 21.11 Optic nerve and pathways to the visual cortex and effects of injury at different sites on the visual fields: 1, pathology in the eye – damage to peripheral field; 2, damage to optic nerve – unilateral blindness; 3, damage to optic chiasma (e.g. pituitary tumour) – bitemporal hemianopia; 4, damage to lateral chiasma (e.g. aneurysms) – nasal blindness on same side; 5 and 6, tumours and trauma of unilateral optic tract – blindness of opposite visual field (homonymous hemianopia); 7, cortical damage – may not destroy macular vision

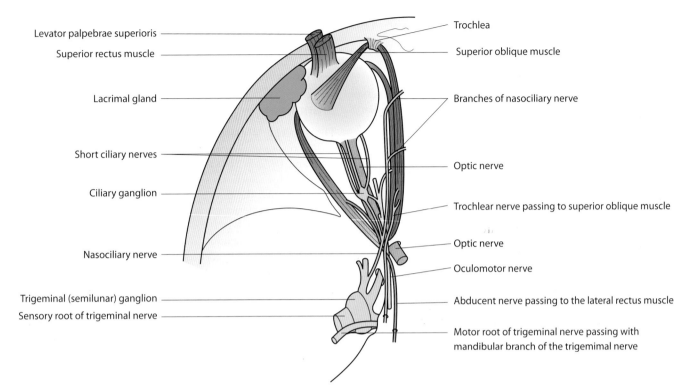

Figure 21.12 Superior view of the left orbit showing IIIrd, IVth and VIth cranial nerves

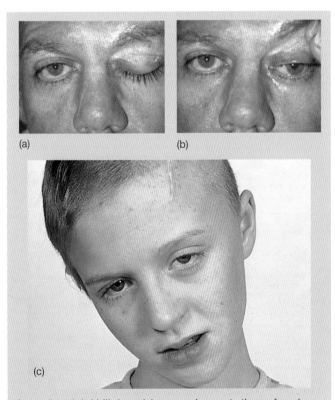

Figure 21.13 (a,b) IIIrd cranial nerve palsy – note the profound ptosis; when examined the eye is deviated downwards and outwards and the pupil dilated due to unopposed sympathetic IVth and VIth cranial nerves control. (c) IVth cranial nerve palsy – note that the child tilts his head to overcome 'double vision' (diplopia) due to loss of action of the superior oblique muscle

CN IV – Trochlear nerve

The trochlear nerve supplies the superior oblique muscle (Fig. 21.12). Emerging from the lower dorsal midbrain, it decussates and passes forwards through the posterior and middle cranial fossae to enter the orbit through the superior orbital fissure.

Relations

In the **posterior cranial fossa** it passes forwards around the midbrain, following the edge of the tentorium, lateral to the oculomotor nerve. In the **middle cranial fossa** it lies in the lateral wall of the cavernous sinus. It traverses the superior orbital fissure outside the tendinous ring and gains the roof of the orbit to supply the superior oblique muscle.

Lesions of this nerve, although rare, may result in 'double vision' (diplopia) and a compensatory tilt of the head (Fig. 21.13c). If the superior oblique muscle is paralysed and no other extraocular muscle is affected, which is rare, diplopia will be found when the patient is looking downwards. The affected eye is pulled downwards only by the inferior rectus and thus in a slightly different direction.

CN V – Trigeminal nerve

The trigeminal nerve conveys sensory fibres and motor fibres to skeletal muscles. The sensory fibres supply the anterior part of the scalp and the dura, the face, nasopharynx, nasal and oral cavities and the paranasal air sinuses. The motor fibres supply the muscles of mastication. The nerve arises in the pons and emerges at the root of the middle cerebellar peduncle as a large sensory and a smaller motor root. It passes forwards to the trigeminal ganglion on the temporal bone in the middle cranial fossa. Ophthalmic, maxillary and mandibular divisions emerge from the ganglion. The motor root passes by the ganglion to join the mandibular division (**Fig. 21.14**).

Ophthalmic division

The ophthalmic division – the smallest division – passes forwards on the lateral wall of the cavernous sinus and, near the superior orbital fissure, divides into lacrimal, frontal and nasociliary nerves, which each pass through the fissure into the orbit (**Fig. 21.12**).

The **lacrimal nerve** traverses the lateral part of the fissure to reach and supply the lacrimal gland, after which it supplies the skin and conjunctiva of the lateral part of the upper lid and adjacent conjunctiva. Parasympathetic secretomotor fibres are carried to the gland by a branch of the zygomaticotemporal nerve.

The **frontal nerve** traverses the superior orbital fissure and then gains the roof of the orbit, where it divides into the supraorbital and supratrochlear nerves. The former leaves the orbit by the supraorbital notch to supply the upper eyelid, frontal sinuses and scalp as far back as the vertex. The supratrochlear nerve supplies the skin of the upper eyelid and medial forehead.

The **nasociliary nerve** traverses the superior orbital fissure to gain the medial wall of the orbit, where it divides into anterior and posterior ethmoidal, infratrochlear and long ciliary nerves:

- **Anterior ethmoidal nerve** – leaves the orbit through a foramen on its medial wall to reach the anterior cranial fossa, where it descends through the cribriform plate to pass through the nose, supplying the anterior cranial fossa dura, ethmoidal air cells, upper anterior nasal cavity and skin of the tip of the nose.
- **Posterior ethmoidal nerve** – supplies the ethmoidal air cells and sphenoidal air sinuses.
- **Infratrochlear nerve** – supplies the medial part of the upper eyelid, conjunctiva and adjacent nose.
- **Long ciliary nerves** – supply the sclera and cornea. Sympathetic fibres are conveyed to the dilator pupillae muscle.

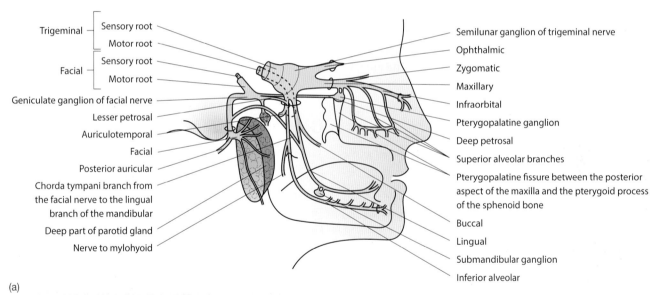

(a)

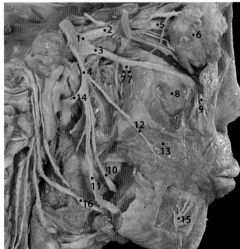

(b)

Figure 21.14 (a) Diagram and (b) dissection of the orbit, cheek and mandible to illustrate the trigeminal nerve branches: 1, trigeminal ganglion in middle cranial fossa; 2, ophthalmic branch to orbit; 3, maxillary branch; 4, mandibular branch; 5, optic nerve; 6, eyeball (globe); 7, superior alveolar nerve; 8, maxillary air sinus; 9, infraorbital nerve; 10, lingual nerve; 11, inferior alveolar nerve; 12, buccal nerve; 13, buccinator; 14, auriculotemporal nerve; 15, mental nerve; 16, hypoglossal nerve (cranial nerve XII)

Ophthalmic herpes zoster (shingles) involving the corneal branch causes sensory loss, ulceration and eventual visual impairment.

Maxillary division

The maxillary division passes forwards through the middle cranial fossa, for a short distance in the cavernous sinus, the foramen rotundum, the pterygopalatine fossa, where the pterygopalatine ganglion is attached to it, and the inferior orbital fissure, where it becomes the infraorbital nerve.

Branches

The **zygomatic nerve** passes forwards on the lateral wall of the orbit and supplies the skin of the temple and cheek. A communication with the lacrimal nerve conveys postganglionic parasympathetic fibres to the lacrimal gland.

The **posterior superior alveolar nerve** branches to supply the upper molar and premolar teeth.

The **infraorbital nerve** is the continuation of the maxillary nerve in the orbit. It lies in the infraorbital groove and canal and emerges at the infraorbital foramen on to the face to supply the lower eyelid and conjunctiva, the side of the nose and the upper lip. Its **anterior superior alveolar branch** supplies the canine and incisor teeth, the side of the nose and the maxillary air sinus. Greater and lesser palatine branches convey sensation from the palate, and the nasopalatine nerves sensation from the floor of the nasal cavity and the anterior palate. Fibres to the pterygopalatine ganglion pass onwards to supply the nose, palate and nasopharynx.

Mandibular division

The mandibular division carries the motor root as well as the sensory fibres of the trigeminal nerve. It leaves the middle cranial fossa via the foramen ovale and divides into **motor branches** to the muscles of mastication (p. 341), tensor tympani and tensor veli palatini. The branches to mylohyoid and the anterior belly of digastric are described below.

The **sensory branches** have a wide distribution. The **meningeal branch** passes through the foramen spinosum to supply the dura of the middle cranial fossa.

The **buccal nerve** passes forwards between the heads of the lateral pterygoid to supply the skin of the cheek and its mucous membrane.

The **auriculotemporal nerve** passes laterally, anterior to the neck of the mandible, and ascends above the parotid gland to the temporal region of the scalp. It carries sensory fibres to the tympanic membrane, external acoustic meatus and auricle, the temporomandibular joint and the temporal region of the scalp. It conveys parasympathetic fibres from the otic ganglion (p. 396) to the parotid gland.

The **inferior alveolar nerve** descends to the mandibular foramen and enters the mandibular canal. It divides to form:

- The **mylohyoid nerve**, which passes forwards close to the mandible to supply the mylohyoid and anterior belly of digastric
- **Dental branches**, which arise in the canal to supply the adjacent gums and teeth

- The **incisor nerve**, supplying the canine and incisor teeth and the central incisor of the opposite side
- The **mental nerve**, which emerges through the mental foramen to supply the skin and mucous membrane of the lower lip and chin.

The **lingual nerve** passes forwards along the side of the tongue, supplying sensory branches to the anterior two-thirds of the tongue, the floor of the mouth and the lingual gum. It receives the chorda tympani branch of the facial nerve about 3 cm below the base of the skull, which carries parasympathetic fibres to the submandibular and sublingual salivary glands and taste fibres from the anterior two-thirds of the tongue.

Damage to the trunk of the mandibular nerve may result from pressure from an aneurysm, infiltration by a tumour and, rarely, injury. This results in (1) paralysis of the muscles of mastication, and (2) loss of sensation on the side of the face. A lower third molar tooth extraction may result in trauma to the lingual nerve and thus loss of sensation to the anterior tongue and reduced salivation if the chorda tympani is also involved.

Pain is frequently referred from one section of the nerve to another; e.g. a patient with a carcinoma of the tongue (supplied by the lingual nerve) may complain of earache in the distribution of the auriculotemporal nerve.

Trigeminal neuralgia is the term given to the condition of severe pain affecting the maxillary and/or mandibular divisions of the nerve, which is often precipitated by touching the area affected. The cause is usually unknown.

CN VI – Abducent nerve

The **abducent nerve** (Fig. 21.12) is a somatic motor nerve. It leaves the inferior border of the pons, passes forwards through the posterior and middle cranial fossae, the cavernous sinus and the orbit, and supplies the lateral rectus muscle.

Relations

In the posterior cranial fossa it lies between the pons and the occiput. It passes through the cavernous sinus to enter the orbit via the superior orbital fissure within the tendinous ring.

This thin nerve is, because of its long intracranial course, susceptible to damage by stretching in patients with raised intracranial pressure, and also in patients with tumours close to the course of the nerve, e.g. pituitary tumours. Paralysis, either partial or complete, results in failure of abduction of the eye and diplopia (Fig. 19.10, p. 319).

CN VII – Facial nerve

The facial nerve (Fig. 21.15) carries motor, sensory and parasympathetic fibres. The motor supply is to the facial muscles; the sensory fibres carry taste sensation from the anterior two-thirds of the tongue to its nucleus in the medulla and the parasympathetic fibres are secretomotor to the submandibular and sublingual salivary glands, the lacrimal gland and the mucous membrane of the nose, pharynx and mouth.

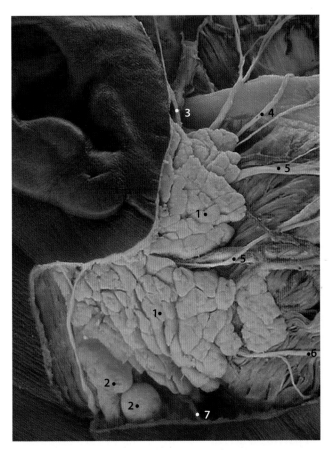

Figure 21.15 Dissection of the facial nerve as it appears on the anterior border of the right parotid gland: 1, parotid gland; 2, lymph nodes; 3, temporal branch; 4, zygomatic branch; 5, buccal branch; 6, mandibular branch (marginal mandibular); 7, cervical branch

Relations

On leaving the pons it passes laterally with the vestibulocochlear nerve through the internal acoustic meatus to the facial ganglion. Next it turns posteriorly to descend through a bony canal in the posterior wall of the middle ear to emerge from the stylomastoid foramen. It then passes into the parotid gland, where it divides into several terminal branches (Fig. 21.15).

Branches

- **Greater petrosal nerve** – carries secretomotor fibres to the pterygopalatine ganglion, leaving the facial nerve at the facial ganglion to join a sympathetic branch from the internal carotid plexus to traverse the sphenoid bone and join the pterygopalatine ganglion.
- Nerve to stapedius muscle.
- **Chorda tympani** – arises above the stylomastoid foramen to pass through the middle ear medial to the tympanic membrane and emerge from the base of the temporal bone to join the lingual nerve about 3 cm below the skull base. It conveys taste fibres from the anterior two-thirds of the tongue and parasympathetic fibres to the submandibular ganglion.
- Nerves to the posterior belly of digastric, stylohyoid, occipitalis and auricular muscles.

- **Motor branches** – temporal, zygomatic, buccal, mandibular and cervical branches supply the muscles of facial expression, buccinator and platysma.

Bell's palsy (Fig. 21.16), the most common cause of facial nerve damage, is of unknown aetiology. Inflammatory swelling of the nerve in the facial canal results in compression of the nerve and partial or complete paralysis. Thus the cheek, lip muscles and orbicularis oculi are paralysed or weakened; food cannot be chewed properly and the eye's lower lid is everted and no longer able to retain the lacrimal fluid within the conjunctival sac. The cornea is at risk of drying and may ulcerate. Virus infections may produce the same clinical picture. Fortunately most cases resolve after 2–3 months.

Other causes of facial nerve paralysis include tumours in the cerebellopontine angle (acoustic neuromata) and strokes causing upper motor neuron lesions of the nerve. The muscles of the upper face above the eyes, like those of the pharynx, larynx and tongue, are bilaterally innervated by upper motor neurons; thus only the lower half of the face is paralysed in a contralateral stroke (a stroke that has affected the cerebral cortex on the side opposite to the paralysis). The peripheral branches of the nerve are vulnerable to injury during surgery on the parotid and submandibular glands.

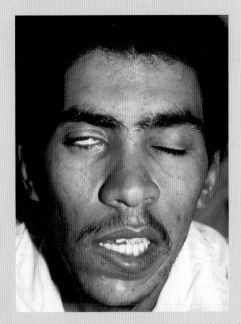

Figure 21.16 VIIth cranial nerve palsy on the right – the patient had been asked to close both eyes tightly

CN VIII – Vestibulocochlear nerve

The vestibulocochlear nerve (Fig. 21.4b) is a sensory nerve of two parts: the vestibular nerve concerned with balance, and the cochlear nerve concerned with hearing. These unite in the internal auditory meatus before passing medially to enter the medulla (see p. 359 for a description of the innervation of the internal ear). The results of injury are also described on p. 358.

CN IX – Glossopharyngeal nerve

The glossopharyngeal nerve has general and visceral sensory, motor and parasympathetic secretomotor fibres. Parasympathetic fibres supply the parotid gland and the motor fibres supply stylopharyngeus.

Relations

The nerve rootlets leave the medulla and join to pass through the jugular foramen with the accessory and vagus nerves and internal jugular vein. The nerve then passes forwards medial to the external carotid artery to pierce the pharyngeal wall between the superior and middle constrictors, to end in the posterior third of the tongue.

Branches

- **Tympanic nerve** – passes to the tympanic plexus in the middle ear and supplies the adjacent mucous membrane.
- Nerve to stylopharyngeus.
- **Sensory branches**, including taste, from the mucous membrane of the oropharynx, tonsil, soft palate and posterior third of the tongue.
- **Sensory branches** from the carotid sinus and body, middle ear and auditory tube.

Lesions affecting the glossopharyngeal nerve alone are rare but the integrity of the nerve can be tested by touching the fauces and posterior tongue. The 'gag' reflex is absent on the side of the lesion (p. 344).

CN X – Vagus nerve

The vagus nerve (Fig. 21.17) has several components: parasympathetic fibres supply the heart, lungs and alimentary canal as far as the splenic flexure; motor fibres supply the striated muscles of the larynx, pharynx and palate; sensory fibres come from the mucous membrane of the palate, pharynx and larynx, and from the heart, lungs and alimentary canal; special sensory fibres (taste) arise from the valleculae and epiglottis; and somatic sensory fibres come from the external acoustic meatus and tympanic membrane.

The nerve emerges from the medulla as rootlets and leaves the skull by the jugular foramen with the glossopharyngeal nerve, accessory nerve and internal jugular vein (Fig. 21.17). It descends the neck and thorax, where it joins with its fellow of the opposite side to form the anterior and posterior vagal trunks, whose branches are distributed throughout the abdomen.

Relations

In the neck the vagus descends in the posterior aspect of the carotid sheath, between the internal jugular vein laterally and the internal and common carotid arteries (Fig. 21.17). It lies on the prevertebral muscles and fascia. In the root of the neck the right nerve descends in front of the subclavian artery to enter the thorax; the left nerve descends between the common carotid and left subclavian arteries.

Branches (in the neck)

- **Auricular nerve** – supplying the external acoustic meatus and tympanic membrane.
- **Pharyngeal nerves** – pass to the pharyngeal plexus to supply the pharyngeal muscles and the mucous membrane of the pharynx.
- **Superior laryngeal nerve** – descends on the lateral wall of the pharynx and divides below the hyoid into external and internal branches, the internal piercing the thyrohyoid membrane to supply the laryngeal mucosa above the vocal cords and the external supplying the cricothyroid muscle.

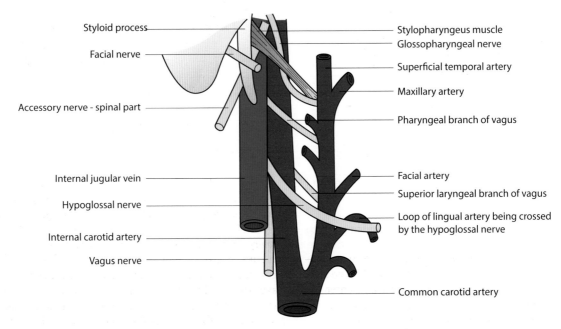

Styloid process — Stylopharyngeus muscle
Facial nerve — Glossopharyngeal nerve
Superficial temporal artery
Maxillary artery
Accessory nerve - spinal part — Pharyngeal branch of vagus
Internal jugular vein — Facial artery
Hypoglossal nerve — Superior laryngeal branch of vagus
Loop of lingual artery being crossed by the hypoglossal nerve
Internal carotid artery —
Vagus nerve — Common carotid artery

Figure 21.17 Lateral view of the last four cranial nerves as they leave the skull

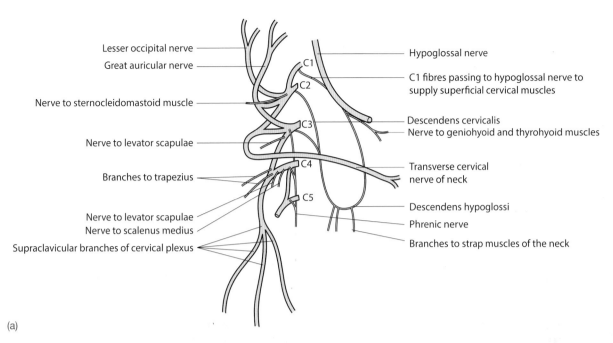

Lesser occipital nerve

Great auricular nerve

Nerve to sternocleidomastoid muscle

Nerve to levator scapulae

Branches to trapezius

Nerve to levator scapulae
Nerve to scalenus medius
Supraclavicular branches of cervical plexus

Hypoglossal nerve

C1 fibres passing to hypoglossal nerve to supply superficial cervical muscles

Descendens cervicalis
Nerve to geniohyoid and thyrohyoid muscles

Transverse cervical nerve of neck

Descendens hypoglossi
Phrenic nerve
Branches to strap muscles of the neck

(a)

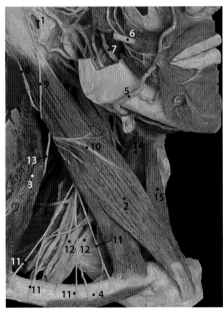

(b)

Figure 21.18 (a) Cervical plexus and links with the XIIth cranial nerve. (b) Dissection of right neck to show the neck triangles and cervical plexus branches: 1, external auditory meatus; 2, sternocleidomastoid; 3, trapezius; 4, clavicle; 5, facial artery overlying mandible; 6, parotid duct; 7, lingual nerve; 8, lesser occipital nerve; 9, great auricular nerve; 10, transverse cervical nerve; 11, supraclavicular nerves; 12, brachial plexus trunks; 13, accessory nerve – spinal part; 14, omohyoid; 15, sternohyoid

- **Right recurrent laryngeal nerve** (Fig. 22.6, p. 375) – loops around the right subclavian artery, and ascends in the groove between oesophagus and trachea to enter the larynx and supply all the intrinsic muscles, apart from cricothyroid, and the mucosa below the vocal folds.
- **Left recurrent laryngeal nerve** – see Fig. 3.6a, p. 57.

Injuries or lesions affect the branches of the nerve much more frequently than the nerve trunk. Injuries are usually the result of surgery or penetrating trauma. Injury to the pharyngeal branches results in difficulty in swallowing and frequent aspiration of food and drink; injury to the superior laryngeal nerve results in cricothyroid paralysis and a weak voice. The recurrent laryngeal nerves are occasionally injured during thyroid surgery and may be invaded by cancers of the thyroid, larynx, oesophagus and lung. Paralysis of the vocal fold results. A simple way to test the integrity of cranial nerves IX, X and XI is to touch the back of the tongue, which causes a 'gag reflex'– the sensory component is via the IXth nerve; the motor movements of the larynx and pharynx are via cranial nerves X and XI. Syringing of the ears may also cause a reflex slowing of the heart via the auricular vagal branches, and lead to heart failure in the elderly. Cleaning the ears with a cotton wool bud may stimulate a cough reflex via the vagus.

For the **vagus nerve** in the thorax and abdomen, see pp. 59 and 162, respectively.

CN XI – Accessory nerve

The accessory nerve has cranial and spinal roots, the cranial root arising from the medullar and the spinal root by rootlets from the first five segments of the spinal cord. The cranial fibres (**Figs. 21.17** and **21.18**) join the vagus to supply the muscles of the pharynx, larynx and oesophagus. The spinal root of the accessory nerve (**Figs. 21.9** and **22.3**, p. 373) conveys motor fibres that supply sternocleidomastoid and trapezius. It arises in the vertebral canal and ascends to pass through the foramen magnum to the posterior cranial fossa. It leaves the cranium via the jugular foramen, passing laterally anterior to the jugular vein into the substance of sternocleidomastoid. It then crosses the posterior triangle of the neck on levator scapulae to reach trapezius.

The subcutaneous course of the spinal root through the posterior triangle of the neck renders it vulnerable to injury during surgery, e.g. lymph node biopsy, in this region. Weakness of trapezius and sternocleidomastoid muscle results. Rotation of the neck is weakened as is shrugging the shoulder.

CN XII – Hypoglossal nerve

The hypoglossal nerve (Figs. 21.17, 21.18 and 19.25, p. 326) supplies all the intrinsic and extrinsic muscles of the tongue except palatoglossus. It emerges from the ventral medulla as 15–20 rootlets and leaves the posterior cranial fossa by the hypoglossal canal to descend behind the carotid sheath before passing forwards around the pharynx to the tongue.

Relations

Below the base of the skull the nerve lies behind the internal carotid artery and vagus nerve on the prevertebral fascia. It passes forwards between the artery and the internal jugular vein, crosses the external carotid artery, the loop of the lingual artery lying on the middle constrictor and the hyoglossus muscle, before ending in the tongue. In this part of its course it is medial to the posterior belly of digastric, submandibular gland and mylohyoid.

It receives motor fibres from the first cervical nerve near to the base of the skull and conveys them through the descendens hypoglossi branch (Fig. 21.18) to supply the geniohyoid and thyrohyoid muscles, before forming the **ansa cervicalis** with branches of the IInd and IIIrd cervical nerves to supply the infrahyoid group of strap muscles.

Injury to the nerve, which may occur during tonsillectomy, produces paralysis of the half of the tongue on the same side as the lesion. When the tongue is protruded it deviates to the paralysed side because of the action of the unparalysed genioglossus on the opposite side (see Fig. 19.26, p. 328). A midbrain lesion may produce a supranuclear paralysis that results in contralateral weakness of the tongue.

MCQs

1. The mandibular branch of the trigeminal nerve supplies the: T/F
  a tensor palati muscle   ( )
  b mylohyoid muscle   ( )
  c posterior belly of digastric   ( )
  d mastoid antrum and air cells   ( )
  e tensor tympani muscle   ( )

Answers
1.
a **T** – By the branch of the mandibular nerve, which also supplies the medial pterygoid muscle.
b **T** – By its nerve to mylohyoid, which comes off the inferior alveolar (dental) nerve.
c **F** – This is supplied by the facial nerve.
d **F** – These are supplied by the glossopharyngeal nerve, as is the middle ear cavity.
e **T** – By the same branch of the mandibular nerve that supplies tensor palati.

2. A patient has an invasive tumour in the cavernous sinus causing pressure on the nerves within the sinus. Presenting signs in the patient may include: T/F
  a a dilated pupil   ( )
  b a drooping eyelid (ptosis)   ( )
  c an eye that cannot abduct from the resting position   ( )
  d a weakness in screwing the eyes up tightly   ( )
  e a deviated eye looking down and laterally   ( )

Answers
2.
a **T** – The nerves found in the sinus are cranial nerves III, IV, VI, the ophthalmic division of V and ...
b **T** – ... sympathetic fibres. Pressure on the IIIrd cranial nerve paralyses all ocular muscles except superior oblique and lateral rectus, and causes ptosis because of paralysis of levator palpebrae superioris. There is paralysis of the ciliary muscle and sphincter pupillae, causing dilatation of the pupil.
c **T** – Because of pressure on the VIth (abducent) cranial nerve and paralysis of lateral rectus.
d **F** – Tight closing of the eyes is a function of orbicularis oculi, which is supplied by the facial nerve. This does not enter the cavernous sinus.
e **T** – This is seen in a lesion affecting the IIIrd cranial nerve. The only muscles then retaining function are the superior oblique and lateral rectus, which together pull the eye downwards and outwards.

SBA

1. A middle-aged man was seen with pain of 2 days' duration over his chin and lower lip. No diagnosis was made, but several days later when vesicles appeared over the same area he was diagnosed with herpes zoster (shingles), a viral infection of cutaneous nerves. Which nerve is affected?
a buccal
b auriculotemporal
c mental
d lesser petrosal
e infraorbital

Answer
c The area affected is supplied by the mental nerve, a branch of the inferior alveolar nerve, itself a branch of the mandibular division of the trigeminal nerve.

2. One day after having a partial thyroidectomy, a patient is noted to have a weak, hoarse voice. What nerve is suspected as having been damaged during the operation?
a ansa cervicalis
b ansa subclavia
c recurrent laryngeal
d internal branch of the superior laryngeal
e external branch of the superior laryngeal

Answer
c It is likely that the recurrent laryngeal nerve has been damaged by being either divided or caught in a ligature on the inferior thyroid artery. The nerve lies in close proximity to the artery and great care must be exercised to identify the nerve and gently separate it from the artery before the artery is divided.

EMQs

Each question has an anatomical theme linked to the chapter, and a list of 10 related items (A–J) placed in alphabetical order: these are followed by five statements (1–5). Match **one or more** of the items A–J to each of the five statements.

Cranial nerves
A. Abducent
B. Facial
C. Glossopharyngeal
D. Hypoglossal
E. Olfactory
F. Optic
G. Trigeminal
H. Trochlear
I. Vagus
J. Vestibulocochlear

Match the following statements with the nerve(s) in the above list.
1. Required to whistle
2. Initiates the gag reflex
3. Required for a lateral gaze
4. Approximates the vocal folds
5. Pushes food around the oral cavity

Answers
1 B; 2 C; 3 A; 4 I; 5 BDG

APPLIED QUESTIONS

1. Why may babies who have a forceps delivery present with temporary facial palsies?

   1. *The mastoid process is rather undeveloped at birth, as the air sacs are still rudimentary and, consequently, the facial nerve is very exposed as it exits the stylomastoid foramen. It can be palpated in the newborn and, if trapped beneath forceps during delivery, a temporary facial palsy may result.*

2. How do you straighten the external auditory meatus in an adult or in an infant when trying to see the tympanic membrane?

   2. *The external auditory meatus is S-shaped: the first part passes forwards and upwards, the second is slightly backwards, and the longest third part runs forwards and slightly downwards. To straighten out this canal in the adult, gentle traction is applied in an upwards and backwards direction on the pinna, which is part of the cartilaginous canal. In the infant, pulling downwards and backwards is more rewarding.*

3. A young child presents in your clinic with a perforation of the eardrum and a large swelling in the mastoid region. Two days later he is brought into the clinic obviously very ill, drowsy and, from the mother's description, having just had convulsions. What has happened to his infection?

   3. *In children an untreated otitis media may spread to the mastoid air cells. From here the infection may well break through the superior wall of the mastoid and into the cranial cavity, affecting the meninges and temporal lobe and causing meningitis or a temporal lobe abscess. If the posterior wall of the mastoid antrum is invaded, the sigmoid dural venous sinus may be infected, causing a thrombosis, with serious consequences. Meningitis, cerebral abscess and venous sinus thrombosis can all cause the symptoms and signs described.*

Bailey & Love · Essential Clinical Anatomy · Bailey & Love · Essential Clinical Anatomy
ential Clinical Anatomy · Bailey & Love · Essential Clinical Anatomy · Bailey & Love
ley & Love · Essential Clinical Anatomy · Bailey & Love · Essential Clinical Anatomy

Chapter 22

The neck

SUPERFICIAL FASCIA

The **superficial fascia**, a fatty layer between the skin and the deep fascia, contains the platysma muscle beneath which lie the external jugular veins and tributaries (**Fig. 22.1**). The **platysma** is a broad sheet of muscle extending over the pectoral muscles and the lower border of the mandible, where it blends with the facial muscles. The **deep fascia** is complex and consists of the investing layer of cervical fascia, prevertebral and pretracheal fascia and the carotid sheath.

The **investing layer of cervical fascia** forms a 'polo neck' collar around the deep structures of the neck; posteriorly it is attached to the ligamentum nuchae and splits to enclose trapezius and sternocleidomastoid. Superiorly it is attached to the superior nuchal lines, the mastoid processes and the inferior body of the mandible. It splits to form a sheath around

the parotid gland that is attached above to the zygomatic arch. Inferiorly the fascia is attached to the manubrium sterni (where it is pierced by the exterior jugular vein), clavicles, acromial processes and spines of the scapulae, and between the scapulae it descends over the postvertebral muscles.

The **prevertebral fascia** is a tough membrane that lies anterior to the prevertebral muscles and the cervical and brachial plexuses. Superiorly it attaches to the base of the skull; inferiorly it blends with the anterior longitudinal ligament in front of the 4th thoracic vertebra. Laterally it covers the postvertebral muscles on the floor of the posterior triangles, blends with the cervical fascia and then envelops the subclavian artery, which carries it into the arm as the **axillary sheath**. It covers the muscles in the floor of the posterior triangle. The cervical nerve roots, cervical plexus and brachial plexus lie deep to the fascia. The lymph nodes of

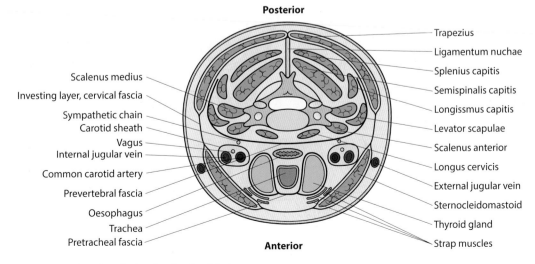

Posterior

- Trapezius
- Ligamentum nuchae
- Splenius capitis
- Semispinalis capitis
- Longissmus capitis
- Levator scapulae
- Scalenus anterior
- Longus cervicis
- External jugular vein
- Sternocleidomastoid
- Thyroid gland
- Strap muscles

- Scalenus medius
- Investing layer, cervical fascia
- Sympathetic chain
- Carotid sheath
- Vagus
- Internal jugular vein
- Common carotid artery
- Prevertebral fascia
- Oesophagus
- Trachea
- Pretracheal fascia

Anterior

Figure 22.1 Transverse section of neck showing the fascial planes

the posterior triangle and the accessory nerve lie superficial to it.

The **pretracheal fascia** lies deep to the infrahyoid strap muscles. It is attached superiorly to the hyoid bone and the thyroid cartilage, and splits to surround the thyroid gland. Laterally it blends with the carotid sheath and descends to fuse with the fibrous pericardium.

The **carotid sheath**, a condensation of the fascias of the neck, is attached to the base of the skull around the carotid canal and below it fuses with the fibrous pericardium. It encloses the internal jugular vein, the common and internal carotid arteries and the vagus nerve The cervical sympathetic trunk lies posteriorly between the sheath from the prevertebral fascia. The sheath lies deep to a line joining the sternoclavicular joint and the tragus of the ear.

The investing layer of cervical fascia serves to define the spread of infection in the soft tissues of the neck. Pus originating behind the prevertebral layer, e.g. from a cervical vertebra, may thus spread laterally to present behind the sternocleidomastoid. Infections arising posterior to the prevertebral fascia may also spread inferiorly posterior to the pharynx and oesophagus to enter the posterior mediastinum. Infections in the space behind the pharynx (retropharyngeal space) may also spread down to the superior mediastinum. The anaesthetist injects local anaesthetic deep to the **prevertebral sheath** when undertaking a brachial plexus block.

THE TRIANGLES OF THE NECK

Each side of the neck is divided, descriptively, by sternocleidomastoid into anterior and posterior triangles (Figs. 22.2–22.4). The **posterior triangle** is bounded by sternocleidomastoid anteriorly, trapezius posteriorly and the clavicle inferiorly (Fig. 22.3). It is floored by the prevertebral fascia over splenius capitis, levator scapulae and scalenus medius, and part of scalenus anterior, and is crossed by the posterior belly of omohyoid. It contains the spinal portion of the accessory nerve and, below the prevertebral fascia, branches of the cervical plexus, the upper and middle trunks of the brachial plexus, lymph nodes and the subclavian artery. The **anterior triangle** (Fig. 22.4), bounded laterally by sternocleidomastoid, superiorly by the body of the mandible and anteriorly by the midline, contains structures related to the floor of the mouth, the larynx, the pharynx and the trachea (Fig. 22.4c).

Care is required during surgical dissection in the posterior triangle to avoid damaging the spinal accessory nerve (Fig. 22.3). Note that its surface marking is between its emergence about a third of the way down the posterior border of sternomastoid to its exit from the triangle about a third of the distance from the anterior border of the trapezius (Figs. 22.3 and 22.4a). It is particularly at risk during lymph node dissection since the nodes are frequently adherent to the nerve. Paralysis of the trapezius results in an inability to retract or elevate the shoulder.

Sternocleidomastoid

Sternocleidomastoid is enclosed by the cervical fascia. Inferiorly it is attached by two heads to the upper surface of the manubrium sterni and the upper surface of the medial third of the clavicle. Superiorly it is attached to the mastoid process and the lateral half of the superior nuchal line (Fig. 22.2). The cervical plexus lies deep to the upper half of the muscle and the carotid sheath lies deep to its lower half. The lower end of the internal jugular vein lies deep to the muscle and is accessible to needle or catheter between the manubrial and clavicular heads.

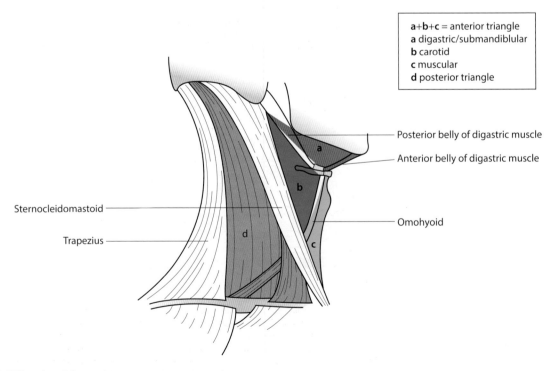

a+b+c = anterior triangle
a digastric/submandiblular
b carotid
c muscular
d posterior triangle

Posterior belly of digastric muscle
Anterior belly of digastric muscle
Omohyoid
Sternocleidomastoid
Trapezius

Figure 22.2 Triangles of the neck

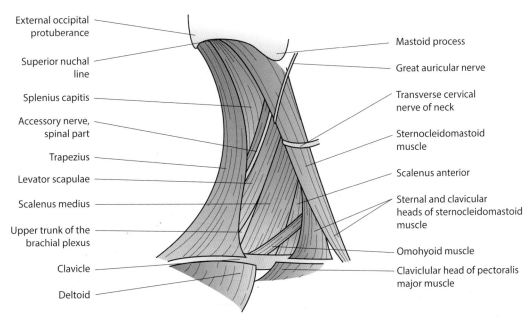

Figure 22.3 Right posterior triangle of the neck showing the muscles and accessory nerve

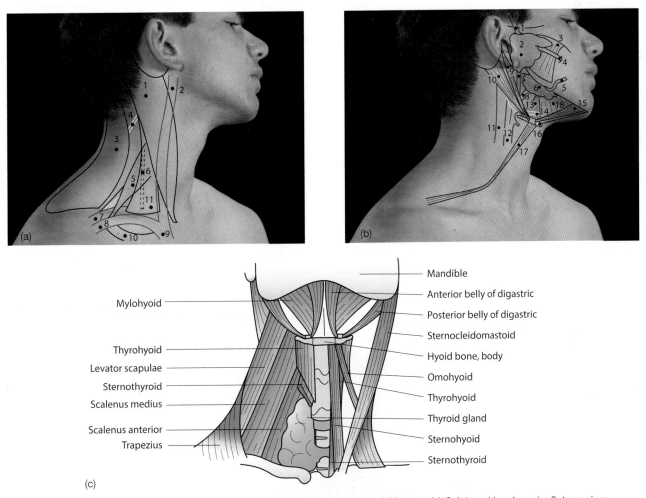

Figure 22.4 (a) Surface anatomy showing the superficial neck contents: 1, sternocleidomastoid; 2, internal jugular vein; 3, trapezius; 4, accessory nerve – spinal part; 5, scalenus anterior; 6, phrenic nerve; 7, axillary artery; 8, axillary vein; 9, brachiocephalic vein; 10, 1st rib; 11, sternocleidomastoid – clavicular head. (b) Deeper structures: 1, superficial temporal artery; 2, parotid gland; 3, masseter; 4, parotid duct piercing buccinator; 5, facial artery; 6, submandibular gland; 7, external carotid artery; 8, origin of facial artery; 9, stylohyoid; 10, digastric – posterior belly; 11, internal jugular vein; 12, common carotid artery; 13, hyoglossus; 14, hypoglossal nerve; 15, digastric – anterior belly; 16, hyoid bone; 17, omohyoid; 18, mylohyoid. (c) Anterior view – left superficial muscles and right deep muscles

Functions

Each muscle turns the chin to the opposite side and laterally flexes the neck to its own side (as in looking under a table); together the muscles extend the altlanto-occipital joints and flex the cervical spine (as in jutting out the chin). When the head is fixed by the extensor muscles of the back, sternocleidomastoid, by raising the upper thorax, is an accessory muscle of inspiration.

Nerve supply

This is via the spinal accessory nerve and branches from the IInd and IIIrd cervical nerves.

Birth injury occasionally causes tearing of the sternocleidomastoid muscle; the subsequent fibrosis and contraction of the muscle results in wry neck (torticollis), a flexion deformity of the neck that produces a tilt and rotation of the neck to the side of the affected muscle and restricted rotation to the opposite side. Idiopathic torticollis is a common condition. The patient awakes to find the neck pulled uncomfortably to one side due to spasm of the sternomastoid or trapezius muscles. It is usually short-lived and of unknown aetiology.

Trapezius

The trapezius is described on p. 193.

THE EXTENSOR MUSCLES OF THE NECK

Those extensor muscles attaching the shoulder girdle to the trunk are described on p. 194 and those that extend the vertebral column on p. 177.

Splenius capitis passes upwards and laterally from the ligamentum nuchae and spines of the upper thoracic vertebrae to the mastoid process and the lateral part of the superior nuchal line. It lies deep to sternocleidomastoid.

Semispinalis passes upwards and medially from the transverse processes to the spines above. Its upper part, **semispinalis**

capitis, attaches to the occiput between the superior and inferior nuchal lines.

It is this muscle that, when hypertrophied, gives the 'bull neck' to rugby prop forwards or linebackers in American football.

Suboccipital muscles

Rectus capitis posterior minor and major and obliquus capitis superior originate from the atlas and axis to be attached below the inferior nuchal line of the occiput (Fig. 22.5 and Fig. 18.9b, p. 308). Obliquus capitis inferior passes from the transverse process of the atlas to the spine of the axis. These muscles extend the skull at the atlanto-occipital joints and rotate it at the atlantoaxial joints. They are all supplied by the posterior ramus of cervical nerve I and are the fine movement adjustors of head tilting and nodding.

The **ligamentum nuchae** is a strong ligament connecting the occipital bone and all the cervical spines.

Prevertebral and scalene muscles

The prevertebral and scalene muscles (Fig. 22.6) lie in front of the cervical and upper thoracic vertebrae, covered by the prevertebral fascia. Rectus capitis anterior and lateralis, longus capitis and longus coli each pass between the skull and the vertebrae and between vertebrae.

Scalenus anterior is attached superiorly to the anterior tubercles of the 3rd to 6th cervical vertebrae and inferiorly to the scalene tubercle on the 1st rib. It is the key surgical landmark for the anatomy of the root of the neck (Fig. 22.6). Its anterior surface is crossed by the phrenic nerve and prevertebral fascia separates it from the sympathetic trunk, the subclavian vein and the carotid sheath. It lies in front of scalenus medius, the dome of the pleura and the subclavian artery.

Scalenus medius is attached superiorly to the posterior tubercles of the 2nd to 7th cervical vertebrae and inferiorly to the upper surface of the 1st rib behind the subclavian artery.

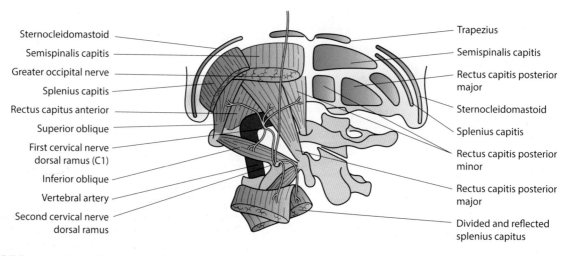

Sternocleidomastoid
Semispinalis capitis
Greater occipital nerve
Splenius capitis
Rectus capitus anterior
Superior oblique
First cervical nerve dorsal ramus (C1)
Inferior oblique
Vertebral artery
Second cervical nerve dorsal ramus

Trapezius
Semispinalis capitis
Rectus capitis posterior major
Sternocleidomastoid
Splenius capitis
Rectus capitis posterior minor
Rectus capitis posterior major
Divided and reflected splenius capitus

Figure 22.5 Posterior view of the upper neck showing the suboccipital muscles

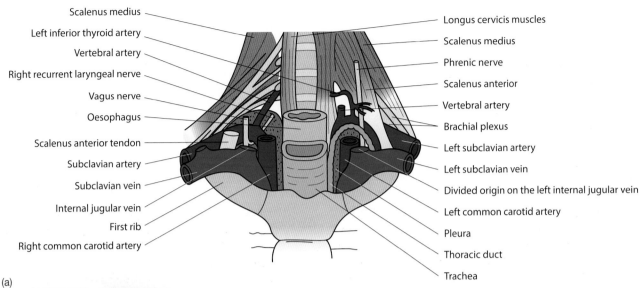

(a)

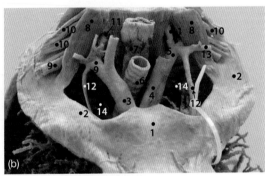

(b)

Figure 22.6 (a) Root of the neck showing relations to scalenus anterior (right scalenus anterior removed). (b) Dissection of the root of the neck to show major relationships: 1, manubrium; 2, 1st rib; 3, brachiocephalic trunk; 4, left common carotid artery; 5, left subclavian artery; 6, trachea; 7, oesophagus; 8, scalenus anterior; 9, right subclavian artery; 10, brachial plexus trunks; 11, vertebral artery; 12, internal thoracic artery; 13, suprascapular artery; 14, apex of lungs, segmental bronchi

Functions

The prevertebral and scalene muscles are weak flexors of the head and neck and the scalenes help to raise and fix the upper two ribs.

They are used as accessory muscles of inspiration, especially in patients with chronic obstructive airways disease and asthma.

Nerve supply

This is via the anterior rami of the cervical nerves.

Scalenus anterior syndrome is one of the conditions that come under the heading of 'thoracic outlet syndrome', where, owing to abnormalities or after trauma, this muscle and its fibrous attachments may cause pressure on the subclavian artery or brachial plexus, which lie immediately posterior to the muscle's insertion on to the 1st rib. The resultant problems include cold hands due to diminished blood flow and hand weakness due to pressure on the T1 nerve, which supplies all of the intrinsic hand muscles.

The infrahyoid muscles

The infrahyoid muscles (**Fig. 22.4c**) comprise four pairs of 'strap' muscles enclosed in a fascial sheath in the anterior neck:

- **Thyrohyoid** is attached superiorly to the body and greater horn of the hyoid bone and inferiorly to the body of the thyroid cartilage.

- **Sternohyoid** is attached superiorly to the body of the hyoid and inferiorly to the back of the manubrium sterni and adjacent clavicle.
- **Omohyoid** has superior and inferior bellies united by an intermediate tendon, which is tethered to the medial end of the clavicle by a fascial sling. Superiorly it is attached to the body of the hyoid and inferiorly to the lateral end of the superior border of the scapula by the suprascapular notch.
- **Sternothyroid** is attached superiorly to the thyroid cartilage and inferiorly to the back of the manubrium and first costal cartilage. It lies deep to sternohyoid.

These muscles fix or depress the hyoid bone during swallowing and speech. They are supplied by the anterior rami of the upper three cervical nerves, via the loop of the ansa cervicalis (**Fig. 21.18**, p. 367).

THE THYROID GLAND

This is a bilobed endocrine gland (**Fig. 22.7**) that lies on each side of the trachea and oesophagus, like a bow tie in both position and shape. Each lobe is joined to the other by a communicating isthmus anterior to the trachea. It is enclosed in pretracheal fascia. Each lobe is about 5 cm long and lies between the level of the thyroid cartilage and the sixth tracheal ring. The isthmus lies on the second and third tracheal rings. Occasionally a pyramidal lobe is found arising from its upper border and passing towards its origin at the root of the tongue.

Relations

Superficial to it lie the strap muscles, the cervical fascia and sternocleidomastoid; on its medial side are the larynx and trachea and, deep to these, the pharynx and oesophagus. The recurrent laryngeal nerves approach the medial surface of the gland and ascend lying medially between the trachea and the oesophagus behind the pretracheal fascia. They pass behind the cricothyroid joint to supply the laryngeal muscles. This is a relationship of considerable importance; the proximity of the nerves to the thyroid gland places them at risk of damage during thyroid surgery. The external laryngeal nerve descends to reach the cricothyroid muscle. Posteriorly are the carotid sheath and its contents, the parathyroid glands and the prevertebral fascia.

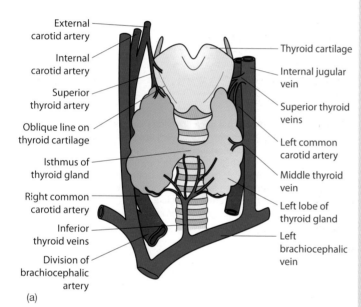

External carotid artery
Internal carotid artery
Superior thyroid artery
Oblique line on thyroid cartilage
Isthmus of thyroid gland
Right common carotid artery
Inferior thyroid veins
Division of brachiocephalic artery
(a)

Thyroid cartilage
Internal jugular vein
Superior thyroid veins
Left common carotid artery
Middle thyroid vein
Left lobe of thyroid gland
Left brachiocephalic vein

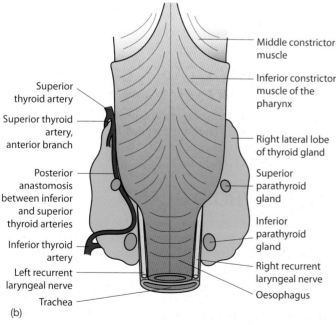

Superior thyroid artery
Superior thyroid artery, anterior branch
Posterior anastomosis between inferior and superior thyroid arteries
Inferior thyroid artery
Left recurrent laryngeal nerve
Trachea
(b)

Middle constrictor muscle
Inferior constrictor muscle of the pharynx
Right lateral lobe of thyroid gland
Superior parathyroid gland
Inferior parathyroid gland
Right recurrent laryngeal nerve
Oesophagus

Figure 22.7 Thyroid gland and its relations: (a) anterior view; (b) posterior view

Blood supply

This is from the superior and inferior thyroid arteries, which lie close to the external and internal laryngeal nerves as these approach the gland. The superior and middle thyroid veins drain to the internal jugular vein, and the inferior thyroid veins drain by a common trunk to the left brachiocephalic vein.

Lymphatic drainage

Drainage is to pretracheal, paratracheal and inferior deep cervical nodes.

Thyroglossal cysts are found along the path of descent of the thyroid during its development, that is, from the tongue base down to the upper trachea (Fig. 22.8).

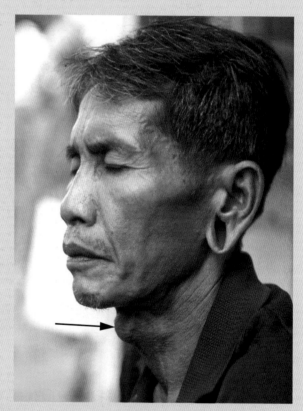

Figure 22.8 A subhyoid thyroglossal cyst (arrow) in an Iban inhabitant of Borneo

Goitre is a non-specific term used to describe enlargement of the thyroid. There are numerous causes, but the most common worldwide is a dietary deficiency of iodine (Fig. 22.9), which is found particularly in regions distant from the sea. A large goitre may extend down into the superior mediastinum and then cause difficulties in breathing (Fig. 22.10). Thyroidectomy for thyrotoxicosis (overactivity of the gland) involves the removal of the anterior three-quarters of the thyroid lobes, thus avoiding inadvertent removal of the parathyroid glands. Attention to the recurrent laryngeal nerve is essential to avoid damage during clamping of the inferior thyroid arteries.

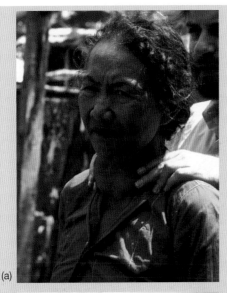

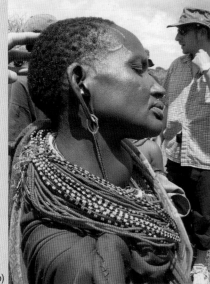

Figure 22.9 Goitre due to iodine deficiency in land-locked developing countries: (a) highlands of Borneo; (b) Samburu region, northern Kenya

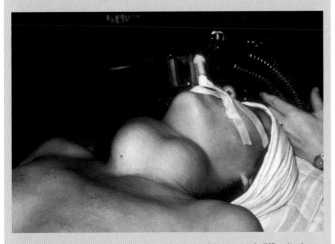

Figure 22.10 Goitre causing breathing problems and difficulty in swallowing (dysphagia)

THE PARATHYROID GLANDS

The parathyroid glands (Fig. 22.7b) are four small endocrine glands situated behind the lateral lobes of the thyroid gland and within its capsule. There is a superior and an inferior gland on each side. Whereas the superior glands are relatively constant in position, behind the middle of the thyroid lobe, the lower glands, although usually located behind the lower lobe, may occasionally be found outside the pretracheal fascia in the neck or even in the superior mediastinum. Each gland is oval and about 3–6 mm in length. They have a rich blood supply from the superior and inferior thyroid arteries. The superior and inferior glands develop from the fourth and third pharyngeal arches, respectively. They secrete parathormone and play an important role in calcium metabolism.

THE TRACHEA

The trachea (Fig. 20.10, p. 346, and see p. 63) begins at the larynx at the level of the 6th cervical vertebra and cricoid cartilage and descends through the neck and thorax to its bifurcation into the two bronchi at the level of the sternal angle, at T4/T5. It is about 10 cm long and 2 cm in diameter, and is covered by the pretracheal fascia. Its walls are formed of fibrous tissue reinforced by 15–20 incomplete cartilaginous rings, which are each completed posteriorly by fibroelastic tissue and smooth muscle.

Relations

In the neck the trachea lies anterior to the oesophagus, with the recurrent laryngeal nerve lying laterally in the groove between them. Anteriorly are the infrahyoid muscles and cervical fascia, and it is crossed by the thyroid isthmus and the left brachiocephalic vein. Laterally are the lateral lobes of the thyroid gland, the inferior thyroid artery and the carotid sheath. For relations in the thorax see p. 63.

Lymphatic drainage

Drainage is to the pretracheal, paratracheal and tracheobronchial nodes.

Nerve supply

There are branches of the sympathetic trunk, with parasympathetic branches from the vagus via the recurrent laryngeal nerve and the pulmonary plexuses (p. 71). Sensory fibres are carried in the recurrent laryngeal nerves.

Tracheostomy is the surgical term applied to the making of an opening into the trachea. It is usually created to assist respiration or overcome upper respiratory tract obstruction. It involves separating the strap muscles and excising a small 6–8 mm diameter portion of the third/fourth tracheal ring below the thyroid isthmus. A tracheostomy tube is then inserted into the trachea and retained by neck straps (Fig. 22.11a). Currently the simpler procedure of cricothyroidotomy, or 'mini-trach', is recommended for emergencies. A thin cannula is inserted through a wide needle passed through the cricothyroid membrane just above the cricoid cartilage. This may be followed if necessary by a formal surgical tracheostomy (Fig. 22.11b).

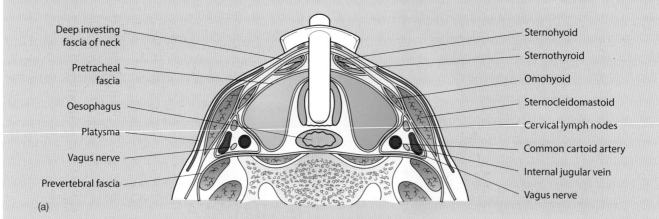

Deep investing fascia of neck
Pretracheal fascia
Oesophagus
Platysma
Vagus nerve
Prevertebral fascia
(a)

Sternohyoid
Sternothyroid
Omohyoid
Sternocleidomastoid
Cervical lymph nodes
Common cartoid artery
Internal jugular vein
Vagus nerve

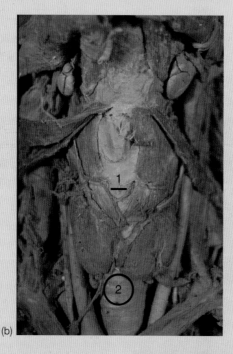

(b)

Figure 22.11 (a) Cross-section of the neck at the level of the fourth tracheal ring (showing a tracheostomy tube in place). (b) Dissection of the neck to show the anatomy and the position of: 1, cricothyroidotomy; 2, tracheostomy

THE OESOPHAGUS

This part of the alimentary tract (**Figs. 22.1, 22.6** and **22.7b**) begins at the level of the 6th cervical vertebra behind the cricoid cartilage, as a continuation of the pharynx. It descends through the neck, thorax and diaphragm, inclining slightly to the left, to enter the stomach in the abdomen at the level of the 10th thoracic vertebra. Its upper end is about 15 cm from the incisor teeth and it is about 25 cm long. Its course in the chest is described on p. 27.

Relations

In the neck the oesophagus lies anterior to the prevertebral fascia and muscles and posterior to the trachea (**Figs. 22.1** and **22.6**), with the recurrent laryngeal nerves, in the groove between the oesophagus and trachea (**Fig. 22.7b**). The lobes of the thyroid gland and the common carotid artery are lateral to it and the thoracic duct ascends for a short distance along its left side.

Blood supply

This is from the inferior thyroid artery, from branches from the aorta, and from the left gastric artery. Venous blood drains to the inferior thyroid, azygos and left gastric veins. The communication between the azygos and left gastric veins in the wall of the oesophagus and upper stomach forms a clinically important portosystemic anastomosis (see p. 103).

Lymphatic drainage

Drainage is to the deep cervical nodes, the posterior mediastinal nodes and, via the left gastric nodes, the coeliac nodes.

Nerve supply

Sympathetic supply is from the thoracic sympathetic chain and greater splanchnic nerves. Parasympathetic fibres are derived from the vagus, from the recurrent laryngeal nerve for the upper oesophagus and from the oesophageal plexus for the middle and lower oesophagus.

Oesophageal varices are caused by portal hypertension (see p. 103). These arise in the submucosa around the gastro-oesophageal junction (**Fig. 22.12**) and, if the overlying mucosa is eroded, will bleed to cause haematemesis.

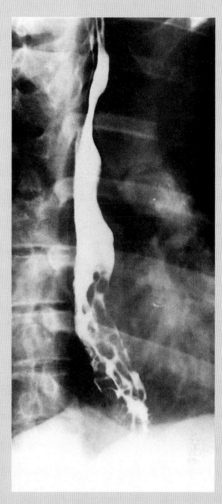

Figure 22.12 Barium swallow showing a normal upper oesophagus and multiple large filling defects in the lower oesophagus (varices)

DEVELOPMENT OF THE PHARYNGEAL ARCHES

Structures of the lower face and neck are formed by the pharyngeal apparatus, which consists of the pharyngeal arches, clefts, pouches and membranes. The pharyngeal arches are U-shaped loops or blocks of embryonic tissue that are stacked on top of each other and surround the future oral cavity and pharyngeal region of the cranial foregut (Fig. 22.13). Each arch has a mesodermal core, covered externally by ectoderm and internally by endoderm. Neural crest cell migration is essential to the correct formation of the arches; defective migration may therefore lead to arch defects that can be accompanied by defects in other organs or systems. Initially six arches develop in a craniocaudal direction. Arches 5 and 6 are relatively small and rudimentary, such that only four arches are visible externally; the fifth arch regresses soon after formation, and the sixth arch fuses with the fourth (Fig. 22.14).

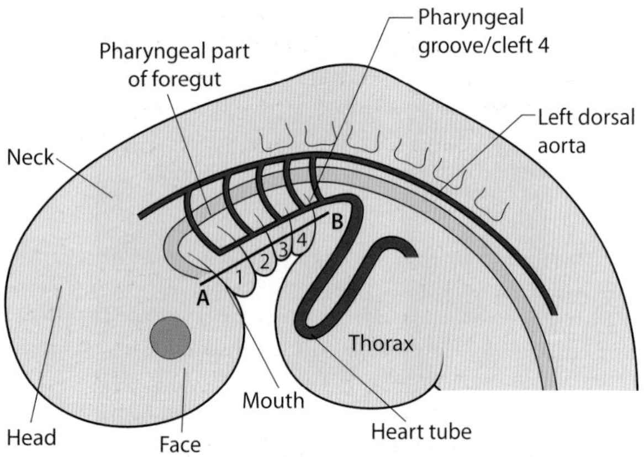

Each pharyngeal arch initially gives rise to, or is associated with:

- a correspondingly numbered aortic arch artery, not all of which persist (See Fig.2.31, p. 48)
- muscles of the face, head and neck
- a cranial nerve
- cartilaginous tissues, some of which later become skeletal
- ligamentous tissues.

The tissues derived from the pharyngeal arches undergo growth, movement and/or regression. In some cases, remnants of pharyngeal arch-derived cartilage or bone can persist as cervical or branchial vestiges that form a firm, palpable, subcutaneous mass situated in the lower neck, close to sternocleidomastoid (Fig. 22.15). Knowledge of the tissue derivatives of each arch (Table 22.1 and Fig. 22.14) helps to explain the normal innervation patterns of some head and neck structures, the potential locations of ectopic tissues or tissue remnants, and the patient observations or symptoms associated with pha-

Figure 22.13 The position of the pharyngeal arches shown relative to the aortic arch arteries and the pharyngeal part of the gut tube (left lateral view). Line A-B relates to Figs. 22.14 and 22.17. Only arches 1-4 are visible externally as arch 5 quickly regresses and arch 6 joins with arch 4

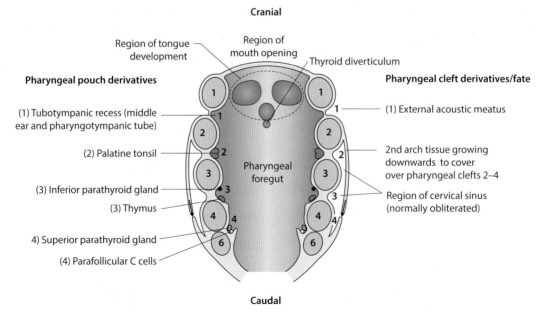

Figure 22.14 The developing pharyngeal arches viewed as if cut from the embryo (along line A-B in Fig 22.13) and viewed from posteriorly. The pharyngeal grooves/clefts are located on the external surface (labeled on right side of figure) and the pharyngeal pouches on the internal surface (labeled on left side of figure) of the pharyngeal arches. Arch 6 is small and fused to arch 4, hence only 4 arches are visible externally

ryngeal arch developmental defects. For example, first pharyngeal arch syndromes such as Treacher Collins or Pierre Robin can produce facial defects that may involve the palate, mandible, zygoma, eye region and ears, and can also be accompanied by conductive hearing loss due to auditory meatus atresia and maldevelopment of the malleus and incus. Alternatively, defective development of the third and fourth pharyngeal pouches can result in DiGeorge syndrome, in which the thymus and parathyroid glands are absent and cardiac outflow defects are often present.

The tissues of a given pharyngeal arch are innervated by a single cranial nerve. In practice this means that the muscle tissue derived from a given arch will retain its cranial nerve innervation no matter where its final location (Table 22.1). Each arch is also initially associated with its correspondingly numbered aortic arch artery, which passes from the aortic sac to the ipsilateral dorsal aorta. The aortic arch arteries quickly remodel and move out of the pharyngeal arches to form much of the great vessel vascular tree (see Figs. 2.31 and 2.33, p. 48).

Pharyngeal grooves or clefts

The externally located indentations between each pharyngeal arch are the pharyngeal clefts or grooves, and the internally located indentations are the pharyngeal pouches (Fig. 22.14). Only the first pharyngeal groove persists as a permanent structure, the external acoustic meatus. Additional remnants of the first groove can form auricular sinuses or cysts, which are located on the lateral aspect of the face, in a triangular region anterior to the tragus (Fig. 22.15). The remaining grooves become covered by a downwards growth of tissue from the second pharyngeal arch. The platysma muscle develops within this downgrowth and serves as an approximate indicator of the location of the downgrowth in the neck. The cervical sinus, the region located between the downgrowth of the second pharyngeal arch and the outer surface of the lower arches and grooves, usually disappears. Its persistence can result in an external cervical/branchial sinus, which opens on to the lower anterior neck along the anterior border of sternocleidomastoid and can discharge cellular debris and/or mucoid material (Fig. 22.18); alternatively, it can produce a cervical/branchial fistula, which passes from the lower or lateral neck to the palatine tonsillar sinus via the interval between the internal and external carotid vessels (Figs. 22.14 and 22.18). In adolescence or adulthood, remnants of cervical sinus tissue can form painless cervical/branchial cysts, which are often located along the anterior border of sternocleidomastoid, in close proximity to the mandible (Fig. 22.16).

TABLE 22.1 The tissue derivates and nervous innervation of the pharyngeal arches, pouches and grooves.[1] Via both the superior and recurrent laryngeal nerves arising from CNX.[2] Other 'non-arch cartilage-derived' bones associated with the maxillary and mandibular prominences arise from arch 1-associated tissues including the maxilla, zygoma, vomer, mandible and squamous temporal bone.

Arch	Associated cranial nerve	Cartilage and skeletal derivates	Muscular derivates	Ligamentous derivates (derived from the arch cartilage)	Pharyngeal pouch and derivates	Pharyngeal groove and derivates
1	V2 and V3	1st arch (Meckel's) cartilage[2] – Malleus – Incus	Muscles of mastication Tensor veli palatini Tensor tympani Digastric (anterior belly) Mylohyoid	Sphenomandibular ligament Anterior ligament of malleus	Pouch 1 – Tympanic cavity – Mastoid antrum – Pharyngotympanic tube	Cleft 1 – External acoustic meatus
2	VII	2nd arch (Reichart's) cartilage – Stapes – Styloid process – Lesser horn of the hyoid	Muscles of facial expression Stapedius Stylohyoid Digastric (posterior belly)	Stylohyoid ligament	Pouch 2 – Tonsillar fossa – Lining of palatine tonsillar crypts	
3	IX	3rd arch cartilage – Greater horn of the hyoid	Stylopharyngeus	None	Pouch 3 – Inferior parathyroid gland – Thymus	Clefts 2–4 – Obliterated with the cervical sinus
4 & 6	X[1]	4th arch cartilage – Laryngeal cartilages (not the epiglottis)	Intrinsic laryngeal muscles Pharyngeal muscles (except stylophayrngeus) Striated oesophageal muscle Levator veli palatini	None	Pouch 4 – Superior parathyroid gland – Parafollicular/ C-cells of thyroid gland (from ultimopharyngeal body)	

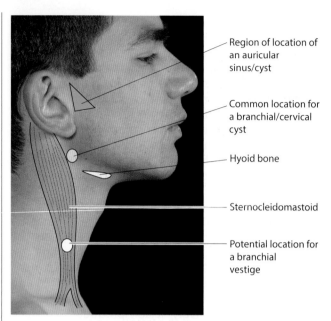

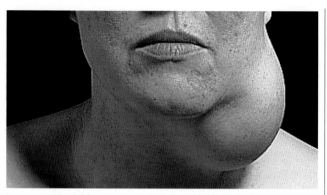

Figure 22.15 Common location for a branchial vestige (white), branchial/cervical cyst (yellow) and an auricular sinus (green)

Figure 22.16 A large cervical/branchial cyst located in the left anterior triangle of the neck on the anterior border of sternocleidomastoid. The cyst formed from tissue remnants within the region of the embryological cervical/branchial sinus (Fig. 22.14)

Pharyngeal pouches

The pharyngeal pouches are the internally located indentations between each pharyngeal arch. The endoderm lining the four paired pharyngeal pouches contributes to the formation of key head and neck structures (Table 22.1). Once formed, certain pouch-derived tissues migrate to their final position; for example,

the thymus and inferior parathyroid glands migrate inferiorly. The inferior parathyroid glands may therefore become situated in ectopic locations anywhere along a route from the bifurcation of the common carotid artery to the superior or anterior mediastinum, including within the thymus and alongside the trachea or oesophagus (Figs. 22.17 and 22.18), a knowledge of which is important during surgical localization. Accessory thymic tissue may also be located long the latter route. The parathyroid gland derived from the third pharyngeal pouch becomes more inferior than the parathyroid gland derived from the fourth pouch as it descends with the thymus. The superior and inferior parathyroid glands usually become associated with

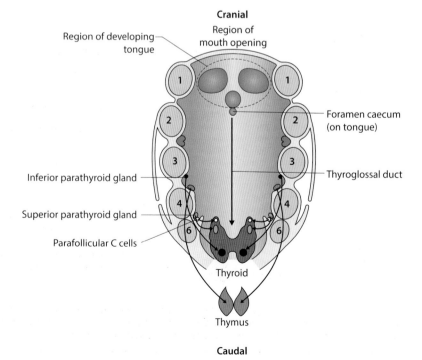

Figure 22.17 Origin and the caudal migration of the thymus, parathyroid glands and thyroid gland. The developing pharyngeal arches are viewed as if cut from the embryo (along line A-B Fig 22.13) and viewed from posteriorly. Accessory/ectopic thyroid gland and thymic tissue can sit anywhere along the original route of descent of each gland/organ (shown by arrows). Ectopic inferior parathyroid gland tissue can be located alongside or within the thyroid or thymus glands, in the superior mediastinum or close to the carotid arteries in the neck

the posterior aspect of the thyroid gland (Fig. 22.7b), where they are at risk of removal in total thyroidectomy.

Thyroid gland

The thyroid gland initially develops as an outgrowth from the pharyngeal floor (the thyroid primordium) in the region of the developing tongue, the original position of which is marked by the foramen caecum of the developed tongue (Figs. 22.17–22.19). The thyroid gland descends the neck and passes anterior to the developing hyoid to reach its final position around the trachea and larynx, where it develops its bilobar shape. Incomplete descent of the thyroid can result in it sitting in a more superior position in the neck, e.g. sublingually. During its descent the thyroid maintains a connection to the tongue via the hollow midline thyroglossal duct. The thyroglossal duct normally disappears, but its persistence can lead to the formation of thyroglossal cysts or sinuses anywhere along its route, infrahyoid cysts being most common (Fig. 22.19). The thyroglossal duct normally connects to the hyoid bone so the surgical excision of thyroglossal cysts or sinuses may also require removal of the midline hyoid. The pyramidal lobe of the thyroid often develops in the distal part of the thyroglossal duct and therefore extends superiorly along the midline of the larynx, from the thyroid isthmus towards the hyoid. Ectopic thyroid gland tissue can be located in several positions relative to the tongue, either on its oral surface, within its muscle mass (lingual thyroid) or in a sublingual location in the upper anterior neck.

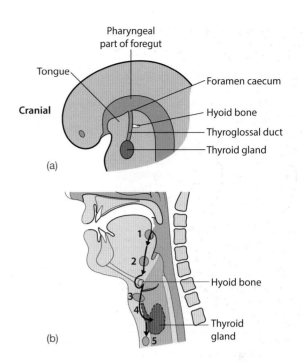

Figure 22.19 Position of the thyroglossal duct and the route of descent of the thyroid gland (midline sagittal view). (a) The position and connections of thyroglossal duct in the tongue and neck. (b) Ectopic thyroid gland tissue or thyroglossal duct cysts can appear anywhere along the original course of the thyroglossal duct. Note the connection of the thyroglossal duct to the midline of the hyoid bone. 1, ectopic lingual thyroid; 2, suprahyoid/lingual thyroglossal duct cyst; 3, infrahyoid thyroglossal duct cyst; 4, pyramidal lobe of thyroid; 5, superior mediastinal thyroid gland

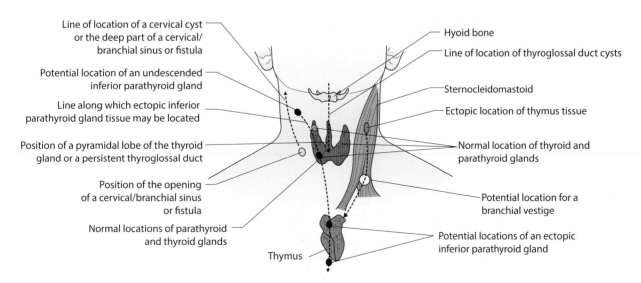

Figure 22.18 Routes of migration of the thymus, parathyroid glands and thyroid gland, and the potential locations of ectopic/accessory tissues, cysts, sinuses, fistulae and branchial vestiges in the neck and mediastinum (anterior view). Black oval, inferior parathyroid gland; green oval, superior parathyroid gland; blue, thymus; red, thyroid; yellow, branchial sinus/fistula opening

MCQs

1. The thyroid gland: **T/F**

a is limited superiorly by the attachment of   (___)
   the sternohyoid muscle
b has the recurrent laryngeal nerve ascending   (___)
   medial to the lateral lobes
c possesses an isthmus that lies on the fifth   (___)
   and sixth tracheal rings
d is enclosed by the pretracheal fascia   (___)
e receives a blood supply from the middle   (___)
   thyroid artery

Answers

1.

a **F** – *The thyroid's upper limit is the oblique line on the thyroid cartilage, to which the sternothyroid muscle is attached.*

b **T** – *The nerve is an important relation to note in thyroidectomy as it lies close by the inferior thyroid vessels.*

c **F** – *The isthmus lies on the second and third thyroid rings.*

d **T**

e **F** – *There is no middle thyroid artery; the gland is supplied by the superior and inferior thyroid arteries.*

2. Fascial planes in the neck are of   **T/F**
   considerable surgical importance. Features
   of the neck fasciae include the:

a superficial fascia contains platysma,   (___)
   external and anterior jugular veins
b pretracheal fascia extends as far as the   (___)
   fibrous pericardium
c prevertebral fascia extends from the base of   (___)
   the skull to the axilla
d investing layer of deep cervical fascia lies   (___)
   deep to the parotid gland
e sympathetic chain lies between the carotid   (___)
   sheath and the investing layer of deep
   cervical fascia

Answers

2.

a **T** – *The superficial fascia contains the veins and the decussating fibres of platysma.*

b **T** – *The pretracheal fascia extends from the cricoid and thyroid cartilages down to the pericardium. It binds the thyroid gland to the larynx.*

c **T** – *The prevertebral fascia lies posterior to the oesophagus, covering the vertebrae and prevertebral muscles from the base of the skull down to the posterior mediastinum. Laterally it also covers the scalene muscles, and where the brachial plexus and subclavian artery leave the neck, the axillary sheath is formed.*

d **F** – *The investing layer of deep cervical fascia lies like a polo neck collar extending from the mandible, zygomatic arch, mastoid process and superior nuchal line above to the manubrium, clavicle, acromion and scapular spine below. It splits to encase the parotid gland, and this explains the pain that acute enlargement of the parotid causes, especially in mumps infections.*

e **F** – *The sympathetic chain lies posterior to the carotid sheath but anterior to, or embedded within, the prevertebral fascia.*

SBA

1. A 3-year-old child is brought to clinic. His mother says that his neck 'has been twisted' since birth. When questioned she says that the birth was a prolonged and difficult one. Examination reveals that the child has a posture with a continuously tilted head; the right ear is pulled downwards towards the right shoulder with his face turned upwards and to the left. Which of the following muscular structures is most likely to have been damaged during birth?

a scalenus anterior
b sternocleidomastoid
c omohyoid
d trapezius
e platysma

Answer

b *The sternocleidomastoid muscle is occasionally injured during a prolonged birth with a cephalic presentation; this was especially seen when forceps were more commonly used in delivery. It is likely that during this child's difficult birth the right sternocleidomastoid was stretched and some fibres were torn, resulting in scarring and subsequent shortening of the muscle.*

2. A patient was admitted with a severe head injury. Recovery over the following 3 weeks was slow and it was decided that a tracheostomy should be performed. At which level of the tracheal cartilages is it desirable to create the tracheostomy?

a first and second
b second and third
c third and fourth
d fourth and fifth
e fifth and sixth

Answer

c *Fewer complications attend this procedure if it is carried out at the level of the third and fourth tracheal cartilages. Here the trachea is wider and the lower border of the isthmus of the thyroid gland, which usually lies at the level of the second cartilage, is not obstructing the surgical field.*

EMQs

Each question has an anatomical theme linked to the chapter, and a list of 10 related items (A–J) placed in alphabetical order: these are followed by five statements (1–5). Match **one or more** of the items A–J to each of the five statements.

Muscles of the neck
A. Levator scapulae
B. Mylohyoid
C. Omohyoid
D. Posterior belly of digastric
E. Scalenus anterior
F. Scalenus medius
G. Sternocleidomastoid
H. Sternohyoid
I. Sternothyroid
J. Trapezius

Answers
1 E; 2 GJ; 3 B; 4 B; 5 BCDH

Match the following statements with the muscles in the above list.
1. Crossed by the phrenic nerve
2. Supplied by the accessory nerve
3. Supplied by the trigeminal nerve
4. Lies deep to the submandibular gland
5. Attached to the hyoid bone

APPLIED QUESTIONS

1. Why does the thyroid gland move on swallowing?

1. Part of the pretracheal fascia forms the sheath of the thyroid gland and can be seen lying between the two sternohyoid muscles when the investing layer of deep cervical fascia has been incised. Superiorly, it is attached to the oblique line of the thyroid cartilage and the arch of the cricoid. Having enclosed the gland, it passes inferiorly to enclose the inferior thyroid veins and then blend with the posterior surface of the pericardium at the bifurcation of the trachea. Thus, when the laryngeal skeleton ascends during swallowing, so must the thyroid gland and any swelling within it.

2. What are the contents and surface markings of the carotid sheath?

2. The carotid sheath is a fascial tube surrounding the common and internal carotid arteries and internal jugular vein. Lying within it posteriorly is the vagus nerve. The sheath is in close connection with the prevertebral fascia, with the sympathetic chain intervening. The surface markings are a thick band some 1.5–2 cm wide from the sternoclavicular joint to the tragus of the ear. The division of the common carotid lies at the upper border of the thyroid cartilage at about C4 vertebral level.

ARTERIES OF THE NECK

The subclavian artery

The right subclavian artery (**Figs. 23.1** and **22.6**, p. 375) arises from the brachiocephalic artery behind the sterno-clavicular joint, passes laterally behind scalenus anterior and arches over the apex of the lung and the 1st rib to become the axillary artery at the lateral border of the rib. The left artery arises from the arch of the aorta, arches over the lung and enters the arm as its continuation, the axillary artery.

Relations

Right side – medial to scalenus anterior it lies behind the right common carotid artery, vagus nerve and internal jugular vein and anterior to the pleura and lung. The right recurrent laryn-geal nerve hooks behind it. Laterally the artery lies on the 1st rib, behind its vein. The lower trunk of the brachial plexus and scalenus medius lie behind its lateral part.

Left side – in the thorax the artery lies behind the left common carotid artery, left vagus and left phrenic nerves. The oesophagus, trachea and left recurrent laryngeal nerve lie medial and the left pleura and the lung lateral. In the root of the neck the relations are similar to those of the right side, except that the left recurrent laryngeal nerve does not hook round it and the thoracic duct and phrenic nerve cross ante-rior to it (**Figs. 3.6a**, p. 57, and **22.6**, p. 375).

Branches

The vertebral and internal thoracic arteries and thyrocervical trunk arise in the root of the neck medial to scalenus anterior, and the costocervical trunk arises behind scalenus anterior.

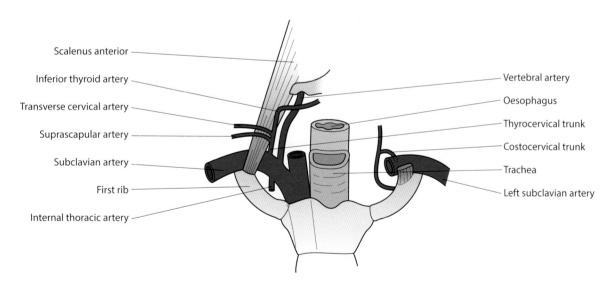

Scalenus anterior

Inferior thyroid artery

Transverse cervical artery

Suprascapular artery

Subclavian artery

First rib

Internal thoracic artery

Vertebral artery

Oesophagus

Thyrocervical trunk

Costocervical trunk

Trachea

Left subclavian artery

Figure 23.1 Root of the neck with the clavicle removed showing the subclavian artery and its branches

- **Vertebral artery** – ascends medially to the transverse process of the 7th cervical vertebra and continues its ascent through the foramina transversaria of the upper six cervical vertebrae (**Figs. 23.2b–c**). It turns medially behind the lateral mass of the atlas (**Fig. 22.5**, p. 374) and, piercing the dura, enters the skull via the foramen magnum. It unites with its fellow in front of the brainstem to form the basilar artery. The artery is surrounded by a sympathetic plexus derived from the inferior cervical ganglion. Within the vertebral foramina it is accompanied by the vertebral vein. In the neck it supplies the spinal cord and vertebral muscles; in the posterior cranial fossa it supplies the upper spinal cord and hindbrain, and sends an important contribution to the circle of Willis (p. 434 and **Fig. 25.7**).
- **Internal thoracic artery** – descends behind the costal cartilages 1 cm lateral to the sternal border to supply anterior intercostal arteries to each intercostal space.

It is often used by cardiac surgeons for coronary artery bypass grafting (CABG).

- **Thyrocervical trunk** – a short vessel that divides to form the inferior thyroid, transverse cervical and suprascapular arteries (**Fig. 23.1**). The tortuous **inferior thyroid artery** ascends medially behind the common carotid artery and sympathetic trunk to gain the lower pole of the thyroid gland. It supplies the thyroid gland, oesophagus, trachea, pharynx and larynx. The **transverse cervical** and **suprascapular arteries** pass laterally over the scalene muscles to join the anastomosis around the shoulder joint and supply the muscles of the shoulder girdle.
- **Costocervical trunk** – passes back over the dome of the pleura to reach the neck of the 1st rib, where it divides into deep cervical and upper two intercostal arteries.

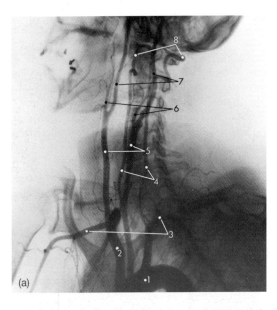

(a)

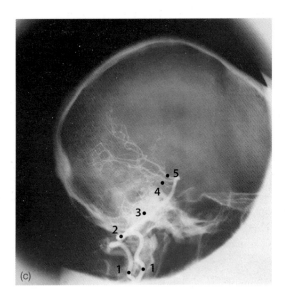

(c)

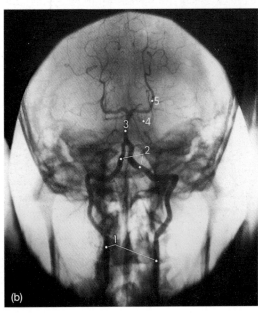

(b)

Figure 23.2 (a) Aortogram showing the subclavian and carotid vessels: 1, aortic arch; 2, brachiocephalic artery; 3, subclavian artery; 4, vertebral artery; 5, common carotid artery; 6, external carotid artery; 7, internal carotid artery; 8, vertebral artery winding around atlas. (b) Vertebral angiogram, anteroposterior view. The contrast material has been introduced into a vertebral artery. The contralateral artery is also demonstrated since the material is introduced under pressure and some passes retrogradely down to the other side: 1, vertebral arteries in transverse foramina; 2, vertebral arteries on basiocciput; 3, basilar artery; 4, superior cerebellar artery; 5, posterior cerebral artery. (c) Vertebral angiogram, lateral view: 1, vertebral artery; 2, looping of artery around transverse process of atlas; 3, basilar artery; 4, superior cerebellar artery; 5, posterior cerebral artery

The common carotid artery

On the **right** side the artery arises, behind the sternoclavicular joint, from the brachiocephalic artery (**Figs. 23.3** and **22.6a**, p. 375). It ascends the neck and divides into internal and external carotid arteries at the upper border of the thyroid cartilage. The artery gives no branches before its bifurcation. On the **left** the artery arises from the aortic arch, ascending the superior mediastinum and neck to bifurcate at the same level. The **carotid sinus**, a dilatation of the upper end of the artery, contains receptors and is sensitive to blood pressure changes. It contains, on its posterior wall, the **carotid body**, a small neurovascular structure that functions as a chemoreceptor. Both structures are richly innervated by the glossopharyngeal nerve.

In the neck (**Fig. 22.11a**, p. 378) both arteries lie within the carotid sheath, with the vagus nerve posterior and the internal jugular vein lateral. The sheath is covered anterolaterally by the infrahyoid and sternocleidomastoid muscles; posteriorly it lies on the prevertebral muscles and sympathetic trunk. To its medial side are the trachea and oesophagus and, in the groove between them, the recurrent laryngeal nerve (**Fig. 22.6a**, p. 375). Higher in the neck the larynx, pharynx and thyroid gland lie medial to the artery.

In the thorax the left artery lies anterior to the vagus and phrenic nerves and the left subclavian artery. Medially are the trachea and brachiocephalic artery and anterolaterally the left pleura and lungs.

The **carotid pulse** must be checked during cardiopulmonary resuscitation. It is found deep to the anterior border of the sternomastoid at the level of the upper border of the thyroid cartilage. The surface marking of the common carotid is along a line joining the sternoclavicular joint and the upper border of the thyroid cartilage. The carotid bifurcation is a common site of **degenerative arterial disease**; thrombosis or embolism may occur in this region. The turbulent blood flow thus produced may be detected with a stethoscope as audible abnormal carotid sounds (bruits). Reduced blood flow may have serious effects on cerebral function. The atherosclerotic plaque (**Fig. 23.4a**) deposited in these vessels may be removed surgically (carotid endarterectomy) to reduce the risk of a cerebrovascular accident.

The **carotid sinus** responds to raised arterial pressure by increasing the parasympathetic outflow of the vagus nerve and thereby slowing the heart rate. Pressure on the sinus may, in responsive individuals, cause fainting as a result of slowing of the heart rate and a reduction in blood pressure.

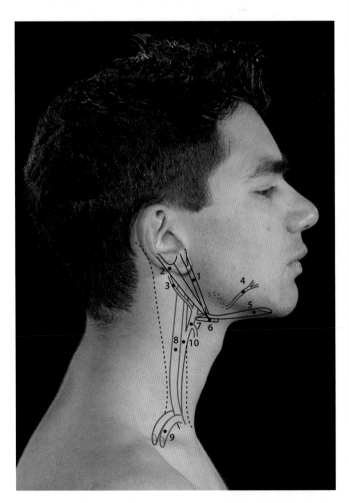

Figure 23.3 Surface anatomy of the lateral neck: 1, stylohyoid; 2, digastric – posterior belly; 3, occipital artery; 4, facial artery; 5, digastric – anterior belly; 6, hyoid bone; 7, external carotid artery; 8, internal jugular vein; 9, subclavian vein; 10, common carotid artery

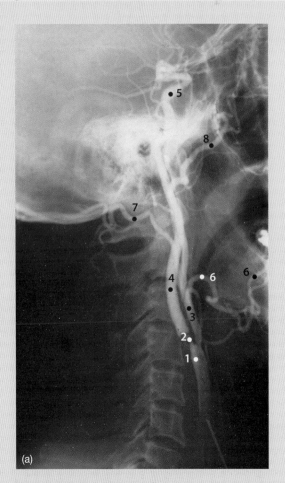

Figure 23.4 (a) Carotid angiogram showing stenosis of the carotid artery: 1, common carotid artery; 2, stenosis at origin of internal carotid artery; 3, external carotid artery; 4, internal carotid artery in neck; 5, internal carotid artery within cavernous sinus; 6, facial artery; 7, occipital artery; 8, maxillary artery. (*continued*)

This knowledge can be of benefit to some patients who have infrequent supraventricular tachycardia, as a gentle carotid massage may return their pulse to normal.

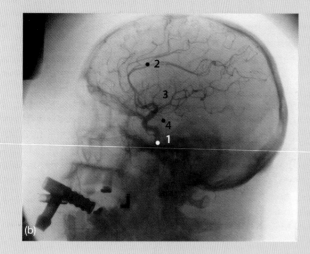

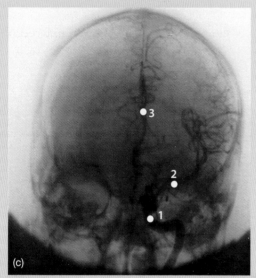

Figure 23.4 (*continued*) (b) Left carotid angiogram, lateral view, arterial phase – contrast material has been introduced into the common carotid artery in the neck; part of the anaesthetic tube can be seen in the lower left corner: 1, internal carotid artery; 2, anterior cerebral artery; 3, middle cerebral artery; 4, posterior communicating artery. (c) Left carotid angiogram, anteroposterior view – contrast material has been introduced into the common carotid artery in the neck: 1, internal carotid artery; 2, middle cerebral artery; 3, anterior cerebral artery

The external carotid artery

This supplies most structures in the upper neck and the face (Figs. 21.17, p. 366 and 19.25b, p. 327). It arises from the carotid bifurcation at the upper border of the thyroid cartilage and ascends, anterior to the internal carotid, to enter the parotid gland, where it ends at the level of the neck of the mandible by dividing into the maxillary and superficial temporal arteries.

Relations

In the neck it lies on the lateral wall of the pharynx, at first anteromedial and then lateral to the internal carotid artery. It begins deep to sternocleidomastoid but, as it ascends anterior to the muscle, it is crossed by the lingual and facial veins, the hypoglossal nerve, stylohyoid and the posterior belly of digastric. In the parotid gland the artery lies deep to the retromandibular vein and the facial nerve.

Branches

These are widely distributed:

- The **superior thyroid artery** (Fig. 22.7, p. 376) descends with the external laryngeal nerve to the upper pole of the thyroid gland; its superior laryngeal branch pierces the thyrohyoid membrane and supplies the larynx.
- The **ascending pharyngeal artery** ascends on the lateral wall of the pharynx, supplying it and the tonsil and soft palate.
- The **lingual artery** (Fig. 19.25, p. 326) arises at the level of the hyoid and passes forwards deep to hyoglossus into the tongue. It initially lies on middle constrictor and, deep to hyoglossus, is crossed by the hypoglossal nerve. It supplies the suprahyoid muscles, tonsil, soft palate, submandibular and lingual salivary glands and tongue.
- The **facial artery** (Fig. 19.25, p. 326) arises close to the lingual artery and arches over the submandibular gland to loop around the inferior border of the mandible just below the anterior border of masseter muscle, where it can easily be palpated. Its origin lies on the middle and superior constrictor muscles; lateral to the submandibular gland it lies medial to the mandible. It then ascends across the face, sending branches to the lips and nose, to reach the medial angle of the eye. It supplies the tonsil, soft palate and submandibular gland, and the lower and middle thirds of the face.

The **occipital artery** arises level with the facial artery and passes back below the posterior belly of digastric. Medial to the mastoid process it ascends over the back of the skull to reach the vertex. The greater occipital nerve lies medial to it. It supplies the posterior neck and scalp.

The **posterior auricular artery** passes back with the posterior belly of digastric to gain the lateral scalp and auricle, which it supplies.

The **superficial temporal artery**, a terminal branch of the external carotid, is formed behind the neck of the mandible within the parotid gland. It emerges and ascends over the posterior zygomatic arch just in front of the cartilaginous tragus to gain the skin of lateral scalp. It supplies the auricle, scalp and, by its transverse facial branch, the face.

This artery is often used by anaesthetists to feel the pulse in an unconscious patient who is well covered by drapes during a surgical procedure. In elderly individuals it occasionally becomes inflamed and tender (temporal arteritis); this can be treated with steroids.

The **maxillary artery** (Fig. 20.4, p. 341), the other terminal branch of the external carotid, arises in the parotid behind the neck of the mandible and passes forwards through the infratemporal fossa and pterygomaxillary fissure to enter the pterygopalatine fossa, where it divides into terminal branches. These accompany the branches of the pterygopalatine ganglion and supply the nose, palate and pharynx. The infraorbital branch supplies branches to the upper teeth; other branches supply the muscles of mastication. The **middle meningeal artery** ascends via the foramen spinosum to the middle cranial fossa, where it divides into anterior and posterior branches, the anterior passing medial to the pterion (p. 305). The artery supplies the dura and bone of the middle cranial fossa and the skull vault.

The middle meningeal artery may be damaged in lateral skull fractures, and intracranial bleeding then results in an extradural haemorrhage and clot formation. This may produce a rapid life-threatening rise in intracranial pressure. Surgical access to the vessel can be gained by drilling through the bone (a burr hole) at the pterion, about 3.5 cm behind and 1.5 cm above the zygomaticofrontal suture.

The **inferior alveolar artery** enters the mandibular canal, from where it supplies the gums and teeth of the lower jaw.

Haemorrhage from this artery after a lower molar tooth extraction may cause distress and worry, especially if the patient has any abnormality of clotting or bleeding time.

The internal carotid artery

This has no branches in the neck, but supplies the greater part of the brain and the contents of the orbit via its ophthalmic branch. It arises from the common carotid at the upper border of the thyroid cartilage (Fig. 21.18, p. 367), ascends to the skull base and, passing through the carotid canal in the temporal bone, enters the middle cranial fossa. Here it passes forwards through the cavernous sinus, exits from its roof and turns back before dividing, by the anterior clinoid processes, into anterior and middle cerebral arteries (see p. 434 and Fig. 24.7).

Relations in the neck

It is surrounded by a sympathetic plexus derived from the superior cervical ganglion. In the neck the artery lies within the carotid sheath, medial to the internal jugular vein, anterior to the vagus nerve, lateral to the pharynx and anterior to the prevertebral muscles. The external carotid artery is, at first, anteromedial and, later, lateral to it, and is separated from it by styloglossus and stylopharyngeus muscles and the glossopharyngeal nerve (Fig. 21.18, p. 367). In the temporal bone the artery lies below the floor of the middle ear, and on entering the middle cranial fossa it passes over and across the foramen lacerum. Within the cavernous sinus it is crossed, on its lateral side, by the abducent nerve. The oculomotor, trochlear, ophthalmic and maxillary nerves lie in the lateral wall of the sinus. The internal carotid artery leaves by the roof of the sinus lateral to the optic chiasma and nerve. It gives branches to the pituitary gland and the meninges, ophthalmic and posterior communicating arteries and its terminal branches and the anterior and middle cerebral arteries (Fig. 23.4).

VEINS OF THE FACE AND SCALP

The **facial vein** is formed at the medial angle of the eye by the union of the supraorbital and supratrochlear veins. It descends obliquely in the superficial fascia to be joined by the anterior branch of the retromandibular vein below the mandible. It drains the anterior scalp and superficial tissues of the face. It communicates with the cavernous sinus by the ophthalmic veins and with the pterygoid venous plexus by the deep facial vein and also with the diploic veins.

The **pterygoid venous plexus** lies around the lateral pterygoid muscle, drains the infratemporal region and communicates with the cavernous sinus by the ophthalmic veins. It drains to the retromandibular vein.

The **retromandibular vein** is formed behind the neck of the mandible by the union of the superficial temporal and maxillary veins. It descends through the parotid gland lateral to the external carotid artery and medial to the facial nerve. Below the gland it divides into anterior and posterior divisions, the anterior joining the facial vein and the posterior joining the posterior auricular vein to form the external jugular vein.

The veins of the back of the scalp drain into the suboccipital venous plexus and thence into the vertebral veins, which are tributaries of the brachiocephalic veins.

VEINS OF THE NECK

The **subclavian vein** (Fig. 22.6a, p. 375) is a continuation of the axillary vein. It commences at the outer border of the 1st rib and ends at the medial border of scalenus anterior, where it joins the internal jugular vein to form the brachiocephalic vein. Its main tributary is the often-visible external jugular vein. Lateral to scalenus anterior the vein lies anterior and inferior to its artery; passing the front of the muscle it crosses the phrenic nerve to end behind the clavicle.

Internal jugular vein

The internal jugular vein drains the intracranial region, the head and the neck (Figs. 23.6 and 22.4a, p. 373). It begins in the jugular foramen in the skull base as a continuation of the sigmoid venous sinus (p. 436), and descends in the neck to behind the medial end of the clavicle. There it is joined by the subclavian vein to form the brachiocephalic vein.

Relations

The internal jugular vein lies within the carotid sheath, the vagus nerve behind it and the internal or common carotid medial to it (Fig. 22.11a, p. 378). Deep cervical lymph nodes surround it. In the skull base it is lateral to the last four cranial nerves. In the neck it lies anterior to the sympathetic chain, the prevertebral muscles, the phrenic nerve and, inferiorly, the subclavian artery. It is crossed anteriorly by the accessory nerve, the posterior belly of digastric and the omohyoid muscle. Further laterally, from above downwards, are the styloid process and its muscles, the sternocleidomastoid muscle and the medial end of the clavicle.

Tributaries

Remember that all these venous channels are very variable. Tributaries are:

- Branches of the **pharyngeal plexus** of veins

- **Facial vein** – which enters the internal jugular vein opposite the hyoid bone
- **Lingual vein**
- **Superior and middle thyroid veins**
- In addition, the **thoracic duct** may enter the left vein and the much smaller **right lymphatic duct** the right vein.

Right ventricular contractions cause pulsations in the internal jugular vein because there are no valves in the veins between it and the heart. With the patient sitting at a 45 degree angle these may be visible at the level of the sternal notch. In mitral valve stenosis, which results in increased pressure in the right ventricle, the pulsations are higher in the neck and more visible. The external jugular vein will, when the venous pressure is raised, become prominent.

Internal jugular vein catheterization is performed to obtain accurate venous pressure readings in a critically ill patient. The vein is gained by needle puncture, either directly through the sternocleidomastoid halfway down the neck or through the gap between the two heads of the muscle just above the sternoclavicular joint. It does not really matter which of the central veins is cannulated, as all are fast-flowing and valveless. The origin of the left brachiocephalic and the lowest portion of the left internal jugular vein are, however, used only as a last resort, as the thoracic duct is in danger during cannulation.

Subclavian vein catheterization is a favoured method of placing a 'central line' to administer drugs or intravenous nutrition or to measure central venous pressure. The right vein is preferred and is entered just below the middle of the clavicle with a needle aimed at a point just behind the suprasternal notch (Fig. 23.5).

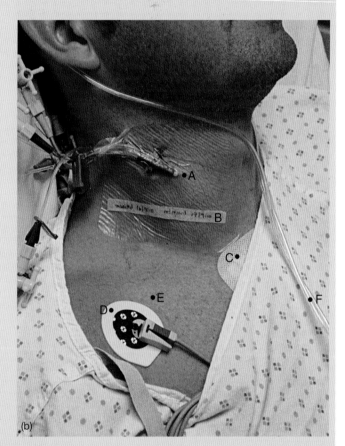

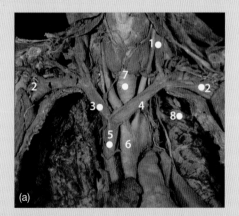

Figure 23.5 (a) Dissection of the neck veins: 1, internal jugular vein; 2, subclavian vein; 3, right brachiocephalic vein; 4, left brachiocephalic vein; 5, superior vena cava; 6, aorta; 7, trachea; 8, lung. (b) Postoperative patient with an internal jugular venous line. A, Line inserted into the right internal jugular vein. On insertion the point of the needle is directed at the V between the sternal and clavicular heads of the sternocleidomastoid muscle and passed backwards into the vessel. B, Date of insertion and when the line is to be removed or replaced. C, Dressing over the midline sternotomy incision. D, ECG electrode. E, Point of entry for a right subclavian line; the needle is directed at the back of the sternoclavicular joint. F, Tube delivering nasal oxygen

External jugular vein

The external jugular vein (Fig. 23.6) is formed behind the angle of the mandible by the union of the posterior auricular vein and the posterior branch of the retromandibular vein. It descends over sternocleidomastoid muscle and pierces the cervical fascia, above the midclavicle, to enter the subclavian vein.

Anterior jugular vein

The anterior jugular vein begins below the hyoid near to the midline and descends laterally deep to sternocleidomastoid to enter the external jugular behind the clavicle. The **jugular arch** unites the two anterior veins just above the sternum.

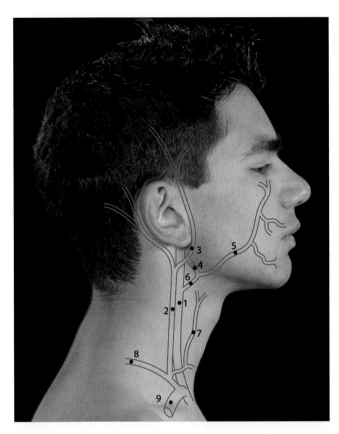

Figure 23.6 Surface anatomy of the neck veins: 1, internal jugular vein; 2, external jugular vein; 3, superficial temporal vein; 4, retromandibular vein, anterior branch; 5, facial vein; 6, retromandibular vein, posterior branch; 7, anterior jugular vein; 8, posterior branch of external jugular vein; 9, subclavian vein

LYMPHATIC DRAINAGE OF THE HEAD AND NECK

The lymph nodes of the head and neck are divided into two groups: a circular chain of nodes around the base of the skull, and the deep and superficial cervical chains accompanying the large veins of the neck (Fig. 23.7).

The **circular chain** consists of seven groups of nodes lying along the upper attachment of the deep cervical 'polo neck' fascia. All are palpable when enlarged.

- **Occipital** – around the occipital artery; drain the posterior scalp and adjacent neck.
- **Posterior auricular** – on the mastoid process; drain the external acoustic meatus, the posterior auricle and the adjacent scalp.
- **Superficial parotid** – in front of the tragus; drain the external meatus, the front of the auricle and the adjacent scalp.
- **Deep parotid** – within the parotid gland; drain the anterior scalp, infratemporal region, orbit, lateral eyelids, upper molar teeth, external acoustic meatus and parotid gland.
- **Retropharyngeal** – between the pharynx and the upper cervical vertebrae; drain the upper pharynx and adjacent structures.
- **Submandibular** – between the mandible and submandibular gland; drain the anterior nasal cavities, tongue, teeth and gums, submandibular and sublingual glands, and all the face apart from the lateral eyelids and the medial part of the lower lip and chin.
- **Submental** – behind the chin on mylohyoid; drain the tip of the tongue, the floor of the mouth and the lower lip and chin.

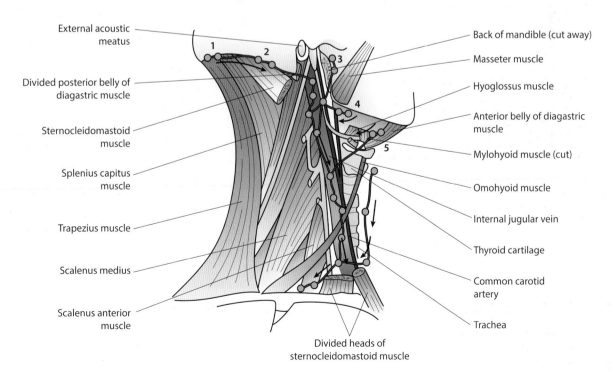

Figure 23.7 Lymphatic drainage of the head and neck. Structures from the head drain to a circle of nodes around the skull base: 1, occipital; 2, posterior auricular; 3, parotid; 4, submandibular; 5, submental. These nodes then drain along the deep cervical chain (internal jugular vein) or superficial chain (anterior jugular vein [shown] and external jugular vein [not shown])

Efferent vessels pass from all these groups to the deep cervical lymph chain, except for the superficial parotid group, which drains to the superficial cervical chain of nodes.

The **deep cervical chain** lies around the internal jugular vein. The lower part of the chain extends laterally above the clavicle. Named nodes in the chain are the:

- **Jugulodigastric** – behind the mandible; drains the tonsil and lateral part of the tongue.
- **Jugulo-omohyoid** – between the internal jugular vein and the superior belly of omohyoid; drains the tongue via the submental and submandibular nodes.
- **Para- and pretracheal** – lie along the inferior thyroid vessels; drain the trachea and thyroid gland. Efferent vessels may pass to mediastinal tracheobronchial nodes.

The **deep cervical chain** drains most of the circular chain of nodes and receives direct efferents from the salivary and thyroid glands, tongue, tonsil, nose, pharynx and larynx. The efferents from the deep cervical chain form the jugular lymph trunk, which, on the left, joins the thoracic duct and, on the right, joins the right lymph duct (p. 71) or, occasionally, opens separately into the internal jugular or subclavian veins.

The **superficial cervical chains** lie along the external and anterior jugular veins. The former drains the superficial parotid nodes and those of the side of the neck and drains itself into the subclavian lymph trunk; the latter accepts drainage from the superficial tissues in the front of the neck and drains to the external jugular chain or the deep cervical chain.

Enlargement of the lymph nodes may follow any infection in the head and neck. The most common nodes to enlarge are the jugulodigastric nodes of the deep cervical chain as a result of nasopharyngeal or tonsillar infections. Cancers of structures around the mouth, larynx and pharynx often produce cervical lymph node enlargement as a result of metastatic spread (Fig. 23.8).

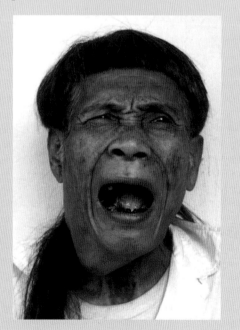

Figure 23.8 Enlarged submandibular nodes due to oral carcinoma caused by betel nut chewing, evidenced here by the red or blackened teeth

NERVES

Cervical plexus

The **cervical plexus** (Fig. 21.18, p. 367) is formed from the ventral rami of the upper four cervical nerves. It lies on scalenus medius and is covered anteriorly by scalenus anterior, prevertebral fascia and the internal jugular vein.

- **Cutaneous branches** – these supply the front and sides of the neck together with parts of the scalp, face and upper chest (Fig. 23.9).
- **Lesser occipital nerve** (C2) – supplies skin over the posterior auricle and the mastoid region.
- **Great auricular nerve** (C2, C3) – supplies skin over the lower auricle and the parotid region of the face.
- **Transverse cervical nerve** (C2, C3) – supplies skin over the anterior and lateral regions of the neck.

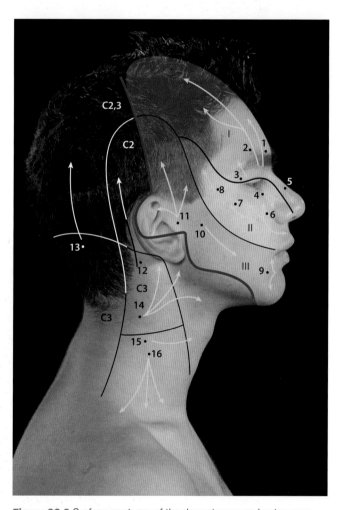

Figure 23.9 Surface anatomy of the dermatomes and cutaneous nerves of the head and neck (the red line divides the cervical plexus from the trigeminal innervation): 1, supratrochlear; 2, supraorbital; 3, lacrimal; 4, infratrochlear; 5, external nasal; 6, infraorbital; 7, zygomaticofacial; 8, zygomaticotemporal; 9, mental; 10, buccal; 11, auriculotemporal; 12, lesser occipital; 13, greater occipital; 14, great auricular; 15, transverse cervical; 16, supraclavicular. Trigeminal nerve divisions: I, ophthalmic; II, maxillary; III, mandibular (see p. 372 for more details)

- **Supraclavicular nerves** (C3, C4) – supply skin above and below the clavicle (**Fig. 23.10**).
- **Communications** with the hypoglossal nerve – fibres from C1 are carried by the hypoglossal nerve to geniohyoid and thyrohyoid, and also contribute to the upper loop of the **ansa cervicalis**, which supplies the infrahyoid muscles.
- **Muscle branches** – to the prevertebral muscles, sternocleidomastoid, trapezius and levator scapulae.
- **Dorsal rami** of the cervical nerves – supply each side of the midline posteriorly. The largest nerve, the **greater occipital** (C2), supplies much of the back of the scalp.

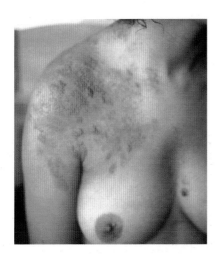

Figure 23.10 This painful case of herpes zoster (shingles) involves the C2, C3 and C4 nerves – note that the C4 nerve covers the anterior chest with blisters, but ends quite sharply as the lower part of the chest wall is innervated by the T1 and T2 spinal nerves

- **Phrenic nerve** (C3, C4, C5) – descends through the neck and thorax to supply a motor function to the diaphragm, and a sensory supply to the pleura, pericardium and peritoneum. The nerve winds around the lateral border of scalenus anterior and passes down its anterior surface. It is here covered by prevertebral fascia and crossed by the internal jugular vein, transverse cervical and suprascapular arteries, and subclavian vein.

Relations in the thorax

The phrenic nerve's cervical origins explain why pain originating in the parietal pleura, pericardium or the peritoneum underlying the diaphragm is often referred to the shoulder region (p. 57). The clinical causes are many, but a ruptured abdominal viscus or intraperitoneal blood that irritates the peritoneum, from, for example, a burst appendicitis or ectopic pregnancy, may present as shoulder tip pain.

THE AUTONOMIC SYSTEM

Sympathetic nervous system in the neck

The cervical sympathetic trunks lie on the prevertebral fascia and muscles deep to the carotid sheath. Each trunk has three ganglia and is continuous below with the ganglionated thoracic trunk (Fig. 23.11). Preganglionic fibres arise mainly in the first thoracic segment; postganglionic fibres are distributed as visceral, spinal and vascular branches.

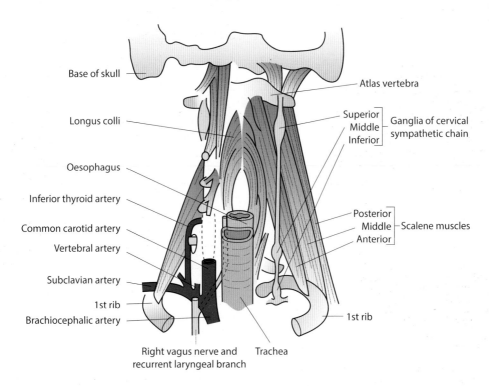

Base of skull

Longus colli

Oesophagus

Inferior thyroid artery

Common carotid artery

Vertebral artery

Subclavian artery

1st rib

Brachiocephalic artery

Right vagus nerve and recurrent laryngeal branch

Trachea

Atlas vertebra

Superior
Middle   Ganglia of cervical
Inferior   sympathetic chain

Posterior
Middle   Scalene muscles
Anterior

1st rib

Figure 23.11 Cervical sympathetic ganglia

The **superior cervical ganglion** (Fig. 23.11) lies opposite the second and third cervical transverse processes behind the angle of the mandible. Its postganglionic fibres pass:

- With the branches of the external carotid artery
- With the internal carotid artery and its intracranial branches
- To the pharyngeal and cardiac plexuses
- To the upper four cervical nerves as grey rami communicantes.

The **middle cervical ganglion** is at the level of the 6th cervical vertebra and cricoid cartilage. Postganglionic fibres pass:

- With the inferior thyroid artery
- To the cardiac plexus, with a loop to the inferior ganglion – the ansa subclavii – that passes round the artery
- To the 5th and 6th cervical nerves as grey rami communicantes.

The **inferior cervical ganglion** lies opposite the 7th cervical vertebra. In half the population it combines with the first thoracic ganglion to form a stellate ganglion on the neck of the 1st rib. Postganglionic fibres pass:

- With the vertebral artery
- To the 7th and 8th cervical nerves as grey rami communicantes, to the cardiac plexus and a loop to the middle ganglion – the ansa subclavii.

Vascular insufficiency presenting as ischaemia of the fingertips may be benefited by a surgical sympathectomy (removal of the second and third thoracic ganglia). Great care is required for the procedure, as injury to the sympathetic trunk or ganglia in the neck or upper thorax may, if it affects the inferior cervical ganglion, cause **Horner's syndrome**: pupillary constriction as dilator pupillae is paralysed; partial drooping of the upper eyelid (ptosis) because the smooth muscle raising the upper eyelid is paralysed; flushing of the face, because of vasodilatation; and a lack of sweating of the facial skin because the secretomotor fibres are inactive.

Parasympathetic nervous system in the head and neck

Postganglionic fibres pass from the nuclei of the oculomotor, facial, glossopharyngeal and vagus nerves (cranial nerves III, VII, IX and X) and synapse either in four ganglia in the head – the ciliary, pterygopalatine, submandibular and otic – or in the walls of the organs they supply (Fig. 21.14, p. 363). The ganglia carry sympathetic and somatic fibres in addition to their parasympathetic content.

The **ciliary ganglion** is in the orbit posterolateral to the optic nerve. Parasympathetic fibres are derived from the oculomotor branch to the inferior oblique muscle. Postganglionic fibres pass to sphincter pupillae and ciliary muscles via the short ciliary nerves; sympathetic fibres from the superior cervical ganglion pass to the eyeball and sensory fibres from the eyeball are conveyed in the nasociliary nerve.

The **pterygopalatine ganglion** is in the eponymous fossa suspended from the maxillary nerve by small branches. Parasympathetic fibres arrive from the facial nerve in the middle ear via its greater petrosal branch. Postganglionic fibres supply the lacrimal gland and glands of the nose, palate and nasopharynx; sympathetic fibres are derived from the superior cervical ganglion via the internal carotid plexus and supply the nose, palate and nasopharynx. Sensory fibres from the nose, palate and nasopharynx are conveyed via the ganglion to the maxillary nerve.

Because of its distribution this ganglion is often referred to as the ganglion of 'hay fever', because its stimulation causes most of the features of the disease, namely watering eyes, running nose and itching palate and back of the mouth.

The **submandibular ganglion** lies lateral to hyoglossus, suspended from the lingual nerve. Parasympathetic fibres coming from the facial nerve in its chorda tympani branch 'hitch-hike' a ride to the ganglion with the lingual nerve; postganglionic fibres supply the submandibular and lingual salivary glands and other glands in the buccal mucosa. Sympathetic fibres are derived from the superior cervical ganglion and are conveyed by the facial nerve to glands in the floor of the mouth; taste fibres may pass through the ganglion.

The **otic ganglion** lies medial to the mandibular nerve on tensor veli palatini. Parasympathetic content is from the glossopharyngeal nerve via the tympanic plexus and the lesser petrosal nerve. Postganglionic fibres pass with the auriculotemporal nerve to the parotid gland; sympathetic fibres come from the superior cervical ganglion to the parotid gland.

Parasympathetic fibres directly from the glossopharyngeal nerve supply the oropharyngeal mucosal glands and glands of the posterior third of the tongue; similar fibres directly from the vagus supply the glands of the larynx, laryngopharynx, oesophagus and trachea.

MCQs

		T/F
1.	**The vertebral artery:**	
a	arises from the second part of the subclavian artery, from behind scalenus anterior	(___)
b	lies anterior to the inferior thyroid artery	(___)
c	passes through the foramen transversarium of C7	(___)
d	lies anterior to the lateral mass of the atlas	(___)
e	meets its opposite artery to form the basilar artery, on the clivus	(___)

Answers

1.

a **F** – *The vertebral artery is a branch of the first part of the subclavian artery.*

b **F** – *It lies posterior to the inferior thyroid artery.*

c **F** – *It normally passes through the C6 foramen transversarium, although its veins often pass through that of C7.*

d **F** – *It passes posterior to the mass of the atlas and then enters the foramen magnum to join its opposite number ...*

e **T** – *... and form the basilar artery on the anterior surface of the medulla, lying on the basiocciput/basisphenoid (clivus).*

		T/F
2.	**Parasympathetic postganglionic fibres are carried by the:**	
a	auriculotemporal nerve	(___)
b	long ciliary nerves	(___)
c	greater petrosal nerves	(___)
d	chorda tympani	(___)
e	deep petrosal nerve	(___)

Answers

2.

a **T** – *Parasympathetic fibres are carried in cranial nerves III, VII, IX and X and sacral nerves S2, S3 and S4. The preganglionic fibres are carried by the tympanic branch of the IXth cranial nerve via the tympanic plexus and the lesser petrosal nerve, through the foramen ovale to the otic ganglion. From there postganglionic fibres are carried by the auriculotemporal nerve to the parotid gland, where they are secretomotor.*

b **F** – *The long ciliary nerves are mixed sensory and sympathetic. They accompany the several short ciliary nerves that carry the parasympathetic postganglionic fibres from the ciliary ganglion to the ciliary muscle and sphincter pupillae.*

c **F** – *The greater petrosal nerve carries preganglionic parasympathetic fibres from the facial nerve to the pterygopalatine ganglion. Postganglionic fibres leave the ganglion via the zygomatic and palatine nerves to the lacrimal and palatine glands.*

d **F** – *The chorda tympani carries preganglionic fibres of the facial nerve, but these are destined for the submandibular ganglion and thereafter for the submandibular and sublingual glands.*

e **F** – *The deep petrosal nerve carries mainly sympathetic fibres from the superior cervical ganglion and internal carotid plexus. In the carotid canal the nerve joins with the greater superficial petrosal nerve to form the nerve of the pterygoid canal.*

SBA

1. A young woman was admitted with abdominal pain of 3 hours' duration. She had a distended abdomen, and peritoneal aspiration revealed a haemoperitoneum. She was also complaining of a persistent pain in her shoulders, which the physicians thought was likely to be referred pain. If that were the case, which nerve would be responsible?
a vagus
b intercostobrachial
c greater splanchnic
d suprascapular
e phrenic

Answer
e *A haemoperitoneum causes inflammation of the peritoneum, and in this sick young woman, who has been lying supine in pain for over an hour, it is likely that the extravasated blood has spread to, and inflamed, the subdiaphragmatic peritoneum. The phrenic nerve supplies sensory fibres to the mediastinal and diaphragmatic pleura, the pericardium and, relevant to this case, the peritoneum underlying the diaphragm.*

2. A middle-aged man presented with a cough and some dyspnoea. A chest X-ray showed a lung cancer in the apex of the left lung. Further examination revealed miosis (constriction of the pupil) of his left eye and a partial ptosis of the left eyelid. Dryness of the left side of his face was also noted. What structure may have caused these signs found during the further examination?
a phrenic nerve
b vagus nerve
c plexuses around the arch of the aorta
d cardiopulmonary plexus
e sympathetic chain

Answer
e *Miosis, partial ptosis and dryness of the skin (anhydrosis) constitute a group of symptoms known as Horner's syndrome. The pupil, eyelid and sweat glands are all under control of sympathetic nervous system cells whose cell bodies lie in the cervical sympathetic ganglia – in this patient these have been invaded by the cancer.*

EMQs

Each question has an anatomical theme linked to the chapter, and a list of 10 related items (A–J) placed in alphabetical order: these are followed by five statements (1–5). Match **one or more** of the items A–J to each of the five statements.

Vessels of the neck
A. Common carotid artery
B. External carotid artery
C. External jugular vein
D. Facial artery
E. Internal jugular vein
F. Left subclavian artery
G. Right subclavian vein
H. Superficial temporal artery
I. Superior laryngeal artery
J. Vertebral artery

Answers
1 AEG; 2 F; 3 E; 4 F; 5 B

Match the following statements with the vessel(s) in the above list.
1. Anterior relation of the scalenus anterior muscle
2. Posterior relation of the scalenus anterior muscle
3. Crossed anteriorly by the accessory nerve
4. Crossed anteriorly by the vagus nerve
5. Formed at the level of the upper border of the thyroid cartilage

APPLIED QUESTIONS

1. Why is it dangerous to point the needle posteriorly when performing central venous catheterization into the internal jugular, subclavian or brachiocephalic veins?

2. What is the stellate ganglion, and why might a cervical sympathectomy cause facial and ophthalmic signs (Horner's syndrome)?

---

1. *The immediate posterior relationship of the great veins of the neck is the dome of the pleura and the apex of the lung. Posteriorly this is the level of the neck of the 1st rib. However, as the ribs slope downwards at a 45 degree angle, the pleura extends above the 1st rib anteriorly. Just posterior to the sternocleidomastoid muscle the pleural dome lies some 2–3 cm above the medial third of the clavicle. In this region the dome of the pleura is strengthened by a fascial thickening, the suprapleural membrane (Sibson's fascia). Any catheterization that misses the veins and continues posteriorly may produce a pneumothorax.*

2. *The inferior cervical and first thoracic sympathetic ganglia are often amalgamated to form the cervicothoracic or stellate ganglion just posterior to the origin of the vertebral artery on the neck of the 1st rib. A cervical or upper thoracic sympathectomy removes the sympathetic innervation to the whole of the head and neck on the same side. This leaves the patient with a hot, dry, flushed face with no capacity to sweat (anhidrosis), drooping of the eyelid (ptosis), constriction of the pupil (meiosis) and retraction of the eye (enophthalmos) – i.e. Horner's syndrome. For this reason, when performing thoracic sympathectomies for vascular problems in the upper limb, it is very wise to avoid the stellate ganglion.*

Chapter

24

Neuroanatomy

The **central nervous system** consists of the brain and spinal cord. The emerging cranial and spinal nerves pass through the meninges and form the **peripheral nervous system**. The **autonomic nervous system** overlaps both the central and peripheral nervous systems and is concerned with the innervation of smooth muscle, cardiac muscle and glands.

The central nervous system consists of billions of neurons and their supporting cells, the neuroglia. The **neuron** is composed of a cell body, dendrites and axon. The majority of neuronal cell bodies are found in the cortex of the cerebrum and cerebellum and form the **grey matter**. Deeply placed aggregations of neuronal cell bodies within the cerebrum and cerebellum are called **nuclei**, while those outside of the central nervous system are grouped into **ganglia**. Axons in the central nervous system are typically myelinated and, when massed together, form white matter tracts. **Neuroglia** are the supporting cells of the neurons and are important in maintaining an appropriate homeostatic internal milieu for optimal neuronal function. There are different populations of neuroglia including **astrocytes**, **oligodendrocytes** and **microglia**.

The brain is situated within the cranium and comprises a **forebrain** (prosencephalon), a **midbrain** (mesencephalon) and a **hindbrain** (rhombencephalon). The forebrain consists of the cerebral hemispheres and the diencephalon. The **cerebral hemispheres** provide us with our higher cognitive (thinking) and executive functions (decision-making), alongside our ability to execute and control movement, interpret the various sensory modalities, learn and remember new tasks and apply an emotional and visceral response to these functions.

The deeper placed **basal ganglia** (corpus striatum) aid higher motor structures in the initiation, planning and control of movements. The central part of the forebrain, consisting mainly of the **thalamus** and **hypothalamus**, provides an essential integrative function in providing sensory and motor information to the higher cortical centres. It also regulates important homeostatic and endocrine mechanisms to main-

tain our internal milieu and control basic behavioural drives such as appetite, thirst, thermoregulation and reproduction.

The hindbrain consists of the **pons, medulla oblongata** and **cerebellum**. The midbrain along with the pons and medulla oblongata makes up the brainstem. The brainstem forms a central axis connecting the forebrain with the spinal cord and cerebellum. It also houses the **reticular activating system**, which is vital for our consciousness, and contains important groups of nuclei that control the cranial nerves. The cerebellum is another motor structure that provides a mechanism of providing feedback to ongoing movements for their correction and for maintaining effective balance and posture.

A series of interconnected cavities that contain **cerebrospinal fluid** (CSF) are present within the brain and form the ventricular system (see Chapter 25). The cavities consist of the two lateral ventricles and the third and fourth ventricles, all of which contain the choroid plexus that continuously produces CSF. The ventricular system is continuous with the **subarachnoid** space, surrounding the brain and spinal cord, and CSF can be reabsorbed into the venous system in this space.

THE CEREBRAL HEMISPHERES

The cerebrum is composed of two cerebral hemispheres that lie on either side of the mid-sagittal plane, with the outer convexity covered superiorly by the skull vault. It sits inferiorly on the anterior and middle cranial fossae and the superior aspect of the tentorium cerebelli. The cerebral hemispheres are incompletely separated by the **median longitudinal fissure**, within which lies the falx cerebri, a fold of dura. The two cerebral hemispheres are joined by a broad band of white matter, the **corpus callosum**. Specific **sulci** and **gyri** can be clearly visualized on all three surfaces: the lateral surface, which lies against the calvarium; the medial surface, which is hidden away in the interhemispheric fissure; and the inferior surface, which sits on the base of the skull.

Surface anatomy of the cerebral hemispheres

The cerebral hemispheres have an outer layer of **grey matter**, the cerebral cortex, and an inner layer of subcortical **white matter**. The cortex is greatly convoluted, producing the ridges of the brain, the **gyri**, which are separated by **sulci**. A deeper sulcus can be termed a **fissure**. These folds greatly increase the cortical surface area, with approximately two-thirds of the total surface area hidden from view in the sulci. The cerebral cortex can be classified macroscopically, based on its function and general topography, and microscopically, according to its degree of lamination on a histological level.

On a topographical level, each hemisphere has a **frontal**, a **parietal**, a **temporal** and an **occipital** lobe. The frontal and occipital poles are the anterior and posterior extremities of the hemisphere. The anteroinferiorly placed temporal pole lies in the middle cranial fossa underneath the frontal lobe.

Lateral surface

On the lateral convexity of the hemisphere (Fig. 24.1), two main fissures – the deep **Sylvian fissure** and the central **Rolandic sulcus** – provide useful anatomical landmarks. The Sylvian fissure extends posteriorly and superiorly, separating the frontal and parietal lobes from the temporal lobe. The Sylvian fissure has two further rami, the anterior and horizontal rami, that extend into the inferior frontal gyrus, dividing it into three parts: the pars orbitalis, pars triangularis and pars opercularis.

The margins of the Sylvian fissure overlap the deeply placed **insula**, an area of cortex that becomes submerged during enlargement of the hemispheres. The **central** (Rolandic) sulcus passes anteroinferiorly from the superior border towards the Sylvian fissure, separating the frontal lobe from the parietal lobe. The posterior boundary of the parietal and temporal lobes with the occipital lobe is not distinct on the lateral convexity, but a line between the occipitoparietal sulcus and the pre-occipital notch can be used as a rough guide.

Medial surface

On the medial surface of the cerebral hemisphere (Fig. 24.2), the cut corpus callosum provides a prominent feature that can be clearly identified. The **cingulate gyrus** lies above the **corpus callosum**, bounded by the callosal sulcus below and the cingulate sulcus above. The central sulcus extends for a short distance on to the medial surface into the **paracentral lobule**.

The posterior aspect of the medial surface contains the **calcarine sulcus** and **parieto-occipital sulcus**. The parieto-occipital sulcus provides a clearer boundary between the parietal and occipital lobes. The **precuneus** is the medial aspect of the parietal lobe that is bounded by the parieto-occipital sulcus posteriorly and the central sulcus anteriorly. The **cuneus** of the occipital lobe is bounded by the parieto-occipital sulcus anteriorly and the calcarine sulcus posteroinferiorly; it plays a key role in receiving visual information from the optic tract.

Inferior surface

The temporal, occipital and frontal lobes can be seen on the inferior surface of the brain (Figs. 24.3 and 24.4). On the medial aspect of the inferior temporal lobe lies the **parahippocampal gyrus**, which is continuous with the **lingual gyrus** posteriorly and the uncus anteriorly. The **fusiform gyrus** is separated medially from the parahippocampal gyrus by the **collateral sulcus** and laterally from the inferior temporal gyrus by the occipitotemporal sulcus. The uncus is bounded laterally by the **rhinal sulcus**, which is usually continuous posteriorly with the **collateral sulcus**. On the inferior aspect of the frontal lobe, the olfactory bulb and tract sit in the **olfactory sulcus**. This sulcus separates the **gyrus rectus** medially from the short irregular **orbital gyri** laterally.

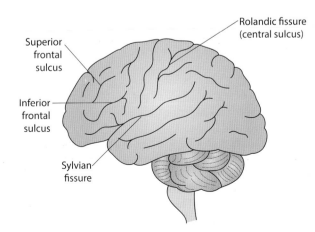

Figure 24.1 The lateral surface of the brain

Superior frontal sulcus

Inferior frontal sulcus

Sylvian fissure

Rolandic fissure (central sulcus)

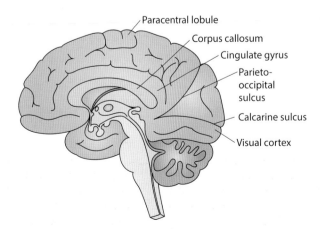

Figure 24.2 The medial surface of the brain

Paracentral lobule

Corpus callosum

Cingulate gyrus

Parieto-occipital sulcus

Calcarine sulcus

Visual cortex

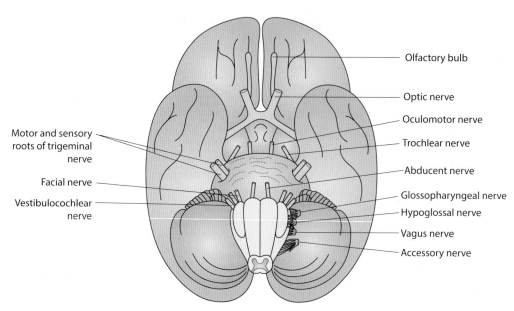

Figure 24.3 The inferior surface of the brain

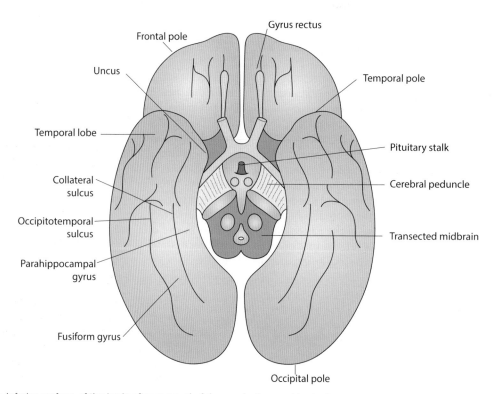

Figure 24.4 The inferior surface of the brain after removal of the cerebellum and brainstem

Specific lobes of the hemispheres

Frontal lobe

The frontal lobe is anterior to the central sulcus and is involved in motor function, eye movement, speech, higher cognitive function and behaviour. Immediately anterior to the central sulcus is the **precentral gyrus**. The **superior, middle** and **inferior frontal gyri** are separated by the superior and inferior frontal sulci. The medial frontal gyrus is a continuation of the superior frontal gyrus on the medial surface of the frontal lobe.

The primary motor cortex lies anterior to the central sulcus in the precentral gyrus. It contains the **pyramidal Betz cells**, which are critical in controlling discrete movements on the contralateral side of the body via the **pyramidal tract (corticospinal tract)**. The primary motor cortex is arranged somatotopically into regional areas as demonstrated on the motor homunculus (a picture of body parts drawn on the brain's surface).

The premotor cortex and supplementary motor areas are anterior to the precentral gyrus. The premotor cortex is involved when preparing to undertake complex movements. On electrical stimulation, it does not produce discrete movements. The premotor cortex extends on to the medial surface of the cerebral hemisphere and constitutes the supplementary motor area, which functions in the planning and organization of movement sequences. Both the premotor cortex and supplementary area are organized in a somatotopic fashion and have direct contributions to the pyramidal tract (see below).

The frontal eye field, anterior to the premotor cortex, within the middle frontal gyrus, is involved in conscious conjugate eye movements. Clinically, a destructive lesion (e.g. an ischaemic stroke) involving the frontal eye field causes a deviation of gaze towards the side of the lesion; this is in contrast to a stimulatory lesion (i.e. focal seizure), which causes deviation of gaze away from the side of the lesion.

The inferior frontal gyrus of the dominant hemisphere is involved in language and contains the motor speech area. This is known as **Broca's area**, after Paul Broca, the 19th-century French physician who made the observation that speech disturbances were associated with lesions in this area.

The prefrontal cortex is anterior to the premotor cortex and determines our personality and higher cognitive and executive functions. The prefrontal cortex has extensive **association** fibres that connect with the temporal, parietal and occipital lobes, and **commissural** fibres projecting to a homologous area in the contralateral prefrontal cortex.

Temporal lobe

The temporal lobe contains a considerable part of the limbic system, speech and auditory areas and multiple association areas, giving it a wide range of functions. The primary auditory cortex is located in the **transverse temporal gyrus (Heschl's gyrus)** of the superior temporal gyrus. It receives auditory information from the cochlea via the medial geniculate nuclei. Further auditory processing areas are located in the **superior** and **middle** temporal gyri. The speech area (**Wernicke's area**) involved in the understanding of written and spoken language lies in the dominant posterior aspect of the superior temporal gyrus.

The hippocampus and amygdala form part of the limbic system and are discussed further below.

Parietal lobe

The parietal lobe is a sensory processing area. The **postcentral gyrus** is the primary **somatosensory** cortex, receiving the terminal axons of the spinothalamic, dorsal column and trigeminothalamic pathways. Much like the primary motor cortex, the primary somatosensory cortex is arranged somatotopically, with various areas receiving greater or smaller representations depending on the extent of their innervation.

Behind the postcentral gyrus lie the **superior** and **inferior parietal lobules**, separated from one another by the intraparietal sulcus. The **supramarginal gyrus** and **angular gyrus** of the inferior parietal lobule can be identified by tracing a line posteriorly along the Sylvian fissure and superior temporal sulcus, respectively. The functions of the lobules can be appreciated by considering their dysfunction. A lesion in the superior parietal lobule results in contralateral sensory neglect and astereognosis. A lesion in the dominant inferior parietal lobule can produce a constellation of features known as Gertsmann's syndrome (right-to-left disorientation, dyslexia, dysgraphia, dyscalculia and finger agnosia).

Occipital lobe

The occipital lobe is concerned with visual processing. The primary visual (**striate**) cortex receives afferent visual information from the lateral geniculate nucleus via the optic radiations. It is located on the medial aspect of the occipital lobe, bordering the **calcarine sulcus**. The striate cortex receives its afferent innervation in an organized fashion. Visual information from the superior and inferior parts of the retina project to the striate cortex above and below the calcarine sulcus, respectively. The remainder of the occipital lobe contains the second, third and fourth visual association areas, which are involved in processing and interpreting images, alongside projecting information to other cortical, subcortical and brainstem structures.

Insular lobe

The functions of the insular cortex (**Fig. 24.5**) remain largely unknown but it is thought to be involved in emotion, regulation of the autonomic nervous system, taste, sensory processing and interoceptive awareness (an awareness of one's own bodily sensations). The insula lies in the depths of the Sylvian fissure, covered by the **opercula** ('operculum' meaning 'lid') of the frontal, parietal and temporal lobes. Once the opercula have been removed, the insular cortex can be visualized. It is divided into an anterior and posterior part by the obliquely running **central** insular **sulcus** and is circumferentially surrounded by the **circular sulcus**. The anterior part has short gyri and the posterior part typically has two long gyri.

The white matter

White matter fibres are categorized according to their origin and destination. **Association** fibres have varying lengths, long or short, and unite widely separated or adjacent gyri in the same hemisphere. **Commissural** fibres cross the midline to join the two hemispheres. **Projection** fibres ascend from, or descend to, lower parts of the central nervous system.

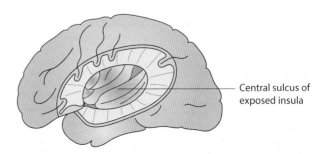

Central sulcus of exposed insula

Figure 24.5 Lateral cortex removed around the Sylvian fissure to show the sunken insula

Association fibres

Short association fibres (Fig. 24.6) join areas of adjacent cortex that are in close proximity. Long association fibres are larger fibre tracts that link different lobes together within the ipsilateral hemisphere.

The **cingulum** is located deep to the cingulate gyrus and follows the curve of the corpus callosum posteriorly before projecting to the parahippocampal gyrus. The **uncinate fasciculus** is a bidirectional tract that connects the orbitofrontal cortex to the anterior temporal lobe and is in close proximity to the **inferior fronto-occipital** fasciculus. The inferior fronto-occipital fasciculus and **superior longitudinal** fasciculus are important tracts that connect the frontal, parietal, temporal and occipital lobes. The **arcuate** fasciculus connects the language areas in the frontal

and temporal lobes and is in close proximity to the superior longitudinal fasciculus. The **inferior longitudinal** fasciculus connects the occipital lobe to the temporal lobe.

Projection fibres

Projection fibres (Fig. 24.7) either start from or end in the cerebral cortex and connect it with lower lying parts of the central nervous system. Many of the projection fibres cross the midline (decussate) and terminate on the contralateral side, but some remain on the side ipsilateral to their origin. Fibres form well-defined layers including the **corona radiata** and **internal capsule**. The corona radiata consists of subcortical white matter that contains ascending and descending projection fibres. The corona radiata is continuous ventrally with the internal capsule.

Internal capsule

The internal capsule (Fig. 24.8) is located between the lentiform nucleus laterally and the thalamus and caudate nucleus medially. In horizontal section, the internal capsule is V-shaped. It is formed of an **anterior limb** (between the head of the caudate nucleus and the lentiform nucleus), an apex (the **genu**) pointing medially, a **posterior limb** (lying between the thalamus and the lentiform nucleus) and **sublenticular** and **retrolenticular parts**.

The anterior limb carries frontopontine fibres (from the frontal lobe to the pons) and thalamocortical fibres (from the medial and anterior thalamic nuclei to the frontal cortex). The genu contains motor corticonuclear fibres that project onto cranial nerve nuclei in the brainstem. The posterior limb contains the corticospinal fibres of the pyramidal tract and ascending somatosensory fibres from the ventral posterior nuclei of the thalamus to the somatosensory cortex in the postcentral gyrus.

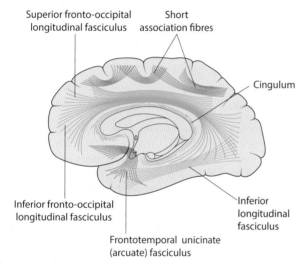

Figure 24.6 Association fibres of the cerebal hemisphere

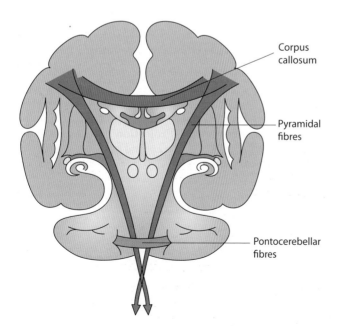

Figure 24.7 Projection fibres (purple) pass from the motor cortex through the internal capsule to the brainstem and spinal cord, the majority decussate (section taken at level B in Fig. 24.8)

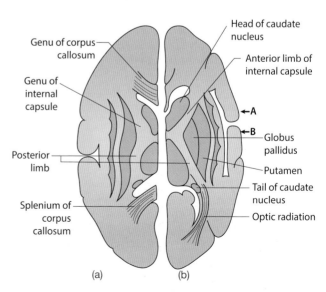

Figure 24.8 Horizontal sections of the brain: (a) through the genu and splenium of corpus callosum; (b) at a deeper level through the optic radiation. Arrow A relates to the coronal section in Fig. 24.10 and arrow B to Fig. 24.7

The sublenticular part contains the auditory radiation from the medial geniculate nucleus to the superior temporal gyrus. The retrolenticular part contains the optic radiation from the lateral geniculate nucleus to the visual cortex.

Commissural fibres

The two cerebral hemispheres are joined together by commissural fibres (Fig. 24.9), including the **corpus callosum**, **anterior commissure** and **hippocampal commissure**. The **posterior** and **habenular commissures** are white matter commissural tracts that belong to the diencephalon.

Corpus callosum

The corpus callosum is a broad band of white matter fibres joining corresponding and non-corresponding cortical areas of the hemispheres. It lies at the base of the median longitudinal fissure and forms the roof of the lateral ventricles. In mid-sagittal section it has the shape of a hook lying horizontally with its bend anteriorly and its point projecting postero-inferiorly. The pointed portion located anteriorly is known as the **rostrum**; this fuses with the lamina terminalis inferiorly. The bend is the **genu**, the horizontal part is the **body** and the expanded part posteriorly is the **splenium**.

The corpus callosum extends laterally into each hemisphere; the anterior fibres pass forwards into the frontal poles and form the **forceps minor**. A thick posterior bundle of fibres, known as the **forceps major**, passes backwards into the occipital poles.

Anterior commissure

The anterior commissure is a white matter tract embedded within the lamina terminalis, and is in close proximity to the columns of the fornix. The anterior commissure projects laterally into the temporal lobe structures. It permits the interhemispheric transfer of olfactory, visual, gustatory and auditory information between the temporal lobes.

Hippocampal commissure

The hippocampal commissure (commissure of the fornix) is located on the undersurface of the corpus callosum where the two crura meet to form the fornix. The hippocampal commissure joins the two hippocampal formations and associated structures.

The cerebral cortex

At a histological level, there are two broad types of cortex based on evolutionary lineage: the older **allocortex** and the newer neocortex. The allocortex is composed of three layers and is found in the olfactory system and hippocampus. The neocortex has six layers (I–VI) and runs parallel to the cerebral surface. The neocortex is not uniformly homogeneous, the layers varying in their microscopic appearance, thickness and neuronal and glial populations. The thickness of the neocortex can vary between 1 and 4 mm. There are two types of neuronal population: the larger **pyramidal** neurons and the smaller **non-pyramidal** (**granular, stellate**) neurons.

Layer I, the outer molecular layer, is composed of axons from other cortical areas and the dendrites of more deeply placed neurons. Layers II and IV are the internal and external granular layers containing granular and stellate neurons. Layer IV is the site of termination for the thalamocortical projection neurons. Layers III and V, which form the external and internal pyramidal layers, contain pyramidal neurons. Layer III contains the neurons that contribute to the commissural, association and projection fibres. The very large pyramidal (Betz) cells of the primary motor cortex are found in layer V. The innermost (multiform) layer VI is composed of pyramidal and non-pyramidal neurons and is adjacent to the subcortical white matter. Corticothalamic neurons originate from this layer.

An early histological classification of the cortex at the turn of the 20th century was derived by Korbinian **Brodmann**, a German psychiatrist and neuroanatomist. He classified cortical areas based on differences in cytoarchitecture, and many of these areas have now been associated with specific functions. Notable areas are summarized in Table 24.1.

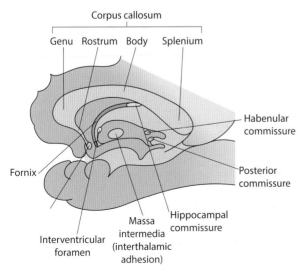

Corpus callosum

Genu   Rostrum   Body   Splenium

Habenular commissure

Fornix

Posterior commissure

Interventricular foramen

Massa intermedia (interthalamic adhesion)

Hippocampal commissure

Figure 24.9 Commissural fibres

TABLE 24.1 Major functional cortical areas and their corresponding Brodmann areas

Brodmann area	Cortical area
1, 2, 3	Primary somatosensory cortex
4	Primary motor cortex
6	Premotor cortex, supplementary motor area
8	Frontal eye field
9, 10, 11, 12	Prefrontal areas
17	Primary visual cortex (striate cortex, calcarine sulcus)
41	Primary auditory cortex (Heschl's gyrus)
44, 45	Broca's area (inferior frontal gyrus)

THE BASAL GANGLIA

The basal ganglia are deep subcortical nuclei that are involved in the initiation and control of voluntary movements, forming part of the extrapyramidal system. The basal ganglia play a role in cognition, learning and reward. Parkinson's disease and Huntington's chorea are familiar diseases associated with pathology of the basal ganglia. The basal ganglia can be considered as the corpus striatum, substantia nigra and subthalamic nucleus. The **corpus striatum** is composed of the **caudate** and the lentiform nucleus. The **lentiform nucleus** is further subdivided into the **putamen** and **globus pallidus**. The putamen and caudate nucleus are known together as the **striatum**.

Caudate nucleus

The caudate nucleus (**Figs. 24.10** and **24.11**) is C-shaped in lateral view and consists of an expanded head, narrow body and tail. The head of the caudate lies anterior to the interventricular foramen of Munro and forms the lateral wall of the lateral ventricle. It projects posteriorly as the body before becoming the tail and turning inferiorly and subsequently anteriorly, forming the roof of the temporal horn. The tail is in contact with the amygdala. The head of the caudate is largely separated from the lentiform nucleus by the anterior limb of the internal capsule, but anterior to this they are connected and form the **ventral striatum** (known as the **nucleus accumbens**).

Lentiform nucleus

The lentiform nucleus, composed of the putamen and globus pallidum, is roughly lens-shaped with its lateral surface facing the external and extreme capsule, claustrum and insula. Its medial surface faces the genu of the internal capsule. Anteromedially it is united across the anterior limb of the internal capsule to the head of the caudate nucleus.

The putamen forms the external aspect of the lentiform nucleus and is continuous with the caudate anteriorly to form the striatum. Although anatomically distinct from the caudate, they share functional similarities and receive the

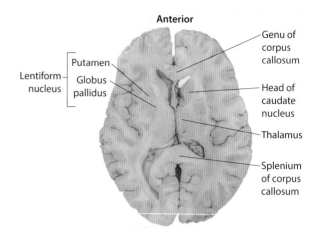

Figure 24.11 Horizontal section of the brain showing the basal ganglia

cortical input to the basal ganglia and dopaminergic innervation from the substantia nigra. The globus pallidus, deep to the putamen, is formed of external and internal parts. The major outflow from the basal ganglia to the cortical motor areas arises from the internal part of the globus pallidus via the ventrolateral nucleus of the thalamus.

Subthalamic nucleus and substantia nigra

These structures, considered functionally to be part of the basal ganglia, are discussed further in their relevant sections. The subthalamic nucleus is part of the subthalamus of the diencephalon and is a target for deep brain stimulation in the treatment of Parkinson's disease. The **substantia nigra** is located within the midbrain and consists of the **pars compacta** and **pars reticularis**. The nigrostriatal tract originates from the pars compacta and densely innervates the striatum. Degeneration of the pars compacta results in the classical features of Parkinson's disease: pill-rolling tremor, bradykinesia, rigidity and postural instability.

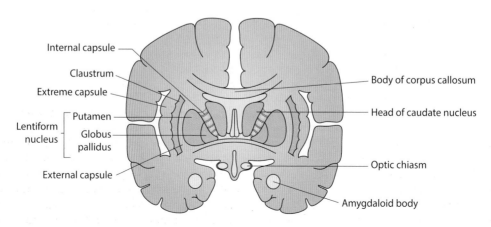

Figure 24.10 Coronal section of the brain showing the basal ganglia. Section taken at level A in Fig. 24.8

THE LIMBIC SYSTEM

The word 'limbic' is derived from the Latin *limbus*, meaning border. The French physician Paul Broca named the structures bordering the medial surface of the brain as the **limbic lobe**. It is now understood that these structures determine our emotional and visceral responses to stimuli and contribute to learning and memory. Multiple structures in the temporal and frontal lobes and diencephalon comprise the limbic system. This includes the **amygdala**, **hippocampus**, **fornix**, specific **nuclei** of the **hypothalamus** and **thalamus**, **cingulate gyrus** and the **septal area**. The anatomy of the **olfactory system** is also considered with the limbic system, given the intricate link between odour and its influence on emotion and behaviour throughout our evolutionary history, alongside the olfactory system's close anatomical interactions with medial temporal lobe structures.

The hippocampus

The hippocampal formation (Figs. 24.12 and 24.13) is a group of structures that includes the **hippocampus** proper, the **dentate gyrus**, the **subiculum** and the **entorhinal cortex**. Within this, the hippocampus is composed of the hippocampus proper and the dentate gyrus and is a cylindrical nuclear mass forming the floor of the temporal horn of the lateral ventricle. It consists of a head anteriorly, body and a tail posteriorly. The head of the hippocampus is closely juxtaposed to the amygdala anteriorly. The hippocampus proper is also known as the **cornu ammonis** because of its resemblance to a ram's horn, and contains nuclear layers CA1–CA4.

The main inflow of information to the hippocampus is via the entorhinal cortex on the inferomedial aspect of the temporal lobe. The entorhinal cortex is widely connected with cortical and subcortical structures and provides a channel for sensory information to enter the hippocampus via the perforant path.

The main outflow from the hippocampus passes into the **fimbria**, a white matter structure lying on the ventricular surface on the hippocampus that eventually becomes the fornix. The **fornix** is a complex three-dimensional, C-shaped structure composed of the crura, the body and its pillars. The left and right crura curve around the thalamus and run anteriorly along the inferior aspect of the splenium of the corpus callosum, and join together to the form the cylindrical **body** of the fornix. Fibres decussating at this point form the **hippocampal commissure**. The body of the fornix then passes inferiorly to form two pillars (or **columns**), which form the anterior boundary of the interventricular foramen of Munro, and splits into precommissural and postcommissural fibres based on whether it passes anterior or posterior to the anterior commissure. The precommissural bundle enters the septal area.

The larger postcommissural bundle, passing posteriorly to the anterior commissure, passes into the **mammillary body**. The mammillary bodies project to the anterior thalamic nuclei via the mamillothalamic tract. The anterior thalamic nuclei subsequently project to the cingulate gyrus, which is connected to the hippocampus via the cingulum. This completed nuclear ring is known as the **Papez circuit**. In 1937

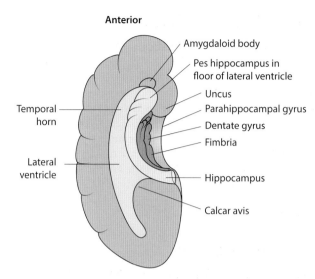

Anterior

Figure 24.12 Horizontal section through the hemisphere viewed from above, showing the lateral ventricle extending into the temporal lobe and exposing the hippocampus

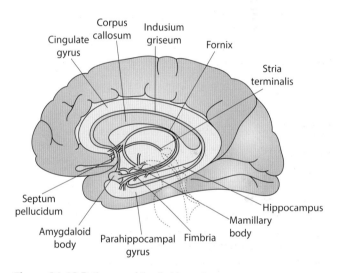

Figure 24.13 Pathways of the limbic system

The American neuroanatomist James Papez initially hypothesized that these interconnected structures were involved in emotion, but it is now widely accepted that its role is in memory formation.

The amygdala

The **amygdala** is an almond-shaped structure in close proximity to the uncus of the temporal lobe, situated at the tail of the caudate nucleus and overlying the anterior extremity of the inferior horn of the lateral ventricle. It is composed of two main nuclear groups: the central nucleus and the basolateral nucleus. The amygdala receives an array of sensory information from cortical association areas and the hippocampus as well as a rich innervation from ascending monoaminergic fibres from the brainstem.

The **stria terminalis** is the major output of the amygdala. It is a narrow bundle running alongside the thalamostriate vein that follows the course of the caudate on the lateral wall of the lateral ventricles. The stria terminalis finishes in the hypothalamus and the **bed nucleus** of the stria terminalis, a collection of nuclei situated around the anterior commissure and the septal area of the cortex. Other, more direct, efferent pathways exist from the amygdala, including the ventral amygdalofugal pathway and direct connections with other cortical, subcortical and brainstem structures.

Direct electrical stimulation of the amygdala can produce intense behavioural, emotional and visceral responses.

The septum

The septum consists of the **septum pellucidum** and the **septal area.** The septum pellucidum is a thin membrane that lies between the anterior horns of the lateral ventricles, extending from the fornix inferiorly to the corpus callosum superiorly. The septal area is considered to be part of the limbic system and consists of a group of paramedian nuclei located inferiorly to the rostrum of the corpus callosum and anteriorly to the lamina terminalis. The septal area receives afferent fibres from the amygdala, the hippocampus via the fornix, the hypothalamus and, via an ascending input, the brainstem. The septal area can influence behaviour via connections to the hypothalamus and the brainstem.

The **medial forebrain bundle** is a projection from the septal area into various hypothalamic nuclei and the midbrain tegmentum. The **stria medullaris thalami** receives contributions from the septal area that are continuous along the lateral walls of the third ventricle posteriorly and into the **habenular nuclei**. The habenular nuclei modulate brainstem function through the **fasciculus retroflexus**.

The olfactory system

The olfactory nerve is unusual compared with other cranial nerves as it is a direct extension of the central nervous system without a peripheral component. This is similar to the optic pathway, but the olfactory system bypasses the thalamus and enters directly into cortical and subcortical structures.

Specialized olfactory epithelium is located in the superior aspect of the nasal cavity. Olfactory nerve cells project their axons through the cribriform plate of the ethmoid bone to synapse with second-order **mitral cells** in the **olfactory bulb**. The olfactory bulb is located in the olfactory sulcus of the orbital surface of the frontal lobe and continues posteriorly as the **olfactory tract**. The mitral cell axons project posteriorly in the olfactory tract. As it approaches the anterior perforated substance, at the level of the optic chiasm, the tract becomes progressively flatter and triangular in shape and is known as the **olfactory trigone**.

The olfactory tract divides into two structures, the medial and lateral olfactory striae. The medial olfactory stria passes to the septal area and the contralateral olfactory bulb. The lateral olfactory stria passes laterally towards the primary olfactory cortex located on the inferomedial aspect of the

temporal lobe and terminates in multiple structures including the piriform cortex, amygdala and entorhinal cortex. The olfactory cortex has further projections to the orbitofrontal cortex, the insula, the thalamus (dorsomedial nucleus) and other limbic structures.

THE DIENCEPHALON

The diencephalon is composed of four components that surround the third ventricle: the **thalamus, hypothalamus, epithalamus** and **subthalamus**.

Thalamus

Function

The thalamus is the largest part of the diencephalon and has an important integrative function for sensory and motor modalities. Other functions include roles in consciousness, the sleep/wake cycle and memory formation. The thalamus receives multiple inputs from the spinal cord, brainstem, cerebellum and basal ganglia and relays this to the relevant cortical areas in the cerebral hemispheres to allow appropriate processing. There is reciprocal innervation between the thalamus and cerebral cortex, which is referred to as corticothalamic and thalamocortical projections.

Anatomy

The two thalami are large nuclear masses situated on either side of the superior aspect of the third ventricle (**Fig. 24.14**). Each thalamus is egg-shaped, having a larger posterior end (**Fig. 24.15**). Its long axis is almost at right angles to that of the brainstem. The narrow anterior end, the **anterior tubercle**, forms the posterior margin of the interventricular foramen. The posterior end projects backwards and laterally over the midbrain as the **pulvinar**. There are two small swellings on its

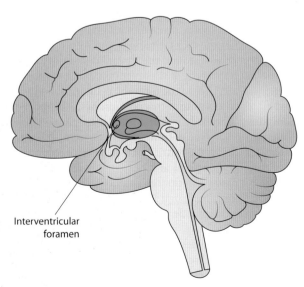

Interventricular foramen

Figure 24.14 The medial surface of the brain, outlining the position of the thalamus in green

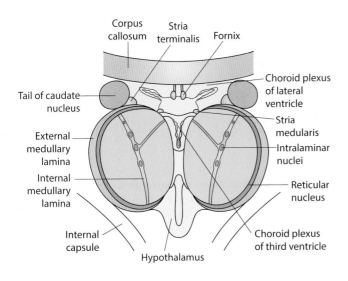

Figure 24.15 Coronal section of the brain through the two thalami

posterior surface, the **medial** and **lateral geniculate bodies**, which act as relay stations for the auditory and optic radiations, respectively. A thin sheet of white matter incompletely covers the thalamus on the dorsal surface, as the **stratum zonale**, and on the lateral surface as the **external medullary lamina**.

A band of white matter, the **internal medullary lamina**, passes through each thalamus and further splits it into groups: the **medial**, **lateral** and **anterior** groups of **nuclei** (Fig. 24.16). Within the internal medullary lamina are further nuclei termed **intralaminar nuclei**.

The arched upper surface of the thalamus is related medially to the **stria medullaris thalami**, a fibre bundle passing from the septal area to the habenula. The superolateral surface of the thalamus forms the floor of the lateral ventricle and is closely related to the stria terminalis (a fibre bundle originating from the amygdala), the thalamostriate vein and the caudate. The medial surfaces of the thalami form the lateral walls of the third ventricle. The lateral surface is applied to the posterior limb of the internal capsule, which separates

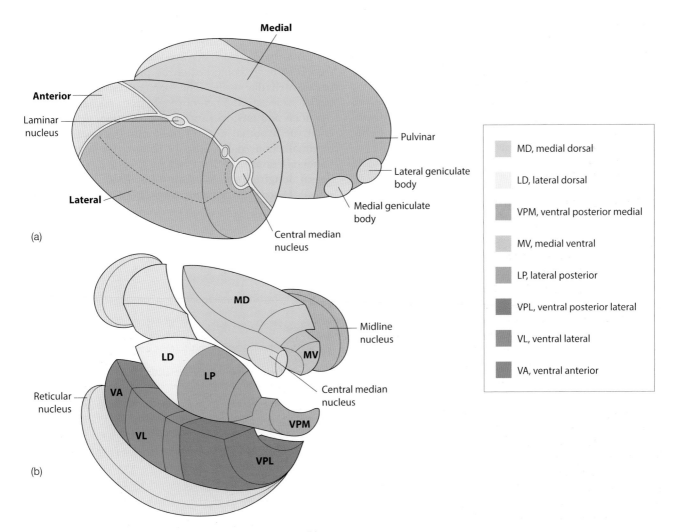

Figure 24.16 The thalamic nuclei (a), shown in exploded view (b)

it from the lentiform capsule. Between the internal capsule and external medullary lamina lies a thin sheet of grey matter known as the **reticular nucleus** of the thalamus.

Nuclei

As described above, each thalamus can be anatomically divided into lateral, medial and anterior nuclear masses. Other nuclei include the lateral and medial geniculate nuclei, intralaminar nuclei and reticular nucleus of the thalamus.

The lateral mass consists of the lateral dorsal, ventrobasal and pulvinar nuclei. The ventrobasal nucleus consists of the **ventroposterior**, **ventrolateral** and **ventroanterior** nuclei. The ventroposterior nuclear complex is of particular importance for receiving sensory information. The ventral posterior medial nucleus receives the trigeminothalamic tract, conveying sensory information from the orofacial structures. The ventral posterior lateral nucleus receives the dorsal column and spinothalamic pathways. The ventrolateral and ventroanterior nuclei receive motor information from the basal ganglia and cerebellum and project this to the motor cortex.

The anterior and medial nuclear masses are associated with the limbic system. The anterior nucleus is involved in memory and forms part of Papez's circuit. It receives fibres from the **mammillothalamic tract** and projects to the cingulate cortex. The medial mass consists mainly of the **dorsomedial nucleus** and is involved in emotional responses. It connects the hypothalamus, olfactory cortex and amygdala with the prefrontal cortex.

The medial geniculate nucleus is a relay station in the auditory pathway, receiving fibres from the lateral lemniscus; its efferents form the auditory radiation, which passes to the transverse temporal gyrus (primary auditory cortex). The lateral geniculate nucleus receives fibres from the optic tract and its efferents form the optic radiation that passes to the striate cortex in the occipital lobe.

The reticular nucleus is a thin layer of inhibitory neurons veiled over the lateral surface of the thalamus. Thalamocortical and corticothalamic neurons pass through the reticular nucleus, thus allowing modulation of thalamocortical activity.

Hypothalamus and pituitary gland

Hypothalamus

The hypothalamus plays an integral role in maintaining homeostasis, influencing reproductive behaviour and emotional responses (Fig. 24.17). This is achieved through the regulation of the autonomic nervous system, orchestrating the majority of the endocrine system via the **pituitary gland** and controlling thermoregulation, hunger and thirst.

The hypothalamus forms the floor and inferolateral wall of the third ventricle. At its anterior aspect is the optic chiasm and behind this is an elevation, the **tuber cinereum**, which gives rise to the infundibulum (pituitary stalk). Two small elevations, the **mammillary bodies**, lie behind the tuber cinereum and separate it from the **posterior perforated substance** and the **cerebral peduncles**. The **hypothalamic sulcus** on the lateral wall of the third ventricle is a groove that separates the thalamus from the hypothalamus.

The anterior columns of the fornix fan out into the hypothalamus, dividing each side into **medial** and **lateral** parts. The medial parts are composed of the **preoptic**, **supraoptic** and **paraventricular** nuclei. The supraoptic and paraventricular nuclei project to the neurohypophysis to release antidiuretic hormone and oxytocin into the circulation. Afferent fibres enter the hypothalamus via the fornix (hippocampus), stria terminalis (amygdala), anterior limb of the internal capsule (cerebral cortex), medial forebrain bundle (septal area) and **dorsal longitudinal fasciculus** (multiple brainstem structures). Descending efferent fibres from the hypothalamus

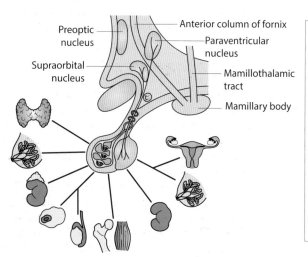

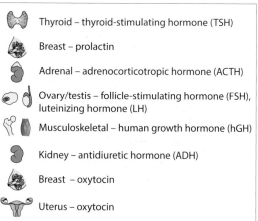

Figure 24.17 The hypothalamus and its target organs

project to the brainstem via the dorsal longitudinal fasciculus, medial forebrain bundle and mamillotegmental tract. Ascending fibres from the hypothalamus include the **mamillothalamic fasciculus**.

Pituitary gland

The pituitary gland (hypophysis cerebri) is an endocrine gland situated in the sella turcica of the body of the sphenoid bone (Fig. 24.18). It is bounded laterally by the cavernous sinuses. It is somewhat spherical in shape and is connected to the hypothalamus by the **infundibulum**. The infundibulum passes through a sheet of dura, the diaphragm sellae, which covers the pituitary gland.

The pituitary gland is composed of the **adenohypophysis** and **neurohypophysis**, which have different embryological origins and functions. The adenohypophysis develops as an ectodermal outpouching of **Rathke's pouch** in the oral cavity, projecting towards the infundibulum. The neurohypophysis derives from the infundibulum, a part of the diencephalon.

The adenohypophysis consists of the **pars distalis** (the anterior lobe), **pars tuberalis** and **pars intermedia**. The pars distalis synthesizes, stores and releases growth hormone, adenocorticotropic hormone, luteinizing hormone, follicle-stimulating hormone, prolactin and thyroid-stimulating hormone. Hypothalamic neurons release peptide hormones into the **median eminence** of the tuber cinereum and pass through the hypothalamo-hypophyseal portal system to the adenohypophysis. These hormones have either inhibitory or stimulatory actions on the pars distalis. The pars intermedia sits between the pars distalis and pars nervosa. The pars tuberalis wraps around the infundibular stalk.

The neurohypophysis is a continuation of the hypothalamus and is composed of the **pars nervosa** (posterior lobe, neural lobe), **infundibular stalk** and median eminence. Neurons in the **supraoptic** and **paraventricular nuclei** of the hypothalamus project their axons through the hypothalamo-hypophyseal tract into the pars nervosa and release antidiuretic hormone and oxytocin into the circulation.

Pituitary tumours are mainly benign adenomas derived from the adenohypophysis. Their clinical effects are derived from over- and underproduction of pituitary hormones (most commonly overproduction of prolactin from prolactinomas) and mass effects on local structures. Lateral extension may compress cavernous sinus structures, resulting in cranial nerve palsies. Superior extension can compress the optic chiasm, causing a bitemporal hemianopia, or more rarely produce an obstructive hydrocephalus from compression of the third ventricle. Pituitary tumours can be surgically resected through a trans-sphenoidal endoscopic approach.

Epithalamus

The epithalamus is situated at the posterior wall of the third ventricle between the posterior ends of the thalami. It comprises the **pineal gland**, **habenular nuclei** and **commissure**, **stria medullaris thalami** and **posterior commissure**.

The pineal gland is an endocrine gland composed of melanocytes that secrete melatonin: it plays an important role in the sleep/wake cycle and comprises one of the circumventricular organs (see Chapter 25). It is attached to the posterior aspect of the third ventricle by its pineal stalk.

The habenula is composed of medial and lateral habenular nuclei with each side connected by the habenular commissure. Afferent fibres from the thalamus project into the habenular nuclei via the stria medullaris thalami. The habenular output is extensive, including the **fasciculus retroflexus** to the brainstem; its exact functions remain obscure. The posterior commissure unites the superior colliculi and pretectal areas and plays a role in the pupillary light reflexes.

Subthalamus

The subthalamus adjoins the midbrain, lying behind the hypothalamus and above the posterior perforated substance between the cerebral peduncles. It contains the **subthalamic nucleus**, the rostral extensions of the **red nucleus** and the **substantia nigra**, and traversing fibre bundles including the sensory fasciculi that ascend to the thalamus. The subthalamic nucleus is involved in the control of motor function and is described further with the basal ganglia.

THE CEREBELLUM

The cerebellum (meaning little brain; Fig. 24.19) fills the larger part of the posterior cranial fossa, lying posterior to the brainstem, and is separated from the overlying cerebrum by the tentorium cerebelli. The cerebellum is involved in the coordination and timing of movement, maintenance of posture and motor learning.

The cerebellum has three surfaces named according to the structure it faces: the superior (tentorial), anterior (petrosal) and inferior (suboccipital) surfaces. The cerebellum consists of two **lateral hemispheres** and the midline, worm-like **vermis**. Two prominent fissures separate the cerebellum into distinct lobes. The **primary fissure** runs transversely on the superior surface, dividing the cerebellum into anterior and

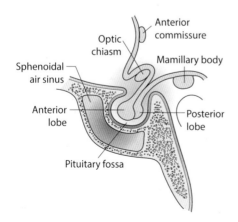

Figure 24.18 The pituitary gland

Labels on figure:
- Optic chiasm
- Anterior commissure
- Sphenoidal air sinus
- Mamillary body
- Anterior lobe
- Posterior lobe
- Pituitary fossa

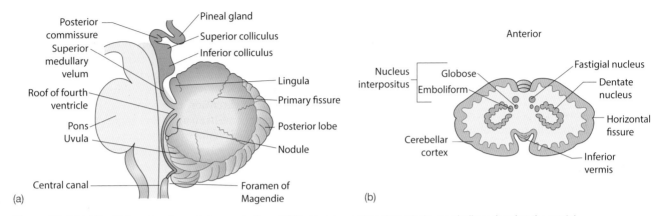

Figure 24.19 (a) Sagittal section through the cerebellum. (b) Transverse section through the cerebellum showing the nuclei

posterior lobes. The **posterolateral fissure** separates the **flocculonodular lobe** from the remainder of the cerebellum. The **nodulus** is the most caudal part of the vermis and the **flocculi** are two small lobules lying either side of it.

The cerebellum can be further classified into lobules, although a full description of the lobules is beyond the scope of this book. However, the **cerebellar tonsils**, located inferomedially and projecting inferiorly towards the foramen magnum, have considerable clinical relevance. Tonsillar herniation through the foramen magnum in the setting of acutely raised intracranial pressure is known as coning and represents a pre-terminal event.

The cerebellum is connected to the brainstem by three pairs of fibre bundles known as the **cerebellar peduncles**. The **superior**, **middle** and **inferior** cerebellar peduncles connect to the midbrain, pons and medulla, respectively, providing conduits for afferent and efferent fibres to enter and exit the cerebellum.

A mid-sagittal section shows a thin layer of outer grey cortical mater with subcortical white matter forming a tree-like appearance known as the **arbor vitae**. The outer grey matter

is greatly convoluted, with the sulci running in parallel; the ridges between these are known as **folia**, given their leaf-like appearance. The histological arrangement of the cerebellar cortex is highly uniform, with three layers: the inner **granular**, middle **Purkinje** and outer **molecular layers**.

There are two types of afferent fibres into the cerebellum: **mossy fibres** and **climbing fibres.** The only source of climbing fibres into the cerebellum is from the inferior olivary nucleus in the medulla, and these fibres terminate directly on Purkinje cells. Mossy fibres are the terminal fibres from the spinal cord, vestibular system and pontine nuclei, and these terminate on the inner granule cells. Purkinje cell axons provide the only efferent output of the cerebellum and project to the deep cerebellar nuclei. There are **four pairs of nuclei**: the large lateral dentate nucleus, the interpositus nuclei (composed of the globose and emboliform nuclei) and the medial fastigial nucleus.

The structure and (dys)function of the cerebellum can be more easily understood by considering its phylogenetic classification into the archicerebellum, paleocerebellum and neocerebellum, as summarized in Table 24.2.

TABLE 24.2 Phylogenetic classification of the cerebellum with its anatomical correlates, associated deep cerebellar nuclei, afferent and efferent output and function

	Archicerebellum	Paleocerebellum	Neocerebellum
Terminology	Vestibulocerebellum	Spinocerebellum	Cerebrocerebellum (pontocerebellum)
Anatomical location	Flocculonodular lobe	Vermis and paravermis	Cerebellar hemispheres
Peduncle input	ICP	ICP, SCP	MCP
Input	Vestibular nucleus (ICP)	Dorsal spinocerebellar tract (ICP) Ventral spinocerebellar tract (SCP)	Corticopontine-cerebellar fibres (MCP)
Deep cerebellar nucleus	Fastigial nuclei	Globose/emboliform nucleus (interposed nuclei)	Dentate nuclei
Output	To: Reticular nuclei (influence reticulospinal tract) Vestibular nuclei (vestibulospinal tract) Thalamus (ventral nuclei)	Via SCP to: Red nucleus (contralateral)	Via SCP to: Thalamus (contralateral ventrolateral nucleus) Red nucleus (contralateral)
Function	Trunk balance and equilibrium, vestibulo-ocular reflex	Muscle tone and posture	Muscle coordination

ICP, inferior cerebellar peduncle; MCP, middle cerebellar peduncle; SCP, superior cerebellar peduncle.

The **archicerebellum** (vestibulocerebellum) is the oldest part of the cerebellum and corresponds anatomically to the flocculonodular lobe. It functions to maintain balance and coordinate eye movements with head movement via the vestibulo-ocular reflex. The vestibular nuclei project via the inferior cerebellar peduncle into the ipsilateral flocculonodular lobe. The output from the archicerebellum is via the **fastigial** and **vestibular nuclei**. The fastigial nuclei influence descending vestibulospinal and reticulospinal tracts and consequently modulate the postural and neck musculature. The vestibular nuclei project to the cranial nerves influencing eye movements. Lesions of the archicerebellum therefore result in postural and gait ataxia and nystagmus.

The **paleocerebellum** (spinocerebellum) functions to coordinate the muscular tone and posture of the body and limbs. Anatomically, this represents the vermis, excluding the nodulus, and the paravermis. The cuneocerebellar and dorsal and ventral spinocerebellar tracts of the spinal cord provide unconscious proprioceptive information to the spinocerebellum. Output from the spinocerebellum is via the **interposed nuclei**. These in turn project through the superior cerebellar peduncle to the contralateral red nucleus of the midbrain and the thalamic ventrolateral nucleus via the cerebellorubral and cerebellothalamic fibres. Damage to the spinocerebellum results in lack of muscle agonist and antagonist coordination, causing gait ataxia and dysmetria.

The **neocerebellum** (cerebrocerebellum, pontocerebellum) is anatomically correlated to the cerebellar hemispheres. The cerebral cortex provides the greatest number of afferent fibres into the cerebellum through the corticopontine-cerebellar pathway and passes through the contralateral middle cerebellar peduncle these into the cerebellum. The **dentate nucleus** of the cerebellum receives the efferent projections of the neocerebellum and projects through the superior cerebellar peduncle to the contralateral red nucleus and ventrolateral thalamus, with subsequent cortical projections. The neocerebellum can therefore indirectly influence descending cortical motor output. A range of clinical signs can be seen with cerebellar hemisphere pathology, through loss of fine motor control, correct timing and correction of movements. These signs include intention tremor, dysmetria, dysdiadochokinesia and ataxia.

It is vital to recall that the different parts of the body are represented on the ipsilateral cerebellar cortex. Cerebellar clinical signs are therefore ipsilateral to the side of the lesion, this is in sharp contrast to cerebral pathology, which manifests itself on the contralateral aspect of the body.

THE BRAINSTEM

The brainstem is formed of the **midbrain**, **pons** and **medulla**, continuous rostrally with the diencephalon and caudally with the spinal cord (**Figs. 24.20** and **24.21**). As previously described, the brainstem is connected to the cerebellum by three pairs of cerebellar peduncles. The brainstem can be considered to have three roles:

- To house the IIIrd to XIIth cranial nerve nuclei and their central connections
- To provide a conduit for ascending and descending tracts between the spinal cord, cerebellum and cerebrum
- As the location of the reticular formation.

The structure of the brainstem can be further broken down into the **tectum**, **tegmentum** and **ventral motor tracts**. The tectum is only present in the midbrain, dorsal to the cerebral aqueduct, and consists of the superior and inferior colliculi. The tegmentum of the brainstem contains cranial nerve nuclei, a range of ascending and descending tracts and the reticular activating system. The tegmentum of the pons and medulla forms the floor of the fourth ventricle while in the midbrain it lies ventral to the cerebral aqueduct. Ventral to the tegmentum lie the descending pyramidal tracts, starting as the **cerebral peduncles** (crus cerebri) in the midbrain, the **pons basis** of the pons and the **pyramids** of the medulla.

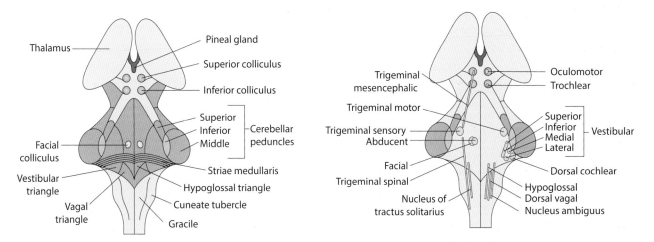

Figure 24.20 Posterior views of the brainstem after removal of the cerebellum

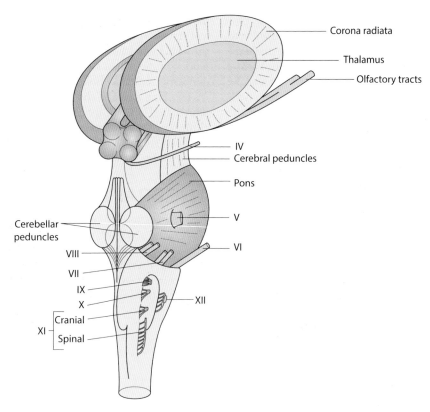

Figure 24.21 Oblique view of the posterior brainstem showing the cranial nerves

The midbrain

The midbrain (**Figs. 24.22** and **24.23**) is a short narrow region that joins the forebrain to the hindbrain through the opening in the tentorium cerebelli. The **cerebral aqueduct** runs through the midbrain and provides a useful landmark for identifying its subdivisions: the tectum and cerebral peduncles. The **tectum** is dorsal to the cerebral aqueduct. The **cerebral peduncles** are composed of the dorsally placed **tegmentum** and the ventral crus cerebri. The aqueduct is surrounded by **periaqueductal grey matter** that plays a role in the modulation of pain.

The tectum is composed of the **superior** and **inferior colliculi** and the pretectal area. The tegmentum contains the **nuclei** of the **IIIrd**, **IVth** and part of the **Vth** cranial nerves, the **substantia nigra** and the **red nucleus** alongside ascending sensory pathways. The ventral crus cerebri contain the descending corticospinal and corticobulbar neurons.

Nuclei

The oculomotor and Edinger-Westphal nuclei

The oculomotor nucleus is at the level of the superior colliculus, ventral to the cerebral aqueduct. It is a complex of multiple nuclei that supplies all the extraocular muscles except the superior oblique and lateral rectus, and provides parasympathetic fibres to the iris. The parasympathetic fibres

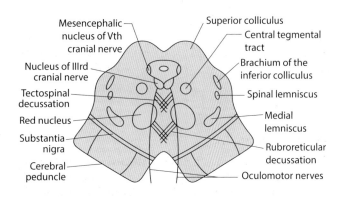

Figure 24.22 The upper midbrain

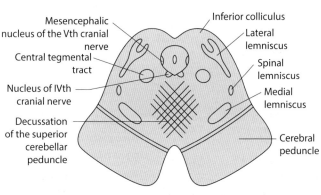

Figure 24.23 The lower midbrain

arise from the Edinger–Westphal nucleus, which is dorsally situated, adjacent to the oculomotor nucleus complex. The somatic and parasympathetic fibres pass ventrally and exit the midbrain on the medial aspect of the cerebral peduncles into the interpeduncular fossa.

Trochlear nucleus

The trochlear nucleus is in a similar position to the oculomotor nucleus but at the level of the inferior colliculus. Its efferent fibres are unusual as they decussate in the substance of the midbrain, exit from its dorsal surface and wrap around the lateral aspects of the midbrain before passing ventrally. The trochlear nucleus controls the superior oblique muscle.

Substantia nigra

The substantia nigra (Latin for black substance) is located within the tegmentum at its junction with the crus cerebri. It is composed of two components: the **pars compacta** and the **pars reticularis**. The neurons of the pars compacta contain neuromelanin, providing the substantia nigra with its pigmented appearance. The pars compacta projects heavily to the caudate and putamen and forms the nigrostrial tract. The substantia nigra is considered as part of the basal ganglia, and loss of the neurons in the pars compacta is implicated in the aetiology of Parkinson's disease.

Red nucleus

The red nuclei are a pair of oval nuclear masses that are more prominent in the upper tegmentum and are dorsal to the substantia nigra complex. The nuclei receive afferents from the cerebellum and motor cortex. The red nucleus has two outputs: to the inferior olive and the spinal cord. It projects to the inferior olive in the medulla via the descending central tegmental tract. The rubrospinal tract crosses over at the level of the midbrain prior to its descent into the spinal cord; its function in humans remains unclear.

Superior and inferior colliculi

The paired superior and inferior colliculi are four elevations clearly noted on the dorsal surface of the midbrain. Collectively, they can be referred to as the **corpora quadrigemina** and are functionally involved in vision and hearing.

The **superior colliculus** is involved in vision and associated visual reflexes. It receives afferent fibres from the optic tracts and the visual cortex in the occipital lobe. Its main output is the tectospinal tract. This functions to integrate ocular movement with head and neck movement. The **pretectal area**, composed of multiple nuclei, is just rostral to the superior colliculus and plays an important role in the pupillary light reflex. It receives afferent fibres from multiple areas including the optic tract. The pretectal area in turn projects to the parasympathetic Edinger–Westphal nuclei to control pupillary constriction.

The **inferior colliculus** receives the lateral lemniscus and is therefore integral to the ascending auditory pathways. Its efferent fibres pass through the inferior brachium to the medial geniculate nucleus of the thalamus.

White matter tracts

Crus cerebri

The crus cerebri is ventrolateral to the tegmentum and is continuous with the internal capsule rostrally and the pons basis and medullary pyramids caudally. The crus cerebri contains the descending corticospinal and corticonuclear tracts. The corticonuclear fibres terminate on cranial nerve nuclei throughout the brainstem. Corticopontine fibres from the frontal and temporal lobes also pass through the crus cerebri and terminate on pontine nuclei. These fibres are organized into specific bundles within the crus cerebri.

Ascending sensory pathways

Ascending within the lateral tegmentum are the medial, spinal, trigeminal and lateral lemnisci. The medial, spinal and trigeminal lemnisci pass into the ventroposterior nucleus of the thalamus. The medial lemniscus contains proprioceptive fibres from the dorsal column. The spinal lemniscus contains pain and temperature fibres from the spinothalamic tract and the trigeminal lemniscus contains the trigeminothalamic tract. The lateral lemniscus contains auditory fibres passing into the inferior colliculus as described above.

Pons

The pons (Figs. 24.24 and 24.25) is located between the midbrain and medulla oblongata. Its ventral surface is convex and has a clear transverse demarcation with the medulla. The **trigeminal** nerve emerges from the lateral mid-pons at the junction of the pons and middle cerebellar peduncle. The **abducens**, **facial** and **vestibulocochlear** nerves emerge, from medial to lateral, at the pontomedullary junction. The dorsal surface of the pons forms the upper part of the floor of the fourth ventricle.

In transverse section, the pons has a dorsal tegmental part and a ventral basilar part (the pons basis). The pontine tegmentum is a continuation of the midbrain tegmentum and contains the nuclei of the Vth–VIIIth cranial nerves, the lemnisci of the ascending sensory pathways, the trapezoid body and the medial longitudinal fasciculus.

The pons basis is in continuity with the crus cerebri and medullary pyramids and contains the descending corticospinal fibres, which are split into small scattered bundles, alongside the corticonuclear and corticopontine fibres. The corticopontine fibres terminate in multiple pontine nuclei that give rise to pontocerebellar fibres. These fibres traverse the pons, cross the midline and sweep dorsally to form the **middle cerebellar peduncle** and enter the contralateral cerebellar hemisphere.

Nuclei

Trigeminal nucleus

The trigeminal nucleus comprises a group of motor and sensory nuclei situated in the mid-pons region in the dorsolateral tegmentum. The motor nucleus is located medial to the chief sensory nucleus in the pons and controls the muscles of

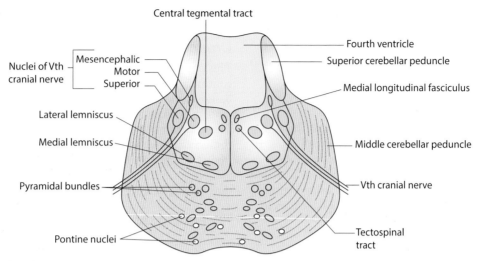

Figure 24.24 The closed pons

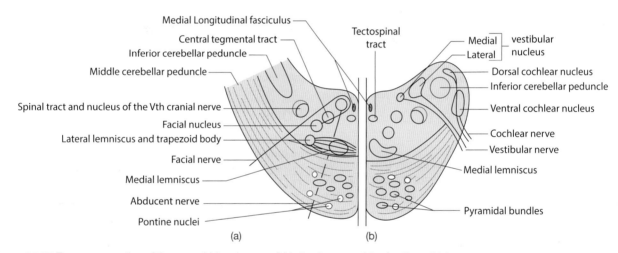

Figure 24.25 Transverse section of the pons. (a) Lower pons. (b) Lateral recess of the fourth ventricle

mastication. The sensory nucleus is composed of three parts that extend cranially and caudally within the brainstem:

- The principal (chief) sensory nucleus, located within the pons, is the largest of the three nuclei and receives fibres conveying the sensory modalities of touch and pressure from oral and facial structures.
- The mesencephalic trigeminal nucleus, located within the midbrain, receives proprioceptive fibres from the muscles of mastication.
- The spinal trigeminal nucleus, extending caudally from the pons into the medulla and upper cervical spinal cord, receives pain and temperature fibres from oral and facial structures via the trigeminal nerve and also the facial, glossopharyngeal and vagal nerves.

The chief sensory and spinal trigeminal nuclei project to the contralateral ventral posteromedial thalamus via the trigeminothalamic tract. This forms the trigeminal lemniscus. The mesencephalic nucleus has connections with the trigeminal motor nucleus and functions to aid controlling bite force and the jaw jerk reflex.

Abducent nucleus

The abducent nucleus supplies the ipsilateral lateral rectus muscle. It is a small motor nucleus that is situated near the midline in the dorsal tegmentum just under the floor of the fourth ventricle. Its fibres pass ventrally and caudally through the pons to emerge at the pontomedullary junction.

Facial motor nucleus and superior salivatory nucleus

The facial motor nucleus supplies the muscles of facial expression, stapedius, the posterior belly of the digastric and the stylohyoid. The nucleus is located in the lateral tegmentum, caudal to the trigeminal motor nucleus. Its fibres pass dorsomedially and sweep around the abducent nucleus before passing ventrolaterally and emerging at the pontomedullary junction. The close relationship between the facial motor fibres wrapping around the abducent nucleus forms the internal genu of the facial nerve; this can be noted as a slight elevation on the floor of the fourth ventricle, known as the facial colliculus.

Prior to exiting the pons the special visceral efferent fibres are joined by preganglionic parasympathetic fibres from the superior salivatory nucleus that supply the lacrimal, submandibular and sublingual glands. The superior salivatory nucleus is located in the caudal pontine tegmentum.

Vestibular and cochlear nuclei

The cochlear nerve fibres project to the cochlear nucleus, which forms part of the complex polysynaptic and bilateral ascending auditory pathways. The cochlear nucleus consists of ventral and dorsal cochlear nuclei containing the second-order neurons. The nuclei are located in the dorsolateral tegmentum close to the floor of the fourth ventricle. Efferent fibres from the cochlear nuclei can ascend uncrossed or can decussate in a compact body, the trapezoid body. The ascending fibres run within the lateral lemniscus, which projects to the inferior colliculus. The cochlear nuclei have a close association with the superior olivary nucleus.

The vestibular nucleus is a complex of multiple smaller nuclei that are located within the dorsolateral caudal pons and rostral medulla near the lateral part of the floor of the fourth ventricle. Its major input is the vestibular portion of the vestibulocochlear nerve. The vestibular nuclei have multiple efferent projections including to the cerebellum (vestibulo-cerebllar tract) and spinal cord (vestibulospinal tract), as well as to cranial nerve nuclei controlling the extraocular muscles via the medial longitudinal fasciculus.

White matter tracts

Numerous white matter tracts traverse the pons, either longitudinally or horizontally. The corticospinal tract and transverse pontine fibres in the pons basis have already been discussed, and the trapezoid body and lateral lemniscus have been described with the cochlear nuclei. The ventral spinocerebellar tract ascends through the lateral tegmentum into the midbrain prior to passing through the **superior cerebellar peduncle** and entering the cerebellum. Other ascending tracts that pass through the pons, including the spinocerebellar tracts, medial longitudinal fasciculus and medial lemniscus, are described below.

Medulla oblongata

The medulla oblongata (Figs. 24.26–24.28) narrows rapidly between the pons and the foramen magnum, where it

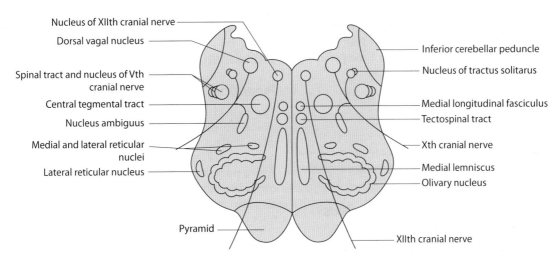

Figure 24.26 Transverse section through open medulla at the level of the olivary nucleus

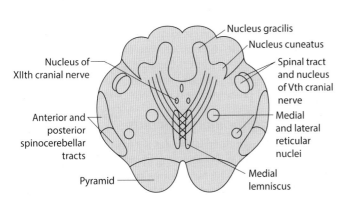

Figure 24.27 The medulla at the level of decussation of the medial lemniscus

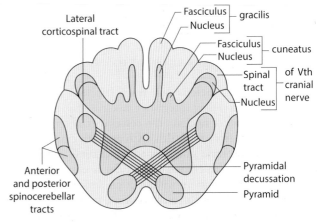

Figure 24.28 The medulla at the level of decussation of the pyramids

becomes continuous with the spinal cord. The upper part of the medulla, the **open medulla**, forms the lower half of the floor of the fourth ventricle. The lower part, the **closed medulla**, has a narrow central canal and resembles the structure of the spinal cord.

On its ventral surface, the anterior median fissure begins at the lower edge of the pons and continues caudally along the spinal cord. The fissure is flanked by two large eminences, the **pyramids**. Lateral to the pyramids lie the **olives**, separated by the anterolateral sulcus. The olives provide a useful reference for the exit of the medullary cranial nerves, with the **hypoglossal** rootlets exiting medial to the olive in the anterolateral sulcus. The **glossopharyngeal** and **vagus** nerves, and the cranial part of the **accessory cranial nerve**, exit laterally to the olive in a craniocaudal order. The dorsal surface of the medulla is described later with the anatomy of the fourth ventricle (see Chapter 25, p. 430). The posterior median sulcus of the spinal cord continues rostrally on to the medulla to the level of the obex, the inferior recess of the fourth ventricle. Either side of the sulcus lie the **gracile** and **cuneate tubercles**, which are separated by the posterior intermediate sulcus.

The internal structure of the medulla can be considered as being the dorsal tegmentum and the ventral pyramids. The medullary tegmentum is continuous with the tegmentum of the midbrain and pons and contains the nuclei of the IXth–XIIth cranial nerves, olivary nuclei, ascending sensory tracts and 'vital centres' involved in homeostasis. The pyramids contain the descending corticospinal tracts of the pyramidal tract.

Nuclei

Hypoglossal nucleus

The hypoglossal nucleus lies near the midline on the dorsal tegmentum of the medulla. It forms the hypoglossal trigone on the floor of the fourth ventricle.

Dorsal motor nucleus of the vagus, nucleus tractus solitarius and nucleus ambiguous

These three nuclei are considered together given their close relation and interconnection with the glossopharyngeal, vagal and accessory nerves:

- The **dorsal motor nucleus** of the vagus nerve lies lateral to the hypoglossal nucleus and forms the vagal trigone. This contains the preganglionic parasympathetic fibres of the vagus nerve that supply the thoracic and abdominal viscera.
- The **solitary nucleus** and **tract** (nucleus tractus solitarius) is a complex integrative nucleus that is lateral to the dorsal motor nucleus. It receives special sensory afferents of taste from the VIIth, IXth and Xth cranial nerves, alongside thoracic and abdominal visceral afferents via the IXth and Xth cranial nerves. The nucleus tractus solitarius has connections with multiple structures including the reticular formation and the dorsal motor nucleus.
- The **nucleus ambiguus** lies ventrolateral to the dorsal motor nucleus and the nucleus tractus solitarius. It contains the cell bodies of the special visceral efferent fibres for the glossopharyngeal, vagal and cranial portion of the accessory cranial nerves.

Gracile and cuneate nuclei

The gracile and cuneate nuclei are situated on the dorsal aspect of the medulla within their respectively named **tubercles**. Primary-order neurons of the dorsal column pathway synapse in these nuclei on to second-order neurons, which decussate as internal arcuate fibres prior to ascending as the medial lemniscus to the thalamus and cerebral cortex. The accessory cuneate nucleus lies lateral to the cuneate nucleus and receives proprioceptive information from the neck. Its efferents form the cuneocerebellar tract, which passes into the ipsilateral cerebellar hemisphere via the **inferior cerebellar peduncle**.

Olivary nucleus

The olivary nucleus is a large, irregular cup-shaped structure forming the prominence on the anterolateral surface of the medulla. It is composed of the **superior** and **inferior olivary nuclei**. The superior olivary nucleus is located in the pons and is composed of multiple nuclei involved in the central auditory pathways. The inferior olivary nucleus provides the only source of climbing fibres to the cerebellum via the **olivocerebellar pathway**.

White matter tracts

Pyramidal tract

The pyramids are large bundles of fibres forming prominences on each of side of the midline on the ventral medullary surface. Each is a convergence of the descending corticospinal tract fibres that have traversed the pons basis. Approximately 80 per cent of the fibres decussate into the contralateral lateral corticospinal tract. The uncrossed fibres continue in the ipsilateral anterior and lateral corticospinal tract.

Internal arcuate fibres and medial lemniscus

Many of the fibres that cross the midline in the open medulla are termed internal arcuate fibres. This contains the second-order neurons of the dorsal column medial lemniscal pathway and the olivocerebellar fibres running from the inferior olivary nucleus into the cerebellum. The medial lemniscus is a continuation of the internal arcuate fibres that contain the second-order neurons from the gracile and cuneate nuclei. It ascends through the pons and midbrain and its axons synapse in the **ventral posterolateral nucleus** of the **thalamus**.

Medial longitudinal fasciculus

The medial longitudinal fasciculus is a white matter tract containing ascending and descending fibres that extend throughout the brainstem. The medial longitudinal fasciculus is close to the midline dorsally in the medulla and retains its midline position as it ascends but becomes increasingly ventral. It connects the cranial nerve nuclei controlling eye movements and the vestibular nucleus. This permits coordination of eye movements with movement of the head, and plays a role in the **vestibulo-ocular reflex**.

Spinocerebellar tract

The spinocerebellar tracts are composed of a dorsal and a ventral component and are described in further detail on p. 433.

The reticular formation

The reticular formation is considered to be phylogenetically ancient given its role in controlling cardiovascular and respiratory function. It also has a range of functions related to awareness, consciousness, modulation of pain and motor function. It is an extensive, polysynaptic, **ill-defined neuronal network** forming the central core of the brainstem that is present throughout the tegmentum of the midbrain, pons and medulla.

Anatomically the reticular formation can be organized into three longitudinal columns: **median**, **paramedian** and **lateral**. Despite being an ill-defined network, various nuclei can be discerned within the reticular formation. Certain nuclei have specific neurotransmitters that project widely across the forebrain and have a wide range of functions related to consciousness, awareness, movement, learning and reward. For example, the **pedunculopontine** nucleus contains cholinergic neurons, the locus **coeruleus** in the dorsal pons contains noradrenergic neurons, and serotinergic neurons are present in the raphe nuclei. Certain nuclei in the pons and medulla are considered to be cardiovascular and respiratory centres.

The reticular formation has a wide range of afferent inputs from the spinal cord, cerebellum, cranial nerves and forebrain structures. It has major ascending and descending outputs that are known as the **reticular activating system** and the **reticulospinal tract**, respectively. The ascending reticular activating system is vital for achieving consciousness and connects the brainstem to the thalamus, through which it can influence various cortical structures. Various nuclei in the pons and midbrain contribute to the ascending reticular activating system and damage to these structures can result in impaired consciousness. The descending medial and lateral reticulospinal tracts originate from the medulla and caudal pons. Their functions vary from the control of posture and limb movement to the modulation of pain.

THE SPINAL CORD AND SPINAL NERVES

Spinal cord anatomy

External anatomy

The spinal cord is the cylindrical caudal continuation of the medulla oblongata that is deeply encased within the vertebral column. It extends caudally from the foramen magnum and terminates as the conus medullaris at the boundary of the 1st and 2nd lumbar vertebrae in adults; there is, however, a variation in the level of termination.

The spinal cord is approximately 40–50 cm in length and has variable anteroposterior and transverse diameters. It has **cervical** and **lumbar enlargements** to account for the increased number of sensory and motor neurons of the upper and lower limbs. Longitudinal grooves are present on the surface of the spinal cord. The ventral median fissure and dorsal median sulcus split the spinal cord into left and right halves. The spinal cord is covered by the three layers of meninges forming the thecal sac. The thecal sac extends beyond the level of the conus medullaris and ends at the second sacral vertebral level.

The conus medullaris is the cone-shaped caudal end of the spinal cord. From the apex of the conus, a fibrous extension, the **filum terminale**, continues caudally (see Chapter 25, p. 432). The filum terminale internum passes through the lumbar cistern and penetrates the caudal aspect of the thecal sac, becoming the filum terminale externum. This continues through the sacral canal, exiting the sacral hiatus and inserting into the dorsal aspect of the first coccygeal segment.

Internal anatomy

In transverse section, the inner grey and outer white matter are clearly visible (Fig. 24.29). The grey matter is butterfly-shaped and within its centre lies the small **central canal**. The grey matter on each side consists of **three columns**, known as the ventral (anterior), lateral and dorsal (posterior) horns, that contain a range of neuronal cell bodies. There is further subclassification of defined neurons into 10 layers (**Rexed laminae**). Layers I–VI comprise the dorsal horn, layer VII the lateral horn and layers VIII–X the ventral horn.

The **ventral horn** contains the large motor neurons that supply voluntary striated muscles. The **dorsal horn** contains the terminal axons of primary-order sensory neurons and the cell bodies of the second-order sensory neurons that project cranially. The ventral and dorsal horns extend throughout the length of the spinal cord. The **lateral horns** are only present in the thoracic, upper lumbar and sacral cord. Preganglionic sympathetic efferent neurons are present in the lateral horns from the **L1 to T2** spinal cord segments. In the **S2–S4** segments, the lateral horns are again present and contain the preganglionic **parasympathetic** efferent neurons. Axons

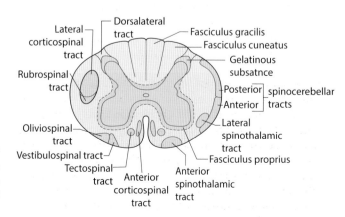

Figure 24.29 Transverse section of the spinal cord

from cell bodies within the grey matter are able to decussate to the contralateral side of the cord in the grey matter lying ventral and dorsal to the central canal.

The white matter surrounds the grey matter and consists of fibres that ascend and descend along the length of the cord. These fibres are divided into anatomical columns: the anterior, posterior and lateral funiculi. Each funiculus contains a range of tracts. The main tracts are summarized in Table 24.3, where they are considered further.

Spinal nerve anatomy

The spinal cord consists of **31 segments** corresponding to pairs of spinal nerves that exit at each segmental level: 8 cervical, 12 thoracic, 5 lumbar, 5 sacral and 1 coccygeal. The direction of the spinal nerves exiting the spinal cord varies based on the development of the spinal cord and vertebral column. The longitudinal growth of the vertebral column is greater than that of the spinal cord *in utero*. This results in the more caudal spinal nerves having to traverse a greater distance to exit at their corresponding vertebral level. Lumbar and sacral spinal nerves must continue inferiorly, beyond the conus medullaris, forming the **cauda equina** within the **lumbar cistern** of the thecal sac.

The 31 spinal nerves are formed by the **ventral** and **dorsal root**s leaving and entering their respective ventral and dorsal horns. Each root consists of multiple rootlets. The dorsal root houses the cell bodies of the first-order sensory neurons, forming a swelling in the root called the **dorsal root ganglion**. The joining of the ventral and dorsal roots forms the **spinal nerve** proper, which passes a short distance through the **intervertebral foramen** before it branches into its ventral and dorsal rami. The ventral ramus is the largest of the two rami and forms the cervical, brachial and lumbosacral plexus and intercostal nerves supplying the arms, legs and anterolateral trunk. The dorsal ramus supplies the muscles and skin of the back.

Descending and ascending tracts of the spinal cord (Table 24.3)

Descending tracts

The descending tracts (Fig. 24.30b) originate from supraspinal structures and control voluntary and involuntary muscle movements, tone, posture and reflexes as well as aspects of thermoregulation and visceral function. The descending

TABLE 24.3 Summary of the main ascending and descending tracts

Ascending tracts	Descending tracts
Corticospinal (pyramidal) tracts:	Dorsal column
Lateral corticospinal tract	Spinocerebellar tracts:
Ventral corticospinal tract	Ventral spinocerebellar tract
Extrapyramidal tracts:	Dorsal spinocerebellar tract
Rubrospinal tract	Spinothalamic tract:
Tectospinal tract	Lateral spinothalamic tract
Vestibulospinal tract	Ventral spinothalamic tract
Reticulospinal tract	

motor systems are subdivided into the **pyramidal** and **extrapyramidal** systems. The pyramidal system (**corticospinal tract**) arises from the cerebral cortex and controls voluntary movements. The extrapyramidal system consists of multiple tracts arising from various locations within the brainstem.

Pyramidal tract

The corticospinal tract has two components within the spinal cord: the larger **lateral** tract controlling fine distal movements of the limbs, and the smaller **ventral** corticospinal tract controlling the proximal limb and axial musculature. These tracts originate from large pyramidal **Betz cells** in the primary motor cortex of the precentral gyrus, alongside input from the premotor area. They are also known as **upper motor neurons**. Lower motor neurons are located within the ventral horn grey matter and innervate voluntary skeletal muscle. The corticospinal tract is accompanied by corticonuclear and corticopontine fibres in the forebrain, midbrain and hindbrain to supply the cranial nerves and pontine nuclei.

The descending axons of the pyramidal tract pass through the posterior limb of the internal capsule in a somatotopically organized fashion. The fibres continue caudally into the crus cerebri and pons basis prior to entering the medullary pyramids, the latter giving its name to the tract. The majority (approximately **90 per cent**) of the axons **decussate** in the pyramids to enter the lateral funiculus, forming the lateral corticospinal spinal tract. The remainder continue as an ipsilateral tract through the pyramids into the ventral corticospinal tract. Fibres of the ventral tract, on reaching their appropriate spinal cord segment, can either remain on the same side or decussate. The upper motor neuron axons terminate predominantly on interneurons in the ventral horns of the spinal cord, by which they can influence lower motor neurons that control movement and reflex activity. A small proportion of descending axons terminate directly on the lower motor neurons.

Extrapyramidal tracts

The extrapyramidal tracts are separate from the pyramidal system as they do not pass through the medullary pyramids. They consist of descending tracts that control a range of subconscious and involuntary movements. These tracts include the rubrospinal, tectospinal, vestibulospinal and reticulospinal tracts.

The function of the **rubrospinal tract** is not clear in humans and it appears rudimentary. It is of greater importance in vertebrates that use limbs and fins for locomotion, sharing similarities with the corticospinal tract. The tract originates from the magnocellular neurons of the red nucleus in the midbrain. The fibres cross over in the ventral tegmental decussation prior to descending through the brainstem and entering the lateral funiculus of the spinal cord, ventral to the lateral corticospinal tract. In humans, the fibres terminate in the upper cervical segments of the spinal cord, although they extend to lumbar and sacral levels in other animals.

The **tectospinal tract** is important in controlling head and neck movements in response to visual stimuli. The tract originates from the superior colliculus, which receives input from the visual cortices and direct information from the optic pathways. The tectospinal tract decussates at the level of the superior colliculi in the dorsal tegmental decussation. It descends through the brainstem, in close proximity to the medial longitudinal fasciculus, and enters the anterior funiculus, terminating in the upper cervical spinal cord.

The **vestibulospinal tract** is composed of the medial and lateral tracts. It is involved in the maintenance of posture through exerting its influence predominantly on large extensor muscle groups of the neck, trunk and limbs.

- The medial vestibulospinal tract originates from the medial and lateral vestibular nuclei and descends bilaterally, in a similar position to the medial longitudinal fasciculus and tectospinal tract. It enters the anterior funiculus and terminates in the cervical segments of the spinal cord. It can function to influence head and neck movements.

- The lateral vestibulospinal tract arises from the lateral vestibular nucleus. It descends ipsilaterally into the anterior funiculus of the spinal cord, terminating in the cervical, thoracic, lumbar and sacral cord segments. The tract has an antigravity effect by influencing axial and proximal limb musculature.

The **reticulospinal tract** originates from various nuclei of the reticular formation in the medulla and pons. It controls a range of functions including initiation of limb movement, control of muscle tone and posture and modulation of pain perception. The medial and lateral reticulospinal tracts both descend bilaterally. The medial tract is in the anterior funiculus and the lateral tract is in the lateral funiculus.

Ascending tracts

The ascending tracts (**Fig. 24.3a**) provide the conduits for various **sensory** modalities to pass through the spinal cord and into higher structures.

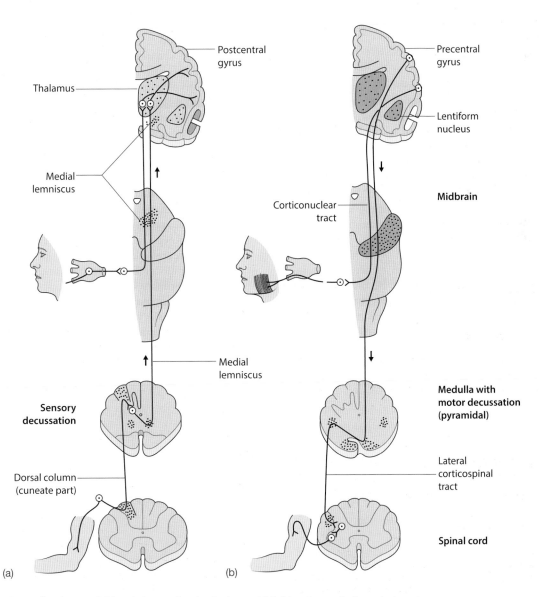

Figure 24.30 Ascending (sensory) (a) and descending (motor/pyramidal) (b) pathways in the spinal cord

Dorsal column

The dorsal column pathway conveys sensory neurons of proprioception, touch, vibration and two-point discrimination to higher centres. The dorsal column pathway consists of the **fasciculus gracilis** and **fasciculus cuneatus**, which are separated by the posterior intermediate sulcus. Primary-order neurons from the skin enter the dorsal horn and project their axons directly into the ipsilateral dorsal column pathway.

The fasciculus gracilis originates at the caudal end of the spinal cord and extends rostrally throughout the length of the cord. It receives sensory input from the lower limbs and lower thorax. The fasciculus cuneatus originates at the 6th thoracic segment of the cord and is lateral to the fasciculus gracilis. It receives sensory input from the upper limbs and upper thorax.

The primary-order axons terminate in the dorsal column nuclei of the medulla, the **nucleus gracilis** and **nucleus cuneatus**. From there, second-order neurons decussate as the internal arcuate fibres and ascend in the **medial lemniscus** to the **ventral posterolateral** nucleus of the **thalamus**. Tertiary-order neurons in the thalamus then continue rostrally to the primary somatosensory cortex.

Spinothalamic tract

The spinothalamic tract is a three-order neuronal system transmitting temperature, nociceptive, crude touch and pressure information to the contralateral somatosensory cortex. It consists of a **lateral** and a **ventral tract**. The lateral tract, located in the lateral funiculus, conveys temperature and nociception, while the ventral tract in the anterior funiculus is responsible for light touch and pressure.

Second-order neurons form the origin of the spinothalamic tract and arise from multiple laminae in the dorsal horn of the spinal cord, receiving axonal projections from primary-order neurons that have their cell bodies in the dorsal root ganglia. The second-order fibres decussate at the level of origin and ascend in either the lateral or the ventral tract. The lateral tract becomes the **spinal lemniscus** in the brainstem, and the ventral tract joins the **medial lemniscus** of the dorsal column pathway. Both tracts synapse on to tertiary-order neurons in the **ventral posterolateral nucleus** of the **thalamus** and continue to the primary somatosensory cortex.

Spinocerebellar and cuneocerebellar tract

The spinocerebellar and cuneocerebellar tracts are **ipsilateral** pathways that transmit proprioceptive and cutaneous information from the trunk and limbs to the cerebellum. These tracts terminate as mossy fibres in the cerebellar vermis and paravermis. The **dorsal** and **ventral spinocerebellar tracts** are responsible for the lower limbs and thorax, while the cuneocerebellar tract is the upper limb equivalent of the dorsal spinocerebellar tract. There are subtle functional differences between the dorsal and ventral tracts. The dorsal tract provides precise information about the position of individual muscles while the ventral tract is less specific, conveying the position of the entire limb.

The dorsal spinocerebellar tract is located in the lateral funiculus originating in the midlumbar spinal cord segments. It ascends ipsilaterally and its axons pass through the inferior cerebellar peduncle into the cerebellum. Axons of the dorsal spinocerebellar tract originate in Clarke's column (dorsal nucleus). Clarke's column is in the grey matter of the spinal cord extending from the C8 to L2 spinal segments. Primary-order neurons in the dorsal column transmitting information from Golgi tendon organs and muscle spindles have collateral branches that synapse in Clarke's column. Primary-order neurons entering the spinal cord below L2 ascend before reaching Clarke's column.

The ventral spinocerebellar tract is located in the lateral funiculus. Its fibres originate from the lumbosacral spinal cord segments in laminae V–VII. The fibres decussate and ascend in the contralateral tract, ventral to the dorsal spinocerebellar tract. The fibres then continue rostrally through the medulla and pons before passing through the superior cerebellar peduncle to the cerebellum and decussate again in the cerebellar white matter. The two decussations ensure that the information from primary-order neurons entering a spinal cord segment still projects to the ipsilateral cerebellar hemisphere.

The **cuneocerebellar tract** is the upper limb equivalent of the dorsal spinocerebellar tract . Clarke's nucleus is absent above C8, so primary order neurons ascend in the cuneate fasciculus and synapse in the accessory cuneate nucleus of the medulla. The accessory cuneate nucleus projects its fibres into the cerebellum, forming the cuneocerebellar tract. (Note that the accessory cuneate nucleus is not to be confused with the cuneate nucleus of the dorsal column pathway.)

DEVELOPMENT OF THE CENTRAL NERVOUS SYSTEM

An understanding of the anatomy of the central nervous system is greatly facilitated by a knowledge of its terminology and embryology. The brain (encephalon) is composed of a forebrain (**prosencephalon**), midbrain (**mesencephalon**) and hindbrain (**rhombencephalon**). The forebrain is subdivided into the telencephalon and the **diencephalon**. The telencephalon is composed of the two cerebral hemispheres and the basal ganglia. The diencephalon consists of the thalamus, hypothalamus, subthalamus and epithalamus. The midbrain is located between the forebrain rostrally and the hindbrain caudally. The hindbrain is subdivided into the **metencephalon** (pons and cerebellum) and **myeloencephalon** (medulla oblongata) and is continuous caudally with the spinal cord as it passes through the foramen magnum.

Neural tube formation

The formation of the neural tube during the 3rd–4th weeks of embryogenesis is the result of the ectoderm folding medially (Fig. 24.31). The cephalic part of the tube is wider and forms the rest of the brain, the remainder becoming the spinal cord. A failure of the neural tube to close, either cranially or caudally, results in a wide range of neural tube defects (including **spina bifida** and **anencephaly**).

The neural tube differentiates into three layers: the internal **ventricular** (ependymal) **layer** lining the cavity of the tube; an intermediate **mantle layer**; and an external **marginal layer**. The ependymal layer forms the lining of the ventricles of the brain and central canal of the spinal cord. The marginal layer develops into the white matter neuronal fibre tracts, while the mantle layer forms the grey cellular matter. The mantle layer develops into **ventral** (basal) and **dorsal** (alar) **plates**, thickenings that become a range of motor and sensory structures in the brain and spinal cord.

In the cranial region of the neural tube, two constrictions divide the tube into three primitive vesicles that form the forebrain, midbrain and hindbrain (Fig. 24.32). **Cephalic**, **cervical** and **pontine** flexures of the tube are formed in response to the development and expansion of the neural tube. Initially, the cephalic (mesencephalic) flexure forms in the midbrain region and the cervical flexure is at the junction of the brain and spinal cord.

The spinal cord

The spinal cord forms from the caudal part of the neural tube. Three **columns**, ventral, lateral and posterior, develop in the mantle layer around the spinal canal (Fig. 24.33). The ventral column forms the ventral horns of the spinal cord, containing motor neurons. Behind this is the lateral column and this, together with the ventral column, forms the **basal plate**. The

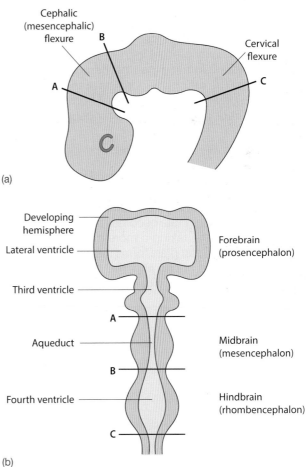

(a)

(b)

Figure 24.32 (a) The primitive neural tube. The cephalic flexure is in the region of the future midbrain and the cervical flexure at the junction of the brain and spinal cord. (b) The neural tube in longitudinal section. Lines A, B and C correspond in the two figures

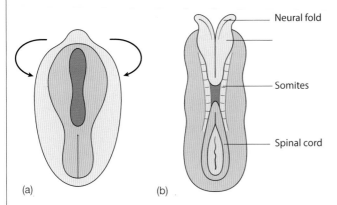

(a)   (b)

Figure 24.31 (a) Primitive embryonic disc. (b) 23 day embryo; folding of the disc to produce the neural tube

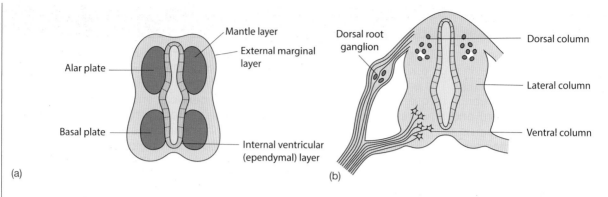

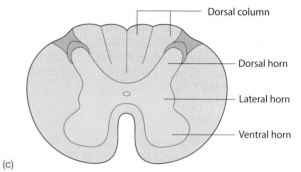

Figure 24.33 (a) The alar and basal plates of the neural tube. (b) The peripheral nerves attached to the spinal cord. (c) The adult form of the spinal cord dorsal root ganglion; The basal plate gives rise to the ventral (motor) column while the alar plate forms the dorsal and lateral columns and the dorsal root ganglion

lateral column does not extend through the length of the cord and is only present in the thoracolumbar and sacral segments, forming part of the autonomic nervous system. The **alar plate** consists of the dorsal column, which develops into the dorsal horn. The dorsal horn has a predominantly sensory function.

The hindbrain

The basal and alar plates of the brainstem are separated by a longitudinal groove, the sulcus limitans. Unlike the spinal cord, which retains its ventral–dorsal orientation of the plates, the alar plate becomes laterally displaced with the basal plate, taking a more medial position in the brainstem. The alar plate forms the cerebellum (Fig. 24.34),the pontine nuclei and the afferent (sensory)

nuclei of the cranial nerves. The basal plate forms the efferent nuclei of the cranial nerves. The cavity of the hindbrain becomes the **fourth ventricle**.

In the brainstem, the columnar arrangement within the spinal cord is present alongside three additional columns: the **special visceral afferent** and **efferent columns** and the **special somatic afferent column**. These columns are discontinuous throughout the length of the brainstem. This functional classification is simplistic but provides a mechanism for understanding the internal structure of the brainstem (see Table 24.4 for a summary).

The basal plate contains three columns: general somatic efferent, special visceral efferent and general visceral efferent. The general somatic efferent column

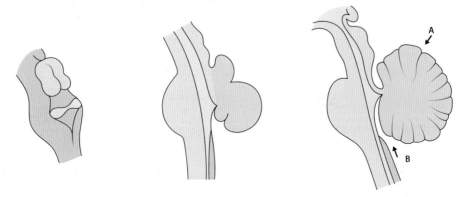

Figure 24.34 The cerebellum develops from the alar plate on the cranial lip of the pontine flexure. Arrow A, primary fissure; arrow B, overlap of the cerebellum over the open part of the fourth ventricle

TABLE 24.4 The functional columns of the brainstem and their associated brainstem nuclei and modalities (functions)

	Column	Brainstem nuclei	Associated cranial nerve nuclei	Modalities
Basal plate	General somatic efferent	Oculomotor nucleus Trochlear nucleus Abducent nucleus Hypoglossal nucleus	III IV VI XII	Eye movement Tongue movement
	Special visceral efferent	Trigeminal motor nucleus Facial motor nucleus Nucleus ambiguus	V VII IX, X XI (cranial part)	Muscles of mastication Muscles of facial expression Pharyngeal, palate and laryngeal musculature Sternocleidomastoid and trapezius
	General visceral efferent	Edinger–Westphal nucleus Superior salivatory nucleus Inferior salivatory nucleus Dorsal motor nucleus of the vagus	III VII IX X	Pupillary constriction Lacrimation and salivation Salivation Control of viscera
Alar plate	General visceral afferent	Nucleus tractus solitarius	IX, X	Visceral afferents from the carotid and aortic bodies and thoracic and abdominal viscera
	Special visceral afferent	Nucleus tractus solitarius	VII, IX, X	Taste
	General somatic afferent	Trigeminal sensory nucleus	V, VII, IX, X	General sensory modalities from the oral cavity, face, nose, pharynx and larynx
	Special somatic afferent	Vestibular and cochlear nuclei	VIII	Balance and hearing

consists of the motor neurons that control the muscles of the eye (extraocular muscles) and the tongue. The special visceral efferent (branchiomotor, branchial) column supplies muscles derived from the pharyngeal arches (Fig. 24.35). The general visceral efferent column provides parasympathetic innervation to parasympathetic ganglia of the head and controls pupillary constriction, lacrimation and the production of saliva. It is also the source of the vagus nerve, which provides the parasympathetic innervation of the thoracic and abdominal viscera.

The alar plate contains four columns: general visceral afferent, special visceral afferent, general somatic afferent and special somatic afferent. The general visceral afferent column receives a wide range of information from the viscera and the carotid and aortic bodies. The special visceral afferent column carries the sensation

of taste. The general somatic afferent column receives the sensory modalities of pain, temperature, general sensation and proprioception of the face, nose, oral cavity, ears, pharynx and larynx. The special sensory column receives fibres responsible for the special senses of hearing and balance.

The midbrain

The midbrain connects the forebrain to the hindbrain and joins the pons and medulla to form the brainstem (Fig. 24.36). The basal plates of the midbrain become the motor nuclei of the midbrain and form the **cerebral peduncles** that contain large descending motor tracts. The alar plates develop into specific structures that are discussed further throughout this chapter: the red nucleus, the substantia nigra and the superior and inferior colliculi. The cavity of the midbrain becomes increasingly narrowed during its development to form the **cerebral aqueduct**, joining the third ventricle to the fourth ventricle.

The forebrain

The forebrain develops from the most rostral primitive vesicle. As it proceeds through its development it forms the telencephalon and the diencephalon on each side. The cavity of this vesicle forms the **lateral and third ventricles**.

Two large outgrowths develop from the sides of the vesicle that form the cerebral hemispheres; these are the sites of the future cerebral cortex (Fig. 24.37). The cavities within these outgrowths become the lateral

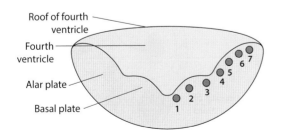

Figure 24.35 Differentiation of the alar and basal plates in the floor of the fourth ventricle. Nuclei: 1, somatic efferent; 2, special visceral efferent; 3, general visceral efferent; 4, general visceral afferent; 5, special visceral afferent; 6, general somatic afferent; 7, special somatic afferent

ventricles and remain continuous with the third ventricle via the interventricular foramen. The cerebral hemispheres enlarge in a lateral, a caudal and then a ventral direction. As a result, the hemispheres, lateral ventricles and other structures, including the caudate nucleus and hippocampus, become elongated and C-shaped.

The diencephalon can be considered to have dorsal and ventral portions and contains a central cavity that forms the third ventricle. The dorsal portion on each side forms the thalamus and epithalamus while the ventral portion forms the hypothalamus (Fig. 24.38). The pituitary gland has dual origin from the brain and the foregut (Fig. 24.36a).

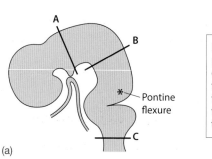

Formation of the pituitary gland by a downgrowth from the forebrain and upward fold (Rathke's pouch) from the primitive foregut

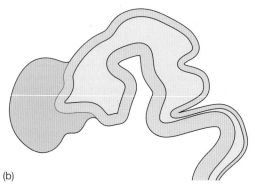

Figure 24.36 (a) The neural tube flexures and their further development, showing the pontine flexure in the region of the hindbrain. The asterisk shows the site of development of the cerebellum in the alar plate. Lines A, B and C correspond to Fig 24.34. (b) Cut-away wall showing cavity

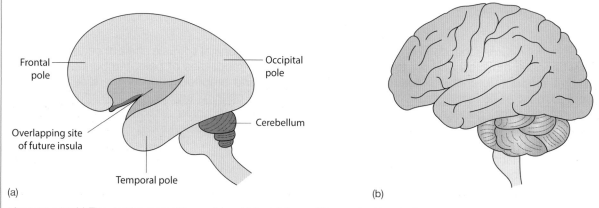

Figure 24.37 (a) The development (5th month) and (b) adult form of the cerebral hemispheres

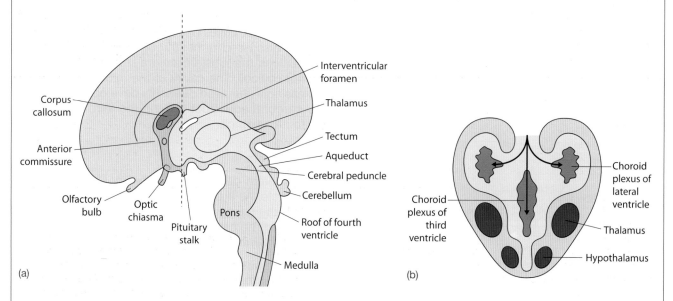

Figure 24.38 (a) The developing diencephalon and choroid plexus (3rd month). (b) A transverse section taken along the dashed line in part (a)

MCQs

1. The ventral posterior lateral nucleus of the thalamus: T/F
a   receives sensory fibres from the face   (____)
b   is a relay station for auditory fibres   (____)
c   lies anterior to the pulvinar   (____)
d   receives sensory fibres from the upper limb   (____)
e   lies adjacent to the anterior limb of the internal capsule   (____)

Answers
1.
a **F** – *trigeminal fibres pass to the ventral posterior medial nucleus*
b **F** – *these fibres relay in the medial geniculate body of the thalamus*
c **T**
d **T** – *dorsal column and spinothalamic tracts end in the nucleus*
e **F** – *it is adjacent to the posterior limb of the internal capsule*

2. The Papez circuit: T/F
a   is part of the limbic system   (____)
b   is concerned with memory function   (____)
c   decussates primarily through the corpus callosum   (____)
d   projects to the septal nuclei   (____)
e   projects predominantly to the postcentral gyrus   (____)

Answers
2.
a **T** – *it lies adjacent to the midline, extending laterally in the floor of the temporal horn of the lateral ventricle*
b **T** – *although Papez originally thought it was concerned with emotion*
c **F** – *decussating is through the fornix and anterior commissure*
d **T** – *both the fornix and stria terminalis project to this area*
e **F** – *this is the primary sensory cortex*

SBA

1. The primary optic pathways pass through the:
a   anterior limb of the internal capsule
b   corpus callosum
c   genu of the internal capsule
d   posterior limb of the internal capsule
e   medial geniculate body

Answer
1.
d *The optic radiation passes from the lateral geniculate body to the visual (striate) cortex in the occipital lobe. The anterior limb of the internal capsule carries thalamocortical fibres to the frontal lobe and the posterior limb carries sensorimotor fibres. The corpus callosum is an interhemispheric commissure and the medical geniculate body is an auditory relay station.*

2. The primary motor cortex is situated in the:
a   precentral gyrus
b   superior frontal gyrus
c   postcentral gyrus
d   superior temporal gyrus
e   cingulate gyrus

Answer
2.
a *The superior frontal gyrus is a secondary motor area, while the postcentral gyrus is the primary sensory cortex. The superior temporal gyrus contains the auditory cortex and the cingulate gyrus is part of the limbic system.*

3. The primary sensory cortex is situated in the:
a   precentral gyrus
b   superior frontal gyrus
c   postcentral gyrus
d   superior temporal gyrus
e   cingulate gyrus

Answer
3.
c *The precentral gyrus is the primary motor cortex and the superior frontal gyrus a secondary motor area. The superior temporal gyrus contains the auditory cortex, while the cingulate gyrus is part of the limbic system.*

4. Fibres from the fasciculus gracilis pass to the:
a   dorsomedial nucleus of the thalamus
b   pulvinar of the thalamus
c   ventral posterolateral nucleus of the thalamus
d   ventral posteromedial nucleus of the thalamus
e   lateral nucleus of the thalamus

Answer
4.
c *The dorsomedial nucleus has connections with the hypothalamus, olfactory cortex, amygdala and prefrontal cortex. The ventral posterolateral nucleus is part of the auditory and visual relay pathways and the ventral posteromedial nucleus is a relay station for trigeminal nerve fibres. The lateral nucleus relays fibres from the basal ganglion and cerebellum to the motor cortex.*

EMQS

Each question has an anatomical theme linked to the chapter, and a list of 10 related items (A–J) placed in alphabetical order: these are followed by five statements (1–5). Match one or more of the items A-J to each of the five statements.

1. Cranial nerve nuclei
A. Eighth
B. Eleventh
C. Fifth
D. Fourth
E. Ninth
F. Seventh
G. Sixth
H. Tenth
I. Third
J. Twelfth

Answers
1 E; *2* EFH; *3* ABEHJ (C and G also have extensions into this area); *4* A; *5* H

Match the following statement to the appropriate cranial nerve nuclei in the the above list.
1. Innervates fibres from the carotid sinus
2. Carries taste fibres
3. Situated in the medulla oblongata
4. Sends efferent fibres through the inferior cerebellar peducle
5. Supplies the cricothyroid muscle

2. Cranial nerve nuclei
A. Abducent
B. Accessory
C. Facial
D. Glossopharyngeal
E. Hypoglossal
F. Oculomotor
G. Trigeminal
H. Trochlear
I. Vagus
J. Vestibulocochlear

Answers
1 D; *2* H; *3* CDFI; *4* G; *5* F

Match the following statement to the appropriate cranial nerve nuclei in the above list.
1. Carry taste fibres from the posterior third of the tongue
2. Situated in the caudal midbrain or at the level of the inferior colliculus
3. Carries parasympathetic fibres
4. Projects to the ventral posterior medial nucleus of the thalamus
5. Concerned with the pupillary light response

APPLIED QUESTIONS

1. A 27-year-old woman attends her doctor with a 3-day history of a left facial weakness, with forehead sparing; she is otherwise well. What is the nerve damage?

   1. *Given the forehead sparing, this is a lower motor neuron pattern of injury to the facial (VII) nerve known as Bell's palsy. The upper part of the face is not involved in a cortical (upper motor neuron) lesion as it is bilaterally innervated.*

2. A 60-year-old man presents with acute onset of weakness of his left arm and leg, and a left hemiparesis with a facial droop. What is the most common cause of this condition?

   2. *This is most likely an ischaemic stroke of the anterior circulation. It is more common in those with atherosclerotic and embolic risk factors*

3. A 36-year-old woman is thrown off her horse and presents with weakness of her legs and sensory loss below her umbilicus. What level of spinal cord injury has she sustained?

   3. *The vertebral and associated spinal injury is at the level of the 10th thoracic vertebra.*

Bailey & Love · Essential Clinical Anatomy · Bailey & Love · Essential Clinical Anatomy
essential Clinical Anatomy · Bailey & Love · Essential Clinical Anatomy · Bailey & Love
iley & Love · Essential Clinical Anatomy · Bailey & Love · Essential Clinical Anatomy

Chapter **25**

The ventricular system, the meninges and blood supply of the cranial cavity

THE VENTRICULAR SYSTEM

The ventricular system (Fig. 25.1) comprises **two lateral ventricles**, the **third ventricle**, the **cerebral aqueduct** (of Sylvius), the **fourth ventricle** and the **spinal canal**. The ventricular system is filled with **cerebrospinal fluid** (CSF), which is produced by epithelium of the **choroid plexus**; this choroid plexus is present in the lateral, third and fourth ventricles. The epithelium has a rich blood supply and invaginates into the ventricular cavities. The CSF flows through the ventricular system and exits into the subarachnoid space via the two **lateral foramina** of Luschka and the **medial foramen** of Magendie, located in the fourth ventricle. The CSF passes from the **subarachnoid spaces** into the dural venous sinuses via the **arachnoid granulations**.

Lateral ventricle

The lateral ventricles are C-shaped cavities located within the cerebral hemispheres. The frontal (anterior) horns extend anteriorly from the **interventricular foramen** and are separated by a thin translucent membrane known as the septum pellucidum. The occipital (posterior) horns project posteriorly into the occipital lobes, and the temporal (inferior) horns project to within 2–3 cm of the temporal poles. The body of the lateral ventricle extends from the interventricular foramen to the splenium of the corpus callosum.

Interventricular foramen of Monro

The lateral ventricles are connected to the third ventricle via the interventricular foramen of Monro. The anterior and

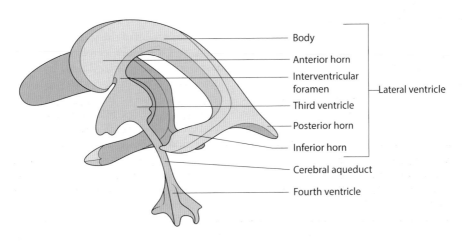

Figure 25.1 Diagrammatic representation of the ventricular system of the brain

posterior boundaries of the foramina are formed by the fornix and thalamus, respectively. The choroid plexus from the lateral ventricle passes through the foramen and is continuous with the choroid plexus within the third ventricle.

Third ventricle

The third ventricle is a vertical slit-like cavity located in the midline of the diencephalon. The lateral walls are formed by the hypothalamus inferiorly and the thalamus superiorly, and are divided by a shallow groove (the hypothalamic sulcus) running from the interventricular foramen to the cerebral aqueduct. The ventricular surfaces of the thalami are interconnected by the **massa intermedia** in approximately 75% of people. The roof is formed by thin membranes and the body of the fornix, and is the location of the choroid plexus of the third ventricle. The floor is formed by multiple structures including the optic chiasm, infundibulum, tuber cinerum and mammillary bodies. Either side of the optic chiasm lie the supraoptic recess anteriorly and infundibular recess posteriorly.

The **lamina terminalis** and **anterior commissure** form the anterior wall of the third ventricle. The posterior wall has multiple recesses (pineal and suprapineal recesses) and is formed from the pineal gland, habenular complex and commissure, the posterior commissure and the cerebral aqueduct posteroinferiorly.

Cerebral aqueduct of Sylvius

The cerebral aqueduct connects the third ventricle to the fourth ventricle. It originates at the posterior wall of the third ventricle and passes through the midbrain between the dorsal tectum and ventral tegmentum to enter the superior aspect of the fourth ventricle.

Fourth ventricle

The fourth ventricle is the cavity of the hindbrain. It communicates superiorly with the third ventricle via the cerebral aqueduct and is continuous inferiorly with the central canal of the spinal cord. When looked at from behind, the floor of the ventricle is diamond-shaped and bounded superolaterally by the superior cerebellar peduncles, inferolaterally by the inferior cerebellar peduncles and inferiorly by the **gracile** and **cuneate tubercles**. The inferior point of the floor is known as the **obex**.

The diamond-shaped floor of the ventricle is formed superiorly by the pons and inferiorly by the medulla. A **median sulcus** grooves its length, and a number of ridges, the striae medullares, pass transversely across it into the **lateral recesses**. On either side of the median sulcus, below the striae medullares, a small depression, the **inferior fovea**, is present. Two diverging sulci descend from the fovea to divide the area below the striae into a medial **hypoglossal triangle**, an intermediate **vagal triangle** and a lateral vestibular area. These overlie their respective cranial nerve nuclei. Superior to the striae medullares, one on each side of the median sulcus, is an elevation, the **facial colliculus**. The colliculus is formed by facial nerve fibres arching over the abducent nucleus. Lateral to this is a rostral extension of the vestibular area.

The roof of the cavity extends backwards into the cerebellum; it is formed superiorly by a glial sheet (the **superior medullary velum**) stretching between the superior cerebellar peduncles, and inferiorly by a thin ependymal sheet (the **inferior medullary** velum) between the inferior cerebellar peduncles. The inferior medullary velum is invaginated by blood vessels and pia mater and forms the **choroid plexus** of the ventricle. The lateral angles of the roof are evaginated to form the lateral recesses that pass forwards around the inferior cerebellar peduncles. The fourth ventricle is continuous with the subarachnoid space. A lateral opening in each tip of the lateral recesses (**foramina of Luschka**) and a median opening (**foramen of Magendi**) in the inferior medullary velum allow CSF to pass from the ventricular system into the cerebellopontine and cerebellomedullary cisterns, respectively.

Circumventricular organs

The circumventricular organs are midline structures located around the third and fourth ventricles. They consist of the **subfornical organ, subcommissural organ, organum vasculosum** of the lamina terminalis, **median eminence, neurohypophysis, area postrema** and **pineal gland**. They lack a blood–brain barrier, thereby allowing blood-borne products to come into contact with the central nervous system. The functions of the circumventricular organs are varied and involve water and fluid homeostasis alongside regulation of other endocrine functions.

THE MENINGES

Three membranes form a protective covering around the brain and spinal cord: an outer, dense, fibrous **dura mater** lining the inside of the cranium; an inner, delicate, vascular **pia mater** covering the brain; and, between them, an intermediate, delicate, avascular **arachnoid mater**. The dura and arachnoid mater are separated by a potential subdural space and the arachnoid and pia by a wider **subarachnoid space** that contains the CSF.

The dura mater

The cranial dura is in two layers: the outer, endocranial layer is the periosteum of the inner surface of the bones of the cranium, and the inner, cerebral layer is continuous with that of the spinal cord (Fig. 25.2). In most areas the two layers are adherent, but in places they separate to enclose the dural venous sinuses. The inner layer is folded to project into the cranial cavity. These folds form the falx cerebri and tentorium cerebelli, both of which act as baffle plates to reduce excessive brain motion during rapid movement of the head. Smaller folds create the falx cerebelli and the diaphragma sellae.

The **falx cerebri** lies in the mid-sagittal plane separating the two cerebral hemispheres. It is attached anteriorly to the vault of the skull to the crista galli, the midline protuberance between the cribriform plates of the ethmoids, and posteriorly to the internal occipital protuberance. It is sickle-shaped, being narrower anteriorly. Posteriorly it blends with the upper surface of the tentorium cerebelli in the midline, where its two layers separate to enclose the straight sinus. The inferior

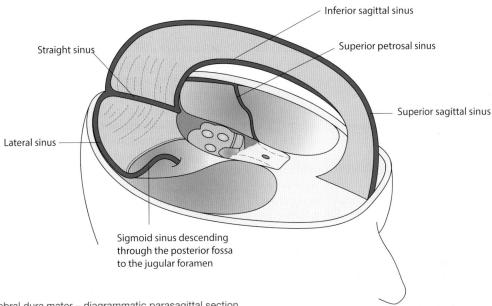

Figure 25.2 Cerebral dura mater – diagrammatic parasagittal section

sagittal sinus lies within its lower free border and the superior sagittal sinus superiorly within its attachment to the skull vault (Fig. 25.2).

The **tentorium cerebelli** roofs the posterior cranial fossa and separates the cerebral hemispheres from the cerebellum. Its free anterior U-shaped border, attached to the anterior clinoid processes, surrounds the midbrain. Its attached border extends from each posterior clinoid process, along the petrous temporal bone and then, inclining posteriorly, to the internal occipital protuberance. The superior petrosal and transverse venous sinuses lie in the attached border and the straight sinus passes backwards along the line of attachment of the falx cerebri to the tentorium cerebelli.

The **diaphragma sellae** is attached to the four clinoid processes and forms a roof for the pituitary fossa. It is perforated in the midline to allow passage of the pituitary (Figs. 25.2 and 25.9a).

The **cerebral layer** of dura forms a sheath around the cranial nerves as they leave the skull. It receives its blood supply from the anterior ethmoidal, middle meningeal, internal carotid and vertebral arteries. It is innervated by meningeal branches of the trigeminal, glossopharyngeal, vagal and upper three cervical nerves. The **spinal dura mater** (Fig. 25.3) is continuous at the foramen magnum with the cerebral layer

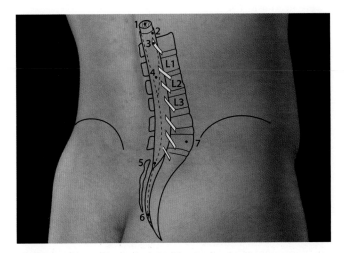

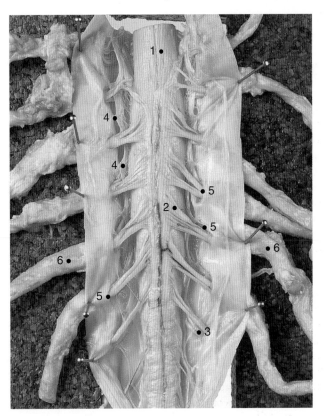

Figure 25.3 Surface anatomy of the spinal canal and contents: 1, spinal cord; 2, dural sac; 3, spinal nerves exiting vertebral canal; 4, conus medullaris (cord ending – L1/L2); 5, termination of dural sac (S2); 6, filum terminale; 7, body of L5

Figure 25.4 Spinal dura mater opened posteriorly: 1, spinal cord; 2, dorsal (posterior) roots; 3, ventral (anterior) roots; 4, dentate ligaments of pia; 5, spinal nerve piercing dura; 6, dural sheath of mixed spinal nerve

of dura mater and extends down to the level of the second sacral vertebra (Fig. 25.3). It is separated from the walls of the vertebral canal by the extradural (epidural) space; this is filled with extradural fat and the internal vertebral venous plexus. The dura is pierced by the ventral and dorsal nerve roots of the spinal nerves, but it ensheaths the nerves as far as the intervertebral foramina.

The arachnoid mater

The arachnoid mater is closely applied to the inside of the cranial and spinal dura mater, and fine trabeculae pass from it to the pia mater. In places the arachnoid mater herniates through the dura, forming **arachnoid villi**, which come into contact with the endothelium of the venous sinuses, especially the superior sagittal sinus and its lateral recesses. Through these villi the CSF is returned to the blood of the venous sinuses. The clusters of villi that appear in later life are known as **arachnoid granulations**; these leave indentations on the skull interior, especially along the path of the superior sagittal sinus.

Skull fractures involving the base of the skull usually tear the dura, and CSF leaks from the nose or ear are common. Vault fractures may injure the middle meningeal vessels and, since these lie between the inner and outer layers of the dura, the inner layer of dura usually remains intact. Bleeding from these vessels will cause extradural haematomas. A midline depressed fracture over the vertex may tear the underlying sagittal sinus. If there is subsequent venous thrombosis, it may interfere with CSF absorption, resulting in increased CSF pressure and, eventually, decreased consciousness and coma.

The pia mater

This is closely applied to the surface of the brain and spinal cord. It contains blood vessels, extends into the sulci of the brain and invests the cranial and spinal nerves and their roots (see Chapter 11). On each side of the spinal cord the pia forms a multiserrated fold, the **ligamentum denticulatum** (Fig. 25.4), running the length of the spinal cord and attached by its serrations, between the spinal nerves, to the dura. These attachments help to stabilize the spinal cord within the dural sheath. At the termination of the conus medullaris, where the cauda equine commences, the pia gives rise to a fibrous band called the **filum terminale**, which passes through the lumbar cistern and anchors the conus to the coccyx.

THE CEREBROSPINAL FLUID

The pia is invaginated by the cerebral arteries, which then lie in a sheath of pia mater. The pia and the ependymal lining of the ventricles are in contact over the roof of the third ventricle and the medial wall of the lateral ventricle. The two layers fuse and are invaginated into the cavity of each ventricle by blood vessels, the **choroid plexuses**. The ependymal cells help produce CSF. Median and lateral apertures in the pia and ependyma of the roof of the fourth ventricle allow CSF to pass from the ventricles to the subarachnoid space.

The arachnoid mater is a thin impermeable membrane supported by the inner layer of the dura mater but separated by a thin layer of fluid in the **subdural space**. Alongside the venous sinuses the arachnoid herniates through the dura mater into the sinuses, forming **arachnoid villi**; these are most frequent in the superior sagittal sinus. Aggregation of these villi occurs in the adult, forming larger **arachnoid granulations** (see also Fig. 25.8) that indent the interior of the vault. The **subarachnoid space**, the space between the pia and the arachnoid mater, is filled with CSF and is narrowest over the cerebral hemispheres.

Larger spaces (**cisterns**) are present where the arachnoid stretches across concavities of the brain; these include the **cerebellomedullary cistern (cisterna magna)** in the angle between the cerebellum and medulla, the **interpeduncular cistern** between the cerebral peduncles and the **pontine cistern** in front of the pons. The **lumbar cistern**, caudal to the end of the spinal cord, contains the cauda equina.

The subarachnoid space extends along the bundles of the olfactory nerve that penetrate the cribriform plate, and along the optic nerve as far as the optic disc in the eyeball.

The cerebellomedullary cistern can be tapped (sampled) for CSF withdrawal by a needle inserted in the midline through the posterior atlanto-occipital membrane and the dura. The lumbar cistern can be punctured by a needle advanced forwards in the midline between the spines of the lumbar vertebrae, normally at the L4/L5 interspace, and a sample of spinal CSF obtained (Figs. 25.5 and 25.6 and p. 180). NB: the spinal cord reaches the 4th lumbar vertebra in children, the adult relationships being due to differential growth of the spinal cord and vertebral column.

Blows to the head cause sudden severe deceleration, producing excessive force on the cranial contents. There are ill-understood changes within the brain that cause a sudden abrupt loss of consciousness immediately after the blow to the head (**cerebral concussion**). In the absence of any visible structural damage and intracranial haemorrhage this loss of consciousness is short-lived. However, **intracranial haemorrhage** is associated with a significant number of usually more severe head injuries.

Extradural haemorrhage between the two layers of dura is usually the result of bleeding from the middle meningeal artery, which is frequently associated with fractures of the temporal bone. This is arterial bleeding and the blood accumulates fairly rapidly, causing compression of the brain and a gradual loss of consciousness. Surgical evacuation of the haematoma and stopping of the haemorrhage is usually achieved through a burr hole drilled in the pterion (p. 305).

A **subdural haematoma** often occurs without any fracture of the skull. It is most common in elderly individuals, in whom some shrinkage of the brain has occurred. The injury may be apparently quite trivial but the smaller brain allows it to be shaken within the cranium, which is followed by a tear in a cerebral vein as it enters the superior sagittal sinus. The venous bleeding is slower than that of arterial trauma, and the results of increasing cerebral compression are thus slower in onset. It is not uncommon for the clinical effects of a subdural haemorrhage to develop 2 or more weeks after the trauma that caused it.

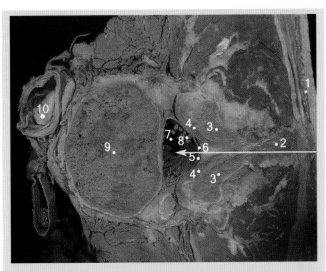

Figure 25.5 Axial dissection to show the anatomy related to lumbar puncture (yellow arrow): 1, skin and subcutaneous tissue, 2, spinous process of lumbar vertebra; 3, laminae of vertebrae; 4, ligamentum flavum; 5, dura mater; 6, epidural (extradural) space; 7, subarachnoid space containing CSF; 8, cauda equina – lumbosacral nerve roots; 9, body of L4 vertebra; 10, aorta

Subarachnoid haemorrhage may follow penetrating brain trauma, but the more common cause is spontaneous bleeding from an aneurysm (swelling) of a cerebral artery. It results in extensive meningeal irritation as the blood spreads under the meninges to cause headache and neck stiffness, progressing to eventual loss of consciousness.

CIRCULATION OF CEREBROSPINAL FLUID

Most of the CSF is produced by the choroid plexuses of the ventricles by secretion from the ependymal cells. Its total volume is about 130 mL, of which 100 mL is in the subarachnoid space and 30 mL in the ventricles. It is produced at a rate of about 20 mL per hour, thus replacing itself approximately three times a day. After flowing through the ventricles the CSF passes into the subarachnoid space through the apertures in the roof of the fourth ventricle, and distributes itself throughout the space around the brain and spinal cord. It is then reabsorbed by the bloodstream, through the arachnoid villi, by direct passage mainly into the superior sagittal sinus or by absorption into perineural lymphatics. Changes in blood pressure have very little effect on CSF pressure, but an increase in venous pressure is followed by a decrease in reabsorption into the cerebral sinuses and an increase in CSF pressure.

If there is disturbance in the balance of the production and reabsorption of CSF, e.g. overproduction, obstruction to its flow or a decrease in its absorption, the ventricles become distended. In a child if the rise in pressure is persistent and long-standing, it causes distraction of the bones of the vault and enlargement of the head, a condition known as **hydrocephalus** (Fig. 18.2, p. 302).

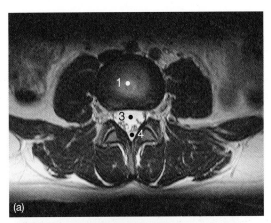

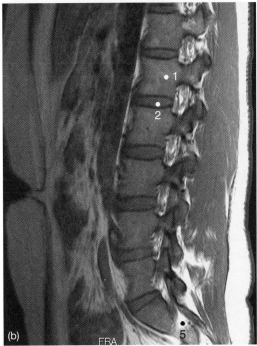

Figure 25.6 MRI of the lumbar region. (a) Axial view. (b) Sagittal view: 1, lumbar vertebral body; 2, intervertebral disc; 3, subarachnoid space with cauda equina; 4, epidural space containing fat, veins and emerging nerve roots; 5, sacral nerve roots in sacral canal

BLOOD SUPPLY OF THE BRAIN AND SPINAL CORD

The skull and spinal dura are unyielding and the brain and the CSF incompressible; the intracranial vascular system is therefore susceptible to any change in intracranial pressure caused by injury, haemorrhage, infection or tumour.

Arterial circulation of the brain

The brain must receive up to 20% of the cardiac output to maintain its metabolic requirements. It is supplied by two **internal carotid arteries** and two **vertebral arteries**. The internal carotid arteries can be considered to be the anterior circulation of the brain, while the vertebral arteries form the posterior circulation; the latter is also referred to as the ver-tebrobasilar system. These four vessels form an anastomotic circle at the base of the brain known as the **circle of Willis** (Fig. 25.7). The anterior and posterior circulations are united by anterior and posterior communicating arteries to complete the anastomotic circle. This has been considered as a mecha-nism of collateral distribution of blood throughout the arterial circulation of the brain, but the circle of Willis can display considerable anatomical variation on an individual level.

Internal carotid artery

The internal carotid artery (**Figs. 21.4a**, p. 357, **23.2**, p. 388, and **23.4c,d**, p. 389) originates from the bifurcation of the common carotid artery. The extracranial portion ascends and enters the **carotid canal**, which passes through the petrous part of the temporal bone. Its extracranial component has no branches. As it runs through the carotid canal it passes over the cartilage-filled foramen lacerum. Once within the cranial vault the internal carotid artery takes an S-shaped course through the **cavernous sinus**, often termed the **carotid siphon**, prior to penetrating the dura mater and entering the subarachnoid space. It then terminates in its two main branches: the **anterior** and **middle cerebral arteries**.

Anterior cerebral artery

The anterior cerebral artery (**Figs. 25.7b,c**) is the smaller ter-minal branch of the internal carotid artery. The anterior cere-bral artery runs anteromedially from the termination of the internal carotid artery until it reaches the **anterior communi-cating artery**, a small artery that joins the two anterior cere-bral arteries. The anterior cerebral artery follows the course of the corpus callosum and sweeps posteriorly within the median longitudinal fissure to supply the medial aspects of the frontal and parietal lobes, including the area of the primary motor cortex controlling lower limb movement. Branches of the anterior cerebral artery include the **callosomarginal** and **pericallosal arteries**. The **recurrent artery** of Heubner (the **medial lenticulostriate artery**) is of particular importance as it supplies the head of the caudate nucleus and the anterior limb of the internal capsule.

Middle cerebral artery

The middle cerebral artery is the largest terminal branch of the internal carotid artery and can be classified surgically into **four parts** (M1–M4). It initially passes laterally from the termination of the internal carotid artery and gives off small **lateral lenticulostriate** branches that supply the putamen, parts of the caudate, and the posterior limb and genu of the internal capsule. The middle cerebral artery then passes from deep to superficial within the Sylvian fissure until its multiple branches reach the cortical surface and supply the majority of the lateral convexity of the cerebral hemispheres.

Other branches of the internal carotid artery

The anterior and middle cerebral arteries are the termi-nal branches of the internal carotid artery, yet there are numerous other arteries arising from the internal carotid artery that require consideration. The **anterior choroidal** artery supplies portions of the optic pathways including the optic tract, lateral geniculate nuclei and optic radiations alongside parts of the basal ganglia, posterior limb of the internal capsule and part of the midbrain cerebral pedun-cles. The **ophthalmic artery** (p. 319) supplies the majority of the orbital structures. There are also direct and indirect hypophyseal branches that supply the pituitary gland. The **posterior communicating artery** is analogous to the anterior

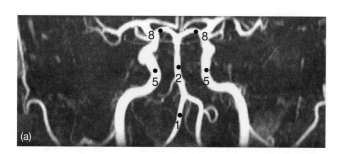

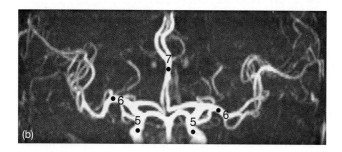

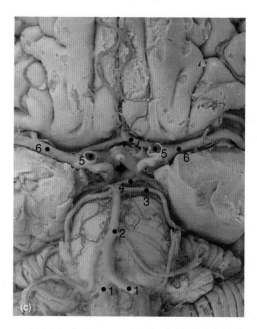

Figure 25.7 Circle of Willis. (a) and (b) MR angiograms; (c) injected dissection. 1, vertebral artery; 2, basilar artery; 3, superior cerebellar artery; 4, posterior communicating artery; 5, internal carotid artery; 6, middle cerebral artery; 7, anterior cerebral artery; 8, posterior cerebral artery

communicating artery and joins the internal carotid artery to the posterior cerebral artery. The posterior communicating artery, like its anterior equivalent, displays considerable anatomical variation.

Vertebral artery

The vertebral artery is the first branch of the subclavian artery and ascends towards the skull through the transverse foramina of the 6th to 2nd cervical vertebrae. It then passes through the foramen magnum, ventral to the brainstem, and joins with its counterpart to form the **basilar artery**. The left vertebral artery is often larger than the right. The **posterior inferior cerebellar artery** and **anterior spinal artery** are important branches of the vertebral artery and are discussed further below.

Basilar artery

The basilar artery is formed by the fusion of the two vertebral arteries. It continues to ascend, giving off the anterior inferior cerebellar artery, small pontine branches and superior cerebellar artery, and terminates in the posterior cerebral arteries.

Cerebellar arteries

Three pairs of cerebellar arteries arise from the vertebrobasilar system: the **superior cerebellar, anterior inferior cerebellar** and **posterior inferior cerebellar arteries**. Each artery supplies a different part of the brainstem, cerebellar peduncle and surface of the cerebellum, and displays considerable anatomical variation.

The posterior inferior cerebellar artery arises from the vertebral artery and takes a convoluted course that supplies the lateral part of the medulla, the inferior cerebellar peduncle and the suboccipital surface of the cerebellum. Occlusion of the posterior inferior cerebellar artery can result in the **lateral medullary syndrome** of Wallenberg. The **posterior spinal artery** is an important branch of the posterior inferior cerebellar artery that supplies the spinal cord. The anterior inferior cerebellar artery arises from the proximal basilar artery and supplies the pons, middle cerebellar peduncle and anterior surface of the cerebellum. The **labyrinthine artery** arises from the anterior inferior cerebellar artery and supplies the inner ear structures. The superior cerebellar artery arises from the distal basilar artery prior to its termination in the **posterior cerebral arteries**. The superior cerebellar artery supplies the midbrain, superior cerebellar peduncle and tentorial surface of the cerebellum.

Posterior cerebral artery

The posterior cerebral artery is the terminal branch of the basilar artery and wraps itself posteriorly around the lateral surface of the midbrain. It then enters the supratentorial compartment and continues posteriorly towards the occipital lobe. Proximally, the posterior cerebral artery is joined by the **posterior communicating artery** from the internal carotid artery. Multiple occipital and temporal cortical branches supply the occipital lobe and inferior temporal lobe. The thalamus receives its blood supply from the posterior cerebral artery via the thalamoperforators.

The presence of occlusive arterial disease in elderly people may mean that, in the event of occlusion by embolus or thrombosis, the arterial anastomoses are not adequate to maintain an adequate circulation to all areas; cerebral ischaemia (inadequate blood supply) occurs and this is marked by the onset of a vascular stroke, or cerebrovascular accident. Haemorrhagic cerebrovascular accidents result from bleeding into the subarachnoid space from an aneurysm, either a congenital 'berry' aneurysm arising in young people from a vessel close to the circle of Willis or, in older people, an acquired aneurysm, the consequence of long-term raised blood pressure.

Venous drainage of the brain

The veins draining the hemispheres are divided into superficial and deep groups, which freely anastomose and drain into the venous sinuses (**Fig. 25.8**).

The **superficial group** of veins comprises the superior, superficial middle and inferior cerebral veins, which drain to the superior sagittal sinus, cavernous sinus and transverse sinus, respectively. Superior and inferior anastomotic veins join the superficial middle cerebral vein to the superior sagittal and transverse sinuses.

In the **deep group** the anterior cerebral vein drains to the deep middle cerebral vein to form the **basal vein** (of Rosenthal), which runs back around the midbrain to join the great cerebral vein. Each **internal cerebral vein** drains midbrain structures. It receives the thalamostriate vein draining the thalamus, and choroidal veins draining the lateral and third ventricles, and then joins its fellow to form the **great cerebral vein**, which opens into the straight sinus.

Dural venous sinuses

The **dural venous sinuses** lie between two layers of cranial dura mater or within a fold of the cerebral layer. They receive venous blood from the brain and communicate via sinuses and emissary veins with veins outside the skull (**Fig. 25.8**). The sinuses may be single or paired.

Single sinuses

- **Superior sagittal sinus** – runs backwards in the upper border of the falx cerebri to the inner occipital protuberance, where it usually turns to join the right transverse sinus. Its walls are invaginated by many arachnoid granulations for reabsorbing CSF.
- **Inferior sagittal sinus** – runs backwards in the lower border of the falx cerebri to join the straight sinus at the attachment of the falx to the tentorium.
- **Straight sinus** – runs in the midline of the tentorium cerebelli to the internal occipital protuberance, where it commonly joins the left transverse sinus.
- **Basilar sinus** – lies on the basal part of the occipital bone.
- **Intercavernous sinuses** – join the cavernous sinus in front and behind the pituitary.

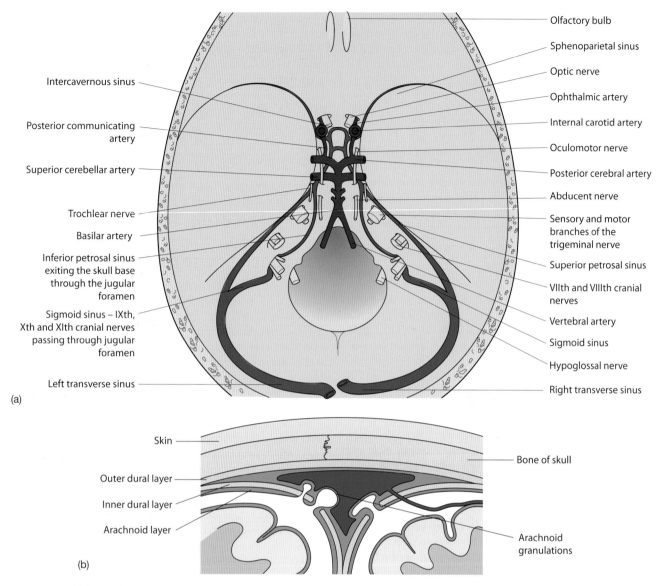

Figure 25.8 (a) Dural venous sinuses. (b) Arachnoid granulations through inner dural layer meeting endothelium of venus sinus for the production of cerebrospinal fluid

Paired sinuses

- **Transverse sinus** – begins at the internal occipital protuberance, the right usually from the superior sagittal sinus and the left from the straight sinus. Each runs in the attached border of the tentorium to the lateral part of the temporal bone, where it becomes the sigmoid sinus. The two transverse sinuses often communicate at the internal occipital protuberance to form the **confluence of the sinuses**.
- **Sigmoid sinus** – a continuation of the transverse sinus beginning at the lateral end of the temporal bone. It curves down and forwards, grooving the inner surface of the mastoid process, to the jugular foramen, and just below this it continues as the internal jugular vein.
- **Cavernous sinus** (Fig. 25.9a) – lies on the body of the sphenoid lateral to the pituitary gland, running from the opening of the carotid canal to the superior orbital fissure. Its roof, in contact with the diaphragma sellae, is under

the hypothalamus. Its lateral wall, related to the temporal lobe, contains the oculomotor, trochlear, ophthalmic and maxillary nerves. The internal carotid artery loops through the sinus to exit its roof anteriorly. The abducent nerve lies in the sinus lateral to the artery. The sinus receives the ophthalmic and superficial middle cerebral veins and the sphenoparietal sinus, and communicates with its fellow on the opposite side via the intercavernous sinuses. It is drained by the superior and inferior petrosal sinuses and the pterygoid venous plexus; eventually, via the transverse sinus, it drains into the internal jugular vein.

The ophthalmic vein, in normal circumstances, drains to the facial vein, but the flow is occasionally retrograde. If a boil in the central facial region around the eye or nose is squeezed, blood (and pus) may be forced into the ophthalmic vein and cavernous sinus, causing infection and thrombosis in the sinus and damage to the IIIrd, IVth, Vth and VIth cranial nerves.

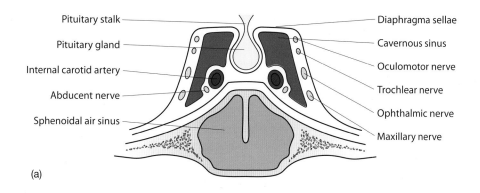

Pituitary stalk

Pituitary gland

Internal carotid artery

Abducent nerve

Sphenoidal air sinus

Diaphragma sellae

Cavernous sinus

Oculomotor nerve

Trochlear nerve

Ophthalmic nerve

Maxillary nerve

(a)

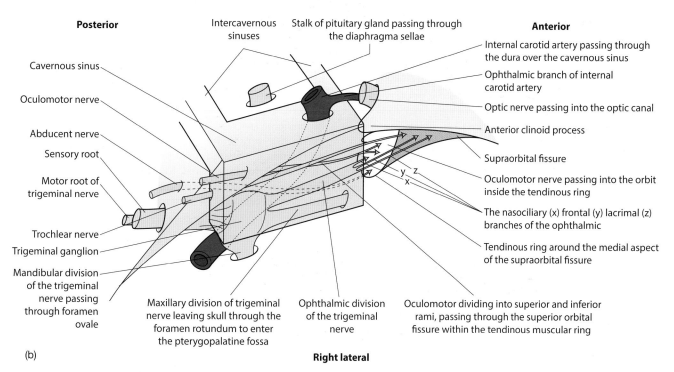

Left lateral

Posterior

Intercavernous sinuses

Stalk of pituitary gland passing through the diaphragma sellae

Anterior

Internal carotid artery passing through the dura over the cavernous sinus

Cavernous sinus

Oculomotor nerve

Abducent nerve

Sensory root

Motor root of trigeminal nerve

Trochlear nerve

Trigeminal ganglion

Mandibular division of the trigeminal nerve passing through foramen ovale

Ophthalmic branch of internal carotid artery

Optic nerve passing into the optic canal

Anterior clinoid process

Supraorbital fissure

Oculomotor nerve passing into the orbit inside the tendinous ring

The nasociliary (x) frontal (y) lacrimal (z) branches of the ophthalmic

Tendinous ring around the medial aspect of the supraorbital fissure

Maxillary division of trigeminal nerve leaving skull through the foramen rotundum to enter the pterygopalatine fossa

Ophthalmic division of the trigeminal nerve

Oculomotor dividing into superior and inferior rami, passing through the superior orbital fissure within the tendinous muscular ring

(b)

Right lateral

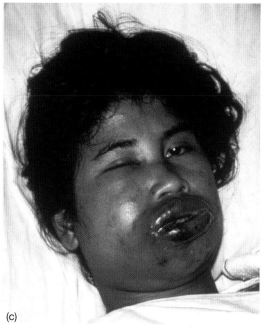

(c)

Figure 25.9 Cavernous sinus. (a) Coronal section. (b) Lateral view showing the abducent nerve passing forwards within the dural coverings of the cavernous sinus and the oculomotor, trochlear and (branches of the) trigeminal nerve in the lateral wall. All except the mandibular branch of the trigeminal nerve pass through the superior orbital fissure into the orbit (see Fig. 19.9, p. 318, for the relations to the tendinous ring). (c) Cavernous sinus thrombosis following infection of the face. Note the extensive swelling of the right cheek.

The **emissary veins** pass through skull foramina, e.g. foramen ovale and foramen lacerum, to unite the intracranial venous sinuses with veins outside the skull. The most constant emissary veins are the condylar, parietal and mastoid.

Diploic veins are present in the frontal, parietal and occipital bones. They drain the diploë and communicate with the veins of the scalp and the dura.

Emissary and diploic veins may be a source of intracranial spread of infection from a scalp wound or abscess.

Arterial circulation of the spinal cord

The arterial supply of the cord is derived from a longitudinal supply that is further reinforced by segmental medullary arteries.

The longitudinal supply is derived from the anterior spinal artery and two posterior spinal arteries. The anterior spinal artery runs along the ventral median surface of the spinal cord and is derived from two small branches of the distal vertebral arteries. The two posterior spinal arteries are branches of the posterior inferior cerebellar artery and run along the dorsolateral surface of the spinal cord. The anterior spinal artery supplies two-thirds of spinal cord while the posterior spinal arteries supply the dorsal columns.

Segmental medullary arteries arise from a range of vessels along the length of the neck and trunk, including the ascending and deep cervical arteries, vertebral artery, posterior intercostal arteries and lumbosacral arteries. The **artery of Adamkiewicz** is of particular importance. This is a large vessel, typically derived from a left-sided posterior intercostal vessel among levels T9–L2, that supplies an extensive number of thoracolumbar spinal cord segments. Damage to the artery of Adamkiewicz may cause an extensive anterior spinal cord syndrome.

Venous circulation of the spinal cord

The venous drainage of the spinal cord is by intrinsic intramedullary veins bringing blood to the pial surface of the cord. These **intramedullary veins** drain into a longitudinal network of **extramedullary veins** running along the surface of the spinal cord. These are known as the **anterior** and **posterior spinal veins**.

The **vertebral venous plexus** runs along the length of the vertebral column and receives the intradural venous supply of the spinal cord. This plexus of veins is **valveless** and consists of internal and external components based on its relation to the vertebral canal. The internal vertebral plexus lies within the epidural space while the external vertebral plexus surrounds the vertebral bodies and neural arch components. Intervertebral veins ultimately drain these systems into **vertebral, posterior intercostal, lumbar** and **lateral sacral veins**. The internal and external plexuses are also in communication with deep pelvic venous structures and cranial dural venous sinuses.

MCQs

1. The cavernous venous sinus is related laterally to the: T/F
- **a** insula ( )
- **b** frontal lobe ( )
- **c** middle meningeal artery ( )
- **d** carotid artery ( )
- **e** pituitary gland ( )

Answers
1.
- **a T –** On the medial aspect of the temporal lobe.
- **b F –** The frontal lobe lies above and anterior.
- **c F –** The middle meningeal artery passes through the foramen spinosum so is not a direct relation.
- **d F –** The carotid artery lies within the cavernous sinus.
- **e F –** The pituitary is situated medially, between the two cavernous sinuses.

2. Cerebrospinal fluid: T/F
- **a** circulation is permitted by a communication between the subarachnoid space and the choroid plexus ( )
- **b** production is mainly by active secretion ( )
- **c** reabsorption is partly through spinal perineural lymph vessels and veins ( )
- **d** is only located in the ventricular system ( )
- **e** circulation is aided by the arachnoid granulations that pierce the inner layer of dura mater ( )

Answers
2.
- **a F –** The communications are in the roof of the fourth ventricle.
- **b T –** The modified ependymal cells of the choroid plexus are involved in this process ...
- **c T –** ... but the main absorption is by the arachnoid granulations in the superior sagittal sinus and its lateral recesses. The spinal contribution is slight ...
- **d F –** ... but also circulates around the spinal cord and brain surface.
- **e T –** These are then in contact with the endothelium of the venous sinuses.

3. The vertebral artery: T/F
- **a** supplies the cerebellum through its superior cerebellar branch ( )
- **b** enters the cranial cavity via the posterior condylar canal ( )
- **c** unites with that of the opposite side in front of the pons to form the basilar artery ( )
- **d** supplies the spinal cord from within the cranial cavity ( )
- **e** supplies the choroidal plexus of the fourth ventricle ( )

Answers
3.
- **a F –** This is a branch of the basilar artery.
- **b F –** The artery passes via the foramen magnum.
- **c T –** The basilar artery is formed at the lower border of the pons.
- **d T –** The anterior spinal artery is a branch of the vertebral and the posterior spinal artery, a branch of the posterior inferior cerebellar artery.
- **e T –** The choroidal artery comes from the posterior inferior cerebellar artery.

EMQs

Each question has an anatomical theme linked to the chapter, and a list of 10 related items (A–J) placed in alphabetical order: these are followed by five statements (1–5). Match **one or more** of the items A–J to each of the five statements.

Vessels of the brain
A. Anterior cerebral artery
B. Basilar artery
C. Cavernous sinus
D. Inferior sagittal sinus
E. Internal carotid artery
F. Middle cerebral artery
G. Posterior cerebral artery
H. Posterior inferior cerebellar artery
I. Posterior superior cerebellar artery
J. Superior sagittal sinus

Match the following statements with the appropriate vessel(s) in the above list.
1. Contributes to the circle of Willis
2. Lies anterior to pons
3. Lateral to the pituitary gland
4. Joins into the straight sinus
5. Gives rise to the ophthalmic artery

Answers
1 AEFG; 2 B; 3 CE; 4 DJ; 5 E

Meninges
A. Anterior spinal artery
B. Arachnoid granulations
C. Arachnoid mater
D. Cauda equina
E. Choroid plexus
F. Denticulate ligament (ligamentum denticulatum)
G. Fat
H. Filum terminale
I. Mixed spinal nerves in dural sheath
J. Vertebral venous plexus (Batson's)

Match the following statements with the contents of the above list
1. Contents of the epidural space
2. Involved in the formation and drainage of cerebrospinal fluid
3. Formed from the pia mater layer
4. In certain areas herniates through the dura mater
5. Is found only between the L2 and S2 vertebral levels

Answers
1 GIJ; 2 BE; 3 FH; 4 B; 5 D

APPLIED QUESTIONS

1. A small depressed fracture of the skull may cause thrombosis of the superior sagittal sinus. Why may this cause rapid onset of unconsciousness?

1. Thrombosis of the superior sagittal dural venous sinus causes blockage in the normal flow of CSF, as most of this fluid drains via the arachnoid granulations into this sinus. Reduced drainage with continuing production of CSF causes the pressure to rise rapidly, and within a day or so the patient may become comatose. The treatment is to drain off the excess fluid by repeated lumbar punctures until the venous sinus recanalizes.

2. Why may squeezing a boil on the cheek lead to a VIth cranial nerve palsy?

2. Some of the veins on the face, especially the region around the eyes and deep tissues of the cheek, drain via the ophthalmic veins and pterygoid venous plexus into the cavernous dural venous sinus. This lies on each side of the pituitary gland and contains within its walls cranial nerves III, IV, V and VI on their way to the eye. Consequently, pus in the cheek, if squeezed into the veins draining towards the cavernous sinus, may precipitate an abscess, causing cavernous sinus thrombosis. This in turn leads to pressure on the VIth cranial nerve, and a lateral rectus palsy may result.

Index

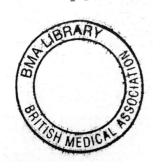